HLA and Disease Associations

Jawahar L. Tiwari and Paul I. Terasaki

HLA and Disease Associations

With 23 Figures

Springer-Verlag
New York Berlin Heidelberg Tokyo

Jawahar L. Tiwari, Ph.D.
UCLA Tissue Typing Laboratory
Center for The Health Sciences
1000 Veterans Avenue
Los Angeles, California
U.S.A.

Paul I. Terasaki, Ph.D.
Professor of Surgery
UCLA Hospital and Clinics
Los Angeles, California
U.S.A.

Library of Congress Cataloging in Publication Data
Main entry under title:
HLA and disease associations
Includes bibliographies and index.
1. Diseases—Causes and theories of causation.
2. HLA histocompatibility antigens—Diagnostic use.
3. Man—Constitution. I. Tiwari, Jawahar L. II. Terasaki,
Paul I. III. Title: HLA and disease associations.
[DNLM: 1. Histocompatibility Testing. 2. HLA Antigens.
WO 680 H6765]
RB152.H5 1985 616.07'1 84-20294

Softcover reprint of the hardcover 1st edition 1985

Typeset by World Composition Services, Incorporated, New York, New York.

9 8 7 6 5 4 3 2 1

ISBN-13: 978-1-4613-8547-9 e-ISBN-13: 978-1-4613-8545-5
DOI: 10.1007/978-1-4613-8545-5

Preface

The human leukocyte antigen (HLA) or tissue types are the products of a rapidly developing field of knowledge within the last 20 years. In the early stages of the research many investigators suspected the existence of a complex series of transplantation antigens, but it was widely believed that these antigens would not be well-defined even in this century. Yet in the last two decades as many as 124 different HLA antigens determined by at least 7 very closely linked genes located on the short arm of chromosome 6 have been identified and subsequently agreed upon by an international nomenclature committee.[1] Extensive international collaboration fueled by the potential clinical application of these antigens to clinical transplantation has advanced the field rapidly. There were nine international histocompatibility workshops held during this period. Although identification of HLA antigens was of primary clinical importance in transplantation and of great basic interest in human genetics and anthropology,[2] a rather unexpected bonus has been the determination that HLA antigens are associated with disease susceptibility to a greater extent than any other known genetic marker in man.

In the past, many genetic polymorphisms have been suspected to be associated with diseases. The most extensively studied markers are blood groups, enzymes, and serum proteins. A comprehensive account of published studies, totalling approximately 1,000, of these markers is available in a book by Mourant et al.[3] Aside from the extensive nature of these studies, one is struck by the data showing only very weak association of diseases with these markers. The relative risk in all of these reports has been less than 2. One of the most thoroughly investigated associations is that of carcinoma of the stomach with blood group A. Analysis of the data on 53,155 patients shows a relative risk of 1.22 indicating that a type A person is only 1.22 times more likely to develop stomach cancer than those who are not type A.[3]

In contrast, the association between HLA-B27 and ankylosing spondylitis has a relative risk of 69. There are many diseases in which relative risk value is greater than 2. Thus, the available data on HLA associations with diseases have far surpassed all the existing knowledge in this field. What is more remarkable is that HLA and disease associations were developed principally in the last 10 years during which approximately 4,000 articles have been published. This burst of activity occurred throughout the world in many different centers, as witnessed by the diverse sources of the bibliography. In many of these diseases the genetic component had long been suspected but now for the first time it has become possible to actually find the genetic inheritance through a well-defined marker.

It was rather surprising that the strength of the association of HLA-B27 with ankylosing spondylitis, first described by our laboratory in 1973[4] and by Brewerton et al.[5] which had been the primary stimulus for the study of other diseases has, in fact, not been exceeded by the many other diseases that have been subsequently found to be associated with the HLA antigens. Thus among more than 530 diseases that have been studied in 4,000 publications, relative risk that is higher than that for ankylosing spondylitis has not been noted. To a certain extent this might be considered to have been somewhat of a disappointment because many of us had expected more diseases to have such a high association. In addition, some diseases that "theoretically" should have been associated with HLA have not yielded the expected association. Instead a rather obscure disease, ankylosing spondylitis, continues to be the disease with the strongest association.

Despite these disappointments, from the research work of the past 12 years, the actual degree of HLA association with various diseases is gradually becoming clear. Although a given single study may have overstated certain associations, there has now been time enough for their confirmation in many different laboratories and thus a more accurate picture of the degree of association is slowly emerging. In this book we have tried to stay close to the data published by the various authors and have refrained from too many interpretations. An attempt has been made for comprehensive coverage, even in instances where we have had suspicions that the data may not have been completely correct. Associations that are true tend to be validated by subsequent studies in other laboratories and those that are spurious are not confirmed in later reports. Important studies on important diseases tend to be followed up whereas findings that are too suspect tend not to be reinvestigated by others. Thus, we leave the reader to draw his conclusions from the comprehensive data presented in this book.

One of the highlights in the study of HLA and disease was an international symposium held in Paris in 1976.[6] This volume presents many of the associations known up to that time, together with ideas on the mechanisms responsible for these associations. Reviews of the literature have been published by Braun in 1979[7] and by Ryder et al.[8] The present book is meant to be a comprehensive account in which all the articles published on HLA and diseases that we are aware of are included. Many of the studies demonstrating associations with the new HLA-DR locus antigens have been undertaken since the publication of the aforementioned reviews.

We hope that this book will serve as a reference for all those who may wish to initiate studies in this interesting area. We also hope that our colleagues will not be too harsh with us for not offering a study involving a resynthesis or strong interpretation of the literature. Our hope has been to make it easy for the reader to arrive at his own conclusions for each of the disease categories.

References

1. Albert ED, Baur MP, Mayr WR (eds): Histocompatibility Testing 1984. Springer-Verlag, Heidelberg, 1984
2. Dausset J, Colombani J (eds): Histocompatibility Testing 1972. Munksgaard, Copenhagen, 1973
3. Mourant AE, Kopec AC, Domaniewska-Solczak K: Blood Groups and Diseases. Oxford University Press, New York, 1978

4. Schlosstein L, Terasaki PT, Bluestone R, Pearson GM: High association of an HL-A antigen, W27, with ankylosing spondylitis. N Engl J Med 288:704-706, 1973
5. Brewerton DA, Caffrey M, Hart FD, James DCO, Nicholls A, Sturrock RD: Ankylosing spondylitis and HL-A27. Lancet i:904-907, 1973
6. Dausset J, Svejgaard A (eds): HLA and Disease. Munksgaard, Copenhagen, 1977
7. Braun WE: HLA and Disease: A Comprehensive Review. CRC Press, Boca Raton, 1979
8. Ryder L, Anderson E, Svejgaard A (eds): HLA and Disease Registry: Third Report. Munksgaard, Copenhagen, 1979

Contents

Acknowledgments

Many of our colleagues at the UCLA Tissue Typing Laboratory have contributed toward the completion of this four-year project. It is a great pleasure to express our gratitude to all these individuals.

Charles A. Pollock has worked on this project from the beginning when we started the computerized database and literature search. The original programs to analyze the population frequency data stored in the Data General computer was written by him. He continued to provide his enthusiastic support even after accepting a new position outside the university. Various changes and modifications to upgrade this program were made by Yong Cho, Ron Oblea, and Nori Sasaki.

In the later stages of this project it became necessary to utilize the flexibility and the convenience of a wordprocessor and also a letter-quality printer. In the laboratory these facilities were available only on the microcomputers and hence a new set of programs for these computers were written by Kevin Hanson, David Kandasamy, and Dennis Aoki. The final manuscript was produced by these programs.

Dr. Pawel Kaszubowski translated many of the papers without an English abstract and also helped in the interpretation of the clinical data in these reports. Dr. Sarina Cats has kindly read the entire manuscript and provided valuable comments.

The manuscript was typed by Pam Kaisaki and the editorial assistance was provided by Rita Loew.

CHAPTER 1

HLA Nomenclature

In the early stages of HLA research individual laboratories assigned new names to the specificities (antigens) discovered by them. Since some of the antigens were independently discovered in different parts of the world, it was obviously important to agree on a worldwide and uniform nomenclature for the HLA antigens. A World Health Organization (WHO) Nomenclature Committee was formed in 1969 and issued its first report in 1970.[1]

Since that time, the HLA nomenclature committee has met after each of the international workshops and used the data developed by the workshop to update and assign new names for the antigens. These name assignments, formally adopted from the very beginning, have permitted an orderly and rapid development of this field. The membership of the WHO Nomenclature Committee is given below.

E. Albert, Kinderpoliklinik der Universitat, Munchen, Germany.
D. B. Amos, Duke Medical Center, Durham, North Carolina, United States.
W. F. Bodmer, Imperial Cancer Research Fund Laboratories, London, England.
R. Ceppellini, Institute for Immunology, Basel, Switzerland.
J. Dausset, Institut de Recherches sur les Maladies du Sang, Hopital Saint-Louis, Paris, France.
F. Kissmeyer-Nielsen, The University Hospital, Aarhus, Denmark.
W. Mayr, Institut für Blutgruppenserologie, Universitat Wien, Wien, Austria.
R. Payne, Stanford University School of Medicine, Stanford, California, United States.
J. J. van Rood, University of Leiden, Leiden, The Netherlands.
P. I. Terasaki, UCLA School of Medicine, University of California, Los Angeles, California, United States.
R. L. Walford, UCLA School of Medicine, University of California, Los Angeles, California, United States.

Since the HLA system is composed of so many factors, advancements in this field would not have been possible without universal agreement on a common nomenclature and strong international collaboration and cooperation achieved through the nine international workshops.

The current specificities of the HLA system recognized by the WHO committee are given in Table 1.1. The specificities of the HLA-A, -B, -C, and -DR loci are determined by the standard serologic methods. The HLA-D locus specificities are defined by the mixed lymphocyte culture (MLC) reactions using homozygous typing cells. One of the important characteristics of the HLA system is that a given specificity may be divided into several parts with these parts being completely included in the original broad specificity. The broad specificities and the "splits" derived from them are also given in Table 1.1.

TABLE 1.1. Complete Listing of Recognized HLA Specificities

A	B		C	D	DR	DQ	DP
A1	B5	BW48	CW1	DW1	DR1	DQW1	DPW1
A2	B7	B49(21)	CW2	DW2	DR2	DQW2	DPW2
A3	B8	BW50(21)	CW3	DW3	DR3	DQW3	DPW3
A9	B12	B51(5)	CW4	DW4	DR4		DPW4
A10	B13	BW52(5)	CW5	DW5	DR5		DPW5
A11	B14	BW53	CW6	DW6	DRW6		DPW6
AW19	B15	BW54(W22)	CW7	DW7	DR7		
A23(9)	B16	BW55(W22)	CW8	DW8	DRW8		
A24(9)	B17	BW56(W22)		DW9	DRW9		
A25(10)	B18	BW57(17)		DW10	DRW10		
A26(10)	B21	BW58(17)		DW11(W7)	DRW11(5)		
A28	BW22	BW59		DW12	DRW12(5)		
A29(W19)	B27	BW60(40)		DW13	DRW13(W6)		
A30(W19)	B35	BW61(40)		DW14	DRW14(W6)		
A31(W19)	B37	BW62(15)		DW15			
A32(W19)	B38(16)	BW63(15)		DW16	DRW52		
AW33(W19)	B39(16)	BW64(14)		DW17(W7)	DRW53		
AW34(10)	B40	BW65(14)		DW18(W6)			
AW36	BW41	BW67		DW19(W6)			
AW43	BW42	BW70					
AW66(10)	B44(12)	BW71(W70)					
AW68(28)	B45(12)	BW72(W70)					
AW69(28)	BW46	BW73					
	BW47						
		BW4					
		BW6					

The listing of broad specificities in parentheses after a narrow specificity, e.g., HLA-A23(9) is optional. The following is a listing of those specificities that arose as clear-cut splits of other specificities.

Original broad specificity	Splits
A9	A23, A24
A10	A25, A26, AW34
AW19	A29, A30, A31, A32, AW33
A28	AW68, AW69
B5	B51, BW52
B12	B44, B45
B14	BW64, BW65
B15	BW62, BW63
B16	B38, B39
B17	BW57, BW58
B21	B49, BW50
BW22	BW54, BW55, BW56
B40	BW60, BW61
BW70	BW71, BW72
DR5	DRW11, DRW12
DRW6	DRW13, DRW14

The following are the generally agreed on inclusions of HLA-B specificities into BW4 and BW6:

BW4: B5, B13, B17, B27, B38(16), B44(12), BW47, B49(21), B51(5), BW52(5), BW53, BW57(17), BW58(17), BW59, BW63(15).

BW6: B7, B8, B14, BW22, B35, B39(16), B40, BW41, BW42, BW45(12), BW46, BW48, BW50(21), BW54(W22), BW55(W22),BW56(W22), BW60(40), BW61(40), BW62(15), BW64(14), BW65(14), BW67, BW70, BW71(W70), BW72(W70), BW73.

The following specificities are generally agreed to be associated with DRW52 and DRW53:

DRW52: DR3, DR5, DRW6, DRW8, DRW11(5), DRW12(5), DRW13(W6), DRW14(W6).

DRW53: DR4, DR7, DRW9.

References

1. WHO Terminology Report: In Terasaki, PI (ed.), Histocompatibility Testing 1970, pp 49. Munksgaard, Copenhagen, 1970
2. Nomenclature for factors of the HLA system 1984. Tissue Antigens 24:73-80, 1984

Chapter 2

The HLA Complex

History

The history of HLA typing originates in the early attempts to define the types of leukocytes. Although red cell antigens had been known since the time of Landsteiner, early efforts to apply the techniques of red cell typing to detect the antigens on leukocytes were fraught with technical problems. A comprehensive review of these historical methods and techniques is provided by Walford[1] and by Killman.[2]

MAC was one of the earliest antigens defined by leukoagglutination, in 1958 by Dausset.[3] However, as a result of the unreliability of the leukoagglutination test, this specificity could not be clearly shown by the time of the First International Histocompatibility Workshop in 1964.[4] At this workshop the typing methodology used by various laboratories was compared and the microdroplet lymphocytotoxicity test, subsquently adopted as the standard method of typing, was introduced by Terasaki.[5] The development of HLA typing was considerably helped by the introduction of computer programs by van Rood[6] to sort out the antigenic specificities. With the aid of these programs, despite numerous false-positive and false-negative reactions included among the data, certain specificities could be discerned.

The Second Histocompatibility Workshop was organized by van Rood[7] in 1965. At this workshop it was possible, for the first time, to see the association between specificities described independently by the pioneer laboratories. These associations have subsequently been confirmed in the succeeding workshops. Also at this workshop, for the first time, it was noted that the MAC antigen, originally described by Dausset, was also defined independently by five other laboratories. The description of LA-1, -2, and -3 by Payne et al.[8] and confirmed by the workshop is one of the classic descriptions of the allelism in the HLA antigens. Based on the correlations between the specificities, Dausset suggested that we were dealing with products from a single locus.[9] It was, however, the Third International Histocompatibility Workshop, brilliantly organized by Ceppellini,[10] that suddenly placed the various detected antigens into a single locus composed of two series of antigens as suggested by Kissmeyer.[11] The segregation of HLA haplotypes could now be clearly demonstrated in the families.

The international collaboration in HLA research also provided impetus for the formation of the official World Health Organization (WHO) Nomenclature Committee in 1967. The Fourth International Histocompatibility Workshop, organized by Terasaki[12] in Los Angeles, fully established the two HLA-A and -B loci as we know them today. At this workshop, all the laboratories also agreed for the first time to standardize the HLA testing by using the microlymphocytotoxicity tests. This standardization enabled the laboratories to exchange the antisera by mail and compare typing results. The microtest also made it possible to perform many tests with a small quantity of the reagent. One milliliter was sufficient for 1000 tests.

Perhaps the peak of international collaborative effort was reached in 1972 when more than 60 populations of the world were typed for HLA antigens by 75 laboratories. In these genetic studies the same reagent had been shared by all the international laboratories and thus the sera reactivities and the antigen frequencies could be compared with each other. The resulting volume from that workshop[13] still remains the best single source of antigen frequencies among the various populations of the world.

The HLA-C and -D loci were first introduced during the Sixth International Histocompatibility Workshop hosted by Kissmeyer.[14] There, it was shown that the C locus could be separately identified. Tests using the mixed lymphocyte culture (MLC) revealed that there might be a fourth locus (D) very closely linked with the HLA complex. The Seventh International Histocompatibility Workshop in 1977, organized under the leadership of Bodmer,[15] clearly established the D locus and also a new DR locus defined by the serologic methods. The D locus specificities were identified with the use of homozygous typing cells. In these tests an individual positive for a specificity would not show reaction against the homozygous typing cells of that specificity. Thus, a person's cells not reacting with DW2 homozygous cells could be classified as positive for DW2 specificity. Most significantly, despite considerable technical difficulties, the typing of B lymphocytes for their DR specificities was accomplished. In typing for the DR antigens B lymphocytes are first isolated from blood samples and then evaluated by the usual microcytotoxicity test. Because of the initial difficulty encountered in B cell isolation techniques, most of the reactions were similar to those used in the early days of leukoagglutination tests. Nevertheless, 7 specificities for the DR locus were established at that workshop. The letter "R" in DR indicates "related," for this locus was found to be either identical with or similar to the D locus identified by the MLC techniques.

A comprehensive description of the serology and the genetics of HLA loci and their specificities was published in a volume derived from the Eighth International Histocompatibility Workshop organized in Los Angeles in 1980.[16]

The Ninth International Workshop was organized under the chairmanship of Albert and Mayr.[17]

In evaluating the publications on HLA and disease associations, it is important to remember that the HLA antigens known at present have gradually evolved during the last 15-20 years. Perhaps the best measure of the development of these antigens can be obtained from the results of the cell exchange program shown in Tables 2.1 and 2.2. Over the past 10 years, lymphocytes from four persons were sent blindly to over 200 laboratories worldwide on a monthly basis for HLA typing. Sixteen antigens were correctly identified by more than 95% of the laboratories (Table 2.1) and considered to be "well-defined." The "developing" antigens were detected by varying percentages of the laboratories. Table 2.2 provides a measure of reliability of typing for each of the HLA antigens. In some respects, the table represents the developmental history of the HLA antigens in the last 10 years.

The Genes of the HLA Complex

The HLA complex is composed of at least seven closely linked loci located on the short arm of chromosome 6 (Fig. 2.1). These loci are called HLA-A, -B, -C, -D, -DR (for D related), -DP, and -DQ. In addition, complement factors C2, C4, Bf (factor B of properdin), and blood groups Chido and Rogers are also located within this complex. These genes are very tightly linked. The recombination between the adjacent loci is <1% (Fig. 2.1). Two other loci, glyoxalase-1 (GLO) and phosphoglucomutase-3 (PGM-3), are also loosely linked with the HLA complex. One very important characteristic of the HLA genes is that they are highly "polymorphic," i. e., several alleles exist at each locus. This makes HLA an ideal marker for genetic studies.

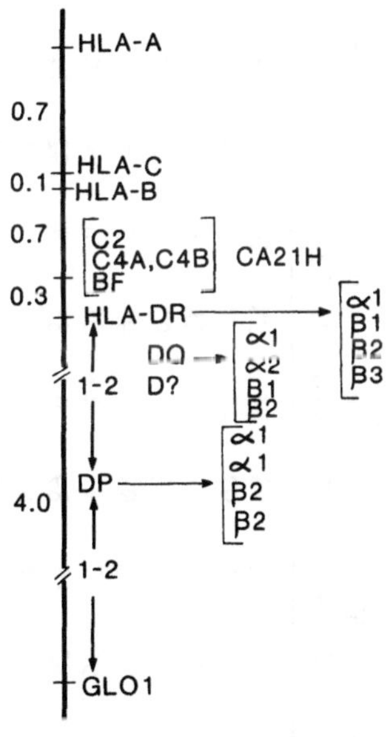

FIGURE 2.1 Map of the HLA region on the short arm of the human chromosome 6. Current evidence suggests that there are 1 α and 2 or 3 β chain genes for HLA-DR, and 2 α and 2 β chains each for HLA-DQ and HLA-DP. The numbers on the left represent the distances between the genes. The orientation and the distance for α and β genes are not known. (Modified from refs. 17 and 29.)

TABLE 2.1. Average Percent Detection of Antigens Tested

	1974		1975		1976		1977		1978		1979		1980		1981		1982		1983		1984[b]	
	No. Times Tested	%	No. Times Tested	%	No. Times Tested	%	No. Times Tested	%	No. Times Tested	%	No. Times Tested	%	No. Times Tested	%	No. Times Tested	%	No. Times Tested	%	No. Times Tested	%	No. Times Tested	%
A1[a]	3	92	2	98	4	98	10	97	6	96	1	97	8	98	14	99	8	99	3	99	3	99
A2[a]	7	96	16	97	10	97	9	98	10	97	11	98	14	98	20	99	18	99	14	99	4	99
A3[a]	1	97	1	98	5	98	5	97	6	97	6	94	9	99	10	99	4	97	4	99	0	—
A9[a]	3	94	12	96	11	97	9	97	15	96	15	98	14	99	15	99	12	97	24	98	4	99
A10[a]	3	97	11	98	9	95	7	99	11	98	4	95	9	98	6	97	11	94	5	83	1	99
A11[a]	3	96	7	97	4	98	6	96	9	96	12	97	4	98	10	99	2	99	7	99	2	99
AW19	6	82	15	89	6	88	7	92	14	94	20	91	18	91	16	93	21	89	8	87	5	99
AW23 (9)	2	30	7	61	1	61	7	71	3	67	4	72	5	81	3	71	1	73	8	88	0	—
AW24 (9)	1	38	6	66	10	72	2	84	12	82	12	85	9	90	12	90	11	89	16	94	4	96
A25 (10)	0	—	4	69	1	79	2	72	6	78	1	75	2	78	3	85	2	93	0	—	0	—
A26 (10)	1	23	5	62	6	78	5	82	5	88	2	81	7	92	3	92	7	93	4	94	1	93
A28	2	82	3	91	0	—	0	—	2	80	5	84	2	95	3	81	7	94	1	93	4	93
A29 (19)	1	72	3	91	2	92	2	88	6	92	3	93	3	93	4	95	3	96	2	97	0	—
AW30 (19)	4	34	7	54	6	71	4	84	4	87	4	76	1	77	2	79	4	89	2	85	1	86
AW31 (19)	0	—	4	58	7	63	1	62	2	78	12	75	7	70	3	79	3	77	6	77	4	82
AW32 (19)	2	57	4	67	1	83	0	—	2	84	2	73	2	82	3	87	3	89	3	91	0	—
AW33 (19)	0	—	2	16	8	40	4	66	3	67	2	70	3	69	3	75	6	68	3	42	0	—
AW34 (10)	0	—	0	—	2	6	0	—	0	—	1	40	2	47	1	55	1	57	0	—	0	—
AW36	0	—	0	—	0	—	1	25	1	30	1	46	0	—	0	—	1	42	1	46	0	—
B5[a]	1	100	5	84	10	71	7	65	8	88	7	91	4	91	4	97	9	92	14	90	3	97
B7[a]	1	100	2	95	3	98	6	97	4	95	4	95	5	96	10	96	2	98	5	96	1	98
B8[a]	2	90	2	98	1	96	11	96	3	99	2	95	6	96	24	98	14	97	2	98	4	98
B12[a]	1	100	8	97	7	98	4	95	10	96	6	98	6	99	5	97	10	99	6	99	1	100
B13[a]	1	88	2	95	2	96	1	94	4	96	1	95	1	94	1	99	2	99	0	—	0	—
B14[a]	1	92	3	97	1	95	0	—	6	95	3	96	3	97	18	96	9	96	3	88	0	—
B15	1	81	3	87	2	90	2	86	7	89	7	88	5	96	9	83	4	89	2	99	3	94
BW16	4	72	11	73	3	75	3	89	8	83	4	81	7	85	7	92	8	85	2	88	5	87
B17	3	94	1	94	6	86	3	95	1	81	6	92	8	97	6	94	8	96	6	95	1	99
B18	1	87	3	78	2	90	0	—	1	89	1	90	0	—	2	94	3	87	1	95	1	94
BW21	1	70	9	75	2	85	6	88	2	90	3	88	5	91	1	94	2	91	0	—	0	—
BW22	4	51	10	43	5	76	1	100	8	67	6	75	1	84	6	85	2	85	9	86	2	90
B27[a]	2	91	2	98	1	95	1	100	1	96	0	—	0	—	4	97	2	99	2	99	1	99
BW35	5	68	6	76	7	68	5	80	6	87	8	80	9	88	3	87	8	81	8	87	2	91
B37	0	—	4	31	0	—	0	—	1	69	0	—	0	—	2	85	0	—	1	90	0	—

BW38 (16)	0	—	5	16	2	32	2	46	3	71	0	—	3	63	2	83	6	72	0	—	2	72
BW39 (16)	0	—	3	7	1	35	1	39	5	57	4	64	4	67	5	81	2	79	2	81	3	73
B40	1	100	6	95	6	96	2	92	4	95	6	92	13	97	9	95	6	92	8	96	0	—
BW41	0	—	0	—	0	—	0	—	0	—	2	30	2	46	1	56	0	—	2	77	0	—
BW42	0	—	0	—	1	11	0	—	1	22	2	31	2	60	1	72	0	—	3	65	1	65
BW44 (12)	0	—	0	—	0	—	1	16	9	16	5	72	4	88	4	89	9	93	5	95	1	97
BW45 (12)	0	—	0	—	2	20	1	30	1	44	0	—	2	75	1	59	1	81	1	83	0	—
BW46	0	—	0	—	2	12	0	—	0	—	0	—	1	6	0	—	0	—	0	—	0	—
BW47	0	—	0	—	0	—	0	—	0	—	0	—	0	—	0	—	1	27	0	—	0	—
BW48	0	—	0	—	0	—	0	—	0	—	1	18	0	—	2	—	0	—	1	28	0	—
BW49 (21)	0	—	0	—	0	—	0	—	2	39	1	70	2	75	1	21	0	—	0	—	0	—
BW50 (21)	0	—	0	—	0	—	4	24	1	13	2	58	3	71	0	82	2	67	0	—	0	—
BW51 (5)	0	—	0	—	0	—	1	22	3	42	3	55	1	77	4	73	5	78	8	83	3	83
BW52 (5)	0	—	0	—	0	—	3	19	5	31	4	57	3	60	0	—	4	62	6	57	0	—
BW53	0	—	0	—	0	—	0	—	0	—	1	6	0	—	0	—	2	35	3	37	0	—
BW54 (22)	0	—	0	—	0	—	0	—	6	18	1	12	0	—	2	34	1	32	5	56	0	—
BW55 (22)	0	—	0	—	0	—	0	—	0	—	2	5	1	19	4	52	1	53	2	52	2	57
BW56 (22)	0	—	0	—	0	—	0	—	0	—	3	10	0	—	0	—	0	—	2	43	0	—
BW57 (17)	0	—	0	—	0	—	0	—	0	—	1	8	3	26	3	42	5	53	1	60	1	67
BW58 (17)	0	—	0	—	0	—	0	—	0	—	4	8	5	25	2	45	3	47	5	47	0	—
BW59 (8.2)	0	—	0	—	0	—	0	—	0	—	1	6	0	—	0	—	2	22	3	32	1	45
BW60 (40)	0	—	0	—	0	—	0	—	1	8	2	14	7	61	7	65	3	71	4	87	0	—
BW61 (40)	0	—	0	—	0	—	0	—	2	6	2	10	6	30	2	51	3	51	4	46	0	—
BW62 (15)	0	—	0	—	0	—	0	—	3	12	3	19	4	66	3	73	1	82	2	89	2	91
BW63 (15)	0	—	0	—	0	—	0	—	2	12	2	26	1	48	4	47	2	41	0	—	1	68
CW1	0	—	0	—	2	18	2	17	5	21	9	30	2	35	8	29	4	40	8	49	3	33
CW2	0	—	0	—	0	—	2	26	3	35	2	52	6	62	4	59	4	44	8	49	1	19
CW3	0	—	0	—	1	18	6	43	13	37	16	41	15	40	17	34	9	42	15	55	1	31
CW4	0	—	0	—	1	50	6	22	8	16	7	20	10	28	3	37	10	27	8	29	2	42
CW5	0	—	0	—	0	—	0	—	0	—	1	8	0	—	0	—	5	19	4	17	0	—
CW6	0	—	0	—	0	—	3	3	1	3	2	11	1	8	4	15	3	14	0	—	0	—
CW7	0	—	0	—	0	—	0	—	0	—	0	—	0	—	10	8	11	15	6	16	5	17

[a] Well-defined antigens.
[b] Based on cell exchanges for February through April.

TABLE 2.2. Antigen Detection Based on the Cell Exchanges of 1983

Well-Defined Antigens (95–100%)	Developing Antigens		
	80–94%	50–79%	<50%
A1	A10	AW31	AW33
A2	AW19	BW41	AW36
A3	AW23	BW42	BW48
A9	AW24	BW52	BW53
A10[a]	A26	BW54	BW56
A11	A28	BW55	BW58
A29	AW30	BW57	BW59
B7	AW32	CW3	BW61
B8	B5		CW1
B12	B14		CW2
B15	BW16		CW4
B17	BW22		CW5
B18	BW35		CW7
B27	B37		
B40	BW39		
BW44	BW45		
	BW51		
	BW60		
	BW62		

[a]Usually detected by 95-100% of the laboratories. Testing of new variants reduced the average percent of detection to 83%. Data from ref. 18.

Inheritance of HLA

Each person has 2 antigens (alleles) for each locus. Both antigens of a locus are expressed independently, that is, the presence of 1 antigen does not suppress the expression of the other. HLA antigens are therefore codominant. If there are two different antigens on 1 locus, the person is considered heterozygous. On the other hand, if both antigens on that locus are the same the person is homozygous. The entire set of A, B, C, D, and DR antigens located on 1 chromosome is called a "haplotype." Recombination in the HLA region of the chromosome is rare (< 1%, Fig. 2.1) and thus a complete set of antigens located on a chromosome is usually inherited by children as a unit (haplotype).

Figure 2.2 illustrates the segregration of HLA haplotypes in a family. The 2 haplotypes of the father are labelled *a* and *b* and the mother's as *c* and *d*. Each offspring inherits 2 haplotypes—one from each parent. Thus only 4 possible haplotypes—*ac, ad, bc,* and *bd*—can be found in the offspring. It can be calculated that 25% of the offspring will have identical HLA haplotypes. Child 3 in this example can be seen to be homozygous at the C locus for he has inherited CW3 from both parents. Child 5 is a recombinant. As a result of crossing-over between B and DR loci in the father, he has inherited DR4, instead of DR3, on the *a* haplotype from his father. His mother's *c* haplotype does not show recombinations. The segregation of these complete haplotypes will continue in the next generation. An occasional crossing-over has the effect of rearranging the genes on the chromosome to produce new haplotypes in the general population.

Frequencies of HLA Antigens

HLA antigen frequencies are simple counts of each antigen generally converted to percent in a specific population. This population is a group of patients or healthy individuals of a specific race or ethnic group (Caucasian, Chinese, Japanese, etc.). These antigen frequencies are "phenotype" frequencies. For practical purposes, they can be converted to "allele frequencies" (or "gene frequencies") by the use of a simple formula:

$$\text{Gene frequency} = 1 - \sqrt{1 - \text{antigen frequency}}.$$

As an example, in a sample of 629 healthy American Caucasians 138 were B8-positive. The B8 antigen or phenotype frequency in this sample is 138/629 = 0.2194 or 21.94%. The B8 gene or allele frequency is equal to $1 - \sqrt{1 - 0.2194}$ or 11.65%.

HLA-A, -B, -C, and -DR loci antigen frequencies in 7 different populations are given in Table 2.3.

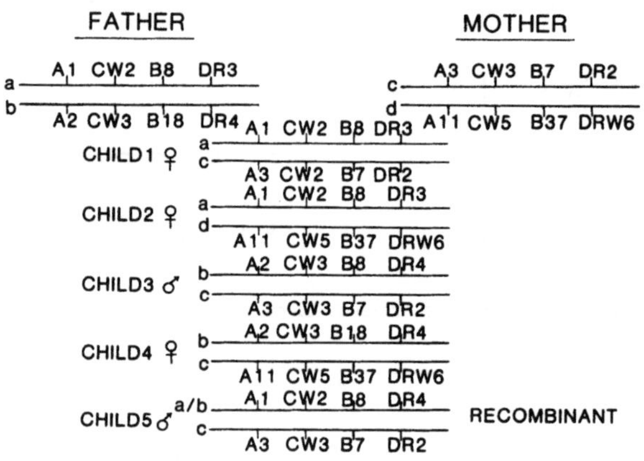

FIGURE 2.2 Segregation of HLA haplotypes in a pedigree.

Racial Variations in Antigen Frequencies

Table 2.3 shows that the frequencies of HLA antigens vary considerably among different races. In fact these antigens show a characteristic distribution in a given racial group. For example, HLA-B8 is relatively high (17.1%) in American Caucasians, drops to 8.5% in Ashkenazi Jews, to 6.0% in Mexicans, 2.9% in American Indians, 0.2% in Japanese and 5.8% in American Blacks. Most of the antigens listed in Table 2.3 show similar trends in different populations.

The worldwide distribution of HLA-B8 is shown in Figure 2.3. These data were obtained from the Fifth International Workshop planned specifically to study the HLA antigen frequencies in various populations of the world. Although the number of individuals sampled from each population was

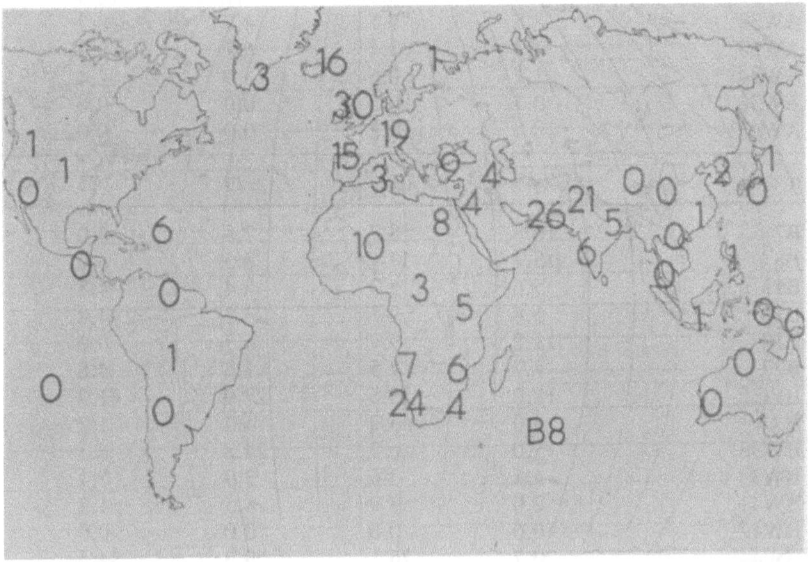

FIGURE 2.3 Worldwide distribution of HLA-B8.

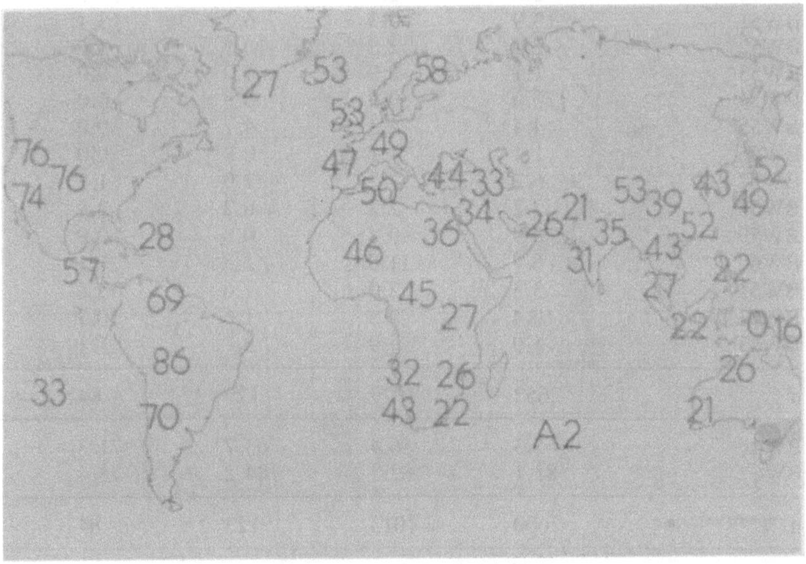

FIGURE 2.4 Worldwide distribution of HLA-A2.

TABLE 2.3. Frequencies of HLA-A, -B, -C, and -DR Loci Antigens

	EUC	NAC	ASH	MEX	AMI	NEG	JPN
A1	27.5	25.7	20.9	18.8	2.9	6.5	1.0
A2	45.3	46.6	40.3	44.3	60.3	27.3	43.2
A3	21.9	26.0	16.3	5.9	2.9	14.2	1.1
A11	11.5	12.5	10.9	7.1	1.5	1.1	17.2
AW23	4.5	5.0	7.0	1.2	1.5	20.4	1.1
AW24	18.2	12.8	19.4	25.9	41.9	5.7	58.5
A25	3.7	4.2	1.6	21.2	0.0	0.8	0.1
A26	7.2	7.2	21.7	11.8	0.0	7.4	18.7
A28	7.7	9.9	7.0	5.9	13.0	16.6	1.1
A29	7.4	8.1	7.8	10.6	4.4	12.3	0.4
AW30	4.7	5.1	5.4	3.5	0.0	28.3	0.3
AW31	5.4	6.2	4.7	12.9	39.0	4.4	15.3
AW32	8.8	7.1	4.7	8.2	4.4	3.0	0.1
AW33	3.3	3.4	6.2	8.2	4.4	9.0	13.1
AW34	1.2	0.5	3.9	2.4	0.0	12.5	1.9
AW36	0.7	0.7	0.0	0.0	0.0	3.3	0.5
AW43	0.0	0.2	0.0	0.0	0.0	1.9	0.0
n	2648	1029	129	85	69	367	949
B7	16.8	18.7	7.8	6.0	1.5	17.0	11.4
B8	15.7	17.1	8.5	6.0	2.9	5.8	0.2
B13	5.6	5.3	5.4	4.8	0.0	1.4	4.0
B14	5.8	9.5	23.3	4.8	1.5	8.0	0.2
B18	11.2	9.7	4.7	0.0	2.9	7.7	0.0
B27	7.7	7.5	1.6	4.8	1.5	3.0	0.8
BW35	18.2	15.6	27.9	41.7	20.3	12.1	14.0
B37	3.0	3.2	4.7	1.2	0.0	0.8	1.1
BW38	5.0	6.2	24.8	8.3	1.5	0.0	0.4
BW39	4.1	3.6	3.9	7.1	21.7	3.6	5.7
BW41	2.0	3.9	8.5	1.2	0.0	2.5	0.7
BW42	0.6	0.6	0.0	0.0	0.0	14.8	1.2
BW44	20.7	26.1	9.3	34.5	5.8	13.7	12.5
BW45	2.2	1.4	0.8	0.0	1.5	7.7	0.3
BW47	0.9	0.4	0.8	0.0	0.0	0.3	0.4
BW48	1.0	1.3	3.1	7.1	4.4	2.2	4.6
BW49	4.5	4.7	0.8	1.2	1.5	4.9	0.6
BW50	2.5	2.6	3.9	14.3	0.0	1.4	0.0
BW51	13.9	9.3	6.2	13.1	43.5	2.7	15.9
BW52	2.9	2.8	10.1	3.6	4.4	1.9	20.5
BW53	1.7	0.9	0.0	0.0	1.5	12.6	0.2
BW54	0.0	0.0	0.8	0.0	0.0	0.0	14.1
BW55	4.4	4.3	4.7	0.0	0.0	1.6	5.8
BW56	1.1	1.1	0.8	0.0	0.0	0.0	2.2
BW57	6.2	7.2	7.0	1.2	0.0	7.7	0.0
BW58	2.2	2.2	6.2	2.4	0.0	20.3	1.7
BW59	0.9	0.8	0.8	0.0	0.0	1.6	4.2
BW60	6.7	11.0	2.3	7.1	18.8	2.7	12.7
BW61	3.3	2.0	1.6	3.6	10.1	0.8	16.8
BW62	10.4	9.5	1.6	10.7	40.6	1.9	16.7
BW63	1.0	1.9	3.1	7.1	2.9	0.6	0.4
n	2652	1029	129	84	69	365	950
BW4	65.3	66.4	63.7	71.3	51.6	65.3	57.6
BW6	83.1	82.3	84.2	78.4	90.7	83.1	87.8
n	2600	1013	127	84	69	359	928

TABLE 2.3. *(continued)*

	EUC	NAC	ASH	MEX	AMI	NEG	JPN
CW1	8.1	6.0	7.0	1.2	20.3	0.1	32.1
CW2	10.0	9.1	5.4	7.1	1.5	22.5	0.7
CW3	19.1	22.6	7.8	19.1	62.3	17.5	46.5
CW4	22.7	20.7	31.0	39.3	14.5	29.3	9.3
CW5	11.7	11.9	6.2	13.1	2.9	5.8	0.2
CW6	15.1	14.9	17.1	10.7	2.9	17.3	1.4
CW7	4.5	6.0	3.9	2.4	0.0	4.7	2.1
CW8	3.8	5.1	9.3	3.6	0.0	0.8	0.2
n	2651	1028	129	84	69	365	950
DR1	13.3	20.0	15.8	8.0	3.0	9.6	12.2
DR2	25.1	25.3	17.3	14.8	46.3	28.5	36.0
DR3	20.4	22.2	13.5	16.0	6.0	31.6	3.2
DR4	18.3	27.3	24.1	28.4	47.8	9.6	41.4
DR5	19.5	19.4	39.0	27.3	3.0	24.8	4.3
DRW6	4.3	7.2	4.5	5.7	7.5	10.2	9.1
DR7	23.4	23.6	27.1	22.7	4.5	18.6	1.0
DRW8	5.4	5.3	5.3	8.0	37.3	10.8	12.6
DRW9	2.2	3.0	3.7	1.1	1.5	5.3	23.0
DRW10	1.4	1.2	1.5	1.1	7.5	3.7	1.2
n	2499	1145	133	88	67	323	884

Abbreviations: EUC, European Caucasian; NAC, North American Caucasian; ASH, Ashkenazi Jews; MEX, Mexican; AMI, American Indian; NEG, Negroes; (American Black); JPN, Japanese.
Data from ref. 16.

somewhat small, a general trend in the distribution of B8 throughout the world can still be seen. The highest frequency is in Scotland and England and decreases to zero in American Indians and some populations of Asia.

In a similar way the worldwide distribution of HLA-A2 is shown in Fig. 2.4. This antigen is one of the most frequent HLA antigens and has a rather high frequency in most races (Table 2.3).

HLA-B27 has a distribution across the northern part of the Northern Hemisphere. The highest frequencies are in North American Indians and Eskimos of Greenland. It is interesting that the South American Indians who represent an earlier wave of migration do not have B27, in contrast to the high frequency in Haida and Bella Coola Indians.

One can also examine the variations in the frequency of an antigen within a narrower geographic area. This type of work has been done in Europe and is shown in Fig. 2.5. The distribution of B8, for example, can be seen as clines in Europe. It shows the highest frequency in Scotland and decreases as populations from the south are sampled. Each of the HLA antigens has characteristic distributions in Europe. Some antigens, for example B5 (Fig. 2.6), show a south to north distribution; the highest frequency is in the Middle East Caucasians and it gradually decreases as one moves northward.

Whether these observed patterns of antigen distribution are the result of population migration or selection has not been resolved, although most of these patterns can be attributed to population migration.

Racial variations in antigen frequencies have significant effects on the strength of disease associations. As an example, approximately 90–95% of ankylosing spondylitis patients from all races and groups are positive for B27 (see Ankylosing Spondylitis). The frequency of B27 is about 50% in American Indians, 10% in Caucasians, and $< 1\%$ in Japanese. The effect of this variation in normal populations of these three races is a relative risk that is highest in the Japanese followed by Caucasian and American Indian groups (see data in Ankylosing Spondylitis).

Some antigens vary between the races but unlike ankylosing spondylitis they do not show a disease association in all races. For example, the frequency of B8 is higher in Caucasians than in Japanese but this antigen is associated with juvenile diabetes mellitus in Caucasians and not in Japanese. The Japanese patients show an association with BW54.

In evaluating the disease association data it is important to consider the time when the study was undertaken. Over the years, as new antisera became available, many antigens were split into component parts. In addition, a certain time interval was necessary to disseminate the well-defined sera even after each of the International Histocompatibility Workshops.

Another measure of reliability of each HLA antigen is the data from the International Cell Exchange.[18] As noted before, this has involved the shipment of four samples of lymphocytes each month over the past 10 years to different laboratories of the world on a "blind" basis. Every month the participating laboratories are required to report the antigens detected on these lymphocytes. Table 2.1 gives the percent recognition of each antigen during the different time periods. It can be noted that antigens such as A2 were readily defined even in 1974 and have continued to be correctly identified by more

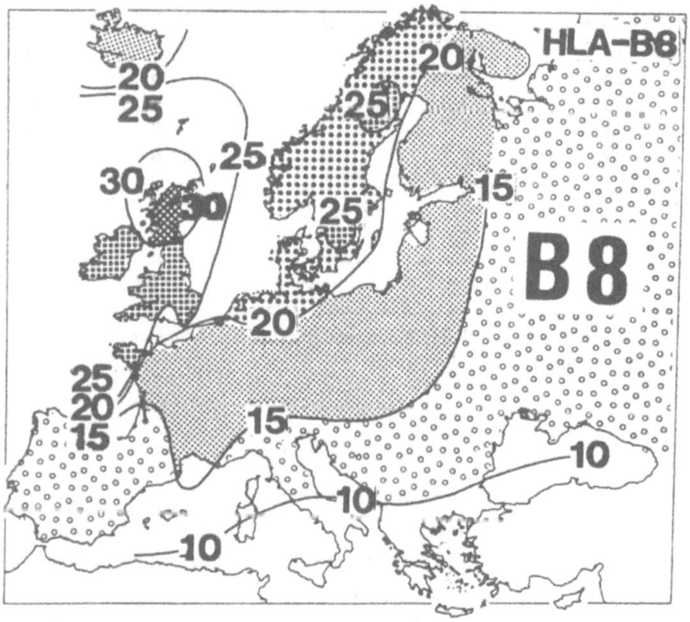

FIGURE 2.5 Distribution of HLA-B8 in Europe. (Modified from ref. 30.)

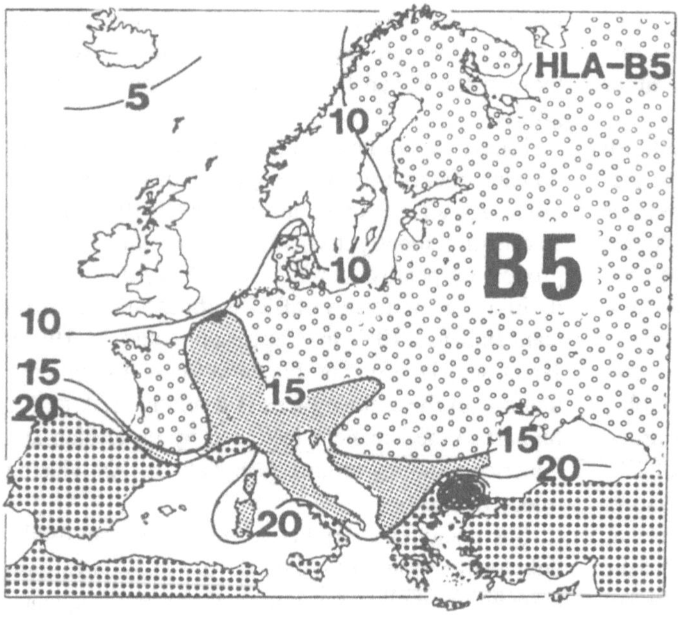

FIGURE 2.6 Distribution of HLA-B5 in Europe. (Modified from ref. 30.).

than 98% of the laboratories during the subsequent years. On the other hand A26 was identified by 23% of the laboratories in 1974 but correct identification reached 93% by 1984. The data in this table are important in evaluating the significance of a given finding for each antigen during each of the time periods. The study done during the period in which the reported antigen was not well defined should be examined carefully according to the laboratory of origin.

From this table it can also be seen that there have been considerable advances in our ability to detect these antigens. It is important to note that even today many specificities are difficult to define accurately. The difficulties will be gradually resolved as better antisera become available.

Cross-Reactivity

The subject of cross-reactivity between HLA antigens has been the subject of numerous studies. Exactly which antigens cross-react with which other ones has become folklore that has accumulated among HLA typers. Usually it is based on the frequency with which two specificities are confused or the frequency with which antibodies having two specificities are encountered. For example, A30 and AW31 can be thought to be cross-reactive since they are difficult to distinguish from each other from available antisera. Anti-HLA-A9 antibodies are much more frequently found than antibodies to AW23 or AW24, thus in the minds of some, there is a strong cross-reaction between these specificities. Cross-reactivity, strictly defined, should be cross-reactions obtained following inhibition or absorption with one specificity upon another.[19] There have actually been very few systematic studies done on cross-reactivity. Clearly there is a quantitative aspect to cross-reactivity, for in some instances it is strong and in other instances very weak. As knowledge of the chemical structure of the antigenic sites develops, a better understanding of cross-reactivity should be possible. Generally speaking, for purposes of disease association studies, typing of the patients with well-defined noncross-reactive antisera provides the clearest answers. For example, HLA-A2 and HLA-A28 are highly cross-reactive. However, antisera that clearly define A2 and those that react only with A28 are known, though rare. With the use of better monospecific antisera, a clear typing can be accomplished by dividing individuals into A2 and A28 types. As much as possible disease studies should be done with the clearly reacting antisera.

Linkage Disequilibrium

Another important characteristic of HLA antigens is the existence of linkage disequilibrium between the alleles of the loci. In a random mating population at Hardy-Weinberg equilibrium[20] the joint frequency of 2 alleles from 2 different loci will be the product of their individual gene frequencies. If the observed value of the joint frequency is significantly different from the expected frequency (the product of the individual allele frequencies) the 2 alleles are said to be in linkage disequilibrium. For example, the gene frequency of A1 in North American Caucasians is 0.138 and that of B8 is 0.090. If there is no preferential association between A1 and B8 then the frequency of the A1-B8 haplotype should be $0.138 \times 0.090 = 0.0124$. However, the data show that the observed value of haplotype A1-B8 in this population is 0.0609.[21] Since there is a difference beween the observed and expected values of haplotype A1-B8, A1 and B8 antigens are said to be in linkage disequilibrium. The measure of linkage disequilibrium is observed haplotype frequency minus expected haplotype frequency. In the case of A1-B8 the linkage disequilibrium value is $0.0609 - 0.0124 = 0.0485$. In population genetics the linkage disequilibrium is also denoted by delta (Δ) or d. In the literature on the population genetics of HLA, linkage disequilibrium values are frequently denoted by Δ values. For A1-B8 the Δ value is positive and thus there is positive linkage disequilibrium between A1 and B8 antigens. As a second example let us consider the haplotype frequency of A1-B7. The gene frequency of B7 from the same table is 0.098 and thus the expected value of this haplotype should be $0.138 \times 0.098 = 0.0135$. The observed value of this haplotype from the same table is 0.0044. The Δ value for A1-B7 is $0.004 - 0.0135 = -0.0091$ and thus there is negative disequilibrium between these 2 antigens in the North American Caucasian population. The method for calculating 3 loci Δ values (e.g., A1-B8-DR2, A1-B7-DR3, etc.) is slightly more complicated. A detailed method for calculating 2 and 3 loci haplotype frequencies and corresponding Δ values is given by Yasuda.[22,23] Tables of 2 and 3 loci haplotype frequencies and Δ values for various races are also available in Histocompatibility Testing 1980.[21] A pictorial representation of linkage disequilibrium between A and B and B and D loci is given in Fig. 2.7 and 2.8. The height of the bars indicate to what extent a given combination is in excess of the random distribution.

It is important to note that the estimated value of linkage disequilibrium (observed minus expected haplotype frequency) may or may not be statistically significant. If it is not significant then the estimated value of Δ is just due to chance or sample variations.[23]

The linkage disequilibrium between 2 loci (e.g., A1-B8) may be the consequence of natural selection[24] for or against a specific gene combination. It may also be due to the fact that the population is only in a transient state and thus has not yet reached the Hardy-Weinberg equilibrium. In the absence of natural selection all linkage disequilibria between linked genes will approach toward zero. When the random mating population is at the Hardy-Weinberg equilibrium, all Δ values will be zero; i.e., the observed values of haplotype frequencies will be equal to their expected values. For very closely linked genes, such as those in the HLA region, the rate of approach to equilibrium is very slow. The detailed mathematical treatment of the genetics of such phenomena and various formulas are available.[20]

Typing Methodology

Earlier methods of typing were based on the use of isolated leukocytes in agglutination tests developed for the typing of red blood cells. However, two specific problems associated with the HLA typing made these techniques difficult to use in routine typing. There are about 1000 red cells to each white cell. To isolate the white cells, one must remove the 1000 red cells and still keep the leukocytes. Within the white cells, lymphocytes have proven to be a much easier cell to handle as compared with the more

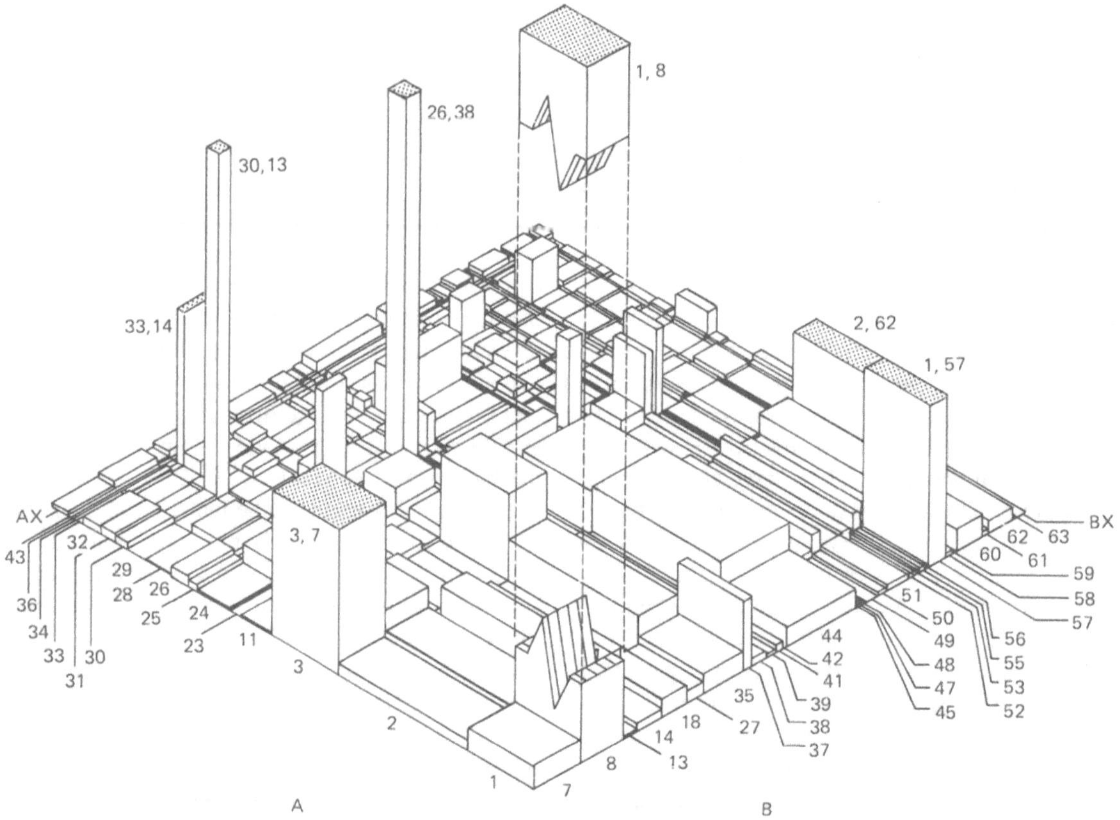

FIGURE 2.7 Linkage disequilibrium between the alleles of HLA-A and -B loci. This figure shows a visualization of the extent of nonrandom occurrence of the haplotype combinations. The tall combinations are the haplotypes that occur much more frequently than would be expected on a random basis. Of interest is the exceptional A1-B8 disequilibrium. AW30-B13 and A26-BW38 haplotypes are also in high linkage disequilibrium.[16]

numerous granulocytes. Isolation of pure lymphocytes for testing was therefore one of the first problems. Furthermore, in comparison with the red cell antigens, there were many more specificities in the HLA system. Thus it was necessary to use a large number of reagents for detecting all these specificities. The microdroplet cytotoxicity test was developed in 1964 [5] to solve these specific problems. It permitted the use of reagents in 0.001-ml quantities and required only 1000 lymphocytes per test. A subcommittee, convened at NIH in 1969, agreed to the uniform test conditions in which 0.001 ml of antisera was incubated with 1000-2000 lymphocytes for 30 min. Then 0.005 ml of rabbit complement was added followed by 1 h of incubation. Because the standard conditions for the microcytotoxicity test were agreed on at the NIH, the test has sometimes been erroneously called the NIH test.

The adoption of the microcytotoxicity test as a uniform standard method of typing in 1969 was one of the reasons for the rapid expansion of HLA typing throughout the world.

Figure 2.9 outlines of the microcytotoxicity test. Machines are now available to "dot" the antisera all at once in the trays and to read the tests semiautomatically. These devices make it possible to process large numbers of antisera and cells.

The HLA-DR locus antigens are typed using the same microcytotoxicity test on B lymphocytes. A great deal of difficulty has been encountered in the isolation of B lymphocytes for DR locus typing. The B lymphocytes were initially isolated by the rosetting of sheep cells.[25] The nylon wool adherence of B lymphocytes has generally proven to be simpler.[26] For typing of patients with various diseases the ox red blood cells coupled with monoclonal Ia antibodies have been shown to be superior.[27]. Use of monoclonal antibodies for isolation of B lymphocytes "B lymphoquick" has made the task considerably easier.

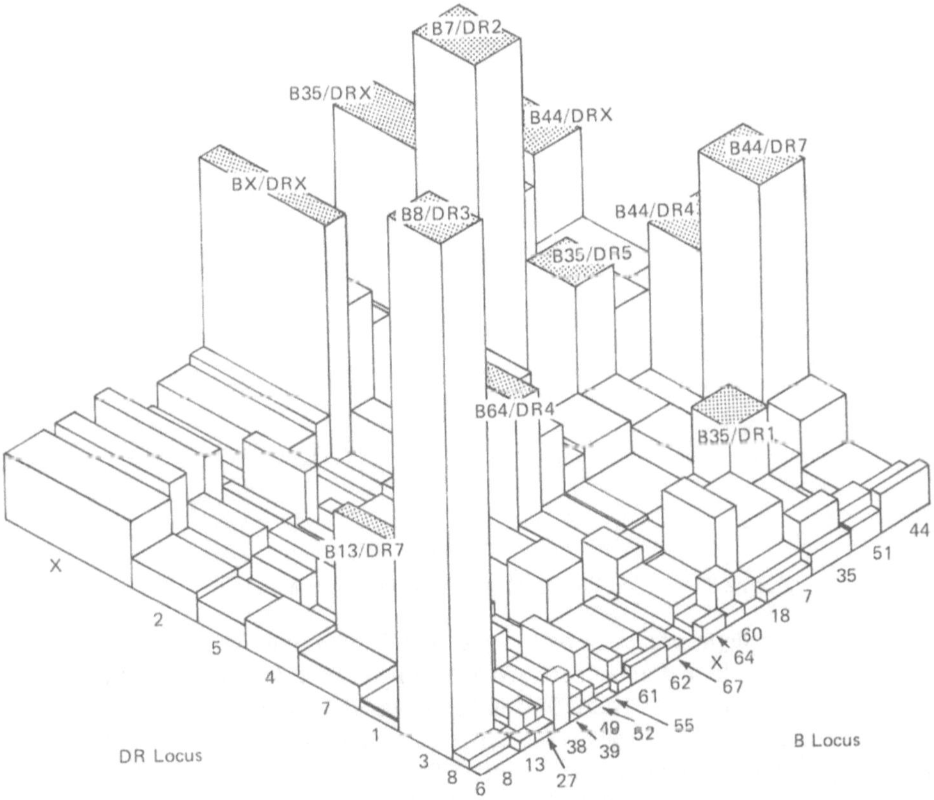

FIGURE 2.8 Linkage disequilibrium between the alleles of HLA-DR and -B loci. Note the high linkage disequilibria between B8-DR3, B7-DR2, and B44-DR7.[16]

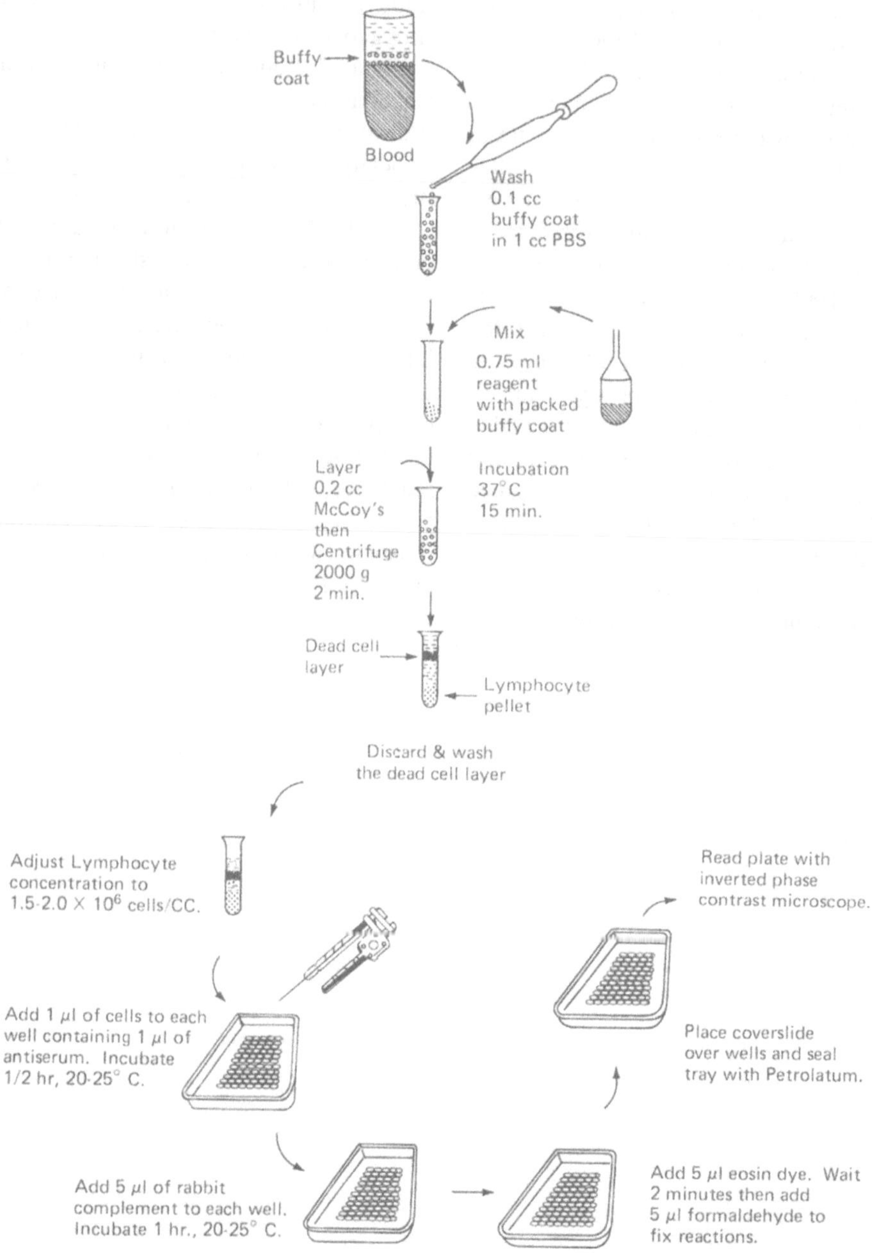

FIGURE 2.9 Microlymphocytotoxicity test procedure.

The HLA-D locus typing is done primarily by using the MLC reaction. In principle, if a given cell does not respond to a known homozygous HLA-D typing cell, then the cell is assumed to have that specificity. Cellular typing for these antigens is technically more difficult than A, B, C, and DR loci typing. Because of these problems relatively small numbers of laboratories are currently using this test. The D locus antigens have been tested in only a small proportion of the diseases studied for HLA associations.

At the Eighth International Histocompatibility Workshop good correspondence between D and DR antigens was shown; e.g., an individual with DR1 antigen also has DW1, and one with DR2 has DW2, etc.[28] D and DR appear to be 2 distinct but very closely linked genes, although the possibility that DR may be the serologic expression of the D locus antigens is not completely ruled out. At present for practical purposes the D and DR loci antigens can be considered to be essentially identical.

Although the microcytotoxicity test is quite simple some errors may result if the test procedure is not followed properly. The most common source of error in HLA typing is in the antisera used for the testing. Some interesting information on this subject can be obtained from the results of the International Cell Exchange.[18] The data in Table 2.1 show the average percent detection of antigens tested "blindly" in more than 250 laboratories from around the world. There are only 16 antigens considered as well-defined antigens, i.e., at least 95% of the laboratories were able to report that antigen correctly over an extended period of time. These results indicate that there are many antigens that still require better definition through the development and identification of "monospecific" antisera. There appears to be a direct relationship between the availability of good monospecific antisera for a specificity and the percent of laboratories accurately identifying that specificity.

References

1. Walford RL: Leukocyte Antigens and Antibodies. Grune & Stratton, New York, 1960
2. Killman S: Leukocyte Agglutinins: Properties Occurrence and Significance. Blackwell, Oxford, 1960
3. Dausset J: Iso-leuco anticorps. Acta Haematol (Basel) 20:156-166, 1958
4. Histocompatibility Testing. National Academy of Sciences, Washington, D. C., 1965
5. Terasaki PI: Microdroplet assay for human blood lymphotoxins. In Histocompatibility Testing, pp 171. National Academy of Sciences, Washington, D.C., 1965
6. van Rood JJ, van Leeuwen A: Leukocyte grouping: A method and its application. J Clin Invest 42:1382-1390, 1963
7. Amos DB, van Rood JJ (eds): Histocompatibility Testing 1965. Munksgaard, Copenhagen, 1965
8. Payne R, Tripp M, Weigle J, Bodmer W, Bodmer J: A new leukocyte isoantigen system in man. Cold Spring Harbor Symp Quant Biol 29:285-295, 1964
9. Dausset J, Ivanyi P, Ivanyi D: Tissue alloantigens in humans: Identification of a complex system (Hu-1). In Histocompatibility Testing 1965, pp 51-62. Munksgaard, Copenhagen, 1965
10. Curtoni ES, Mattiuz PL, Tosi RM (eds): Histocompatibility Testing 1967. Munksgaard, Copenhagen, 1967
11. Kissmeyer-Nielsen F, Svejgaard A, Hauge M: Genetics of the human HL-A transplantation system. Nature 219:1116-1119, 1968
12. Terasaki PI (ed): Histocompatibility Testing 1970. Munksgaard, Copenhagen, 1970
13. Dausset J, Colombani J (eds): Histocompatibility Testing 1972. Munksgaard, Copenhagen, 1973
14. Kissmayer-Nielsen F (ed): Histocompatibility Testing 1975. Munksgaard, Copenhagen, 1975
15. Bodmer WF, Batchelor JR, Bodmer JG, Festenstein H, Morris PJ (eds): Histocompatibility Testing 1977. Munksgaard, Copenhagen, 1977
16. Terasaki PI (ed): Histocompatibility Testing 1980. UCLA Tissue Typing Laboratory, Los Angeles, 1980
17. Albert ED, Baur MP, Mayr WR (eds): Histocompatibility Testing 1984. Springer-Verlag, Heidelberg, 1984
18. Loon J, Takemura S, Terasaki PI: Ten year progress report of the international cell exchange. Tissue Antigens, 24:215-227, 1984
19. Mittal KK, Terasaki PI: Cross-reactivity in the HL-A system. Tissue Antigens 2:94-104, 1972
20. Lee CC: Population Genetics, University of Chicago Press, 1955
21. Baur MP, Danilovs JA: Reference tables for two and three locus haplotype frequencies of HLA-A, B, C, DR, Bf, and GLO. In Terasaki PI (ed): Histocompatibility Testing 1980, pp 994-1210. UCLA Tissue Typing Laboratory, Los Angeles, 1980
22. Yasuda N, Tsuji K: A counting method of maximum likelihood for estimating haplotype frequency in the HL-A system. Jpn J Hum Genet 20:1-15, 1975
23. Yasuda N: Estimation of haplotype frequency and linkage disequilibrium parameter in the HLA system. Tissue Antigens 12:315-322, 1978
24. Bodmer WF, Bodmer JG: Evolution and function of the HLA system. Br Med Bull 34:309-316, 1978
25. van Rood JJ, van Leeuwen A, Keuning JJ, Blusse van Oud Alblas A: The serological recognition of the human MLC determinants using a modified cytotoxicity technique. Tissue Antigens 5:73, 1975
26. Danilovs J, Ayoub G, Terasaki PI: B lymphocyte isolation by thrombin-nylon wool. In Terasaki PI (ed): Histocompatibility Testing 1980, pp 287-288. UCLA Tissue Typing Laboratory, Los Angeles, 1980
27. Cicciarelli JC, Ayoub G, Terasaki PI, Billing R: Improved HLA-DR typing of dialysis patients using monoclonal antibodies. Transplantation 33:558-560, 1982
28. Dupont B, Braun DW Jr, Yunis J, Carpenter CB: HLA-D by cellular typing. In Terasaki PI (ed): Histocompatibility Testing 1980, pp 229-267. UCLA Tissue Typing Laboratory, Los Angeles, 1980
29. Robson EB, Lamm LU: Human Gene Mapping 7: Report of the committee on the genetic constitution of chromosome 6. Cytogenet Cell Genet 37:47-70, 1984
30. Ryder LP, Anderson E, Svejgaard A: An HLA map of Europe. Hum Hered 28:171-200, 1978.

CHAPTER 3

The Data and Statistical Analysis

The Data

The material presented in this book has been taken from the journals listed in *Index Medicus* (covering approximately 2700 journals) and *Current Contents* (covering approximately 1150 journals). The papers published from January 1970 and listed under "Histocompatibility" and "HLA" constitute the database and the bibliography. We have attempted to include all published and available material. Only the publications that could not be obtained easily are excluded. However, these constitute a very small fraction (approximately 5–10%) of the total published material. In addition, the data and reports from the "Histocompatibility Testing" series and "Transplantation Reviews" were generally not included, since most of them had been subsequently published in various forms elsewhere. Also, we have not included *unpublished data* on the HLA antigen frequencies in patients and controls.

We recorded from each paper that contained population data, the numbers of patients and controls in the study and the frequencies of HLA antigens (% positive) in these 2 groups. The frequencies were rounded off to the nearest whole number with the following approximation rule: Any fraction 0.5% or greater is equal to 1.0% and 0.4% or less is equal to zero. Thus, an antigen with a frequency of 18.5% was recorded as 19% and that with 22.4% was recorded as 22%.

When there was more than one report on the same disease from the same author or a group of authors, the original report or the one with the largest sample size is presented in the data tables. The others are listed in the bibliography.

Population Data Analysis

The existing literature on HLA and disease associations consists primarily of population frequencies of HLA antigens in a group of patients and some suitable controls. In some studies families with more than one affected patient have also been typed for HLA antigens. The basic methods for analyzing this type of population data, i.e., for comparing the antigen frequencies in unrelated patients and controls, were developed by Woolf in 1955[1] and later modified by Haldane.[2]

In a typical report on the association between HLA and a disease, a group of unrelated patients are typed for HLA antigens. In addition, a relatively large group (compared to the size of the patient group) of unrelated healthy *control* individuals matched for race, sex, age, and other appropriate variables are also typed for the same antigens using the same antisera. Thus, the HLA antigen frequencies are generated in matched patient and control groups. From these data, the question generally raised is: Is there a significant difference in the frequency of the antigen between patients and controls? If the frequency is significantly increased of decreased in the patients then the antigen is considered as associated with the disease under study.

The method used in this book for analyzing the population data was originally proposed, as mentioned earlier, by Woolf[1] and later modified by Haldane.[2] We will present only an outline of this method. The mathematical details are available in the 2 original papers.[1,2] This method enables us to compare the antigen frequency in patients and controls in a particular study and also in the pooled data from several such studies.

The data analysis with respect to a particular antigen (e.g., A1, A2, etc.) starts with a simple 2 × 2 table containing the number of positive and negative individuals in the patient and control groups:

	Number of Individuals	
	Positive for the antigen	Negative for the antigen
Patients	h	k
Controls	H	K

Testing for the Significant Difference in the Frequency of an Antigen

The incidence of the disease in individuals positive for the antigen will be h/H × some constant and that in individuals negative for the antigen will be k/K × the same constant. The *relative incidence*, X, as defined by Woolf[1] is:

$$X = \frac{h/H}{k/K} = \frac{hK}{Hk} \quad [1]$$

(Since the same constant is present in numerator and denominator it is cancelled out in the ratio of one rate to another.)

In the literature on HLA and disease associations the term "relative risk" has been used to describe the quantity X. To avoid confusion we will also use the term *relative risk* throughout this book.

The relative risk indicates how many times more frequent the disease is in the individuals positive for the antigen than in individuals negative for the antigen.

If the ratios h/k and H/K are similar then the relative risk will be close to unity. It will be < 1 if the antigen is less frequent in the patients. However, the calculated value of X may not be significantly different from unity. Let:

$$y = \log_e X \quad [2]$$

The sampling variance, V, of y is

$$V = \frac{1}{h} + \frac{1}{k} + \frac{1}{H} + \frac{1}{K} \quad [3]$$

and w, the weight of y is

$$w = \frac{1}{v} \quad [4]$$

$$\chi^2_{1\,\mathrm{df}} = wy^2 \quad [5]$$

The statistical significance of the difference of X from unity is tested by this χ^2 with 1 degree of freedom.

If this χ^2 is > 3.84, we conclude that the relative risk is significantly different from 1 and the antigen is associated with the disease. In other words there is a significant difference between the frequency of the antigen in the patient and control groups (however, see the sections on significance and p values below).

In the study of HLA antigens, frequently some of the values for h, k, H, and K are either very small or zero. The small numbers in the above formula will introduce some bias in the estimates of relative risk. Also, when all the patients are positive for an antigen (k = 0) or no individual in the control group is positive for the antigen (H = 0) the relative risk by Woolf's formula is undefined. For such situations Haldane has modified Woolf's formula for relative risk. With this modification the relative risk is:

$$X = \frac{(2h + 1)(2K + 1)}{(2H + 1)(2k + 1)} \quad [6]$$

The value of y is:

$$y = \log_e \frac{(2h + 1)(2K + 1)}{(2H + 1)(2k + 1)} \quad [7]$$

and the sampling variance, V, of y is:

$$V = \frac{1}{h+1} + \frac{1}{k+1} + \frac{1}{H+1} + \frac{1}{K+1} \quad [8]$$

As in Woolf's formula:

$$w = \frac{1}{V} \quad [9]$$

$$\chi^2_{1\,\mathrm{df}} = wy^2 \quad [10]$$

Combining Data from Several Studies

The data from several studies on the same antigen and disease can also be combined by Haldane's formula:

$$Y = \frac{\sum_{i=1}^{n} wy}{\sum_{i=1}^{n} w} \quad [11]$$

In the above expression $\sum_{i=1}^{n} wy$ is the sum of all wy from n studies used in the combined analysis. Similarly $\sum_{i=1}^{n} w$ is the sum of all w from the same n studies.

The estimate of relative risk in the combined data is:

$$X = \mathrm{antilog}_e y \quad [12]$$

The significance of its difference from unity is given by:

$$\chi^2_{1\ \mathrm{df}} = \frac{(\sum_{i=1}^{n} wy)^2}{\sum_{i=1}^{n} w} \qquad [13]$$

The heterogeneity of the combined data is given by:

$$\chi^2_{n-1\ \mathrm{df}} = \sum_{i=1}^{n} wy^2 - \frac{(\sum_{i=1}^{n} wy)^2}{\sum_{i=1}^{n} w} \qquad [14]$$

The heterogeneity χ^2 has $n - 1$ degrees of freedom (n = number of studies).

The analysis of the data presented in this book is based on Haldane's modified formulas.

The Level of Significance and p Values

If the calculated value of χ^2 in Eq. [10] is > 3.84 then it is concluded that the relative risk is significantly different from 1, i.e., the antigen is associated with the disease. The level of significance is reported in terms of probability (p) value. The smaller the p value, the greater the likelihood that the estimated value of relative risk is not different from unity by chance. For biologic data, the generally accepted rule is that, for a difference to be considered significant, the p value must be ≤ 0.05. The p value corresponding to the χ^2 of 3.84 is 0.05 (hence the rule that the calculated value of χ^2 must be > 3.84). It is possible to determine the p value associated with any calculated value of χ^2. Statistical tables and formulas for this purpose are available in many statistics books (for example, see Dixon and Massey[3]). A p value of 0.001 is considered highly significant (for additional details on the analysis of frequency data see Fleiss[4]).

Multiple Comparisons and the Corrected p Value

In studies of the HLA antigens and disease association each individual is tested for several antigens and the same data are used to compare the frequency of all the typed antigens. Because of this multiple comparison, it is probable that an antigen frequency significantly (increased or decreased at a p value of 0.05 may be due to chance alone. To phrase it differently, if the patients and controls are typed for the 92 known antigens of A, B, C, D, and DR loci, one can expect to find, by chance alone, 4–5 antigens significantly increased or decreased in the patients at a p value of 0.05 (or $\chi^2 = 3.84$). Thus the aforementioned rule to accept a frequency deviation as significant if $\chi^2 = 3.84$ will yield many spurious HLA associations. This error can be corrected by the use of the Bonferoni inequality method (for mathematical details see Dunn[5,6]). In this procedure the p values corresponding to the calculated χ^2 for each antigen comparison are "corrected" by multiplying with the number of antigens compared. If any resulting corrected p value for an antigen is still $\leq$ 0.05 then that antigen is considered as significantly associated with the disease. Thus, by adjusting the p values upward this method sets more stringent requirements for accepting an association as statistically significant. As an example let us suppose that 25 antigens were compared in order to search for any association and one antigen was found to be increased in the patients at a calculated p value of 0.003. Because of 25 comparisons this p value, although < 0.05, would not be considered as significant. The corrected p value in this case would be $0.003 \times 25 = 0.075$, a value > 0.05 and thus the antigen would not be considered as significantly associated with the disease.

Another way to correct for the bias due to the multiple comparisons is to do a second study on the same disease and then look for associations with antigens that were found to be significantly increased or decreased at the p value of 0.05 or less in the first study. If the p values in the second study are again $\leq$ 0 0.05 then those antigens are considered as significantly associated with the disease. The second study is done with a specific hypothesis ("Is antigen "A" associated with the disease?") and thus the corrections for multiple comparisons are not necessary.

An Example

A detailed numerical example of the method used in this book is given in Table 3.1.

An Analysis of Primary Association When 2 Antigens of Different Loci Are Associated with a Disease

Several diseases are known to be associated with antigens of 2 different loci. Juvenile diabetes mellitus, for example, is associated with B8, B15, DR3, and DR4 antigens. Similarly, multiple sclerosis shows an association with B7 and DR2 antigens. It is well known from HLA population genetics that linkage disequilibria exist between B8 and DR3 and between B7 and DR2. In such situations, it is interesting and

TABLE 3.1. Association of BW54 with Juvenile Diabetes Mellitus in 4 Studies from Japan

Study	Patients		Controls						Relative Risk					
	n	%+	n	%+	h	k	H	K	$X = \frac{(2h+1)(2K+1)}{(2H+1)(2k+1)}$	$y = \log_e X$	$V = \frac{1}{h+1} + \frac{1}{k+1} + \frac{1}{H+1} + \frac{1}{K+1}$	$w = 1/V$	wy	$\chi^2 = wy^2$
Wakisaka et al.[36]	32	44	76	13	14.080	17.920	9.880	66.120	5.080	1.625	0.226	4.425	7.191	11.685
Okimoto et al.[37]	89	44	128	10	39.160	49.840	12.800	116.200	6.854	1.925	0.126	7.937	15.279	29.412
Kawa et al.[38]	27	63	106	21	17.010	9.990	22.260	83.740	6.178	1.821	0.201	4.975	9.059	16.496
Sakurami et al.[39]	131	36	101	9	47.160	83.840	9.090	91.910	5.445	1.695	0.142	7.042	11.936	20.232
Total												24.382	43.465	77.825

1. Combined estimate of relative risk (X):

$$Y = \frac{\sum_{i=1}^{n} wy}{\sum_{i=1}^{n} w} = \frac{43.465}{24.382} = 1.783$$

$$X = \text{antilog}_e y = \text{antilog}_e\, 1.783 = 5.948$$

2. χ^2 for the significance of relative risk:

$$\chi^2_{1\,\text{df}} = \frac{(\sum_{i=1}^{n} wy)^2}{\sum_{i=1}^{n} w} = \frac{(43.465)^2}{24.382} = 77.484$$

3. χ^2 for the heterogeneity:

$$\chi^2_{3\,\text{df}} = \sum_{i=1}^{n} wy^2 - \frac{(\sum_{i=1}^{n} wy)^2}{\sum_{i=1}^{n} w} = 77.825 - 77.484 = 0.341$$

TABLE 3.2. Association of Celiac Disease with HLA-B8 and DW3

	Patients		Controls		
	+	−	+	−	χ^2
B8	22	6	31	69	17.81
DW3	27	1	27	73	25.89

TABLE 3.3. Analysis of Association Between Celiac Disease and HLA-B8 in the Presence and Absence of DW3

	DW3+		DW3−		
Group	B8+	B8−	B8+	B8-	Total χ^2
Patients	22	5	0	1	
Controls	21	6	10	63	
χ^2	0.11		0.31		0.42

χ^2 for significance = 0.30
χ^2 for heterogeneity = 0.12

important to know if the association is primarily with 1 antigen and the observed association with the other antigen is due only to the linkage disequilibrium with the first antigen. A method used by several investigators is the analysis of association with 1 antigen in the subgroups of patients and controls positive and negative for the other antigen. To illustrate we will consider the data analysis on 28 Dutch patients with celiac disease and 100 controls by Keuning et al.[7] As the data in Table 3.2 show, celiac disease is associated with both B8 and DW3 antigens.

The data were first analyzed (Table 3.3) for an association with B8 in the presence and absence of DW3. As the χ^2 values indicate there was no significant association with B8. The second analysis was done for an association with DW3 in the presence and absence of B8 (Table 3.4). In this case, the calculated value of χ^2 (23.52) is highly significant. Thus it was concluded that celiac disease is primarily associated with DW3; its association with B8 is secondary to that with DW3.

It should be noted that Porta and McHugh[8] have used a complex method of analysis (requiring a computer program) on the data presented above. Their conclusion was that celiac disease is associated with haplotype B8-DW3 (for mathematical details the author's paper[8] should be consulted).

HLA Haplotype Associations with Disease

As discussed in the previous section there are several diseases in which significant associations with antigens of 2 different loci have been found. These antigens are also in strong linkage disequilibrium. Both HLA-B7 and -DR2 are associated with multiple sclerosis in the Caucasian population, and are also in strong linkage disequilibrium. Thus, it is possible that multiple sclerosis might be associated with haplotype B7-DR2.

Terasaki and Mickey[9] have applied a method to calculate A and B loci haplotype frequencies in 32 diseases. The number of patients tested for each disease ranged from 43 to 512. Common haplotypes, such as A1-B8, were not found in acute lymphocytic leukemia, colon cancer, ankylosing spondylitis, rheumatoid arthritis, and prostate cancer. In these diseases more than 100 patients were typed. HLA-A3-B7, another common haplotype, was also absent in psoriasis, ankylosing spondylitis, acute lymphocytic leukemia, carcinoma of the stomach, endometrium, tongue, and larynx. It was found that only certain B27-bearing haplotypes were strongly associated with ankylosing spondylitis.

Thomson and Bodmer[10] have pointed out that because of the third-order linkage disequilibria involving the disease gene and 2 HLA genes it is not easy to detect haplotype associations if an individual antigen association with the disease exists. Later, Porta and McHugh[8] formulated a mathematical approach to solve some of the problems outlined by Thomson and Bodmer[10]. Porta and McHugh[8] applied their method on the data of Keuning et al.[7] on celiac disease and found a significant association with the B8-DW3 haplotype. It should be noted that Keuning et al.[7] concluded, on the basis of their own analysis outlined in the previous section, that the primary association of the disease was with antigen DW3.

The mathematical details and arguments in the methods of Terasaki and Mickey[9], Thomson and Bodmer[10], and Porta and McHugh[8] are more complicated than the methods for detecting single antigen associations. The interested reader should consult the original sources.

Family Data Analysis

The family data in which disease status and family members' HLA types are available has been used to answer questions regarding genetic linkage between a "disease susceptibility gene" and HLA genes. A

TABLE 3.4. Analysis of Association Between Celiac Disease and DW3 in the Presence and Absence of B8

	B8+		B8−		
Group	DW3+	DW3−	DW3+	DW3−	Total χ^2
Patients	22	0	5	1	
Controls	21	10	6	63	
χ^2	8.09		15.52		23.61

χ^2 for significance = 23.52
χ^2 for heterogeneity = 0.09

method for detecting linkage in data from brothers and sisters (sib-pairs) was developed by Penrose[11] in 1935. Variations and modifications of this "sib-pair test" have been used by many investigators. Another linkage test in which probabilities of joint segregation of a disease susceptibility gene and a marker gene, such as HLA, in entire pedigree are compared, was developed by Morton[12,13]. This method, frequently known as the lod score test, has become a standard method for detecting linkage in the pedigree data.

In comparison with the population association studies the data on complete families of patients are insufficient and in most cases inadequate for genetic analysis to determine the inheritance of the disease and its linkage with the HLA complex. However, in diseases such as diabetes, multiple sclerosis, hemochromatosis, and celiac disease, families with multiple cases of the disease have been HLA-typed and some genetic analysis has been done. The methods of statistical analyses and resulting conclusions are variable, however. For example, on the basis of population and family data the inheritance of juvenile diabetes mellitus has been proposed by various authors as recessive, dominant, intermediate, 2 different genes associated with HLA, 2 different genes but only one linked with HLA, 3-allele model, and epistatic (see Juvenile Diabetes Mellitus).

Sib-Pair Test

The sib-pair test for detecting linkage, originally proposed by Penrose in 1935,[11] is based on the principle that, when pairs of sibs are taken at random from a series of families, certain types of sib pairs will be more frequent if there is linkage than if there is independent assortment of the 2 characters studied. Various modifications and variations of this test have been published by many investigators.

A simple sib-pair test was applied to family data on juvenile diabetes mellitus by Cudworth and Woodrow.[14] If one considers the data on a pair of affected sibs from several families typed for HLA antigens then the sib pairs can be classified into 3 categories: (1) those with both haplotypes identical; (2) with one haplotype identical; and (3) with no haplotypes identical. If juvenile diabetes mellitus and HLA haplotypes were segregating independently the expected proportions of the sibs in the 3 aforementioned categories will be 0.25, 0.50, and 0.25, respectively (see Table 3.5).

TABLE 3.5. The Expected Proportions of Sib-Pairs Sharing 2, 1, and 0 Haplotypes

		First member of the affected sib-pair HLA haplotypes			
		ac	*ad*	*bc*	*bd*
Second member of the affected sib-pair	*ac*	*ac/ac**	*ac/ad*†	*ac/bc*†	*ac/bd*‡
	ad	*ad/ac*†	*ad/ad**	*ad/bc*‡	*ad/bd*†
	bc	*bc/ac*†	*bc/ad*‡	*bc/bc**	*bc/bd*†
	bd	*bd/ac*‡	*bd/ad*†	*bd/bc*†	*bd/bd**

* = Sib-pair sharing 2 haplotypes = 4/16 = 0.25
† = Sib-pair sharing 1 haplotypes = 8/16 = 0.50
‡ = Sib-pair sharing 0 haplotypes = 4/16 = 0.25

On the other hand, if HLA and the "juvenile diabetes mellitus gene" are on the same chromosome they will segregate together and thus the number of sib pairs sharing both haplotypes will be more than expected on the basis of independent assortment. In the data of Cudworth and Woodrow[14] on 15 affected sib pairs the following proportions were observed:

	2-Haplotype Identical	1-Haplotype Identical	0-Haplotype Identical
Observed	10	4	1
Expected	3.75	7.50	3.75

There is a significant difference between observed and expected number of sib pairs ($\chi^2_{2\ df}$ = 14.067, $p < 0.001$). These data indicate the existence of linkage between the juvenile diabetes mellitus gene and the HLA complex. This simple sib pair test has been applied in some other diseases and results and references are noted in the sections on individual diseases.

The Method of Lod Scores

The method of lod ("lod" means "log odds," i.e., "log probability ratio") was developed in 1955 by Morton[12] and has become a standard method for detection and estimation of linkage. Unlike the sib-pair test this method utilizes available information from parents and other members of the pedigree. It is more efficient and provides not only a test for the presence of linkage but also an estimate of the recombination (i.e., genetic distance) between the disease gene and the HLA complex. The mathematical details are complex and interested readers should consult Morton's original papers.[12,13] Extensive tables of lod scores are available in the book by Maynard-Smith et al.[15] A very good discussion of the method with specific examples is also given in Cavalli-Sforza and Bodmer.[16]

The family data on HLA and disease associations are generally available in the form of HLA typings and disease status (affected or unaffected) of parents and children. In some cases this information is also available for other members of the pedigree. For each family a set of lod scores are calculated for various recombination values (e.g., 0.0, 0.1, 0.2, . . . 0.5) between the HLA and the disease susceptibility genes. The recombination fraction at which the lod score is maximum is the maximum likelihood estimate of the recombination between the disease susceptibility gene and the HLA gene. A lod score of +3.00 (1000 to 1 odds) is considered as significant evidence in favor of linkage and a score of −2.00 is generally taken as evidence against linkage. If data on several families are available then total lod scores are obtained by adding the scores of individual families. As before, the recombination fraction at which the total score is maximum is the maximum likelihood estimate of the recombination. One advantage of Morton's method is that lod scores from new pedigrees can be sequentially added to the previously collected data. The process can be continued until the maximum score in the total sample reaches +3 or −2 at which point a definite statement regarding the presence or absence of linkage can be made. A detailed example of this procedure is available in Morton's original paper[13] on the detection and estimation of linkage between the genes for elliptocytosis and the Rh blood group. This paper also gives a method for testing heterogeneity among pedigrees.

A very useful and general purpose computer program, called LIPED, has been developed by Ott[17,18] to calculate the lod scores for human pedigrees. The program facilitates the computation of scores for various modes of inheritance, recombination fractions, penetrance values, and complex pedigrees. The family data on several diseases have been analyzed by using this program and results of the analysis and references are noted in the sections on individual diseases.

Other Methods

The existence of antigen associations at the population level and linkage at the family level has generated considerable interest in the analyses of these data. There is no controversy in the analysis of population data. However, a slightly different formula for relative risk has been proposed by Curie-Cohen.[19] Smouse[20] has reported a method for detecting HLA allelic frequency differences between the patients and controls. Nijenhuis[21] has outlined a statistical method to distinguish between various possible explanations for the association between HLA and disease (dominant or recessive disease susceptibility gene, or the HLA antigen itself is responsible for disease susceptibility).

The alternate methods of analyzing family data to detect linkage between HLA and a disease susceptibility gene and to explain the mode of inheritance of this susceptibility gene have been proposed by many investigators (Lalouel and Morton[22], Morton and Lalouel[23], Thomson[24], Suarez et al.[25,26], Suarez[27], Kidd et al.[28], Green and Woodrow[29], De Vries et al.[30], Fishman et al.[31], Thomson and Bodmer[32], Hodge et al.[33], and Day and Simons[34]). The statistical models proposed by these workers incorporate specific features of HLA, such as linkage disequilibria, racial variation, association with 2 or more antigens of the same locus, stronger association with the D/DR antigens, etc. These methods have been applied to data on diseases such as juvenile diabetes mellitus, ankylosing spondylitis, multiple sclerosis, etc. Despite extensive analysis the genetics of the HLA-associated diseases remains unclear. The mathematical details in these methods are considerable and the interested reader should consult the original reference.

Diagnostic Value of HLA Typing

Of all the known HLA associations the association of B27 with ankylosing spondilitis is the strongest. The B27 antigen is present in > 90% of the patients as compared with its frequency of 5-10% in the controls. Thus, B27 typing has been used as one of the diagnostic tests for ankylosing spondylitis. Many reports on the usefulness of this test have appeared in the literature and they are discussed and referred to in the section on Ankylosing Spondylitis. Here we will consider one of the statistical methods used in the evaluation of the predictive value of diagnostic test. The method outlined below is described in detail by Katz.[35] The mathematical basis for the method is Bayes' theorem. The formula incorporates the *prior probability* that a patient has the disease and the frequencies of the "false positive" and "false negative" in the B27 test.

$$\text{PD/A+} = \frac{(1 - \text{FN}) \times \text{PP}}{([1 - \text{FN}] \times \text{PP}) + (\text{FP} \times [1 - \text{PP}])} \quad [15]$$

$$\text{PD/A-} = \frac{\text{FN} \times \text{PP}}{(\text{FN} \times \text{PP}) + ([1 - \text{FP}]\,[1 - \text{PP})]} \quad [16]$$

In the above formulas

PD/A+ = The probability that a patient has the disease given he/she is positive for the antigen.

PD/A− = The probability that a patient has the disease given he/she is negative for the antigen.

FN = Frequency of the false negative, i.e., 1 − frequency of the antigen in the controls.

FP = Frequency of the false positive, i.e., the frequency of the antigen in the controls.

PP = Prior probability of the disease, i.e., the probability that the patient has the disease before the typing for the antigen was performed.

The prior probability of the disease is specified on the basis of clinical evaluation and other tests done to diagnose the disease.

The frequencies of false-positives and false negatives can be defined in terms of antigen frequencies in controls and patients. For example, if only 90% of the Caucasian ankylosing spondylitis patients are positive for B27 then this test has a 10% false-negative frequency. Similarly, if 8% of the normal population is B27 positive then this test also has an 8% false-positive frequency. On the other hand, if all the ankylosing spondylitis patients were positive for B27 and this antigen was completely absent in the normal population then the B27 test would have 0% false-negative and 0% false-positive frequencies.

Since the frequencies of an antigen in patients and controls of a given population are fixed (except for the sampling variation) the probability that a patient has the disease in the presence or the absence of the antigen is dependent on the prior probability of the disease. A specific numerical example of ankylosing spondylitis in a Caucasian population is given in Table 3.6. The probabilities of the disease after the B27 test are tabulated for several values of prior probability. If a physician, after examining a Caucasian patient, is only 50% certain that the patient has ankylosing spondylitis (i.e., prior probability of ankylosing spondylitis is 0.5), then the presence of B27 in the patient will increase the probability to 91.8%. On the other hand, if the test was negative then there is only a 9.8% probability that the patient has the disease.

TABLE 3.6. The Diagnostic Value of B27 Test in Ankylosing Spondylitis

False negative = 10%
False positive = 8%

Prior probability of ankylosing spondylitis	Probability of ankylosing spondylitis in a patient if he/she is: B27+	B27-
0.20	0.738	0.026
0.40	0.882	0.068
0.50	0.918	0.098
0.60	0.944	0.140
0.80	0.978	0.303

The above formulas can be used to evaluate the diagnostic value of HLA typing in any disease associated with an HLA antigen. All population association studies provide data on the frequencies of the antigen in patients and controls of a given population. These data can easily be converted to false-negative and false-positive values. The prior probability of the disease will depend on the physician's evaluation of clinical and other relevant information available on the presence of the disease in that patient.

Interpretation of the Data and the Analysis

The Relative Risk (RR) and χ^2

In this book the basic data in the table for a particular disease are the frequencies (percent positive) of an antigen in the patients and controls from a country/population. For each individual study the relative risk, its significance as measured by the χ^2, and the reference are given on the same line.

If there is more than one study on the same population then for each such group the total number of patients, percent positive, total number of controls, percent positive, the combined estimate of relative risk, its χ^2, and the heterogeneity χ^2 together with its degrees of freedom are also given. These results are printed after the single solid line.

Finally, the results of the combined analysis are also given for each major racial/population group (e.g., all Caucasians, blacks, etc.). The results of these "major groups" are printed after the double solid lines.

As an illustrative example let us consider the data for HLA-A2 in the table for Rheumatoid Arthritis. There are 6 studies on Caucasian patients from the U.S.A. In the first report the frequencies of A2 in 16 patients and 172 controls were 69 and 44 percent, respectively. The estimated relative risk was 2.69. It had a χ^2 of only 3.56 and thus was not significant.

In this group of 6 studies a total of 371 patients and 2127 controls were typed for A2. The frequencies of this antigen in the total patients and the controls were 57 and 49% respectively. The estimate of relative risk for this group was 1.31 with a χ^2 of 5.55. The heterogeneity χ^2 with 5 degrees of freedom was 6.0, indicating no significant heterogeneity in this group.

There were 16 studies on the Caucasian populations from U.S.A., Australia, and Europe. The total number of patients and controls from all these 16 studies were 906 and 7038, respectively. The estimate of the relative risk was 1.33 with a χ^2 of 15.32. The heterogeneity χ^2 for this group was 26.71 with 15 degrees of freedom. These results are printed after the double solid lines.

The Level of Significance

The associations presented in the tables are only those that are statistically significant or "interesting." As a general rule, if an association has a χ^2 of 10.0 or greater in the pooled data (combined estimate of relative risk) we have considered it significant. The χ^2 of 10.0 gives an uncorrected probability of approximately 0.001. For 20 and 25 antigens compared in the study the corrected probabilities will be 0.02 and 0.025, respectively. The χ^2 of 10.0 for cut-off is a reasonable compromise for pooling the data from several studies in which variable numbers of antigens were studied.

In cases where comparison with other antigens or races appeared interesting we have also included associations with χ^2 values of < 10.0 (on rare occasions < 3.84). This was also done in diseases in which only one or 2 studies are available. We hope that these data, although not strictly significant, will serve as the bases for future followup studies.

References

1. Woolf B: On estimating the relation between blood group and disease. Ann Hum Genet 19:251-253, 1955
2. Haldane JBS: The estimation and significance of the logarithm of a ratio of frequencies. Ann Hum Genet 20:309-311, 1956
3. Dixon WJ, Massey FJ: *Introduction to Statistical Analysis*. McGraw Hill, New York, 1973
4. Fleiss JL: *Statistical Methods for Rates and Proportions*. John Wiley & Sons, New York, 1973
5. Dunn OJ: Estimation of the means of dependent variables. Ann Math Stat 29:1095-1111, 1958
6. Dunn OJ: Multiple comparisons among means. Am J Stat Assoc 56:52-64, 1961
7. Keuning JJ, Pena AS, Van Leeuwen A, Van Hooff JP, Van Rood JJ: HLA-DW3 associated with coeliac disease. Lancet i:505-507, 1976
8. Porta J, McHugh R: Detection of HLA haplotype associations with disease. Tissue Antigens 15:337-345, 1980
9. Terasaki PI, Mickey MR: HL-A haplotypes of 32 diseases. Transplant Rev 22:105-119, 1975
10. Thomson G, Bodmer W: HLA haplotype associations with disease. Tissue Antigens 13:91-102, 1979
11. Penrose LS: The detection of autosomal linkage in data which consists of pairs of brothers and sisters of unspecified parentage. Ann Eugen 6:133-138, 1935
12. Morton NE: Sequential tests for the detection of linkage. Am J Hum Genet 7:277-318, 1955
13. Morton NE: The detection and estimation of linkage between the genes for elliptocytosis and the Rh type. Am J Hum Genet 8:80-96, 1956
14. Cudworth AG, Woodrow JC: Evidence for HL-A linked genes in "juvenile" diabetes mellitus. Br Med J 3:133-135, 1975
15. Maynard-Smith S, Penrose LS, Smith CAB: *Mathematical Tables for Research Workers in Human Genetics*. Churchill, London, 1961
16. Cavalli-Sforza LL, Bodmer WF: *The Genetics of Human Populations*. Freeman, San Francisco, 1971
17. Ott J: Estimation of the recombination fraction in human pedigrees: Efficient computation of the likelihood for human linkage studies. Am J Hum Genet 26:588-597, 1974

18. Ott J: A simple scheme for the analysis of HLA linkages in pedigrees. Ann Hum Genet 42:255-257, 1978
19. Curie-Cohen M: A note on relative risks. Tissue Antigens 9:59-61, 1977
20. Smouse PE: Statistical analysis of HLA-disease associations. Prog Clin Biol Res 32:545-551, 1979
21. Nijenhuis LE: Genetic considerations on association between HLA and disease. Hum Genet 38:175-182, 1977
22. Lalouel JM, Morton NE: Complex segregation analysis with pointers. Hum Hered 31:312-321, 1981
23. Morton NE, Lalouel JM: Relation of linkage for irregular phenotype systems. Hum Hered 31:3-7, 1981
24. Thomson G: A two locus model for juvenile diabetes. Ann Hum Genet 43:383-398, 1980
25. Suarez B, Hodge SE, Reich T: Is juvenile diabetes determined by a single gene closely linked to HLA? Diabetes 28:527-532, 1979
26. Suarez BK, Rice J, Reich T: The generalized sib pair JBD distribution: Its use in the detection of linkage. Ann Hum Genet 42:87-94, 1978
27. Suarez BK: The affected sib pair JBD distribution for HLA- linked disease susceptibility genes. Tissue Antigens 12:87- 93, 1978
28. Kidd KK, Bernoco D, Carbonara AO, Daneo V, Steiger U, Ceppellini R: Genetic analysis of HLA-associated diseases: The "illness-susceptible" gene frequency and sex ratio in ankylosing spondylitis. In Dausset J, Svejgaard A (eds):HLA and Disease. Munksgaard, Copenhagen, 1977, pp 72-80
29. Green JR, Woodrow JC: Sibling method for detecting HLA- linked genes in disease. Tissue Antigens 9:31-35, 1977
30. De Vries RRD, Fat RFMLA, Nijenhuis LE, Van Rood JJ: HLA-linked genetic control of host response to *Mycobacterium leprae*. Lancet ii:1328-1330, 1976
31. Fishman PM, Suarez B, Hodge SE, Reich T: A robust method for the detection of linkage in familial diseases. Am J Hum Genet 30:308-321, 1978
32. Thomson G, Bodmer W: The genetic analysis of HLA and disease associations. In Dausset J , Svejgaard A (eds): HLA and Disease. Munksgaard, Copenhagen, 1977, pp 84-93
33. Hodge SE, Rotter JI, Lange KL: A three-allele model for heterogeneity of juvenile onset insulin-dependent diabetes. Ann Hum Genet 43:399-412, 1980
34. Day NE, Simons MJ: Disease susceptibility genes–their identification by multiple case family studies. Tissue Antigens 8:109-119, 1976
35. Katz M: A probability graph describing the predictive value of a highly sensitive diagnostic text. N Engl J Med 291:1115-1116, 1974
36. Wakisaka A, Aizawa M, Matsuura N, Nakagawa S, Nakayama E, Okuno A, et al.: HLA and juvenile diabetes mellitus in Japanese. Lancet ii:970, 1976
37. Okimoto K, Juji T, Ishiba S, Maruyama H, Tokyama H, Kusaka K: HLA-BW54 (BW22-J, J-1) antigens in juvenile onset diabetes mellitus in Japan. Tissue Antigens 11:418-422, 1978
38. Kawa A, Nakazawa M, Kono Y, Sakaguchi S, Nakamura S, Kanekisa T: HLA-BW54 and B5 in Japanese diabetics with juvenile-onset and insulin-dependency (with special reference to the family history). Experientia 24:669-670, 1978
39. Sakurami T, Nagaoka K, Nabeya N, Imura H, Kuno S: Islet-cell antibodies and HLA types in Japanese insulin- dependent diabetics. Endocrinol Jpn 27:149-152, 1980

CHAPTER 4

Mechanisms of HLA and Disease Associations

General Background

The discoveries of HLA associations with certain diseases have been a major breakthrough in our understanding of the genetics of these diseases. We now know that at least part of the genetic basis of the associated diseases lies in the HLA region of chromosome 6. Furthermore, the "disease susceptibility genes" for hemochromatosis, congenital adrenal hyperplasia, and olivopontocerebellar ataxia (Menzel type) are known to be in linkage with HLA and have been mapped on chromosome 6.[1] HLA markers are already providing some useful clinical information regarding these diseases (for references see the individual sections on these diseases). However, it is interesting to note that in the beginning these HLA associations generated high hopes and enthusiasm that the etiology of these diseases will soon be resolved. Yet, surprisingly, a decade after the landmark results on HLA-B27 and ankylosing spondylitis[2,3] we are still searching for the mechanism(s) involved in these associations. Various hypotheses have been proposed but thus far none is supported by clear-cut evidence.

The nature of the mechanisms underlying the empirically observed associations between HLA antigens and diseases has been the subject of much speculation. In a discussion of the association mechanism it is important to recapitulate some of the general characteristics of the available HLA data. The primary data showing the associations are increased frequencies of certain HLA antigens in groups of patients as compared with a sample of normal individuals. Some disease studies of families with more than 1 patient have also demonstrated the disease segregation with an HLA haplotype within a family. However, all the reported pedigrees on a particular disease do not show a consistent segregation pattern. Beyond this, at present there are very little data on humans that can be used as bases for proposing mechanisms for the observed associations. Furthermore, none of the observed associations is absolute. The strongest association to date is that of ankylosing spondylitis with B27 with a relative risk of about 70.0 estimated from the pooled data on all Caucasian patients. With few exceptions, the relative risks of all other associations are in the range of 2.0-15.0. It should also be noted that the diseases that are associated with HLA antigens do not show simple Mendelian segregation in families, have a very weak or no effect on reproduction, and are of unknown etiology. Heterogeneity is another important characteristic of these diseases.

Mechanisms

The proposed mechanisms for the disease associations can be categorized into 2 main groups.

Involvement of HLA Antigens

Receptors
It has been suggested that HLA antigens may act as receptors for pathogenic organisms (e.g., viruses). Thus, it is hypothesized that B27 molecules on the surface of lymphocytes may be the receptors for some organisms responsible for ankylosing spondylitis, Reiter's syndrome, and other B27-associated diseases.

Helenius et al.[4] have presented data showing that the proteins coded for by the HLA-A and -B loci in man and the H-2K and H-2D loci in mice were acting as cell surface receptors for Semliki Forest virus.

However, Oldstone et al.[5] reported that murine F9 and PCC4 teratoma cells, which do not express H2 antigens, can be infected with and readily replicate many types of viruses (Coxsackie B3, Semliki Forest virus, mouse hepatitis, Sindbis, lymphocytic choriomeningitis, Pichinde, vesicular stomatitis, herpes simplex type 1). The extent of infection and replication was the same as for murine F12 teratoma cells and mouse embryo fibroblast, all of which express the H-2 antigens. It was also shown that Daudi cells, which lack HLA antigens, block the replication of Semliki Forest virus (see also Oldstone[6]).

Haspel et al.[7] studied the interaction of HLA antigens with measles virus antigens. The large amounts of virus antigens inserted into the membranes remained physically independent from HLA antigens. HLA antigens appeared neither to serve as receptors for measles virus nor to be incorporated into the maturing virus particle. However, infection of cultured human lymphoblastoid cells with poliomyelitis virus and vesicular stomatitis virus was found to decrease the concentration of HLA antigens.

A study by Couillion and Fellous[8] examined the correlation between specific receptors of 3 enteroviruses (poliovirus II, Coxsackie B3, and echovirus II) and HLA antigens in man-mouse hybrid cells. No correlation was found, suggesting that HLA antigens are not the receptors for these viruses.

Thus most of the data do not support the role of HLA antigens as receptors for the viruses.

Molecular Mimicry

The molecular mimicry hypothesis, originally proposed by Snell,[9] postulates that the molecular structures of infectious agents are similar to those of the HLA antigens on the cell surface. Because of this mimicry the host organism cannot recognize such viruses, bacteria, and parasites as "non-self" and is, therefore, unable to initiate an immune response.

Cross-reaction between 7 HLA antigens and streptococcal M proteins has been described by Hirata and Terasaki.[10] However, this cross-reactivity was not specific; all 7 antigens were inhibited by the M protein. Several recent reports from Australia and England contain very interesting data on the cross-reaction between B27 and *Klebsiella* (see section on Ankylosing Spondylitis). It is somewhat disturbing, however, that despite widespread attempts to repeat these findings confirmatory reports have not appeared in the literature. Molecular mimicry may be a mechanism especially in the case of some of the B27-associated diseases, in which no association with D/DR antigens has been found.

Interaction of HLA Molecules with Nonimmunologic Ligands

Svejgaard and Ryder[11] have postulated that HLA antigens may interfere with ligand–receptor interactions not directly involved in immune reactions. It was hypothesized that some HLA molecules may have structures similar to those on receptors for certain hormones that could cause competition between HLA and receptor molecules for the hormone. Such interactions may, under certain conditions, lead to nonimmunologic diseases, such as hemochromatosis.

A similar hypothesis was also proposed by Mitchell and Nicholls[12] as an explanation of association between HLA and autoimmune diseases. They have postulated that the HLA antigens bind foreign molecules, creating a hapten-carrier relationship that will direct the immune response to the surface of the cells. The HLA antigens on the surface of cells of some solid tissues may bind haptenic material, leading to an immune response directed in part against the tissue.

Viral Modification of HLA Antigens

It has been shown by Doherty and Zinkernagel[13–15] that cytotoxic T cells from mice infected acutely with lymphocytic choriomeningitis virus interact only with H-2-compatible virus-infected cells. Similar results have been observed for vaccinia virus by Koszinowski and Ertl[16] and for ectromelia virus by Blanden et al.[17] Two models have been proposed to explain this phenomenon.[18] The *dual recogniti on* model proposes that T cells have 2 receptor molecules, 1 for the relevant histocompatibility-coded self-marker and the other for the specific viral antigen. The *single recognition or altered self* model postulates that T cells have a single clonally expressed recognition molecule that is specific for either a complex of the antigen plus the histocompatibility-coded self-marker or for a specific structurally modified self-marker.

McMichael et al.[19] have reported HLA restriction of cell-mediated lysis of influenza virus-infected cells. Similar results have also been reported by Dickmeiss et al.[20]

Shaw et al.[21] have shown that in vitro human cytotoxic T cell responses to 2 closely related influenza viruses (HK types A and B) are HLA-restricted.

Involvement of Genes Closely Linked with the HLA Complex

The second group of hypotheses proposes that HLA antigens are not involved in the causation of the disease. They are markers for the "disease susceptibility genes" that are very closely linked with the HLA complex. The observed population associations are due to the existence of linkage disequilibria between the HLA antigens and the alleles for the disease susceptibility genes. As an example, it can be postulated that the association of DR2 with multiple sclerosis (MS) is due to the existence of an MS susceptibility gene very closely linked with the DR locus. The disease susceptibility allele of this locus is in linkage disequilibrium with the DR2 allele of the DR locus. Thus, DR2 is simply a neutral marker for an MS susceptibility allele. The presence of the disease in only a small fraction of the people carrying the marker HLA allele can be explained by the following: (1) Genetic factors not linked with HLA may be contributing toward the disease susceptibility; (2) the disease may be heterogeneous and may have more than 1 etiology; the observed HLA association is only with a subset of affected individuals; (3) environmental factors, such as exposure to viruses, determine whether individuals with disease susceptibility will contract the disease; and (4) if the association is due to a thus-far undetected allele at a closely linked locus, then this allele may occur at a much lower frequency than the one detected at the presently known A, B, C, and D/DR loci.[22,23]

Terasaki and Mickey[24] have proposed "a single mutation hypothesis" for the association between HLA and MS. In this hypothesis there is a MS susceptibility gene in genetic linkage with the HLA complex. Furthermore, this susceptibility gene originated by mutation in a single prehistoric individual who lived in Northern Europe and had HLA-A3, -B7, and -DR2 antigens. The susceptibility gene was transmitted from generation to generation throughout the world so that today all MS patients are the descendants of the original hominoid. Generations of chromosomal crossovers have seperated and recombined the disease gene with other HLA antigens. The introduction of this disease gene into other distinct populations was accomplished by the processes of migration and gene admixture.

Immune Response Genes

It is postulated that disease associations are due to the immune response (Ir) genes closely linked with the HLA complex and in linkage disequilibrium with certain alleles of A, B, C and D/DR loci. Histocompatibility-linked immune response genes have been shown to exist in mouse and other animal species.[25–29]

In the mouse Ir genes have been mapped in the I region of the chromosome.[25–28,30,31] The D/DR loci in humans are believed to be analogous to the I region in the mouse and thus it has been hypothesized that Ir and immune suppression genes also exist in the D/DR region of the HLA complex.

A strong argument in favor of this hypothesis is that some of the diseases known to be associated with the alleles of the B locus now show stronger associations with the alleles of the D/DR loci. For example, the association of MS with DW2/DR2 is stronger than that with B7 and similarly the association of juvenile diabetes with DW3/DR3 and DW4/DR4 is stronger than that with B8 and B15. If the disease susceptibility loci are closer to the D/DR loci then there will be stronger linkage disequilibria with DW2/DR2, DW3/DR3, and DW4/DR4 alleles. In this case the associations with the alleles of the B locus are secondary to those with D/DR alleles.

Another argument supporting this hypothesis is the association of the same disease with 2 different alleles of the same HLA locus. As an example, Grave's disease is associated with B8 in Caucasians and with BW35 in Japanese. If Grave's disease is the same in both populations then these associations can be explained by the different patterns of linkage disequilibria with the disease susceptibility gene in different populations.[32]

Metabolic Genes

It is possible that genes other than those involved in immune response and immune suppression are linked with the HLA complex. These genes may be responsible for the diseases with no apparent immunologic basis. These genes may affect some step(s) in metabolic pathways through enzymes or common precursor substance.

Some other interesting mechanisms have been discussed in a report by Bodmer.[33]

It should be noted that in the most recent report[1] of the Committee on the Genetic Constitution of Chromosome 6 no HLA-linked immune response genes have been assigned to chromosome 6. Only loci for olivopontocerebellar ataxia (Menzel type), congenital adrenal hyperplasia, and hemochromatosis have been assigned to this chromosome. The linkage of these diseases with HLA is confirmed.

References

1. Robson EB, Lamm LU: Human gene mapping 7: Report of the committee on the genetic constitution of chromosome 6. Cytogenet Cell Genet 37:47-70, 1984

2. Schlosstein L, Terasaki PI, Bluestone R, Pearson GM: High association of an HL-A antigen, W27, with ankylosing spondylitis. N Engl J Med 288:704-706, 1973
3. Brewerton DA, Caffrey M, Hart FD, James DCO, Nicholls A, Sturrock RD: Ankylosing spondylitis and HL-A27. Lancet i:904-907, 1973
4. Helenius A, Morein B, Fries E, Simons K, Robinson P, and Schirrmacher V, et al: Human (HLA-A and HLA-B) and murine (H-2K and H-2D) histocompatibility antigens are cell surface receptors for Semliki Forest virus. Proc Natl Acad Sci 75:3846-3850, 1978
5. Oldstone MBA, Tishon A, Dutko FJ, Kennedy SIT, Holland JJ, Lampert PW: Does the major histocompatibility complex serve as a specific receptor for Semliki Forest virus? J Virol 34:256-265, 1980
6. Oldstone MBA: Relationship between major histocompatibility antigens and disease: Possible associations with human arenavirus diseases. Bull WHO 52:479-486, 1975
7. Haspel MV, Pellegrino MA, Lampert PW, Oldstone MBA: Human histocompatibility determinants and virus antigens: Effect of measles virus infection on HLA expression. J Exp Med 146:146-156, 1977
8. Couillion P, Fellous M: Recherche d'une correlation entre is systeme antigenique HL-A et les recepteurs viraux trois enterovirus a l'aide de l'hybridization cellulaire. Soc Biol 168:180-186, 1974
9. Snell GD: The H-2 locus of the mouse: Observations and speculations concerning its comparative genetics and its polymorphism. Folia Biol 14:335-358, 1968
10. Hirata HA. Terasaki PI: Cross-reactions between Streptococcal M proteins and human transplantation antigens. Science 168:1095-1096, 1970
11. Svejgaard A, Ryder LP: Interaction of HLA molecules with non-immunological ligands as an explanation of HLA and disease associations. Lancet ii:547-549, 1976
12. Mitchell NR, Nicholls EM: HLA and the genetics of autoimmune diseases. Med Hypotheses 4:149-155, 1978
13. Doherty PC, Zinkernagel RM: T-cell-mediated immunopathology in viral infection. Transplant Rev 19:89, 1974
14. Zinkernagel RM, Doherty PC: Restriction of in vitro T cell-mediated cytotoxicity in lymphocytic choriomeningitis virus within a syngeneic semiallogeneic system. Nature 248:701-702, 1974
15. Doherty PC, Blanden RV, Zinkernagel RM: Specificity of virus-immune effector T cells for H-2K or H-2D compatible interactions: Implications for H-antigen diversity. Transplant Rev 29:89-124, 1976
16. Koszinowski U, Ertl H: Lysis mediated by T cells and restricted by H-2 antigen of target cells infected with vaccinia virus. Nature 255:552-554, 1975
17. Blanden RV, Doherty PC, Dunlop MBC, Gardner ID, Zinkernagel RM, David CS: Genes required for cytotoxicity against virus-infected target cells in K and D regions of H-2 complex. Nature 254:269-270, 1975
18. Zinkernagel RM: Role of the H-2 gene complex in cell- mediated immunity to infectious disease. Transplant Proc 9:1835-1838, 1977
19. McMichael AJ, Ting A, Zweerink HJ, Askonas BA: HLA restriction of cell-mediated lysis of influenza virus- infected human cells. Nature 270:524-526, 1977
20. Dickmeiss E, Soeberg B, Svejgaard A: Human cell-mediated cytotoxicity against modified target cells is restricted by HLA. Nature 270:526, 1977
21. Shaw S, Shearer GM, Biddison WE: Human cytotoxic T-cell responses to type A and type B influenza viruses can be restricted by different HLA antigens: Implication for HLA polymorphism and genetic regulation. J Exp Med 151:235-245, 1980
22. Bodmer WF and Bodmer JG: Evolution and function of the HLA system. Br Med Bull 34:309-316, 1978
23. McDevitt HO, Bodmer WF: HL-A, immune-response genes, and diseases. Lancet i:1269-1275, 1974
24. Terasaki PI, Mickey MR: A single mutation hypothesis for multiple sclerosis based on the HL-A system. Neurology 26:56-58, 1976
25. Shreffler DC, David C: The H-2 major histocompatibility complex and the I immune response region: Genetic variation, function, and organization. Adv Immunol 20:125- 195, 1975
26. Winchester RJ, Kunkel HG: The human Ia system. Adv Immunol 28:221-292, 1979
27. Benacerraf B, Katz D: The histocompatibility-linked immune response genes. Adv Cancer Res 21:121-173, 1975
28. Gill TH III, Cramer DV, Kunz HW: The major histocompatibility complex–comparison in mouse, man, and the rat. Am J Pathol 90:737-777, 1978
29. Snell GD, Dausset J, Nathenson S: Histocompatibility, Academic Press, New York, 1976
30. Benacerraf B, Germain RN: The immune response genes of the major histocompatibility complex. Immunol Rev 38:70- 119, 1978
31. Snell GD: Recent advances in histocompatibility immunogenetics. Adv Genet 20:291-355, 1979
32. Bodmer WF, Thomson G: Population genetics and evolution of the HLA system. In Dausset J and Svejgaard A (eds): HLA and Disease. Munksgaard, Copenhagen, 1977, pp 280-295
33. Bodmer WF: Models and mechanisms for HLA and disease associations. J Exp Med 152:353s-357s, 1980

CHAPTER 5

Overview

In this chapter we present a summary of the most significant associations and also a list of all the HLA antigens that have been found to be associated with various diseases. We hope that this summary list will provide a convenient reference table for all the investigators interested in this field.

Summary of the Most Significant Associations

A list of the most significant HLA and disease associations are given in Table 5.1. The data in this table were pooled from all available studies on a major race. Thus, for example, there were a total of 2130 Caucasian ankylosing spondylitis patients form 40 independent studies in which the association of HLA-B27 was examined. The frequency of this antigen in 2130 patients was 89%. In the pooled samples of the controls the frequency of B27 was found to be 9%. (The total number of controls from these 40 studies are not given in this table. They can be found in the data table for ankylosing spondylitis.) The combined estimate of relative risk (RR) from these 40 studies was 60.1.

The following figures summarize the data by the country of origin and race. The total number of patients studied from that country is given in the third column. The lower end of the solid bars drawn on the "antigen frequency scale" marks the antigen frequency in the total controls (sample size not given in the diagram). Similarly, the upper end of the bars represents the antigen frequency in the patient population. Thus the lengths of the solid bars in the figure give percent increase of the antigen frequency in the patient population. The numbers near the upper end of each bar are the values of the relative risk estimated from those data.

TABLE 5.1. Some Significant HLA and Disease Associations

Disease	Race	Studies N	Patients No.	Patients %+	Cont. %+	RR
Rheumatoid Arthritis						
B27	C	17	861	16	9	2.0
DR4	C	17	1127	68	25	3.8
BW54	O	3	221	24	11	2.5
DR4	O	5	348	66	39	2.8
DR4	N	3	109	40	10	5.4
Juvenile Rheumatoid Arthritis						
B27	C	15	1146	25	9	3.9
DR5	C	5	422	34	15	3.3
Ankylosing Spondylitis						
B27	C	40	2130	89	9	69.1
B27	O	7	211	85	15	207.9
B27	N	2	33	58	4	54.4
Acute Anterior Uveitis						
B27	C	10	520	47	10	8.2
Reiter's Disease						
B27	C	25	906	80	9	37.1
Juvenile Diabetes Mellitus						
B8	C	39	4322	40	21	2.5
B15	C	36	4052	22	14	2.1
DR3	C	13	1174	46	22	3.3
DR4	C	12	1051	51	25	3.6
BW54	O	8	453	39	11	5.6
DR3	O	4	139	38	14	4.8
DR4	O	4	139	49	25	2.6
B8	N	6	337	19	11	2.4
B15	N	5	299	6	5	2.2
DR3	N	3	135	57	28	3.2
DR4	N	3	135	46	11	6.7
Grave's Disease						
B8	C	18	1445	43	23	2.5
DR3	C	4	333	56	25	3.7
B35	O	3	162	42	14	4.4
Celiac Disease						
B8	C	16	696	68	22	7.6
DR3	C	5	194	79	22	11.6
DR7	C	4	137	60	15	7.7
Narcolepsy						
DR2	C	2	45	100	22	129.8
DR2	O	1	92	100	34	358.1

Disease	Race	Studies N	Patients No.	Patients %+	Cont. %+	RR
Psoriasis Vulgaris						
B13	C	36	2579	19	5	4.1
B17	C	35	2515	19	7	5.3
B37	C	15	804	7	2	3.9
CW6	C	7	353	56	15	7.5
DR7	C	5	296	48	23	3.2
B13	O	5	336	24	8	3.3
B17	O	4	224	12	9	1.9
B37	O	3	206	20	2	8.4
CW6	O	4	262	27	4	8.5
DR7	O	2	148	10	1	7.6
Pemphigus Vulgaris						
A26	CJ	5	117	60	20	4.8
B38	CJ	5	117	59	21	4.6
DR4	CJ	3	62	91	32	14.6
Dermatitis Herpetiformis						
B8	C	14	498	75	22	9.8
DR3	C	4	126	82	20	17.3
Behcet's Disease						
B5	C	6	150	31	12	3.8
B5	O	6	199	68	33	4.5
Idiopathic Hemochromatosis						
A3	C	11	493	72	28	6.7
B7	C	11	493	48	26	2.9
B14	C	10	481	19	6	2.7
Sjögren's Syndrome						
B8	C	6	184	50	24	3.3
DW3	C	4	105	64	24	5.7
Systemic Lupus Erythematosus						
B8	C	17	855	40	20	2.7
DR3	C	9	316	42	21	2.6
Goodpasture's Syndrome						
DR2	C	2	25	88	27	13.8
Multiple Sclerosis						
B7	C	38	4964	37	24	1.8
DR2	C	13	1051	51	27	2.7
Myasthenia Gravis						
B8	C	12	747	44	19	3.3

N = Number of Studies
No. = Number of Patients

C = Caucasian
O = Oriental
N = Negro
J = Jewish

%+ = Percent Positive
RR = Relative Risk

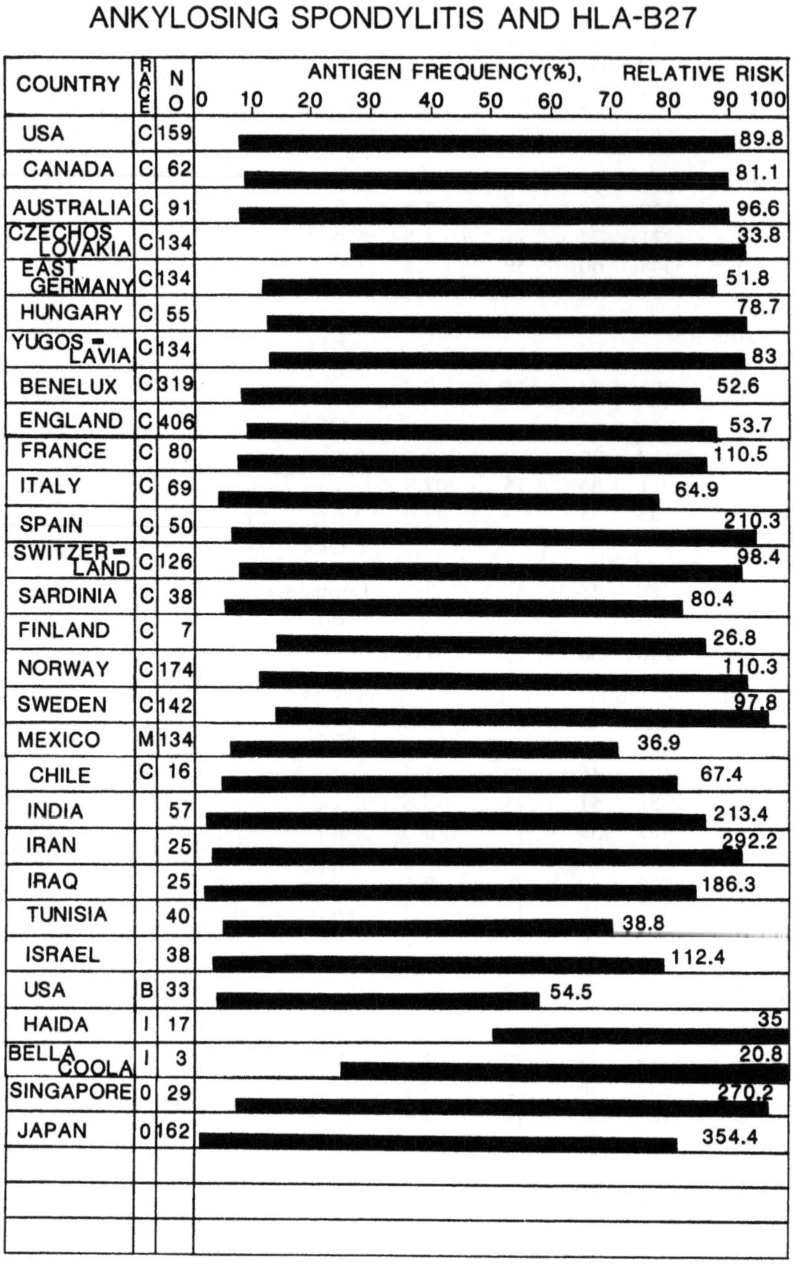

FIGURE 5.1 The strongest association is still between HLA-B27 and ankylosing spondylitis. The frequency of B27 in the control populations is generally < 10%. In the patient groups its frequency is in the 90% range. The only exception for the controls is Haida Indian population of Canada, in which a high frequency of 50% has been found. In Bella Coola Indians of Canada 100% of the patients were found to be positive for B27. Interestingly, in every population studied thus far the antigen B27 is associated with this disease.

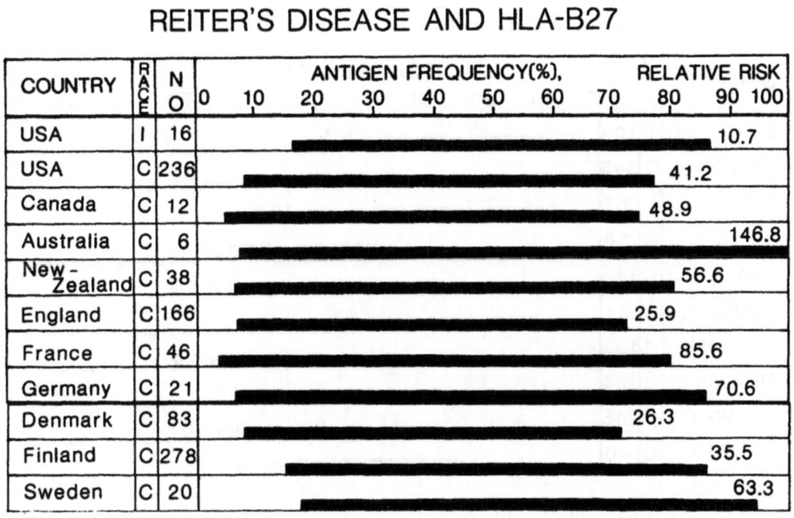

FIGURE 5.2 HLA-B27 is strongly associated with Reiter's disease in all the reported Caucasian populations.

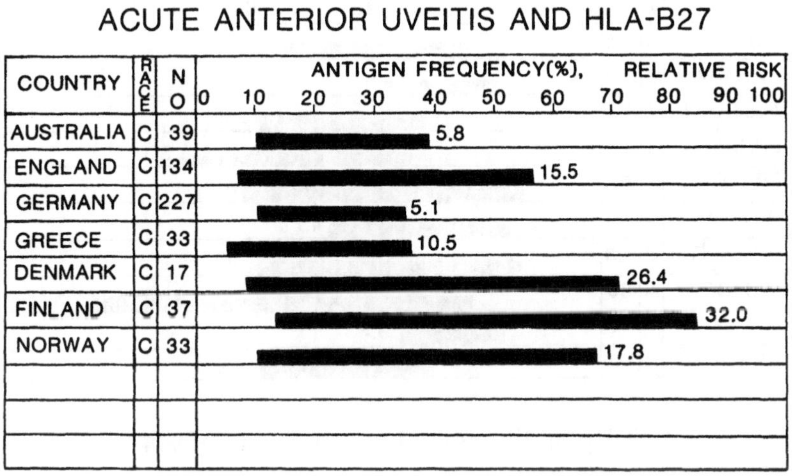

FIGURE 5.3 Acute anterior uveitis is another disease showing strong association with HLA-B27 in various Caucasian populations.

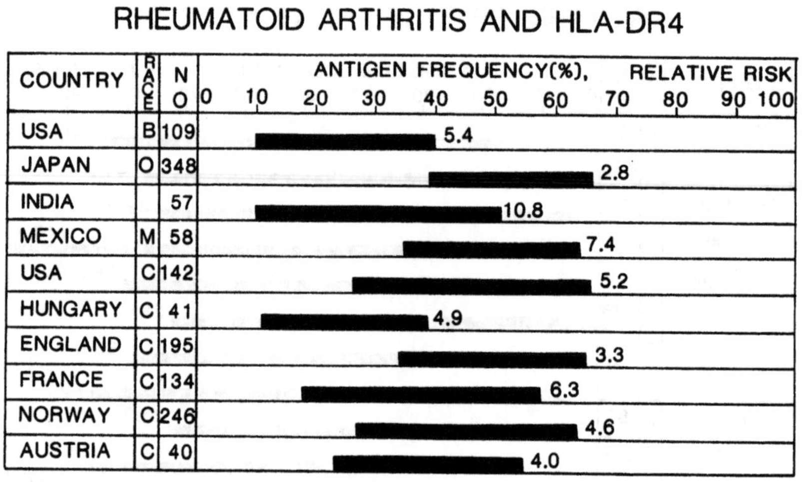

FIGURE 5.4 Rheumatoid arthritis is clearly associated with HLA-DR4 in various races.

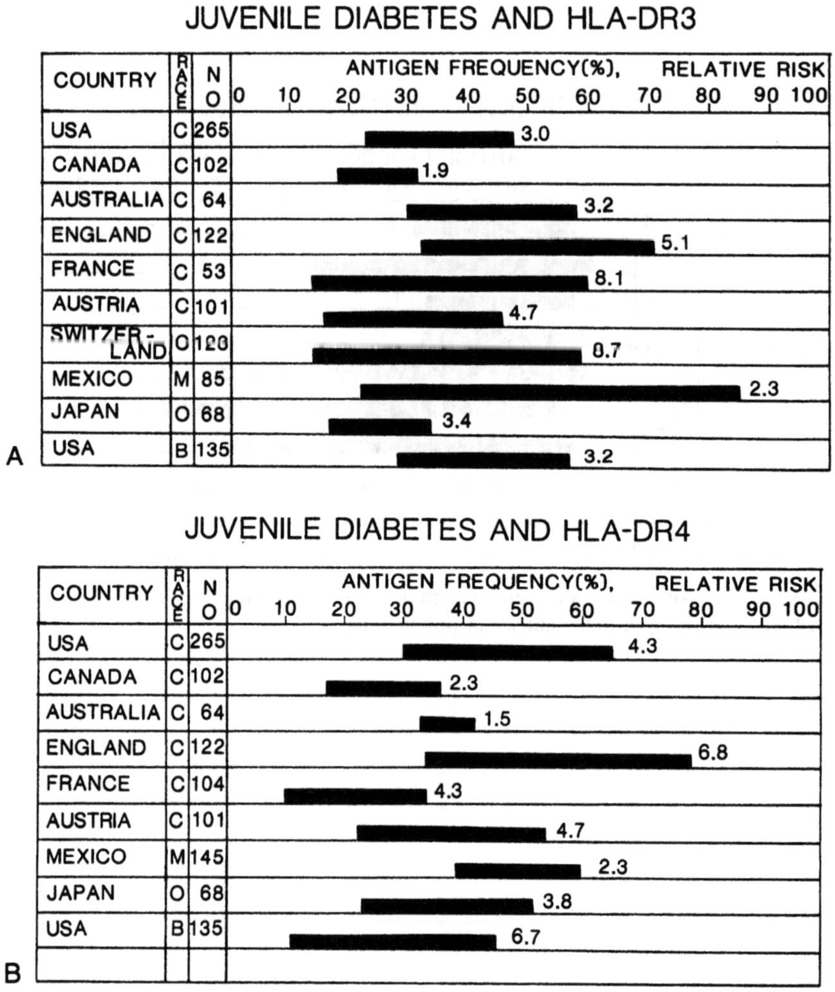

FIGURE 5.5A AND B HLA-DR3 and -DR4 antigens are significantly increased in patients with juvenile-onset diabetes. This dual association along with the significantly reduced frequency of DR2 in patients is a striking feature of this disease.

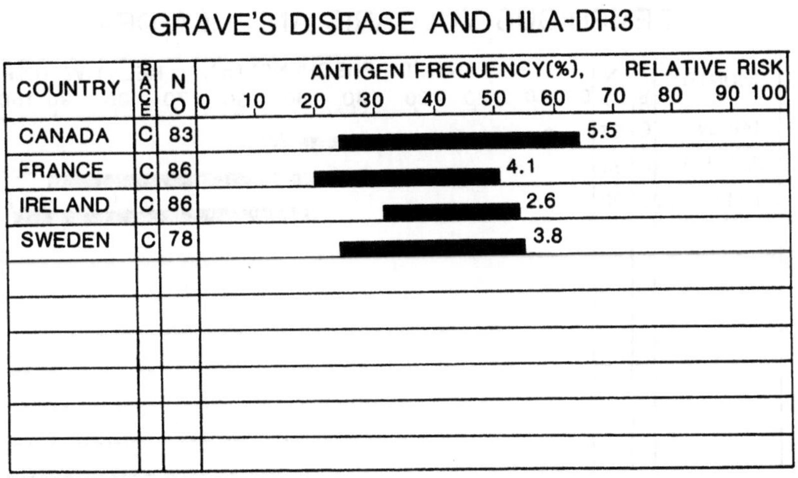

FIGURE 5.6 Grave's disease is associated with HLA-DR3 in 4 caucasian populations.

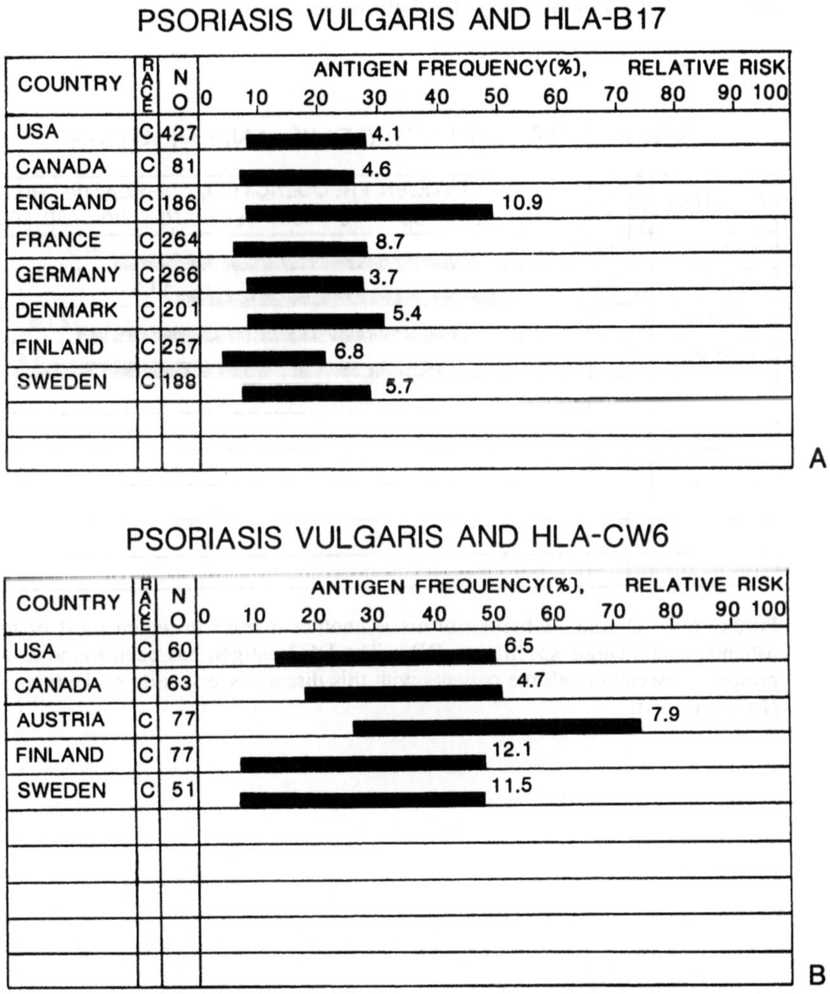

FIGURE 5.7A AND B Psoriasis vulgaris was originally found to be associated with HLA-B13 and -B17. In later studies a stronger association with HLA-CW6 was also observed. It is one of the very few diseases with an association with C locus antigens.

PEMPHIGUS VULGARIS AND HLA-DR4

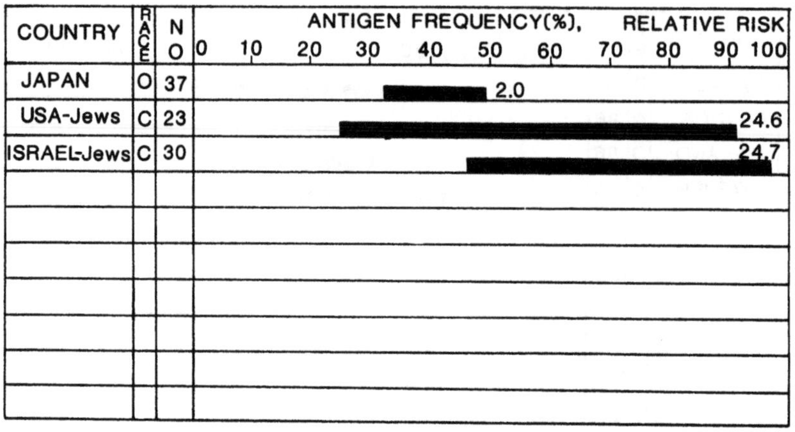

FIGURE 5.8 Pemphigus vulgaris was first shown to be associated with HLA-A11 and later found to be more strongly associated with HLA-DR4. This disease occurs more frequently in Jewish caucasians. It appears that essentially all the patients with the disease have HLA-DR4 antigen.

DERMATITIS HERPETIFORMIS AND HLA-DR3

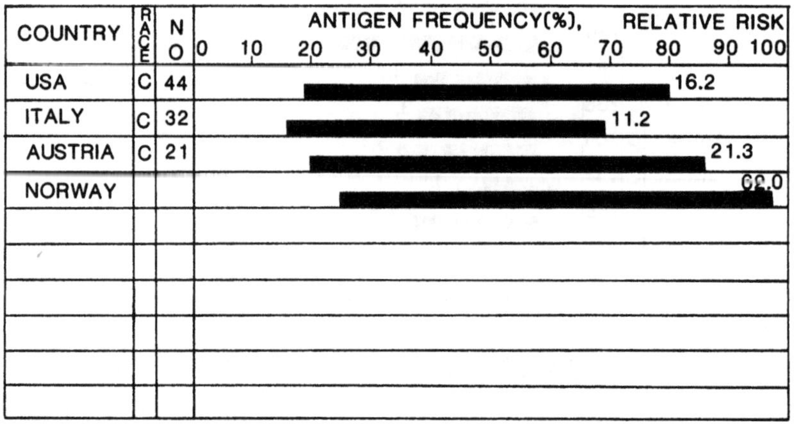

FIGURE 5.9 Dermatitis herpetiformis is another disease in which most of the patients have a single specificity, DR3. The DQ2 antigen has been found to be present in essentially all the patients with this disease (see section on Dermatitis Herpetiformis).

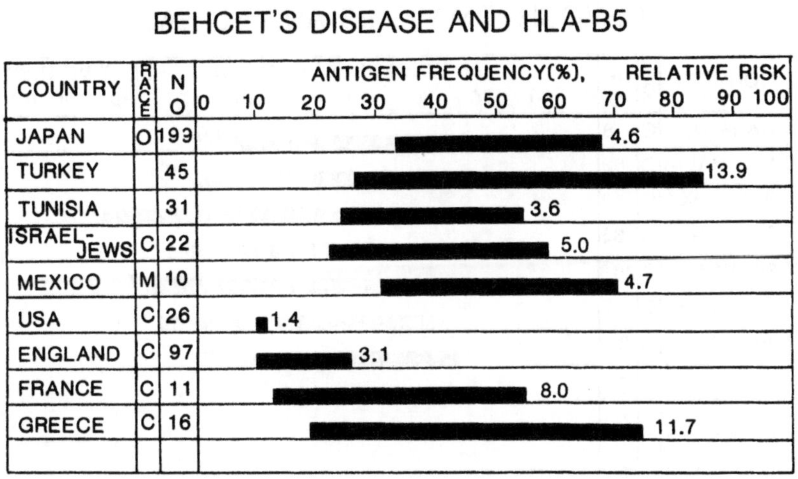

FIGURE 5.10 Behcet's disease and HLA-B5 association was first noted in Japan. It has been confirmed in several other populations from throughout the world.

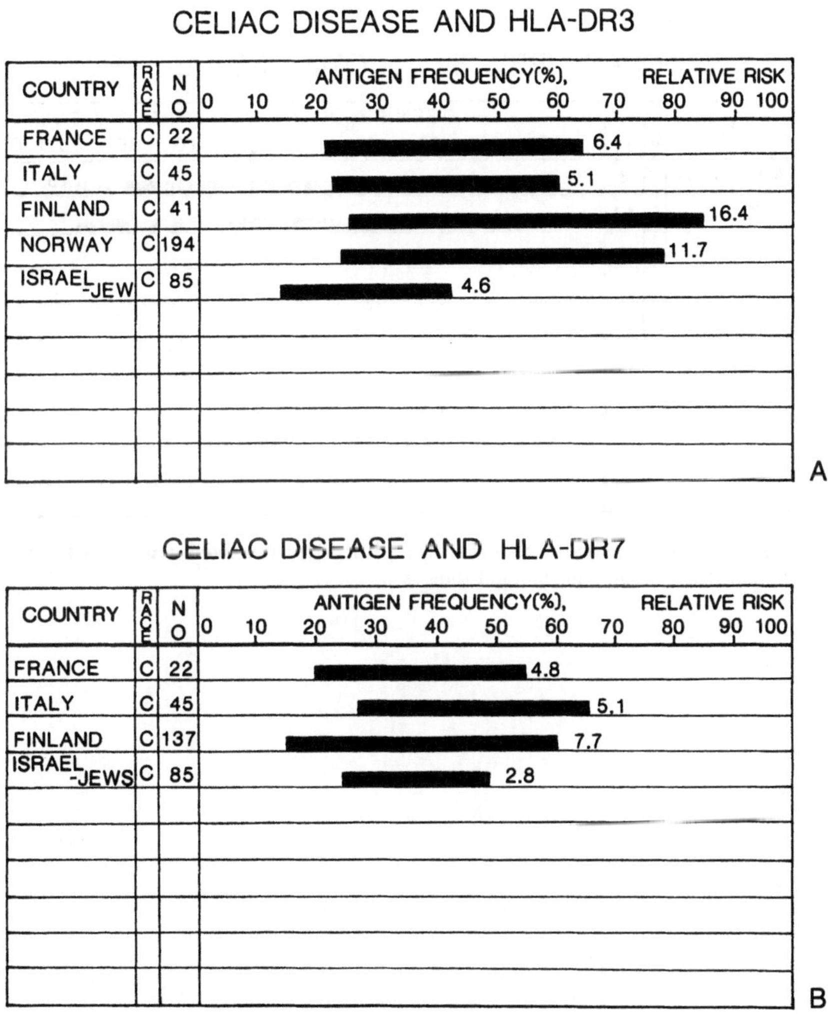

FIGURE 5.11A AND B Two DR locus antigens, DR3 and DR7, are significantly associated with celiac disease.

HEMOCHROMATOSIS AND HLA-A3

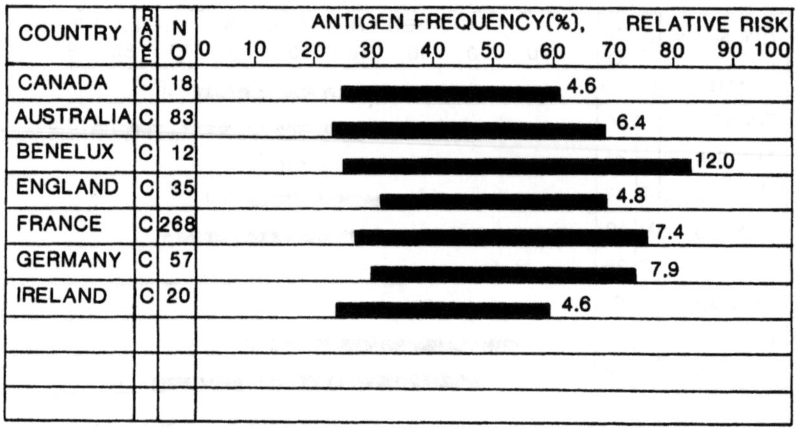

FIGURE 5.12 Hemachromatosis is strongly associated with HLA-A3 in all of the studied Caucasian patients from various countries. The initial and extensive followup studies have been reported from France.

GOODPASTURE'S SYNDROME AND HLA-DR2

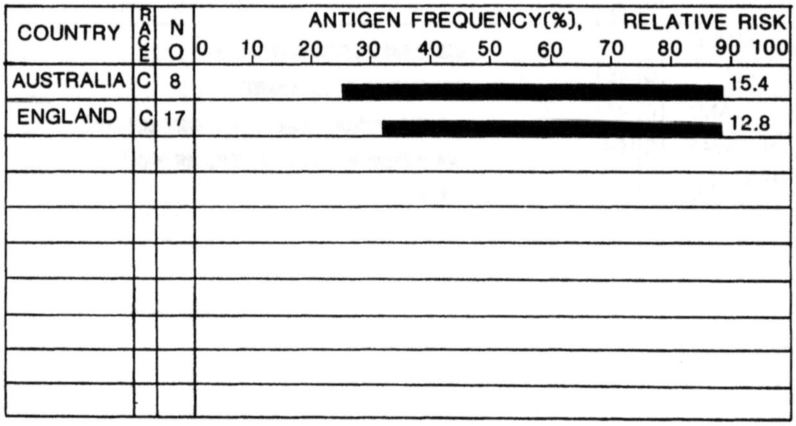

FIGURE 5.13 Goodpasture's syndrome is strongly associated with HLA-DR2 in 2 Caucasian populations studied thus far.

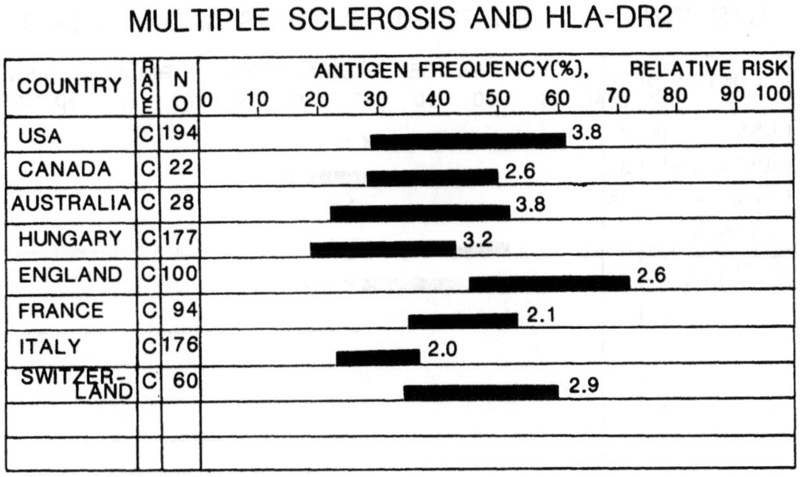

FIGURE 5.14 Multiple sclerosis has been extensively studied in caucasian populations in which a significant association with HLA-DR2 has been found. The earlier data on this disease also showed associations with HLA-A3 and -B7.

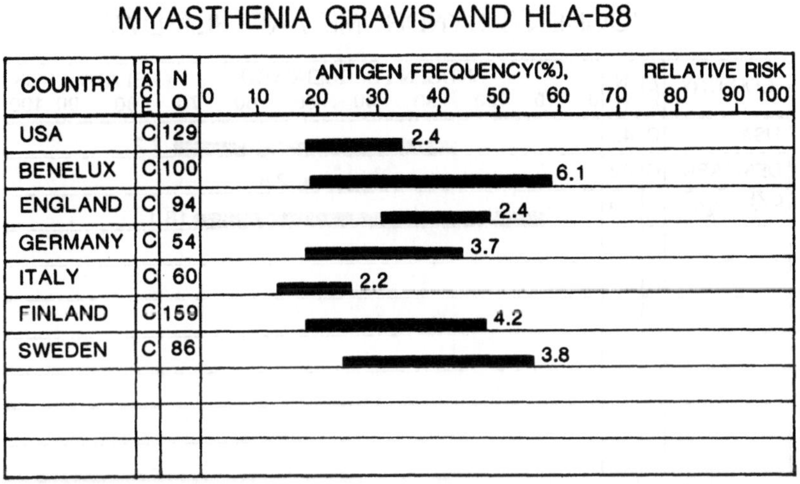

FIGURE 5.15 In several Caucasian populations myasthenia gravis is associated with HLA-B8. A stronger association of this disease with any of the DR locus antigen has not been found.

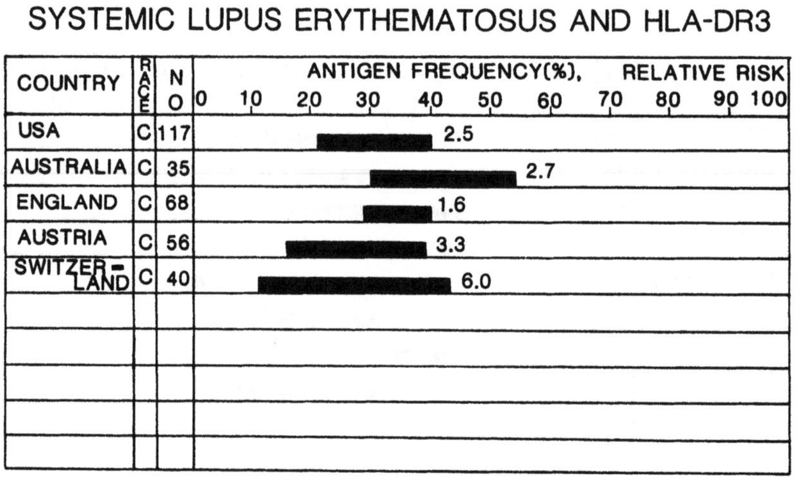

FIGURE 5.16 Systemic lupus erythematosus is associated with DR3. In various studies several other B locus antigens were reported to be associated with this disease but HLA-DR3 association appears to be the strongest.

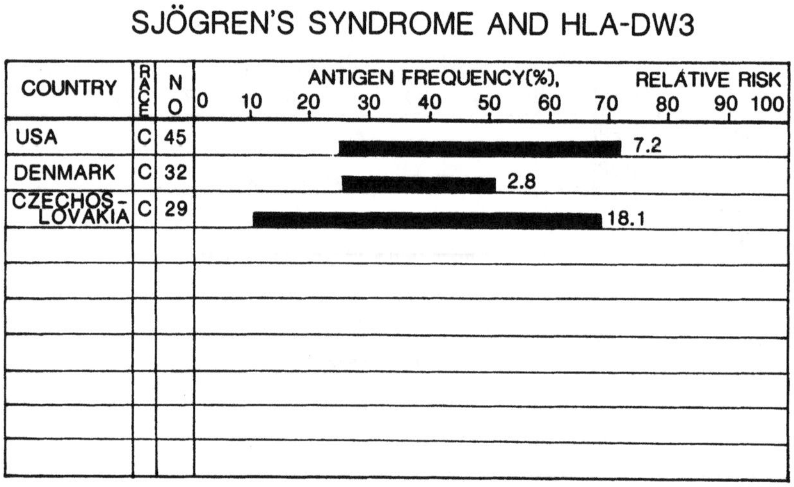

FIGURE 5.17 Sjögren's syndrome has been found to be associated with HLA-DW3.

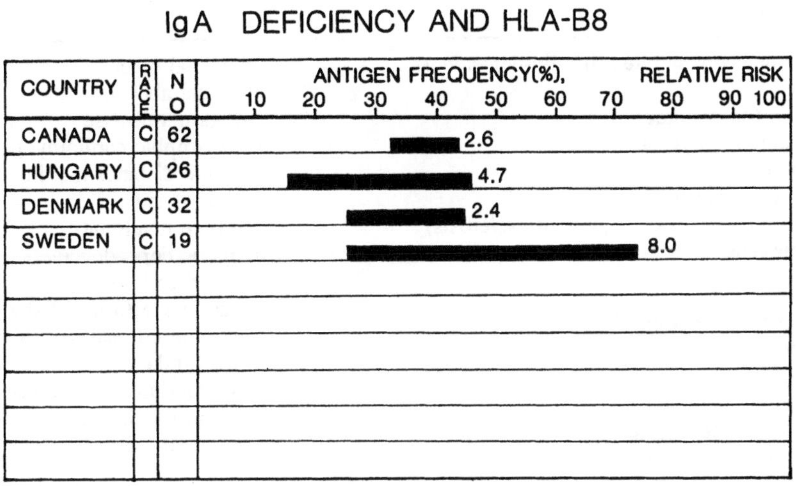

FIGURE 5.18 In 4 caucasian populations HLA-B8 was observed to be associated with IgA deficiency.

HLA Antigens Associated with Diseases

A list of all the HLA antigens that have been found to be associated with various diseases is given in Table 5.2. This list is based on the antigens for which frequency data are given in the tables in the sections on individual diseases. Thus, as discussed in the chapter on The Data and Statistical Analysis, it includes some antigens and diseases that show "interesting" associations ($\chi^2 < 10.0$). On rare occasions an association with a $\chi^2 < 3.84$ was also presented for comparisons in these tables.

TABLE 5.2. HLA Antigens Associated with Diseases

A1	Adrenocortical hyperfunction
	Carcinoma of the liver
	Carcinoma of the prostate
	Celiac disease
	Chronic active hepatitis without hepatitis B surface antigen
	Chronic active hepatitis (unspecified)
	Congenital dislocation of hip
	Dermatitis herpetiformis
	Graves' disease
	Hashimoto's thyroiditis
	Hodgkin's disease
	Myasthenia gravis
	Myasthenia gravis—female
	Myasthenia gravis—male
	Paget's disease
	Paracoccidioidomycosis
	Perthes' disease
	Positive direct Coomb's test
	Psoriasis vulgaris
	Psoriatic arthropathy (unspecified)
	Recurrent herpes labialis
	Vitiligo
A2	Acute lymphatic leukemia
	Aplastic anemia
	Carcinoma of the nasopharynx
	Congenital heart malformation
	Epilepsy
	Hydroxyapatite rheumatism (calcific periarthritis)
	Juvenile rheumatoid arthritis
	Maturity-onset diabetes mellitus (insulin-independent)
	Multiple sclerosis
	Paralytic dementia
	Periodontitis
	Periodontosis
	Raynaud's phenomenon
	Rheumatoid arthritis
	Tendinous calcifications
	Tuberculoid leprosy
	Vitiligo
A3	Adrenocortical hyperfunction
	Amyotrophic lateral sclerosis
	Idiopathic hemochromatosis
	Immune response to Rh(D) antigen
	Lichen planus
	Multiple sclerosis
	Porphyria cutanea tarda
	Rheumatic fever and rheumatic heart disease
A9	Alopecia areata
	Buerger's disease
	Carcinoma of the bladder
	Carcinoma of the ovary
	Carcinoma of the stomach
	Cystinosis
	Habitual abortion

TABLE 5.2. *(continued)*

A9	Juvenile diabetes mellitus (insulin-dependent)
	Leprosy
	Leukemia (unspecified)
	Paracoccidioidomycosis
	Periodontosis
	Rheumatoid arthritis
	Scleroderma (progressive systemic sclerosis)
	Syringomyelia
	Wilms' tumor
A10	Carcinoma of the stomach
	Cedar pollinosis
	Pemphigus vulgaris
	Polymyalgia rheumatica
	Recurrent herpes labialis
	Sudden infant death syndrome
	Vitiligo
A11	Congenital hypothyroidism
	Multiple sclerosis
	Scabies
AW19	Hay fever
	Idiopathic scoliosis
	Immunoproliferative small intestinal disease (Mediterranean abdominal lymphoma)
	Kaposi's sarcoma
	Lepromatous leprosy
	Mycosis fungoides
	Ulcerative colitis
	Varicose veins of lower extremities
AW24	Bullous pemphigoid
	Congenital hypothyroidism
	Leprosy
	Paralytic dementia
A26	Pemphigus foliaceus
	Pemphigus vulgaris
A28	Carcinoma of the prostate
	Erythrodermic psoriasis
	Lichen planus
	Lymphosarcoma
	Schizophrenia
A29	Birdshot retinochoroidopathy
	Carcinoma of the liver
	Porphyria cutanea tarda
	Recurrent herpes labialis
	Subacute sclerosing panencephalitis
AW30	Renal-cell carcinoma
AW31	Mycosis fungoides
	Vitiligo
AW32	Infection with measles
	Malignant choroidal melanoma
	Mycosis fungoides
	Porphyria cutanea tarda
BW4	Atopy (unspecified, includes eczema)
B5	Behcet's disease
	Buerger's disease
	Chronic idiopathic pancreatitis
	Cirrhosis of unknown etiology
	Colorectal adenoma
	Duodenal ulcer
	Habitual abortion
	Hodgkin's disease
	Hypertrophic cardiomyopathy
	Juvenile diabetes mellitus (insulin-dependent)
	Lichen planus
	Multiple myeloma
	Narcotic dependence
	Polycythemia vera
	Pseudopolyarthritis of the spine
	Recurrent corneal herpes (herpetic keratitis)
	Spina bifida
	Systemic lupus erythematosus
	Takayasu's disease
	Ulcerative colitis
B7	Allergy to ragweed
	Atopy (unspecified, includes eczema)
	Buerger's disease
	Celiac disease
	Cystinosis
	Essential homogeneous immunoglobulinemia
	Idiopathic hemochromatosis
	Juvenile diabetes mellitus (insulin-dependent)
	Juvenile rheumatoid arthritis
	Lennox-Gastaut syndrome
	Lepromatous leprosy
	Mixed connective tissue disease
	Multiple sclerosis
	Narcolepsy
	Optic neuritis
	Pemphigus vulgaris
	Pernicious anemia
	Porphyria cutanea tarda
	Presumed ocular histoplasmosis
	Psoriasis vulgaris
	Spinal muscular atrophy
	Steroid-responsive nephrotic syndrome of childhood
	Varicose veins of lower extremities
B8	Acute anterior uveitis
	Adult iridocyclitis
	Alcoholic liver disease
	Allergy to rye
	Carcinoma of the pituitary gland
	Carcinoma of the prostate
	Carcinoma of the salivary gland
	Celiac disease
	Chronic active cryptogenic hepatitis
	Chronic active hepatitis without hepatitis B surface antigen
	Chronic active hepatitis (unspecified)
	Chronic relapsing idiopathic inflammatory polyneuropathy (Guillain-Barre type)
	Congenital adrenal hyperplasia (21-hydroxylase deficiency)
	Dermatitis herpetiformis
	Graves' disease
	Hashimoto's thyroiditis
	Hay fever
	Hodgkin's disease
	Hypercholesterolemia
	Idiopathic Addison's disease

Table 5.2. *(continued)*

B8	Idiopathic autoimmune hemolytic anemia
	Idiopathic membranous nephropathy
	Immune response to platelet group PL^{A1}
	IgD level in serum IgA deficiency
	Juvenile dermatomyositis
	Juvenile diabetes mellitus (insulin-dependent)
	Leprosy
	Maturity-onset diabetes mellitus (insulin-independent)
	Multiple sclerosis
	Myasthenia gravis
	Myasthenia gravis—female
	Myasthenia gravis—male
	Persistent palmoplantar pustulosis (pustulosis palmaris et plantaris)
	Polymyalgia rheumatica
	Positive direct Coomb's test
	Primary sclerosing cholangitis
	Psoriasis vulgaris
	Recurrent herpes labialis
	Renal patients transiently carrying hepatitis B surface antigens
	Scleroderma (progressive systemic sclerosis)
	Sjögren's syndrome
	Steroid-responsive nephrotic syndrome of childhood
	Subacute cutaneous lupus erythematosus
	Systemic lupus erythematosus
	Temporal arteritis (giant cell arteritis, Horton's disease)
	Tuberculosis
	Vertebral ankylosing hyperostosis (Forestier's disease)
	Wegener's granulomatosis
B12	Acute lymphatic leukemia
	Acute poststreptococcal glomerulonephritis
	Alopecia areata
	Buerger's disease
	Carcinoma of the esophagus
	Carcinoma of the liver
	Carcinoma of the ovary
	Carcinoma of the salivary gland
	Congenital neutropenia
	Duodenal ulcer
	Follicular lymphoma
	Hypertrophic cardiomyopathy
	Immunoproliferative small intestinal disease (Mediterranean abdominal lymphoma)
	Malignant rheumatoid arthritis
	Mesangial IgA glomerulonephritis (Berger's disease)
	Multiple sclerosis
	Myasthenia gravis
	Myasthenia gravis—female
	Myasthenia gravis—male
	Psoriasis vulgaris
	Recurrent oral aphthae
	Retinoblastoma
	Seborrheic dermatitis
	Steroid-responsive nephrotic syndrome of childhood
	Uveitis (unspecified)
B13	Chronic idiopathic pancreatitis
	Erythrodermic psoriasis
	Guttate psoriasis
	Neuroblastoma
	Persistent palmoplantar pustulosis (pustulosis palmaris et plantaris)
	Psoriasis vulgaris
	Psoriatic arthropathy (central)
	Psoriatic arthropathy (peripheral)
	Psoriatic arthropathy (unspecified)
	Systemic lupus erythematosus
B14	Idiopathic hemochromatosis
	Juvenile diabetes mellitus (insulin-dependent)
	Keloids and hypertrophic scars
	Leprosy
	Parkinson's disease
B15	Alzheimer's disease
	Benign monoclonal gammopathy
	Cedar pollinosis
	Crohn's disease
	Cryptogenic fibrosing alveolitis
	Erythema multiforme
	Essential homogeneous immunoglobulinemia
	Graves' disease
	Healthy hepatitis B surface antigen carriers
	Juvenile diabetes mellitus (insulin-dependent)
	Juvenile rheumatoid arthritis
	Multiple sclerosis
	Periodontosis
	Rheumatic heart disease
	Scleritis
	Tuberculosis
BW16	Hashimoto's thyroiditis
	Manic-depressive disorder
	Meningococcal infection
	Parkinson's disease
	Psoriasis vulgaris
	Psoriatic arthropathy (central)
	Psoriatic arthropathy (peripheral)
	Psoriatic arthropathy (unspecified)
	Sensorineural hearing loss
B17	Crohn's disease with peripheral arthritis
	Erythrodermic psoriasis
	Guttate psoriasis
	Hyperlipoproteinemia, type IIA
	Leprosy
	Psoriasis vulgaris
	Psoriatic arthropathy (central)
	Psoriatic arthropathy (peripheral and sacroiliitis)
	Psoriatic arthropathy (peripheral)
	Psoriatic arthropathy (unspecified)
	Rheumatic fever and rheumatic heart disease
	Systemic lupus erythematosus
	Tuberculoid leprosy
B18	Alopecia areata
	Balkan endemic nephropathy
	Carcinoma of the ovary
	Hodgkin's disease
	Idiopathic membranous nephropathy

TABLE 5.2. *(continued)*

B18	Juvenile diabetes mellitus (insulin-dependent) Neurogenic paraosteoarthropathy Paralytic dementia Schonlein-Henoch nephritis Sensorineural hearing loss Steroid-responsive nephrotic syndrome of childhood
BW21	Allergy to insulin Carcinoma of the larynx Juvenile diabetes mellitus (insulin-dependent) Leprosy Myasthenia gravis Neuroblastoma Polycythemia vera
BW22	Carcinoma of the prostate Intestinal adenomatous polyposis Juvenile diabetes mellitus (insulin-dependent) Kawasaki's disease Multiple sclerosis Pemphigus vulgaris Rheumatoid arthritis
B27	Acute anterior uveitis Adult iridocyclitis Amyloidosis in rheumatoid arthritis Ankylosing spondylitis Ankylosing spondylitis in inflammatory bowel disease Arthritis (unspecified) Asbestosis Balanitis Chronic brucellosis Crohn's disease Crohn's disease with ankylosing spondylitis Flax byssinosis Granulocytic leukemia Juvenile rheumatoid arthritis Low back pain Meningococcal meningitis Postgonorrhoic arthritis Postsalmonella arthritis Postshigellosis arthritis Postyersinia arthritis Psoriatic arthropathy (central) Psoriatic arthropathy (peripheral) Psoriatic arthropathy (unspecified) Pustular psoriasis Reactive arthritis after *Campylobacter jejuni* enteritis Reiter's disease Rheumatoid arthritis Sacroiliitis Seronegative "spondylitic variant" syndrome Seronegative pauciarticular arthritis Seronegative peripheral arthritis Sexually acquired reactive arthritis Spondylarthritis in chronic brucellosis Ulcerative colitis Uveitis (unspecified) Vertebral ankylosing hyperostosis (Forestier's disease) Whipple's disease
BW35	Atopic dermatitis Azoospermia Capsular glaucoma Carcinoma of the breast Carcinoma of the colon Carcinoma of the rectum Chronic active hepatitis with hepatitis B surface antigen Duodenal ulcer Generalized granuloma annulare Glioma Graves' disease Hydroxyapatite rheumatism (calcific periarthritis) Hyperlipoproteinemia, type IIA Infertility (unexplained) Juvenile diabetes mellitus (insulin-dependent) Keratoacanthoma Mesangial IgA glomerulonephritis (Berger's disease) Mitral valve prolapse Mononucleosis Myasthenia gravis Narcolepsy Periodontosis Persistent palmoplantar pustulosis (pustulosis palmaris et plantaris) Retinoblastoma Schonlein-Henoch nephritis Subacute thyroiditis (de Quervain) Tendinous calcifications Ulcerative colitis Urticaria Venous thromboembolism
B37	Psoriasis vulgaris
BW38	Pemphigus vulgaris Polymyalgia rheumatica Pseudopolyarthritis of the spine Psoriatic arthropathy (central) Psoriatic arthropathy (peripheral and sacroiliitis) Psoriatic arthropathy (peripheral) Psoriatic arthropathy (unspecified)
BW39	Leprosy
B40	Age Alcoholic liver disease Amyotrophic lateral sclerosis Avian hypersensitivity Chronic alcoholic pancreatitis Colorectal adenoma Healthy hepatitis B surface antigen carriers Hemangioma Immune response to vaccinia virus Juvenile rheumatoid arthritis Lepromatous leprosy Leprosy Lichen sclerosus et atrophicus Multiple sclerosis Paralytic dementia Systemic lupus erythematosus

TABLE 5.2. *(continued)*

BW41	Maturity-onset diabetes mellitus (insulin-independent)
BW42	Juvenile diabetes mellitus (insulin-dependent)
BW45	Caplan's syndrome
BW46	Carcinoma of the nasopharynx
	Graves' disease
BW47	Congenital adrenal hyperplasia (21-hydroxylase deficiency)
BW51	Behcet's disease
	Kawasaki's disease
BW52	Buerger's disease
	Carcinoma of the breast
	Graves' disease
	Immune response to *Schistosoma japonicum*
	Juvenile diabetes mellitus (insulin-dependent)
	Takayasu's disease
BW54	Buerger's disease
	Cirrhosis of unknown etiology
	Juvenile diabetes mellitus (insulin-dependent)
	Kawasaki's disease
	Maturity-onset diabetes mellitus (insulin-independent)
	Rheumatoid arthritis
	Vogt-Koyanagi-Harada syndrome
BW57	Psoriasis vulgaris
BW61	Maturity-onset diabetes mellitus (insulin-independent)
CW1	Ankylosing spondylitis
	Atherosclerotic disease
	Sacroiliitis
CW2	Ankylosing spondylitis
CW3	Chronic alcoholism
	Immune response to vaccinia virus
	Juvenile diabetes mellitus (insulin-dependent)
CW4	Juvenile diabetes mellitus (insulin-dependent)
	Narcotic dependence
	Schizophrenia
	Subacute thyroiditis (de Quervain)
	Venous thromboembolism
	Vertebral ankylosing hyperostosis (Forestier's disease)
CW5	Varicose veins of lower extremities
	Venous thromboembolism
CW6	Guttate psoriasis
	Psoriasis vulgaris
	Varicose veins of lower extremities
	Venous thromboembolism
CW7	Chronic active hepatitis without hepatitis B surface antigen
DR1	Carcinoma of the thyroid gland
	Glioma
	Rheumatoid arthritis
DR2	Alcoholic liver disease
	Autoimmune thrombocytopenic purpura
	Buerger's disease
	Goodpasture's syndrome
	Hashimoto's thyroiditis
	Idiopathic hemochromatosis
	Juvenile diabetes mellitus (insulin-dependent)
	Multiple sclerosis
	Narcolepsy
	Pemphigus vulgaris
	Pernicious anemia
	Presumed ocular histoplasmosis
	Recurrent oral aphthae
	Systemic lupus erythematosus
	Takayasu's disease
	Tuberculoid leprosy
	Wegener's granulomatosis
DR3	Acute myeloid leukemia
	Antibodies to native DNA
	Celiac disease
	Chronic active hepatitis without hepatitis B surface antigen
	Chronic active hepatitis (unspecified)
	Chronic relapsing idiopathic inflammatory polyneuropathy (Guillain-Barre type)
	Dermatitis herpetiformis
	Graves' disease
	Guillain-Barre syndrome
	Hashimoto's thyroiditis
	Herpes gestationis
	Idiopathic membranous nephropathy
	Immune response to platelet group PL^{A1}
	IgA deficiency
	Juvenile dermatomyositis
	Juvenile diabetes mellitus (insulin-dependent)
	Myasthenia gravis
	Myasthenia gravis—female
	Myasthenia gravis—male
	Polymyositis
	Primary ovarian failure
	Subacute cutaneous lupus erythematosus
	Systemic lupus erythematosus
	Thygeson's superficial punctate keratitis
DR4	Acute poststreptococcal glomerulonephritis
	Chronic active hepatitis (unspecified)
	Felty's syndrome
	Herpes gestationis
	Hydralazine-induced systemic lupus erythematosus
	Juvenile diabetes mellitus (insulin-dependent)
	Juvenile rheumatoid arthritis
	Melanoma
	Mesangial IgA glomerulonephritis (Berger's disease)
	Multiple sclerosis
	Pemphigus foliaceus
	Pemphigus vulgaris
	Rapeseed oil disease
	Rheumatoid arthritis
	Systemic lupus erythematosus
	Vitiligo
	Vogt-Koyanagi-Harada syndrome

TABLE 5.2. *(continued)*

DR5	Graves' disease Hashimoto's thyroiditis Juvenile rheumatoid arthritis Kaposi's sarcoma Renal-cell carcinoma Scleroderma (progressive systemic sclerosis)
DRW6	Idiopathic hemochromatosis Multiple sclerosis
DR7	Behcet's disease Burkitt's lymphoma Celiac disease Nephrotic syndrome Neurogenic paraosteoarthropathy Psoriasis vulgaris Recurrent herpes progenitalis (HSV-2) Steroid-responsive nephrotic syndrome of childhood
DR8	Juvenile rheumatoid arthritis
DW1	Mixed connective tissue disease
DW2	Allergy to ragweed Juvenile diabetes mellitus (insulin-dependent) Multiple sclerosis Optic neuritis Pernicious anemia Sjögren's syndrome
DW3	Celiac disease Chronic active hepatitis without hepatitis B surface antigen Chronic active hepatitis (unspecified) Chronic relapsing idiopathic inflammatory polyneuropathy (Guillain-Barre type) Dermatitis herpetiformis Graves' disease Hashimoto's thyroiditis Juvenile diabetes mellitus (insulin-dependent) Myasthenia gravis Myasthenia gravis—female Myasthenia gravis—male Sjögren's syndrome Systemic lupus erythematosus
DW4	Juvenile diabetes mellitus (insulin-dependent) Juvenile rheumatoid arthritis Rheumatoid arthritis
DW5	Hashimoto's thyroiditis Juvenile rheumatoid arthritis
DW6	Avian hypersensitivity Cryptogenic fibrosing alveolitis
DW7	Celiac disease Dermatitis herpetiformis Juvenile rheumatoid arthritis Testicular cancer
DW8	Juvenile rheumatoid arthritis
DW12	Graves' disease Immune response to *Schistosoma japonicum*
DW-EI	Psoriasis vulgaris
DW-En	Acute poststreptococcal glomerulonephritis Mesangial IgA glomerulonephritis (Berger's disease)
DW-Wa	Vogt-Koyanagi-Harada syndrome
DHO	Immune response to tetanus toxoid Takayasu's disease
DMA	Psoriasis vulgaris
DYT	Juvenile diabetes mellitus (insulin dependent) Rheumatoid arthritis
Te24	Dermatitis herpetiformis
BFF1	Idiopathic membranous nephropathy Juvenile diabetes mellitus (insulin-dependent)
BFS1	Juvenile diabetes mellitus (insulin-dependent)

CHAPTER 6

Rheumatology and Joint Diseases

Brachymetacarpia

Population Association

Saint-Hillier et al.[1] typed 7 French patients for A and B loci antigens. When compared with a control population of unknown size, they found no significant difference between the 2 groups.

Family Data

Farriaux et al.[2] published data on a 2-generation French family in which the father was affected by brachymetacarpia and the mother was affected by pseudohypoparathyroidism. Three offspring (2 girls and 1 boy) had both of these conditions, 1 girl had only pseudohypoparathyroidism, and 1 boy was normal. The father and 3 affected offspring had the A3-BW5 haplotype in common.

Reference

1. Saint-Hillier Y, Dupond JL, Perol C, Herve P, Betuel H: Les groupes HLA chez malades ayant une brachymetacarpie. Nouv Presse Med 5:1003, 19762. Farriaux JP, Delmas Y, Ropartz C, Fontaine G: Brachymetacarpie-groupe HL-A. Nouv Presse Med 4:589-590, 1975

Congenital Dislocation of Hip

Population Association

Zervas et al.[1] have reported A and B antigen frequencies in 42 unrelated Greek children (8 males and 34 females). These data showed a significant increase of A1 in the patients (Table 6.1).

Reference

1. Zervas J, Zoubopoulos H, Constantopoulos C, Theodorou SD, Toubis M, Fessas Ph: HLA antigens and congenital dislocation of the hip. Tissue Antigens 22:295-297, 1983

Spina Bifida

Population Association

In a report on 32 unrelated cases from Belgium, De Bruyere et al.[1,2] observed a nonsignificant increase in the frequency of B5. Later another report from France by Vannier[3] also showed a similar increase in B5. The data for both studies are given in Table 6.2. The combined sample shows a significant association of B5 with this disease and there is no indication of heterogeneity in the data.

In a third study from Poland, Pietrzyk and Turowski[4] investigated A and B loci antigens in 46 children affected by spina bifida and 13 with spina bifida occulta. These 59 children were from 46 families and thus all were not unrelated. The authors calculated gene frequencies in this sample of 59 patients and compared them with 240 controls. The most interesting result was a significantly increased gene frequency of B27 in the patients: 13.56% vs. 4.79% in the controls. However, since some of the patients in the sample were related, this analysis was incorrect and thus no valid inference can be drawn.

TABLE 6.1. Congenital Dislocation of Hip

	Patients		Controls				
Country/Population	n	%+	n	%+	RR	χ^2	Ref.
HLA-A1							
Greece	42	26	400	52	0.33	9.62	1

Disease Heterogeneity

In an interesting study of correlation between the incidence of spina bifida and HLA antigen frequencies, Feingold et al.[5] reported a significant positive correlation with B5 and BW35. The data on incidence of the disease and HLA frequencies were from published studies from 23 different European and nonEuropean populations.

Family Data

The first report by Amos et al.[6] included a 4-generation Caucasian family from North Carolina. Ninety-eight members of this large pedigree were typed for HLA. An X-ray examination was also performed on all individuals. In this pedigree, 2 forms of spinal abnormalities (spina bifida occulta and asymmetry of the facet joints) were associated with the haplotypes introduced from 2 ancestors. On the basis of the assumption that these 2 abnormalities were due to a single dominant allele, significant evidence ($p < 0.01$) of linkage with HLA was observed. The distance between HLA and the "disease gene" was a 28% recombination unit with a standard error of 0.06.

However, in 3 other reports there was no evidence of linkage with HLA. Bobrow et al.[7] studied 9 families from England in which 11 children were affected with spina bifida and 21 were normal. There were 2 families in which 2 siblings were affected and 2 were normal. The other 7 families had only 1 affected child. The 2 affected siblings of multiple-case families did not have identical haplotypes. In single-case families affected and unaffected siblings had identical haplotypes.

De Bruyere et al.[1] also presented data on 14 multiple-case families. The individuals were affected by spina bifida cystica, spina bifida occulta, and asymmetry of vertebral joint facets. In some families all 3 types were present. In this study, again affected siblings in the same family did not share haplotypes.

Vannier et al.[8] have also studied 33 families with a history of spina bifida with myelomeningocele. The analysis of these data showed an independent segregation between the disease and HLA haplotypes.

Thus, 2 studies[1,7] did not provide evidence of linkage between HLA and spina bifida. The discrepancy between these 2 studies and that of Amos et al.[6] may have resulted from the heterogeneity of the disease and/or variable penetrance and expressivity of the disease gene (also see 9). It is interesting to note that mutant alleles of the T/t locus, linked to the H-2 complex in mice, produce a range of developmental abnormalities including shortening of tail and vertebral anomalies.

References

1. De Bruyere M, Kulakowski S, Malchaire J, Delire M, Sokal G: HLA gene and haplotype frequencies in spina bifida: Population and family studies. Tissue Antigens 10:399-402, 1977
2. Kulakowski S, Delire M, De Bruyere M: Recherche d'une segregation des haplotypes HLA dans une

TABLE 6.2. Spina Bifida

	Patients		Controls				
Country/Population	n	%+	n	%+	RR	χ^2	Ref.
HLA-B5							
BENELUX	32	31	868	16	2.42	5.42	1
France	53	28	412	15	2.23	6.01	3
	85	29	1280	16	2.31	11.41	
	Heterogeneity χ^2 (1 df)					0.02	

etude familiale d'enfants atteints de spina bifida. J Hum Genet 27:205-219, 1979
3. Vannier JP, Cavelier B, Martin JP, Lefort J, Rivat L, Feingold J: HLA, PI, GM and KM phenotypes in a spina bifida population with myelo-meningocele. Tissue Antigens 15:501-504, 1980
4. Pietrzyk JJ, Turowski G: Immunogenetic bases of congenital malformations: Association of HLA-B27 with spina bifida. Pediatr Res 13:879-883, 1979
5. Feingold J, Feingold N, Bois E: Spina bifida and anencephaly: Geographic correlation with the HLA system. Tissue Antigens 15:318-324, 1980
6. Amos DB, Ruderman R, Mendell NR, Johnson AH: Linkage between HL-A and spinal development. Transplant Proc 7:93-95, 1975
7. Bobrow M, Bodmer JG, Bodmer WF, McDevitt HO, Lorber J, Swift P: The search for a human equivalent of the mouse T-locus-negative results from a study of HL-A types in spina bifida. Tissue Antigens 5:234-237, 1975
8. Vannier JP, Lefort J, Cavelier B, Ledosseur P, Assailly C, Feingold J: Spina bifida cystica families X-ray examination and HLA typing. Pediatr Res 15:326-329, 1981
9. Pietrzyk JJ, Turowski G: Family studies on HLA system in children with CNS malformations. Indian J Exp Biol 13:278-284, 1980

Idiopathic Scoliosis

Population Association

In a study of 64 Caucasian patients, Bradford et al.[1] reported an increased frequency of AW19 (Table 6.3). The patients had a lateral curvature of the spine measuring 20° or greater. Patients with a paralytic spine deformity or other known diseases associated with scoliosis were not included.

Disease Heterogeneity

Bradford et al.[1] arbitrarily divided their patients into 2 groups: 29 with severe curvature (50°–79°) requiring surgery and 35 with milder (20°–45°) who had either received no treatment or who had been managed satisfactorily with a Milwaukee brace.

In the nonsurgical group the frequency of A29 was 20% as compared with 3.6% in 218 controls (corrected $p < 0.027$).

Reference

1. Bradford DS, Noreen H, Hallgren HM, Yunis EJ: Histocompatibility determinants in idiopathic scoliosis. Clin Orthop 123:261-265, 1977

Ossification of Posterior Longitudinal Ligament of the Cervical Vertebrae

Population Association

Sonozaki et al.[1] reported A and B loci antigen frequencies in 21 Japanese patients. No significant deviations, when compared with 78 normal controls, were found.

The authors noted that the paravertebral ossifications in this disease are similar to those in ankylosing spondylitis. Thus, it is interesting to note that none of these patients (as well as healthy controls) were positive for B27, an antigen very strongly associated with ankylosing spondylitis (see Ankylosing Spondylitis). This may provide some evidence that these 2 diseases are etiologically different.

Reference

1. Sonozaki H, Seki H, Chang S, Okuyama M, Juji T: Human lymphocyte antigen, HL-A27, in Japanese patients with ankylosing spondylitis. Tissue Antigens 5:131-136, 1975

Dactylitis ("Sausage-Like" Toes)

Population Association

De Ceulaer et al.[1] reported data on 9 patients from the Netherlands. These patients showed a "sausage-like" swelling of 1 or more toes, accompanied by an oligoarthritis, predominantly of the lower extremities. None of the patients had diarrhea, urethritis, conjunctivitis, skin eruption, or nail lesions.

All 9 patients were positive for B27. The authors do not give the frequency of B27 in that control

TABLE 6.3. Idiopathic Scoliosis

	Patients		Controls				
Country/Population	n	%+	n	%+	RR	χ^2	Ref.
HLA-AW19							
U.S.A.	64	33	218	18	2.25	6.67	1

TABLE 6.4. Hydroxyapatite Rheumatism (Calcific Periarthritis)

	Patients		Controls				
Country/Population	n	%+	n	%+	RR	χ^2	Ref.
HLA-A2							
France	38	66	591	44	2.42	6.71	1
HLA-BW35							
France	38	34	591	19	2.23	5.31	1

population. However, this antigen is present in about 7–10% of healthy Caucasians.

Reference

1. De Ceulaer K, Van Der Linden JMJP, Cats A: "Sausage-like" toes (dactylitis) and HLA B27. J Rheumatol Suppl 3, 4:66-69, 1977

Hydroxyapatite Rheumatism (Calcific Periarthritis)

Population Association

The only data available are from a French study[1] on 38 patients in whom A2 and BW35 were increased (Table 6.4). However, the difference was nonsignificant.

Disease Heterogeneity

The patients were divided into 2 categories: 10 with 1 calcification and 28 with 2 or more calcifications. The frequencies of A2 in these 2 groups were 50% and 71%, respectively. This difference was not significant. However, when compared with 591 healthy controls A2 was significantly increased in the patients with 2 or more calcifications (71% vs. 44% in the controls, $p < 0.005$).

Reference

1. Amor B, Cherot A, Delbarre F, Roldan AN, Hors J: Hydroxyapatite rheumatism and HLA markers. J Rheumatol 4(Suppl 3):101-104, 1977

Low Back Pain

Population Association

In a report from Yugoslavia on 652 patients with low back pain (of various origin) that had lasted for more than 3 months, Jajic[1] found a significant increase in the frequency of B27 (Table 6.5).

It is interesting to note that of the 276 patients positive for B27, 128 had ankylosing spondylitis. The association of low back pain, however, would be significant even after excluding the ankylosing spondylitis patients.

See also reference 2.

References

1. Jajic I: The role of HLA-B27 in the diagnosis of low back pain. Acta Orthop Scand 50:411-413, 1979
2. Sagredo JP, Eguren TT, Valverde VR: Antigene d'histocompatibilite HLA-B27 dans les arthrites seronegatives et les lombalgies idiopathiqus. Rev Rhum 47:409-413, 1980

Chondrocalcinosis

Population Association

Nyulassy et al.[1,2] reported data on A and B loci antigens in 13 unrelated Czechoslovakian patients with nonfamilial chondrocalcinosis. When compared with 314 healthy controls, no significant difference in the antigen frequencies was observed. Similar results have also been reported by Reginato et al.[3] in a group of 47 Chilean patients (from Chiloe Island). In this study, however, all the patients were not related and thus the validity of the results is doubtful.

Disease Heterogeneity

The report by Reginato et al.[3] included 10 patients with severe chondrocalcinosis characterized by fibrous or bony ankylosis of the hip and knees along with marked lumbar spine involvement clinically mimicking ankylosing spondylitis. The authors have termed this subgroup as ankylosing chondrocalcinosis. The HLA antigen frequencies in this group

TABLE 6.5. Low Back Pain

	Patients		Controls				
Country/Population	n	%+	n	%+	RR	χ^2	Ref.
HLA-B27							
Yugoslavia	652	42	302	12	5.25	74.57	1

were not significantly different from those in the controls. None of these patients was B27-positive.

Family Data

A family with 4 patients has been reported by Nyulassy et al.[2] There was no evidence of linkage with HLA in this data, however.

See also Hereditary Chondrocalcinosis.

References

1. Nyulassy S, Stefanovic J, Sitaj S, Zitnan D: HL-A system in articular chondrocalcinosis. Arthritis Rheum 19:391-393, 1976
2. Nyulassy S, Stefanovic J, Sitaj S: HL-A homozygosity and calcium pyrophosphate metabolism: Preliminary report. In Kissmeyer-Nielsen F (ed): Histocompatibility Testing 1975, pp 805-808. Munksgaard, Copenhagen, 1975
3. Reginato AJ, Schiapachasse V, Zmijewski CM, Schumacher HR, Fuentes C, Gfaldamez M: HLA antigens in chondrocalcinosis and ankylosing chondrocalcinosis. Arthritis Rheum 22:928-932, 1979

Hereditary Chondrocalcinosis

Population Association

See Chondrocalcinosis.

Family Data

HLA typing of a large 3-generation pedigree from France in which 27 of the 39 members who were affected by diffuse articular chondrocalcinosis did not show any evidence of linkage with HLA.[1,2] In 2 other families investigated by Netter et al.[3] (France) and Reginato et al.[4] (Chile), the disease did not segregate with HLA haplotypes.

Nyulassy et al.[5] investigated 12 patients in 7 families from Czechoslovakia. The haplotype A2-BW5 was present in all but 1 family member of the study group. However, this haplotype was present in both affected and healthy members.

Thus, in these families there was no strong evidence for close linkage between HLA and this disease.

References

1. Gaucher A, Faure G, Netter P, Pourel J, Raffoux C, Streiff F, et al: HLA antigens and hereditary diffuse articular chondrocalcinosis. J Rheumatol 4 (Suppl 3):113-114, 1977 (Abstr)
2. Gaucher A, Pourel J, Faure G, Netter P, Peterschmitt J, Cromer R: Les chondrocalcinoses articulaires diffuses hereditaires. Rev Rhum 44:589-597, 1977
3. Netter P, Faure G, Pourel J, Raffoux C, Janot J, Schooneman F: Chondrocalcinose articulaire diffuse a caractere familial. Nouv Presse Med 4:2814, 1975
4. Reginato AJ, Schiapachasse V, Zmijewski CM, Schumacher HR, Fuentes C, Gfaldamez M: HLA

TABLE 6.6. Perthes' Disease

	Patients		Controls				
Country/Population	n	%+	n	%+	RR	χ^2	Ref.
HLA-A1							
England	50	38	551	35	1.15	0.21	3
West Germany	74	41	1000	29	1.71	4.85	1
Greece	34	65	280	25	5.44	20.55	2
	158	45	1831	30	1.90	14.65	
	Heterogeneity χ^2 (2 df)					10.96	

antigens in chondrocalcinosis and ankylosing chondrocalcinosis. Arthritis Rheum 22:928-932, 1979
5. Nyulassy S, Stefanovic J, Sitaj S, Zitnan D: HL-A system in articular chondrocalcinosis. Arthritis Rheum 19:391-393, 1976

Perthes' Disease

Population Association

An increased frequency in 74 unrelated German children (16 girls and 58 boys) with true Perthes' disease was first reported by Bertrams et al.[1] This antigen was also significantly increased in another study from Greece by Zervas et al.[2] Thompson and Woodrow,[3] however, did not find any significant deviations. In the combined data (Table 6.6) A1 is significantly associated with this disease. Also, there is some evidence of heterogeneity in the data.

References

1. Bertrams J, Schiersmann P, Ritgen G: HLA antigens in Perthes' disease. Tissue Antigens 12:157-158, 1978
2. Zervas J, Theodorou S, Constantopoulos C, Mandale C, Fessas Ph. HLA-A1 probable association with Perthes' disease. Tissue Antigens 20:159-160, 1982
3. Thompson SK, Woodrow JC: HLA antigens in Perthes' disease. J Bone Joint Surg 63:278-279, 1981

Paget's Disease

Population Association

Seignalet et al.[1] have reported an increased frequency of A1 in a sample of 50 French patients (Table 6.7). In other studies from France by Mercier and coworkers[2–4] and also from England (Table 6.7) by Cullen et al.[5], this increase was not evident. Thus, in the present data there is no evidence of a significant association with any HLA-A and -B loci antigens.

Disease Heterogeneity

Mercier et al.[3] grouped their 100 French patients into those with generalized disease (when 3 or more bones were involved) and those with localized disease (when only one or 2 bones were involved). Another classification, based on values for alkaline phosphatase, hydroxyproteinuria, and calcuria, divided cases into progressive and nonprogressive types of disease. The antigen frequencies in these 4 subgroups did not differ significantly from those in the controls.

Family Data

Fotino et al.[6] examined the segregation of HLA haplotypes in 3 multiple-case families. In 3 of the 29 informative children there was evidence of a recombination between the haplotype and the disease locus. The maximum lod score was 2.44 at the recombination value of 10.8%. A lod score of 3.00 is generally considered as significant evidence in favor of linkage and thus these results can be interpreted as indicative of probable linkage with HLA. (The pedigree diagrams are not available in the report.)

References

1. Seignalet J, Simon L, Blotman F: Repartition des antigenes HL-A dans la maladie de paget. Nouv Presse Med 4:2204, 1975
2. Roux H, Mercier P, Maestracci D, Eisinger J, Recordier AM: HL-A et maladie de paget. Rev Rhum Mal Osteoartic 42:661-662, 1975
3. Mercier P, Roux H, Maestracci D, Serratrice G, Seignalet J, Simon L, et al: Paget's disease and HLA antigens. J Rheumatol 4(Suppl 3):113, 1977 (Abstr)

TABLE 6.7. Paget's Disease

	Patients		Controls				
Country/Population	n	%+	n	%+	RR	χ^2	Ref.
HLA-A1							
England	40	40	83	35	1.24	0.31	5
France	50	36	270	20	2.26	6.30	1
	90	38	353	24	1.76	5.20	
	Heterogeneity χ^2 (1 df)					1.41	

4. Mercier P, Maestracci D, Roux H: HL-A et maladie de paget. Nouv Presse Med 4:674, 1975
5. Cullen P, Russel RGG, Walton RJ, Whiteley J: Frequencies of HLA-A and HLA-B histocompatibility antigens in Paget's disease of bone. Tissue Antigens 7:55-56, 1976
6. Fotino M, Haymovits A, Falk CT: Evidence for linkage between HLA and Paget's disease. Transplant Proc 9:1867-1868, 1977

Frozen Shoulder

Population Association

In their first report on 38 patients from England Bulgen et al.[1] found a significant association with B27. However, in a second sample of 40 patients[2] they failed to confirm their earlier report. Similar nonsignificant results were also reported by Stodell and Sturrock[3] on 21 English, by Seignalet et al.[4] on 46 French, and by Noy et al.[5] on 48 Israeli Jewish patients.

References

1. Bulgen DY, Hazleman BL, Voak D: HLA-B27 and frozen shoulder. Lancet i:1042-1044, 1976
2. Bulgen DY, Hazleman BL: Immunoglobulin-A, HLA-B27, and frozen shoulder. Lancet ii:760, 1981
3. Stodell MA, Sturrock RD: Frozen shoulder. Lancet ii:527, 1981
4. Seignalet J, Sany J, Caillens JP, Lapinski H: Lack of correlation between frozen shoulder and HLA-B27. Semin Hop Paris 57:41-42, 1981
5. Noy S, Dekel S, Orgad S, Efter T, Mizrachi Y, Gazit E: HLA-B27 and frozen shoulder. Tissue Antigens 17:251, 1981

Arthritis (Unspecified)

Population Association

Duquesnoy et al.[1] reported a significant increase of B27 in 67 American Caucasian patients (Table 6.8). Meyer et al.[2] have also reported 25 French patients with unclassifiable inflammatory rheumatism. All were positive for B27 (no data on the control group).

See also ref. 3.

References

1. Duquesnoy RJ, Kozin F, Rodey GE: High prevalence of HLA-B27, CW1 and CW2 in patients with seronegative spondyloarthritis. Tissue Antigens 12:58-62, 1978
2. Meyer O, Vignoli M, Ryckewaert A: Unclassifiable inflammatory rheumatism with HLA B27. Rev Rhum Mal Osteoartic 49:11-16, 1982
3. Rose E, Espinoza LR, Osterland CK: Intestinal bypass arthritis: Association with circulating immune complexes and HLA B27. J Rheumatol 4:129-134, 1977

Rheumatoid Arthritis

Population Association

Although there are only 3 studies[1-3] in which a significant association of this disease with B27 was observed, combined data from several independent studies on Caucasian populations showed a significant association with B27 (Table 6.9). It is difficult to determine the influence of erroneous inclusion of ankylosing spondylitis in this diagnosis. The association with A2 in the pooled data (Table 6.9) is also significant.

In a study of 32 Iranian patients by Nikbin et al.,[4] a significant association with A9 was evident (Table 6.9).

In Japanese patients, the disease appears to be associated with BW22 and BW54.

As the frequency data in the Table 6.9 show, the strongest association of this disease is with DR4 and DW4 antigens. These antigens are significantly increased in all the available studies (Table 6.9). Furthermore, the association with DR4 is evident in Japanese, Indians, American Blacks, Venezuelan and Mexican patients. In a study by Nichol et al.[6] on 24 Indian patients DR1 was found to be increased (Table 6.9). This was not confirmed in 2 later reports,[7,8] however.

It is interesting that in Sasazuki's[9] study, DYT,

TABLE 6.8. Arthritis (Unspecified)

Country/Population	Patients n	Patients %+	Controls n	Controls %+	RR	χ^2	Ref.
HLA-B27							
U.S.A.	67	36	306	9	5.65	29.60	1

TABLE 6.9. Rheumatoid Arthritis

Country/Population	Patients n	Patients %+	Controls n	Controls %+	RR	χ^2	Ref.
HLA-A2							
U.S.A.	16	69	172	44	2.69	3.56	64
U.S.A.	104	62	600	52	1.50	3.52	2
U.S.A.	62	64	114	58	1.28	0.59	65
U.S.A.	32	43	200	45	0.93	0.04	35
U.S.A.	119	49	906	48	1.04	0.04	66
U.S.A.	38	61	135	43	2.04	3.81	5
	371	57	2127	49	1.31	5.55	
	Heterogeneity χ^2 (5 df)					6.00	
Australia	38	63	700	50	1.68	2.39	67
Czechoslovakia	40	55	200	46	1.43	1.09	68
USSR	100	40	200	51	0.64	3.21	69
USSR	63	43	600	26	2.15	8.24	70
	163	41	800	32	1.12	0.39	
	Heterogeneity χ^2 (1 df)					11.06	
France	50	44	300	47	0.89	0.15	71
France	56	75	100	50	2.93	8.95	72
	106	60	400	48	1.46	2.66	
	Heterogeneity χ^2 (1 df)					6.45	
Italy	52	54	398	50	1.17	0.29	73
Denmark	47	60	1967	54	1.27	0.64	18
Finland	45	67	326	55	1.63	2.25	3
Finland	44	61	120	45	1.89	3.26	25
	89	64	446	52	1.75	5.42	
	Heterogeneity χ^2 (1 df)					0.09	
	906	55	7038	49	1.33	15.32	
	Heterogeneity χ^2 (15 df)					26.71	
HLA-A9							
Iran	32	56	400	25	3.78	13.34	4
HLA-BW22							
Japan	88	2	104	7	0.33	2.49	19
Japan	67	48	317	24	2.91	15.21	74
Japan	63	2	76	9	0.27	2.88	20
	218	16	497	18	1.78	5.68	
	Heterogeneity χ^2 (2 df)					14.91	
HLA-B27							
Jews (unspecified)	28	14	456	3	5.62	9.50	1
U.S.A.	104	10	600	3	3.65	10.97	2
U.S.A.	16	13	172	7	2.29	1.45	64
U.S.A.	119	8	906	8	1.04	0.01	16
U.S.A.	38	13	135	7	2.05	1.72	5
U.S.A.	30	23	91	7	3.89	5.84	75
	307	11	1904	6	2.08	12.64	
	Heterogeneity χ^2 (4 df)					7.35	

TABLE 6.9. *(continued)*

Country/Population	Patients n	Patients %+	Controls n	Controls %+	RR	χ^2	Ref.
HLA-B27							
Australia	38	19	700	9	2.48	4.83	67
Czechoslovakia	40	18	200	10	2.04	2.47	68
USSR	63	16	600	7	2.60	6.84	70
England	11	9	89	14	0.84	0.04	36
France	56	2	100	10	0.25	3.21	72
France	50	14	300	9	1.71	1.55	71
	106	8	400	9	1.08	0.04	
	Heterogeneity χ^2 (1 df)					4.72	
Italy	52	4	398	5	0.95	0.01	73
Denmark	47	13	1967	9	1.61	1.33	18
Finland	44	20	120	16	1.34	0.45	25
Finland	45	49	326	14	5.85	28.35	3
	89	35	446	15	3.40	21.53	
	Heterogeneity χ^2 (1 df)					7.27	
Norway	48	13	1000	10	1.43	0.74	15
Sweden	60	29	692	17	2.02	5.66	76
	861	15	8396	9	2.03	45.18	
	Heterogeneity χ^2 (16 df)					30.29	
HLA-BW54							
Japan	63	21	76	13	1.75	1.60	20
Japan	88	24	104	12	2.27	4.66	19
Japan	70	26	210	9	3.53	12.59	9
	221	24	390	11	2.53	17.21	
	Heterogeneity χ^2 (2 df)					1.64	
HLA-DYT							
Japan	57	44	205	15	4.41	20.80	9
HLA-DW4							
U.S.A.	80	54	69	16	5.94	21.27	77
U.S.A.	39	36	42	12	3.86	6.15	33
	119	48	111	14	5.14	27.01	
	Heterogeneity χ^2 (1 df)					0.41	
Denmark	36	44	157	17	3.80	11.88	18
	155	47	268	16	4.56	38.52	
	Heterogeneity χ^2 (2 df)					0.78	
HLA-DR1							
India	24	58	31	19	5.46	8.46	6
India	17	0	10	20	0.10	3.62	7
India	40	10	40	8	1.24	0.10	8
	81	22	81	14	1.99	2.66	
	Heterogeneity χ^2 (2 df)					9.52	

TABLE 6.9. *(continued)*

Country/Population	Patients n	Patients %+	Controls n	Controls %+	RR	χ^2	Ref.
HLA-DR4							
U.S.A.—Black	18	39	125	8	7.21	12.68	5
U.S.A.—Black	35	46	49	14	4.96	9.89	24
U.S.A.—Black	56	36	193	10	5.00	20.03	7
	109	40	367	10	5.41	42.25	
	Heterogeneity χ^2 (2 df)					0.34	
Japan	104	63	792	41	2.44	17.40	7
Japan	43	61	222	32	3.28	12.42	9
Japan	63	71	67	42	3.31	10.77	20
Japan	88	71	104	46	2.84	11.89	19
Japan	50	59	144	33	2.89	10.19	78
	348	66	1329	39	2.80	61.80	
	Heterogeneity χ^2 (4 df)					0.86	
India	40	70	40	13	14.12	23.32	8
India	17	6	13	0	2.49	0.51	7
	57	51	53	10	10.77	22.27	
	Heterogeneity χ^2 (1 df)					1.56	
Mexico	41	58	19	5	17.53	12.42	7
Mexico	17	77	180	38	5.01	8.72	5
	58	64	199	35	7.40	19.51	
	Heterogeneity χ^2 (1 df)					1.63	
Venezuela	23	70	30	23	7.15	10.96	79
	81	65	229	33	7.31	0.47	
	Heterogeneity χ^2 (2 df)					1.64	
Caucasians (unspecified)	329	47	662	25	2.66	47.37	7
U.S.A.	38	61	135	14	9.29	30.41	5
U.S.A.	16	56	172	30	2.91	4.53	64
U.S.A.	53	70	68	28	5.80	19.91	77
U.S.A.	35	71	50	40	3.54	7.68	24
	142	66	425	26	5.23	58.35	
	Heterogeneity χ^2 (3 df)					4.18	
Hungary	41	39	66	11	4.93	10.84	7
England	100	74	82	35	5.18	26.40	6
England	95	56	200	34	2.46	12.64	23
	195	65	282	34	3.27	35.70	
	Heterogeneity χ^2 (1 df)					3.35	
France	31	32	116	13	3.14	6.28	80
France	30	53	100	25	3.33	8.16	81
France	17	88	56	20	23.57	20.15	82
France	56	67	100	14	11.95	39.59	72
	134	58	372	18	6.25	63.41	
	Heterogeneity χ^2 (3 df)					10.77	

TABLE 6.9. *(continued)*

Country/Population	Patients n	Patients %+	Controls n	Controls %+	RR	χ^2	Ref.
HLA-DR4							
Austria	40	55	125	23	4.02	13.84	21
Norway	39	67	116	27	5.33	18.48	26
Norway	48	61	200	27	4.16	18.72	15
Norway	132	66	200	27	5.19	46.65	34
Norway	27	54	116	27	3.12	7.16	13
	246	64	632	27	4.60	89.70	
	Heterogeneity χ^2 (3 df)					1.31	
	1127	58	2564	25	3.88	303.78	
	Heterogeneity χ^2 (16 df)					35.04	

a new D locus antigen (somewhat similar to DR4), was also associated with this disease.

Willkens et al.[10] studied 15 American Indian female patients (Yakima Indians from Washington state) for A and B loci antigen frequencies. No significant difference was found between patients and 17 age- and sex-matched controls.

In another study of Chippewa Indians a significant correlation with DR4 was reported by Harvey et al.[11,12]

Disease Heterogeneity

Rheumatoid Factor

Dobloug et al.[13–15] subdivided their patients into groups based on the seropositivity for rheumatoid factor (RF). In 33 RF-positive patients,[14,15] the frequency of DR4 was 61% as compared with only 27% in 15 RF-negative patients ($p < 0.05$). A similar association of RF positivity, severity of the disease, and DR4 was also noted by Jaraquemada et al.[16]. However, in the studies of Engleman et al.,[17] Thomsen et al.,[18] Ueno et al.,[5] Maeda et al.,[19] Nakai et al.,[20] Scherak et al.,[21] Panayi et al.,[22,23] and Stastny[7] this association was not confirmed. Thus, in the existing data, there is no evidence to suggest a significantly higher frequency of DR4 in the patients with RF.

Rheumatoid Factor Titer

Stastny[7] has reported a significant increase of DR4 in 48 patients with "high" titer as compared with 76 patients with "low" titer. This difference, however, was not found in the studies of Nakai et al.[20] and Karr et al.[24]

Sex

The frequencies of DR4 and DW4 were increased in both sexes.[5,7,13,14,18,19,25,26]

Age at Onset

There is no specific HLA association with age at onset.[5,7,13,19,21,23,25]

Agranulocytosis

Schmidt et al.[27,28] reported HLA data on 5 Rheumatoid arthritis (RA) patients who were treated with levamisole. All patients had drug-induced agranulocytosis. Five of these patients were positive for B27. In 2 reports by Mielants and Veys,[29,30] 8 of the 16 patients were positive for B27. Thus, the B27 frequency in these patients was higher than the 7–10% found in Caucasian populations (also see 31).

Functional Scores/Classes

There was no significant difference in the functional capacity between DR4-positive and DR4-negative patients.[5,19,26]

Disease Severity

In 16 patients classified as "severe" by Roitt et al.[16,32] all but 1 (97.76%) were DR4-positive. On the other hand, only 1 out of 13 (7.69%) with "mild" and 5 out of 8 (62.5%) patients with "moderate" disease were positive for DR4. Similar relationships between disease severity and DR4 have also been reported by McMichael et al.[33] However, disease severity as measured by the functional classification of the American Rheumatism Association and histories of gold, *D*-penicillamine, or corticosteroid treatments did not show any association with DR4 in 38 Caucasian, 18 American Black, and 17 Mexican patients studied by Ueno et al.[5] Similar results were also observed by Thomsen et al.,[18] Scherak et al.,[21] and Stastny.[7]

Nodule

There is no HLA difference between patients with and without nodules.[5,18,19,23,33]

Family History

In a study by Panayi et al.[23] 31 patients had a family history of RA. Twenty-four (77%) of these patients were positive for DR4. In the group of 62 patients with no family history of the disease, 27 (44%) had DR4 ($p < 0.04$). However, in another study of 63 Japanese patients by Nakai[20] no association of DR was found with the family history of the disease.

Drug Toxicity

Panayi et al.[23] reported an increase of DR2 and DR3 in patients who developed toxic reactions after treatment with sodium aurothiomalate and/or penicillamine. Twenty-one of 26 patients with DR2 and DR3 developed toxic reactions. There were 16 patients without these antigens and with toxic reactions and 17 without these antigens and without toxic reactions ($p \leq 0.025$). In a subsequent report by the same group of authors,[26] 71 patients who had toxic reactions to sodium aurothiomalate or *D*-penicillamine and 20 without toxicity were studied. Nineteen of 24 patients in whom proteinuria developed were positive for DR3 (79.17%) as compared with 18 out of 67 (26.87%) without proteinuria ($p < 0.00025$). There was no association with DR4, however.

Gran et al.[34] studied 132 patients treated with parenteral gold. The group with DR3 antigen had an 11 times higher risk of developing proteinuria than those without DR3.

Another report by Latts et al.[35] showed a 64.3% frequency of B12 in 14 patients who developed gold toxicity as compared with only 22.2% in 18 patients without such toxicity ($p < 0.035$).

In a report by Karr et al.[24] on 35 American Black and 35 American Caucasian patients, no association between DR antigens and the development of toxic reactions to gold or penicillamine was found. Another study by Nakai et al.[20] on 63 Japanese patients also did not find any association with drug toxicity (also see 19).

Duration of the Disease

Husby et al.[26] found no difference in the mean duration of the disease between DR4-positive and DR4-negative groups.

Serum IgM, IgA, and IgE

Dobloug et al.[14] reported significantly higher concentrations of serum IgM, IgA, and IgE in DR4-positive patients (as compared with DR4-negative patients). Detailed data are available in the report.[14]

Antinuclear Antibody

There was no specific HLA association in the subgroup of patients positive for antinuclear antibody.[21]

Radiological Severity

There was no specific HLA association in patients with severe disease based on X-ray evaluations (stages III and IV).[20,21]

Ankylosing Rheumatoid Arthritis

Calin et al.[36] reported no difference in the reported frequency of B27 in 11 patients with advanced ankylosing RA. Only 1 out of 11 (9%) such patients had B27, a frequency not significantly different from 13.5% found in 89 healthy controls.

Fecal Klebsiella pneumoniae

Ebringer et al.[37] have studied the carriage of fecal *Klebsiella pneumoniae* in 64 patients from England. The incidence of carriage was found to be increased in 16 patients with B7 cross-reacting antigens (B7, BW22, and B27) as compared with 48 patients without these antigens (32%, $p < 0.001$). Interestingly, there were no significant differences for B27 alone and DR4 and DW4 antigens.

Family Data

Khan et al.[38–40] typed 10 multiple-case families. All affected individuals within each family shared 1 haplotype. The second haplotype was usually different. Similar data have also been reported by Nunez et al.[41] In this study, 12 families with 2 or more cases of adult RA were HLA-typed. Except in 2 instances, the individuals affected by the disease had at least 1 HLA haplotype in common. The data from these 2 studies suggest a dominant disease-susceptibility gene linked with HLA.

A report by Zilko et al.[42] on 8 Australian families

showed 2 families in which affected members did not share any haplotype. In 1 family, the 2 affected siblings were HLA-identical. The remaining 5 families had patients sharing 1 haplotype. The authors noted that their analysis of shared haplotypes in siblings did not show a significant difference from the expected segregation ratio.

Strom and Moller[43] have also studied 5 Swedish families with 2 or more members with rheumatoid arthritis. The disease did not segregate with a specific haplotype in 1 family with 4 affected siblings. In 4 other families the affected siblings shared at least 1 haplotype.

In a linkage analysis of 5 multiple-case families (mixture of adult and juvenile RA), Rossen et al.[44,45] reported a maximum lod score of 2.995 at 5% recombination. These data provide some evidence in favor of a disease-susceptibility gene for rheumatoid-like arthritis linked with HLA.

See also refs. 46–63, 83–98.

References

1. Brautbar C, Porat S, Nelken D, Gabriel KR, Cohen T: HLA B27 and ankylosing spondylitis in the Israeli population. J Rheumatol 4(Suppl 3):24-32, 1977
2. Kueppers F, Brackertz D, Mueller-Eckhardt CH: HL-A antigens in sarcoidosis and rheumatoid arthritis. Lancet ii:1425, 1972
3. Isomaki H, Koota K, Martio J, Nissila M, Tiilikainen A: HL-A27 and arthritis. Ann Clin Res 7:138-145, 1975
4. Nikbin B, Davatchi F, Ala F: HLA A9-B5 haplotype in rheumatoid arthritis. J Rheumatol 4(Suppl 3):111, 1977 (Abstr)
5. Ueno Y, Iwaki Y, Terasaki PI, Park MS, Barnett EV, Chia D, Nakata S: HLA-DR4 in Negro and Mexican rheumatoid arthritis patients. J Rheumatol 8:804-807, 1981
6. Nichol FE, Woodrow JC: HLA DR antigens in Indian patients with rheumatoid arthritis. Lancet i: 220-221, 1981
7. Stastny P: Rheumatoid Arthritis. In Teraasaki PI (ed): Histocompatibility Testing 1980, pp 681-686 UCLA Tissue Typing Laboratory, Los Angeles, 1981
8. Mehra NK, Vaidya MC, Taneja V, Agarwal A, Malaviya AN: HLA-DR antigens in rheumatoid arthritis in north India. Tissue Antigens 20:300-302, 1982
9. Sasazuki T, Kaneoka H, Ohta N, Hayase R, Iwamoto: Common HLA haplotypes and their association with diseases in the Japanese population. Transplant Proc 11:1871-1873, 1979
10. Willkens RF, Blandau L, Aoyama DT, Beasley RP: Studies of rheumatoid arthritis among a tribe of northwest Indians. J Rheumatol 3:9-14, 1976
11. Harvey J, Lotze M, Arnett FC, Bias WB, Billingsley LM, Harvey E, et al: Rheumatoid arthritis in a Chippewa band II: Field study with clinical serologic and HLA-D correlations. J Rheumatol 10:28-32, 1983
12. Bias WB, Hsu SH, Pollar MK, Harvey J, Lotze MT, Arnett FC, et al: HLA-DR characterization of a Chippewa Indian subpopulation with high prevalence of rheumatoid arthritis. Hum Immunol 2:155-163, 1981
13. Dobloug JH, Forre O, Thorsby E: HLA-DRW4 and rheumatoid arthritis. Lancet i:548-549, 1979
14. Dobloug JH, Forre O, Kass E, Thorsby E: HLA antigens and rheumatoid arthritis: Association between HLA-DRW4 positivity and IGM rheumatoid factor production. Arthritis Rheum 23:309-313, 1980
15. Forre O, Dobloug JH, Hoyeraal HM, Kass E, Thorsby E: HLA-antigens in rheumatoid arthritis and juvenile rheumatoid arthritis: Increased frequency of the HLA-DRw4 antigen only in sero-positive patient groups. Adv. Inflamation Res 3:195-201, 1982
16. Jaraquemada D, Pachoula-Papasteriadis C, Festenstein H, Sachs JA, Roitt IM, Corbett M, et al: HLA-D and DR determinants in rheumatoid arthritis. Transplant Proc 11:1306, 1979
17. Engleman EG, Sponzilli EE, Batey ME, Ramcharan S, McDevitt HO: Mixed lymphocyte reaction in healthy women with rheumatoid factor. Arthritis Rheum 21:690-693, 1978
18. Thomsen M, Morling N, Snorrason E, Svejgaard A, Sorensen SF: HLA-DW4 and rheumatoid arthritis. Tissue Antigens 13:56-60, 1979
19. Maeda H, Juji T, Mitsui H, Sonozaki H, Okitsu K: HLA DR4 and rheumatoid arthritis in Japanese people. Ann Rheum Dis 40:29-302, 1981
20. Nakai Y, Wakisaka A, Aizawa M, Itakura K, Nakai H, Ohashi A: HLA and rheumatoid arthritis in the Japanese. Arthritis Rheum 24:722-725, 1981
21. Scherak O, Smolen JS, Mayr WR: Rheumatoid arthritis and B lymphocyte alloantigen HLA-DRW4. J Rheumatol 7:9-12, 1980
22. Panayi GS, Wooley PH, Batchelor JR: HLA-DRW4 and rheumatoid arthritis. Lancet i:730, 1979
23. Panayi GS, Wooley P, Batchelor JR: Genetic basis of rheumatoid disease: HLA antigens, disease manifestations, and toxic reactions to drugs. Br Med J 2:1326-1328, 1978
24. Karr RW, Rodey GE, Lee T, Schwartz BD: Association of HLA-DRW4 with rheumatoid arthritis in black and white patients. Arthritis Rheum 23:1241-1245, 1980

25. Pasternack A, Tiilikainen A: HLA-B27 in rheumatoid arthritis and amyloidosis. Tissue Antigens 9:80-89, 1977
26. Husby G, Ghran JT, Ostensen M, Johannessen A, Thorsby E: HLA-DRW4 and rheumatoid arthritis. Lancet i:549, 1979
27. Schmidt KL, Mueller-Eckhardt C, Breithaupt H: HLA-B27, antinuclear antibodies and drug-induced agranulocytosis. Klin Wochenschr 56:1189-1191, 1978
28. Schmidt KL, Mueller-Eckhardt C: Agranulocytosis, levamisole, and HLA-B27. Lancet ii:85, 1977
29. Veys EM, Mielants H, Rosenthal M: Agranulocytosis, levamisole and HLA-B27. Lancet ii:764, 1977
30. Mielants H, Veys EM: B27 and agranulocytosis in rheumatoid arthritis patients treated with levamisole. Acta Rhumatol 3:104-109, 1979
31. Hodinka L, Geher P, Meretey K, Gyodi EK, Petranyi GG, Bozsoky S: Lavamisole-induced neutropenia and agranulocytosis: Association of HLA B27 leukocyte agglutinating and lymphocytotoxic antibodies. Int Arch Allergy Appl Immunol 65:460-464, 1981
32. Roitt IM, Corbett M, Festenstein H, Jaraquemada D, Papasteriadis C, Hay FC, et al: HLA-DRW4 and prognosis in rheumatoid arthritis. Lancet i:990, 1978
33. McMichael AJ, Sasazuki T, McDevitt HO, Payne RO: Increased frequency of HLA-CW3 and HLA-DW4 in rheumatoid arthritis. Arthritis Rheum 20:1037-1042, 1977
34. Gran JT, Husby G, Thorsby E: HLA DR antigens and gold toxicity. Ann Rheum Dis 42:63-66, 1983
35. Latts J, Antel JP, Levinson DJ, Arnason BGW, Meadof ME: Histocompatibility antigens and gold toxicity. J Clin Pharmacol 20:206-209, 1980
36. Calin A, Grahame R, Tudor M, Kennedy L: "Ankylosing rheumatoid arthritis," ankylosing spondylitis and HL-A antigens. Lancet i:874-875, 1974
37. Ebringer R, Colthorpe D, Young A, Corbett M: Increased incidence of faecal *Klebsiella pneumoniae* in patients with HLA B27 CREG antigen and men with rheumatiod arthritis. Br J Med 281:583-585, 1980
38. Khan MA, Kushner I, Ballou SP, Braun WE: Familial rheumatoid arthritis and HLA-DRW4. Lancet i:921-922, 1979
39. Khan MA, Braun WE, Steinberg AG, Kushner I, Dejelo CL, Ballou SP: Clinical and HLA studies in familial rheumatoid arthritis. Arthritis Rheum 23:702-703, 1980
40. Khan MA, Kushner I, Braun WE, Dejelo CL, Ballou SP: Clinical and HLA studies in multiple case families with rheumatoid arthritis. Tissue Antigens 18:136-138, 1981
41. Nunez G, Moore S, Ball GV, Hurd E, Khan MA, Stastny P: The inheritance of HLA haplotypes in families with rheumatoid arthritis. Arthritis Rheum 23:726, 1980
42. Zilko PJ, Feeney D, Christiansen FT, Hawkins BR, Dawkins RL: HLA and GM typing in families with rheumatoid arthritis. Arthritis Rheum 23:767, 1980
43. Strom H, Moller E: HLA and rheumatoid arthritis. A study of five families. Tissue Antigens 18:92-100, 1981
44. Rossen RD, Brewer EJ, Sharp RM, Ott J, Templeton JW: Familial rheumatoid arthritis. J Clin Invest 65:629-642, 1980
45. Rossen RD, Brewer EJ, Sharp RM, Ott J, Templeton JW: Demonstration of a disease susceptibility locus centromeric to HLA-D in a family with multiple cases of seropositive rheumatoid arthritis. Arthritis Rheum 23:739, 1980
46. Dequeker J, Decock T, Walravens M, Van De Putte I: A systematic survey of the HLA B27 prevalence in inflammatory rheumatic diseases. J Rheumatol 5:452-459, 1978
47. Kohno M: SLE and HLA antigens. Nippon Rinsho 36:3143-3146, 1978
48. Gibofsky A, Winchester RJ, Patarroyo M, Fotino M, Kunpel MG: Disease associations of the IA-like human alloantigens. J Exp Med 148:1728-1732, 1978
49. Brackertz D, Mueller-Eckhardt CH, Heinrich D, Kueppers F, Schulz G, Kretschmer V: Histocompatibility antigens of patients with rheumatoid arthritis. Z Immun Forsch BD 146:108-113, 1973
50. Stastny P, Fink CW: HLA-DW4 in adult and juvenile rheumatoid arthritis. Transplant Proc 9:1863-1866, 1977
51. Stastny P, Sittler S, Fink CW: IA-like antigens in rheumatoid arthritis (RA), systemic lupus erythematosus (SLE) and chronic active hepatitis (CAH). Tissue Antigens 10:210, 1977
52. Sachs JA, Brewerton DA: HLA, ankylosing spondylitis and rheumatoid arthritis. Br Med Bull 34:275-278, 1978
53. Stastny P: Mixed lymphocyte culture typing cells from patients with rheumatoid arthritis. Tissue Antigens 4:571-579, 1974
54. Marcolongo R, Contu L: Les antigenes HL-A dans la polyarthrite chronique rhumatismale et la spondylarthrite ankylosante en sardaigne. Nouv Presse Med 3:2023, 1974
55. Calin A: HLA-DRW4, rheumatoid factor, and prognosis in rheumatoid arthritis. Lancet i:873-874, 1979
56. Elson DJ, Crawford DH, Bucknall RC, Allen C, Thompson JL, Epstein MA, et al: Infection with EB virus and rheumatoid arthritis. Lancet i:105, 1979
57. Genth E, Peuckert H, Brude E, Hehl M, Hartl W: HLA-B27-positive oligarthritis. Z Rheumatol 37:313-328, 1978

58. Seignalet J, Clot J, Sany J, Serre H: Les antigens HL-A dans la polyarthrite chronique rhumatismale. Nouv Presse Med 1:2097-2102, 1972
59. Vischer TL, Jeannet M, Boussina I: HL-A27 diagnosis of rheumatic diseases. Lancet i:1001, 1974
60. Cleland LG: HLA B27 and arthritis. Ann Intern Med 87:496, 1977
61. Isomaki H, Nissila M, Koota K, Martio J, Tiilikainen A: HL-A27 and rheumatoid arthritis. Lancet ii:1212-1213, 1974
62. Fink CW, Stastny P: Results of serologic HLA-DR typing in juvenile arthritis and adult rheumatoid arthritis. Arthritis Rheum 23:673, 1980
63. Karsh J, Klippel JH, Mann DL, Reinertsen JL, Moutsopoulos HM, Johnson AH, et al.: Histocompatibility antigens in rheumatiod arthritis. Arthritis Rheum 23:701, 1980
64. Powell TR, Michalski JP, McCombs CC, Danilovs JA, Terasaki PI, Park MS, et al.: HLA-Bw44 and HLA-DRw4 in male Sjögren's syndrome patients with associated rheumatoid arthritis. Clin Immunol Immunopathol 17:463-468, 1980
65. Lies RB, Messner RP, Troup GM: Histocompatibility antigens and rheumatoid arthritis. Arthritis Rheum 15:524-529, 1972
66. Schlosstein L, Terasaki PI, Bluestone R, Pearson CM: High association of an HL-A antigen, W27, with ankylosing spondylitis. N Engl J Med 288:704-706, 1973
67. Morris PJ, Vaughan H, Tait BD, Mackay IR: Histocompatibility antigens (HLA): Association with immunopathic diseases and with response to microbial antigens. Aust NZ J Med 7:616-624, 1977
68. Nyulassy S, Ravingerova G, Zvarova E, Buc M: HL-A antigens in rheumatoid arthritis. Lancet i: 450-451, 1974
69. Govallo VI, Shelepina TA: Immunological studies in carcinogenesis: Distribution of the tissue incompatibility antigens (HL-A) system) in oncological patients. Vopr Onkol 21:13-19, 1975
70. Benevolenskaya LI, Tananov AT, Kutyina RM, Alekseeva LI, Orlov-Morozov AV: Rheumatoid arthritis and HLA antigens. Vopr Reum 3:8-11, 1981
71. Signalet J, Clot J, Sany J, Serre H: HL-A antigens in rheumatoid arthritis. Vox Sang 23:468-471, 1972
72. Dryll A, Debeyre N, Guedi D, Ryckewaert A, Legrand L, Marcelli A, et al: Etude des haplotypes HLA chez 56 patients atteints de polyarthrite rhumatoide classique vus au Centre Viggo Petersen. Rev Rhum 11:669, 1980
73. Marcolongo R , Contu L: HL-A antigens associated with rheumatoid arthritis and ankylosing spondylitis in an ethnic homogeneous population. Biomedicine 23:88-91, 1975
74. Toyoda K, Saito S, Naito S, Konomi K, Yamamoto H, Nobunaga M, et al: HLA antigens in classical and malignant rheumatoid arthritis in Japanese population. Tissue Antigens 10:56-59, 1977
75. Nasrallah NS, Masi AT, Chandler RW, Feigenbaum SL, Kaplan SB: HLA-B27 antigen and rheumatoid factor negative (seronegative) peripheral arthritis: Studies in younger patients with early-diagnosed arthritis. Am J Med 63:379-386, 1977
76. Bjelle A, Cedergren B, Dahlqvist SR: HLA B27 in the population of northern Sweden. Scand J Rheumatol 11:23-26, 1982
77. Stastny P: Association of the B-cell alloantigen DRW4 with rheumatoid arthritis. N Engl J Med 298:869-871, 1978
78. Sakurami T, Ueno Y, Iwaki Y, Park MS, Terasaki PI, Saji H: HLA-DR specificities among Japanese with several autoimmune diseases. Tissue Antigens 19:129-133, 1982
79. Perez-Rojas G, Penchasadeh G, Rodriguez M, Armas P, Bianco N: HLA-DRW4 antigen and B40-CW3-DRW4 haplotype in rheumatoid arhritis. In Terasaki PI (ed): Histocompatibility Testing 1980, p 952. UCLA Tissue Typing Laboratory, Los Angeles, 1981
80. Merciet P, Dallesr R, Roux H: Association HLA-DR et polyarthrite rhumatoide de l'adulte dans le sud de la France. Nouv Presse Med 9:1037, 1980
81. Llorca G, Betuel H, Gebuhrer L, Deslous-Paoli MP, Andre-Fouet E, Bonvoisin B, et al: HLA and rheumatoid arthritis. Rev Rhum Mal Osteoartic 48:691-696, 1981
82. Tongio MM, Asch L, Mayer S, Kuntz JL, Kieffer KD: HLA DRw4 dans la polyarthrite rhumatoide. Rev Rhum 47:667-668, 1980
83. Karr RW, Rodey GE, Lee T, Schwartz BD: Association of HLA-DRw4 rheumatiod arthritis in black and white patients. Arthritis Rheum 23:700-701, 1980
84. Wooley PH, Griffin J, Panayi GS, Batchelor JR, Welsh KI, Gibson TJ: HLA-DR antigens and toxic reaction to sodium aurothiomalate and *D*-penicillamine in patients with rheumatoid arthritis. N Engl J Med 303:300-302, 1980
85. Catalano MA, Carson DA, Stastny P, Freer S, Vaughan JH: Correlation between anti-RANA and anti-EBNA titers in normal subjects with and without HLA-DRw4. Arthritis Rheum 23:1049-1052, 1980
86. Ting A, Mackay LR, Morris PJ: HL-A in autoimmune diseases and infectious mononucleosis. Symp Ser Immunobiol Standard 18:276-281, 1973
87. Klareskog L, Forsum U, Scheynius A, Kabelitz D, Wigzell H: Evidence in support of a self-perpetuating HLA-DR-dependent delayed-type cell reaction in rheumatoid arthritis. Proc Natl Acad Sci USA 79:3632-3636, 1982
88. Forre O, Dobloug JH, Natvig JB: Augmented numbers of HLA-DR-positive T lymphocytes in the

synovial fluid and synovial tissue of patients with rheumatoid arthritis and juvenile rheumatoid arthritis. Scand J Immunol 15:227-231, 1982
89. Sagredo JP, Eguren TT, Valverde VR: Antigene d'histocompatibilite HLA-B27 dans les arthrites seronegatives et les lombalgies idiopathiqus. Rev Rhum 47:409-413, 1980
90. Gran JT, Husby G, Thorsby E: HLA-antigener (human leucocyte antigens) og reumatoid artritt. Tidsskr Nor Laegeforen 23:1350-1352, 1980
91. Poulter LW, Duke O, Hobbs S, Janossy G, Panayi G: Histochemical discrimination of HLA-DR positive cell populations in the normal and arthritic synovial lining. Clin Exp Immunol 48:381-388, 1982
92. Stastny P: The HLA-D region the genetics of rheumatoid arthritis. In Gorini S et al. (eds): Advances in Inflammation Research Vol 3: Rheumatoid Arthritis, pp 41-48. Raven Press, New York, 1982
93. Kay PH, McCluskey J, Christiansen FT, Feeney D, McCann VJ, Zilko PJ, et al: Complement allotyping reveals new genetic markers in rheumatoid arthritis and diabetes mellitus. Tissue Antigens 21:159-160, 1983
94. Khan MA, Kammer G, Dejelo CL, Kushner I, Braun WE, Ballou SP: Study of HLA antigens in familial sporadic rheumatoid arthritis. Tissue Antigens 21:35-38, 1983
95. Calin A: Epidemiology of the rheumatic diseases, with a focus on HLA. Curr Ther Res 30:S15-S23, 1981
96. Sach JA: HLA systems and rheumatic diseases. Curr Top Pathol 71:235-262, 1982
97. Rodriguez MA, Bankhurst AD, Williams Jr RC, Troup GM, Stastny P: Studies on the relationship between HLA DR4 and in vitro IgM rheumatoid factor production. Clin Immunol Immunopathol 27:96-109, 1983
98. Dawkins RL, Christiansen FT, Kay PH, Garlepp M, McCluskey J, Hollingsworth PN, et al: Disease associations with complotypes, supratypes and haplotypes. Immunol Rev 70:5-22, 1983

Juvenile Rheumatoid Arthritis

Population Association

An increased frequency of B27 was first reported by Rachelefsky et al.[1] and Buc et al.[2] Subsequent reports on several patient populations (Table 6.10) confirmed this association. Whether misdiagnosed early-onset ankylosing spondylitis patients had been included remains to be determined. Furthermore, there were also significant associations with A2, B7, and B15 antigens in the analysis of pooled data from these studies (Table 6.10).

In 27 Japanese patients and 181 healthy controls studied by Mitsui et al.,[3,4] B27 was completely absent. However, there was an increased frequency of B40 (Table 6.10).

HLA-D and -DR loci antigens have also been studied in several reports. A report by Stastny and Fink[5] found that, unlike adult rheumatoid arthritis (RA), there was no increase of DW4 in juvenile rheumatoid arthritis (JRA) patients. In a later report[6], these authors observed a moderately significant increase of DW7 and DW8 antigens (Table 6.10). All available data on interesting associations with DW antigens are given in Table 6.10.

DR locus antigen frequencies are available in several reports from the United States and Europe. These data show highly significant associations with DR5 and DR8 (Table 6.10). Interestingly, DW5 was not found to be associated with this disease in the report of Stastny and Fink[6] on 54 patients (Table 6.10).

If we compare the relative risks for B27 and DR5, it is slightly higher for B27 (3.94 vs. 3.30). The estimates for DR5, however, are based on fewer data than for B27.

Disease Heterogeneity

Sex

The sex distribution of B27-positive and -negative patients available in 6 studies[1,7–11] showed a higher frequency of males in B27-positive groups and a predominance of females in the B27-negative group. However, DR5 frequencies studied by Suciu-Foca et al.[12] in 13 male and 27 female patients were not significantly different (also see 13).

Pauciarticular vs. Polyarticular

In the studies of Rachelefsky et al.[1] and Gershwin et al.,[11] B27 was increased in both poly- and pauciarticular types of onset. However, Buc et al.[2] observed that, in a total of 30 patients, 10 had B27 and 9 of these also had the polyarticular form of the disease. The data of Schaller et al.[10] showed that the B27 increase was significant only in the boys with pauciarticular type. All patients with polyarticular and the girls with the pauciarticular disease did not show any association with B27.

Morling et al.[14] have reported that in 38 pauciarticular patients DW5 and DW8 were significantly increased. In the subgroup with polyarticular disease only DW4 was found to be increased.

Forre et al.[13,15] subdivided their patients into pauciarticular (n = 47) and polyarticular (n = 20) types and did not find any difference in the DR antigen frequencies between the 2 groups. All patients in the studies of Glass et al.[16,17] and Suciu-Foca et al.[12] were of pauciarticular onset type and, as the data in Table 6.10 show, DR5 was significantly increased in these patients. Suciu-Foca et al.[12] noted that all patients positive for DR5 were also positive for DW5 and there was no difference between patients and controls with respect to A, B, and C loci antigens (including B27). Stastny and Fink[6] observed an increased frequency of TMo (related to cross-reactive antigens DW7 and DW11) in patients with persistent pauciarticular type of arthritis (46% in the patients vs. 1% in healthy controls). The study of Fink and Stastny[18] in which DR5 was increased in the patients (Table 6.10) did not report the antigen frequencies in various clinical subgroups of patients.

Systemic Onset

Hall et al.[9] found typical systemic disease equally in those with and without antigen B27. Schaller et al.,[10] on the other hand, reported no significant association with B27 and systemic onset JRA. In the data of Stastny and Fink,[6] an increased frequency of DW7 was found in a small sample of 14 patients with this type of disease.

Age at Onset

Rachelfesky et al.[1] reported a lower (average 4.5 years) age at onset in 11 B27-positive patients (as compared with an average of 8.4 years in 15 B27-negative patients). Hall et al.[9] showed that the average age at onset in the B27 positive group was 9.5 years and 7.2 years in the B27 negative group.

Macurova et al.[8] subdivided their patients into groups of younger or older than 9 years of age at the time of the first signs of the disease. B27 was present in 62.5% of the 16 boys in the older group as compared with 26.6% in the younger group (n = 16). In girls, the frequency of B27 was similar in both groups.

Rheumatoid Factor

Forre et al.[13,15] have reported that DR4 was significantly increased in patients positive for rheumatoid factor. However, in 3 other studies there was no significant HLA difference between rheumatoid factor-positive and -negative patients.[1,8,11]

Antinuclear Antibody

In patients positive for antinuclear antibody, a higher frequency of B27[19] and DR5[16,17] has been observed. However, in a third study,[11] there was no HLA (A and B loci) difference between the antibody-positive and -negative groups (also see 13 and 15).

Presence of Uveitis

No specific HLA association was found in a subgroup of patients who also had uveitis.[1,11,19]

Progression of the Disease

In a follow-up study of 46 Caucasian patients by Edmonds et al.,[20,21] 7 patients were found to have developed ankylosing spondylitis. Six of these were positive for B27. There was only 1 female with B27 and ankylosing spondylitis.

Sacroiliitis

There was no specific HLA association in a subgroup of patients with sacroiliitis.[8,19–21]

Patients with Tenosynovitis

Gibson et al.[22] reported an increased frequency of B7 (66%) in 12 patients who also had tenosynovitis. In the total patient population (n = 123), the frequency of B7 was only 19% ($\chi^2 = 11.64$).

Definite vs. Probable Disease

No difference in the frequency of B27 between the 2 groups of patients[9] was demonstrated.

Radiologic Abnormalities

Hall et al.[9] observed that changes consistent with JRA were more commonly seen in patients with B27.

Chronic Iridocyclitis

In the data of Schaller et al.,[10] the frequency of B27 in 13 patients with chronic iridocyclitis was 13% as compared with 8% in 1863 controls. Thus, there was no significant difference between the 2 groups. Forre et al.[13,15] did not find any DR antigen difference between patients with (n = 15) and without (n = 62) a history of iridocyclitis.

Lymphocyte Response to Mitogen

Rola-Pleszczynski et al.[23] have studied proliferative responses to concanavalin A (Con A), phytohemagglutinin (PHA), pokeweed mitogen (PWM), and *Staphylococcus aureus* phase lysate (SL). Patients positive for B27 showed depressed responses to Con A and PWM and higher responses to PHA compared to B27-negative patients and controls.

Other Variables

Gershwin et al.[11] also subdivided their patients into groups based on the presence of fever, positive family history of the disease, and hematologic abnormalities. No significant associations were found.

TABLE 6.10. Juvenile Rheumatoid Arthritis

Country/Population	Patients n	Patients %+	Controls n	Controls %+	RR	χ^2	Ref.
HLA-A2							
U.S.A.	112	66	1863	50	1.93	10.51	10
U.S.A.	123	59	125	42	1.98	7.10	19
U.S.A.	26	65	267	47	2.04	3.01	1
U.S.A.	46	61	1205	48	1.68	2.96	11
	307	62	3460	49	1.90	23.34	
	Heterogeneity χ^2 (3 df)					0.23	
Czechoslovakia	62	63	350	48	1.83	4.66	8
BENELUX	35	64	1000	49	1.82	2.98	38
England	24	67	597	48	2.13	3.24	39
England	66	60	300	48	1.61	3.08	9
	90	62	897	48	1.75	6.01	
	Heterogeneity χ^2 (1 df)					0.31	
	494	62	5707	49	1.85	36.89	
	Heterogeneity χ^2 (7 df)					0.64	
HLA-B7							
U.S.A.	46	0	1205	25	0.03	11.50	11
U.S.A.	123	19	125	26	0.67	1.73	19
U.S.A.	112	22	1863	24	0.91	0.19	10
U.S.A.	26	19	267	26	0.71	0.48	1
	307	17	3460	25	0.73	3.46	
	Heterogeneity χ^2 (3 df)					10.44	
Czechoslovakia	62	13	350	22	0.55	2.39	8
BENELUX	35	3	1000	19	0.19	5.23	38
England	24	21	597	30	0.66	0.75	39
England	66	14	300	27	0.46	4.63	9
	90	16	897	29	0.53	5.00	
	Heterogeneity χ^2 (1 df)					0.39	
	494	15	5707	24	0.63	12.09	
	Heterogeneity χ^2 (7 df)					14.81	
HLA-B15							
U.S.A.	26	11	267	10	1.26	0.15	1
U.S.A.	123	13	125	10	1.33	0.55	19
U.S.A.	46	15	1205	10	1.68	1.66	11
U.S.A.	112	20	1863	9	2.56	14.69	10
	307	16	3460	9	1.94	14.15	
	Heterogeneity χ^2 (3 df)					2.90	
Czechoslovakia	62	8	350	13	0.63	1.02	8
BENELUX	35	23	1000	11	2.51	5.42	38
England	24	4	597	8	0.71	0.21	39
England	66	14	300	17	0.82	0.27	9
	90	11	897	11	0.80	0.45	
	Heterogeneity χ^2 (1 df)					0.03	

TABLE 6.10. *(continued)*

Country/Population	Patients n	Patients %+	Controls n	Controls %+	RR	χ^2	Ref.
HLA-B15							
Finland	47	49	326	26	2.73	10.32	40
	541	17	6033	11	1.70	17.74	
	Heterogeneity χ^2 (8 df)					16.56	
HLA-B27							
Tunisia	20	15	20	0	8.20	3.27	41
U.S.A.	112	26	1863	8	4.07	37.66	10
U.S.A.	26	42	267	6	11.16	27.87	1
U.S.A.	123	15	125	6	2.66	5.12	19
U.S.A.	46	26	1205	8	4.13	17.21	11
U.S.A.	28	25	91	7	4.32	6.74	42
U.S.A.	248	17	283	8	2.33	9.66	43
	583	21	3834	8	3.74	94.60	
	Heterogeneity χ^2 (5 df)					9.65	
Czechoslovakia	62	31	350	8	5.16	24.48	8
Czechoslovakia	34	29	314	9	4.18	12.09	2
	96	30	664	8	4.75	36.41	
	Heterogeneity χ^2 (1 df)					0.16	
BENELUX	35	58	1000	7	18.06	66.56	38
England	24	29	597	9	4.26	10.46	39
England	66	24	300	10	2.86	9.62	9
	90	25	897	9	3.31	19.57	
	Heterogeneity χ^2 (1 df)					0.50	
West Germany	170	36	200	9	5.57	35.41	44
Denmark	48	25	3301	9	3.46	14.30	14
Finland	47	17	326	14	1.31	0.45	40
Norway	77	21	1000	10	2.44	9.28	15
	1146	25	11222	9	3.94	245.21	
	Heterogeneity χ^2 (14 df)					41.68	
HLA-B40							
Japan	27	56	181	19	5.32	15.99	3
HLA-DW4							
U.S.A.	122	9	84	20	0.40	5.06	6
Denmark	48	27	345	19	1.61	1.90	14
	170	14	429	19	0.90	0.17	
	Heterogeneity χ^2 (1 df)					6.80	
HLA-DW5							
U.S.A.	54	6	76	5	1.23	0.09	6
Denmark	48	21	191	6	4.15	10.02	14
	102	13	267	6	2.89	7.95	
	Heterogeneity χ^2 (1 df)					2.16	

TABLE 6.10. *(continued)*

Country/Population	Patients n	Patients %+	Controls n	Controls %+	RR	χ^2	Ref.
HLA-DW7							
U.S.A.	62	31	75	13	2.92	6.38	6
Denmark	48	2	345	18	0.14	7.07	14
	110	18	420	17	1.38	0.76	
	Heterogeneity χ^2 (1 df)					12.69	
HLA-DW8							
U.S.A.	98	26	82	9	3.39	8.11	6
Denmark	48	23	335	8	3.48	10.48	14
	146	25	417	8	3.44	18.59	
	Heterogeneity χ^2 (1 df)					0.00	
HLA-DR4							
U.S.A.	40	33	133	33	1.01	0.00	12
U.S.A.	90	10	85	29	0.28	9.57	18
U.S.A.	45	16	84	25	0.59	1.30	17
	175	17	302	30	0.57	5.54	
	Heterogeneity χ^2 (2 df)					5.33	
Denmark	48	27	260	32	0.80	0.42	14
Norway	77	25	200	27	0.91	0.09	15
	300	21	762	30	0.71	4.42	
	Heterogeneity χ^2 (4 df)					6.96	
HLA-DR5							
U.S.A.	45	62	84	19	6.72	22.22	17
U.S.A.	90	21	85	7	3.34	6.60	18
U.S.A.	40	60	133	22	5.20	19.22	12
	175	40	302	17	5.07	46.77	
	Heterogeneity χ^2 (2 df)					1.28	
West Germany	170	32	200	17	2.28	11.13	44
Norway	77	21	200	9	2.68	7.34	15
	422	34	702	15	3.30	59.41	
	Heterogeneity χ^2 (4 df)					7.11	
HLA-DR 8							
U.S.A.	40	8	133	8	1.09	0.02	12
U.S.A.	90	23	85	8	3.27	6.99	18
U.S.A.	45	20	84	5	4.45	6.71	17
	175	19	302	7	2.69	10.52	
	Heterogeneity χ^2 (2 df)					3.21	
Norway	77	20	200	11	2.03	3.99	15
	252	19	502	9	2.39	14.15	
	Heterogeneity χ^2 (3 df)					3.57	

Family Data

Rossen et al.[24,25] have calculated lod scores for 5 multiple-case families (mixture of adult and JRA). The total maximum lod score for these families was 2.995 at 5% recombination.[25] A maximum lod score of +3.00 is generally considered as evidence in favor of linkage and thus there is evidence for linkage between HLA and JRA. The estimate of recombination between the disease gene and HLA is 5%. Studies of 14 affected sibling pairs by Suciu-Foca et al.[26] have also shown strong evidence of linkage. In these data 6 (43%) shared both parental haplotypes, 7 (50%) shared 1 haplotype, and 1 (7%) had no haplotype in common. On the basis of these results the authors have calculated a dominant mode of inheritance with a gene frequency of 0.1.

See also refs. 27–37 and 45–55.

References

1. Rachelefsky GS, Terasaki PI, Katz R, Stiehm ER: Increased prevalence of W27 in juvenile rheumatoid arthritis. N Engl J Med 290:892-893, 1974
2. Buc M, Nyulassy S, Stefanovic J, Michalko J, Mozolova D: HL-A system and juvenile rheumatoid arthritis. Tissue Antigens 4:395-397, 1974
3. Mitsui H, Juji T, Sonozaki H: Juvenile ankylosing spondylitis, its clinical features and HLA-B27. Arch Orthop Unfallchir 87:31-37, 1977
4. Mitsui H, Juji T, Sonozaki H, Watanabe N: Distribution of HLA-B27 in patients with juvenile rheumatoid arthritis. Pediatrics 60:562, 1977
5. Stastny P, Fink CW: HLA-DW4 in adult and juvenile rheumatoid arthritis. Transplant Proc 9:1863-1866, 1977
6. Stastny P, Fink CW: Different HLA-D associations in adult and juvenile rheumatoid arthritis. J Clin Invest 63:124-130, 1979
7. Veys EM, Coigne E, Mielants H, Verbruggen G: HLA and juvenile chronic polyarthritis. J Rheumatol 4 (Suppl 3):74-77, 1977
8. Macurova H, Ivaskova E, Havelka S, Ivanyi P: HL-A antigens in juvenile rheumatoid arthritis. J Immunogenet 3:229-236, 1976
9. Hall MA, Ansell BM, James DCO, Zylinski P: HL-A antigens in juvenile chronic polyarthritis (Still's disease). Ann Rheum Dis 34:36-38, 1975
10. Schaller JG, Ochs HD, Thomas ED, Nisperos B, Feigl P, Wedgwood RJ: Histocompatibility antigens in childhood-onset arthritis. J Pediatr 88:926-930, 1976
11. Gershwin ME, Opelz G, Terasaki PI, Castles JJ, Gorman TA: Frequency of HLA-DW3 in juvenile rheumatoid arthritis. Tissue Antigens 10:330-336, 1977
12. Suciu-Foca N, Jacobs J, Godfrey M, Woodward K, Khan R, Reed E, et al: HLA-DR5 in juvenile rheumatoid arthritis confined to few joints. Lancet ii:40, 1981
13. Forre O, Dobloug JH, Hoyeraal HM, Thorsby E: HLA antigens in juvenile arthritis. Arthritis Rheum 26:35-38, 1983
14. Morling N, Hellesen C, Jakobsen BK, Platz P, Ryder LP, Svejgaard A, et al: HLA-A B, C, D, DR antigens and primed lymphocyte typing (PLT) defined Dp-antigens in juvenile chronic arthritis. Tissue Antigens 17:433-441, 1981
15. Forre O, Dobloug JH, Hoyeraal HM, Kass E, Thorsby E: HLA-antigens in rheumatoid arthritis and juvenile rheumatoid arthritis: Increased frequency of the HLA-DRw4 antigen only in sero-positive patient groups. Adv Inflammation Res 3:195-201, 1982
16. Glass DN, Wallace K, Litvin DA, Chylack L, Garovoy M, Carpenter CB, et al: Iritis, antinuclear antibody, HLA and pauciarticular onset juvenile arthritis. Arthritis Rheum 23:680, 1980
17. Glass D, Litvin D, Wallace K, Chylack L, Garovoy M, Carpenter CB, et al: Early onset pauciarticular juvenile rheumatoid arthritis associated with human leukocytes: Antigen-DRW5, iritis, and antinuclear antibody. J Clin Invest 66:426-429, 1980
18. Fink CW, Stastny P: Results of serologic HLA-DR typing in juvenile arthritis and adult rheumatoid arthritis. Arthritis Rheum 23:673, 1980
19. Gibson DJ, Carpenter CB, Stillman JS, Schur PH: Reexamination of histocompatibility antigens found in patients with juvenile rheumatoid arthritis. N Engl J Med 293:636-638, 1975
20. Edmonds J, Morris RJ, Metzger AL, Bluestone R, Terasaki PI, Ansell B, et al.: Follow-up study of juvenile chronic polyarthritis with particular reference to histocompatibility antigen W27. Ann Rheum Dis 33:289-292, 1974
21. Edmonds J, Metzger A, Terasaki P, Bluestone R, Ansell B, Bywaters EGL: HL-A antigen W27 in juvenile chronic polyarthritis. Ann Rheum Dis 33:576, 1974
22. Gibson D, Schur PH, Carpenter CB, Stillman JS: Distribution of HL-A antigens in patients with juvenile rheumatoid arthritis (JRA). Arthritis Rheum 18:285, 1975
23. Rola-Pleszczynski M, Pare C, Camerlain M: HLA-B27 positive juvenile rheumatoid arthritis: Altered lymphocyte responses to mitogens and low cytotoxic activity. Clin Immunol Immunopathol 24:102-110, 1982
24. Rossen RD, Brewer EJ, Sharp RM, Ott J, Templeton JW: Familial rheumatoid arthritis. J Clin Invest 65:629-642, 1980
25. Rossen RD, Brewer EJ, Sharp RM, Ott J, Templeton JW: Demonstration of a disease susceptibility

locus centromeric to HLA-D in a family with multiple cases of seropositive rheumatoid arthritis. Arthritis Rheum 23:739, 1980
26. Suciu-Foca N, Godfrey M, Jocobs J, Khan R, Rohowsky C, Foca-Rodi A, et al: Increased frequency of DRW5 in pauciarticular JRA. In Terasaki PI (ed): Histocompatibility Testing 1980, p 953. UCLA Tissue Typing Laboratory, Los Angeles, 1981
27. Sturrock RD, Dick HM, Henderson N, Goel GK, Lee P, Dick WC, et al: Association of HL-A27 and AJ in juvenile rheumatoid arthritis and ankylosing spondylitis. J Rheumatol 1:269-273, 1974
28. Stastny P, Sittler S, Fink CW: IA-like antigens in rheumatoid arthritis (RA), systemic lupus erythematosus (SLE) and chronic active hepatitis (CAH). Tissue Antigens 10:210, 1977
29. Calabro JJ, Repice MM: W27 antigen and juvenile rheumatoid arthritis. N Engl J Med 291:103-104, 1974
30. Rachelefsky GS, Stiehm ER, Terasaki PI: W27 antigen and juvenile rheumatoid arthritis. N Engl J Med 291:104, 1974
31. Havelka S, Macurova H, Hoza J, Ivaskova E, Bardfeld R: Histocompatibility antigens in juvenile rheumatoid arthritis. Cesk Paediatr 32:391-392, 1977
32. Gershwin ME, Terasaki PI, Castles JJ: B cell alloantigens in juvenile rheumatoid arthritis. Tissue Antigens 11:71-73, 1978
33. Raum D, Glass D, Soter NA, Stillman JS, Carpenter CB, Schur PH: Lymphocytotoxic antibodies: HLA antigen associations, disease associations, and family studies. Arthritis Rheum 20:933-936, 1977
34. Veys EM, Coigne E, Mielants H, Verbruggen A: HLA et polyarthrite chronique juvenile. Rev Rhum Mal Osteoartic 43:491-495, 1976
35. Jacobs JC: HLA-B27 associated spondyloarthritis in children. Arthritis Rheum 23:695-696, 1980
36. Arnett FC, Bias WB, Stevens MB: Juvenile-onset chronic arthritis: clinical and roentgenographic features of a unique HLA-B27 subset. Am J Med 69:369-376, 1980
37. Mathon G, Pare C, Menard H, Tetreault L, Camerlain M: Arthrite rhumatoide juvenile et HLA-B27. Can Med Assoc J 123:377-379, 1980
38. Veys EM, Coigne E, Mielants H, Verbruggen A: HLA and juvenile chronic polyarthritis. Tissue Antigens 8:61-65, 1976
39. Dick HM, Sturrock RD, Goehl GK, Henderson N, Canesi B, Rooney PJ, et al: The association between HL-A antigens, ankylosing spondylitis and sacro-iliitis. Tissue Antigens 5:26-32, 1975
40. Nissila M, Elomaa L, Tiilikainen A: HL-A antigens in juvenile rheumatoid arthritis. N Engl J Med 292:430, 1975
41. Hamza M, Houissa R, Ben Ayed H: HLA-B27 et polyarthrites chroniques juveniles. Tunis Med 54:779-782, 1976
42. Nasrallah NS, Masi AT, Chandler RW, Feigenbaum SL, Kaplan SB: HLA-B27 antigen and rheumatoid factor negative (seronegative) peripheral arthritis: Studies in younger patients with early-diagnosed arthritis. Am J Med 63:379-386, 1977
43. Glass DN, Litvin DA: Heterogeneity of HLA associations in systemic onset juvenile rheumatoid arthritis. Arthritis Rheum 23:796-799, 1980
44. Scholz S, Albert E: HLA and diseases: Involvement of more than one HLA-linked determinant of disease susceptibility. Immunol Rev 70:77-88, 1983
45. St Neri TM, Reali G, Savi M, Truog P: Association of HLA-BW39 and DRW8 with a variant of juvenile chronic polyarthritis. In Terasaki PI (ed): Histocompatibility Testing 1980, p 954. UCLA Tissue Typing Laboratory, Los Angeles, 1981
46. Rosenberg AM, Petty RE: Similar patterns of juvenile rheumatoid arthritis within families. Arthritis Rheum 23:951-953, 1980
47. Knowles WC, Bennett PH: HL-A W27 and juvenile rheumatoid arthritis. N Engl J Med 293:1323, 1975
48. Forre O, Dobloug JH, Natvig JB: Augmented numbers of HLA-DR-positive T lymphocytes in the synovial fluid and synovial tissue of patients with rheumatoid arthritis and juvenile rheumatoid arthritis. Scand J Immunol 15:227-231, 1982
49. Reekers P, Schretlen EDAM, Van De Putte LBA: Increase of HLA "DRw6" in patients with juvenile chronic arthritis. Tissue Antigens 22:283-288, 1983
50. Fink CW Stastny P: HLA-DR typing in juvenile arthritis. Adv Inflammation Res 3:191-194, 1982
51. Jacobs JC, Baum J: Juvenile arthritis. Am J Dis Child 136:81-82, 1982
52. Arnett FC, Bias WB, Stevens MB: Juvnile-onset chronic arthritis: Clinical and roentgenographic features of a unique HLA-B27 subset. Am J Med 69:369-376, 1980
53. Calin A: Epidemiology of the rheumatic diseases, with a focus on HLA. Curr Ther Res 30:S15-S23, 1981
54. Sach JA: HLA systems and rheumatic diseases. Curr Top Pathol 71:235-262, 1982
55. Jacobs JC, Berdon WE, Johnston AD: HLA-B27-associated spondyloarthritis and enthesopathy in childhood: Clinical, pathologic, and radiographic observations in 58 patients. J Pediatr 100:521-528, 1982

Malignant Rheumatoid Arthritis

Population Association

Toyoda et al.[1] typed A and B loci antigens in 39 Japanese patients with malignant rheumatoid arthritis (MRA). This sample included 25 definite and 14 suspected MRA cases. B12 was completely absent

TABLE 6.11. Malignant Rheumatoid Arthritis

	Patients		Controls				
Country/Population	n	%+	n	%+	RR	χ^2	Ref.
HLA-B12							
Japan	39	0	317	17	0.06	7.44	1

in the patients compared with 17% in the controls (Table 6.11).

In the same report, 67 rheumatoid arthritis (RA) patients were also studied. In this group, BW22 was significantly increased (see Rheumatoid Arthritis). The frequency of B12 was similar to that in controls. On the basis of this difference, the authors have argued that RA and MRA constitute different clinical diagnostic entities.

Reference

1. Toyoda K, Saito S, Naito S, Konomi K, Yamamoto H, Nobunaga M, et al.: HLA antigens in classical and malignant rheumatoid arthritis in Japanese population. Tissue Antigens 10:56-59, 1977

Seronegative Pauciarticular Arthritis

Population Association

Eastmond et al.[1] studied a group of 26 patients (20 males and 6 females) in which the pattern of arthritis and male predominance was very similar to that observed both in patients with juvenile pauciarticular arthritis who later developed ankylosing spondylitis and in patients with Reiter's syndrome. In this group of 26 patients, the mean age at onset of the arthritis was 29.3 years (range 9–64 years). There were 5 patients who would satisfy the juvenile rheumatoid arthritis criteria.

Antigen B27 was associated with this type of arthritis (Table 6.12).

Joliat et al.[2] reported a similar increase of B27 in 18 Swiss patients with an inflammatory pauciarticular peripheral arthropathy. The antigen was present in 44% of the patients (8/18) compared with a frequency of 6% in a control population of unknown size. Destructive joint changes and deformities were absent in these patients.

Disease Heterogeneity

In the British study[1], mean age at onset, sex ratio, and number of affected joints were similar in 18 B27-positive and 8 B27-negative patients. The knees were equally commonly affected in both groups. The B27-positive patients had more low back or buttock symptoms.

See also ref. 3.

References

1. Eastmond CJ, Rajah SM, Tovey D, Wright V: Seronegative pauciarticular arthritis and HLA B27. Ann Rheum Dis 39:231-234, 1980
2. Joliat G, Ferro A, Jeannet M, Ott H: HLA-B27 antigen in diagnosis of atypical seronegative inflammatory arthropathy. Ann Rheum Dis 35:531-533, 1976
3. Genth E, Peuckert H, Brude E, Hehl M, Hartl W: HLA-B27-positive oligarthritis. Z Rheumatol 37:313-328, 1978

Seronegative Peripheral Arthritis

Population Association

In 109 patients typed for A and B loci antigens, Sebes et al.[1] reported an increase of B27 (Table 6.13).

TABLE 6.12. Seronegative Pauciarticular Arthritis

	Patients		Controls				
Country/Population	n	%+	n	%+	RR	χ^2	Ref.
HLA-B27							
England	26	69	229	12	15.55	37.06	1

TABLE 6.13. Seronegative Peripheral Arthritis

	Patients		Controls				
Country/Population	n	%+	n	%+	RR	χ^2	Ref.
HLA-B27							
U.S.A.	109	23	91	7	3.75	8.86	1

Disease Heterogeneity

In the aforementioned study sacroiliac radiographs were available on 42 patients (18 B27-positive and 24 B27-negative). Sacroiliitis was present in 83% of the B27 positive patients (15/18) but only in 21% of the B27 negative patients (5/24) (χ^2 = 13.70).

Reference

1. Sebes JI, Nasrallah NS, Rabinowitz JG, Masi AT: The relationship between HLA-B27 positive peripheral arthritis and sacroiliitis. Radiology 126:299-302, 1978

Seronegative Chronic Polyarthritis

Population Association

There was no association of B27 in 58 Canadian patients.[1] See also refs. 2 and 3.

References

1. Esdaile JM, Dwosh IL, Urowitz MB, Smythe HA, Falk J: HLA B27 in rheumatoid factor-negative polyarthritis. Ann Intern Med 86:699-702, 1977
2. Kuthan F, Streda A, Parma R, Krepelkova M, Hill Z, Valnickova Z: Diagnostic importance of the incidence of tissue antigen HLA-B27 in some rheumatic diseases. Vnitr Lek 25:578-583, 1979
3. Seignalet J, Clot J, Sany J, Serre H: Les antigenes HL-A dans la polyarthrite chronique rhumatismale. Nouv Presse Med 2:510, 1973

Gonococcal Arthritis

Population Association

In a small sample of 12 American Caucasian patients studied by Morris et al.,[1] none was B27-positive. This 0% frequency was not significantly different from 8% in 1863 controls. No other interesting deviations in A and B loci antigens were observed.

Similar results were also reported by Wagner and Fessel[2] in a sample of 7 American Caucasian and 5 American Black patients from San Francisco. All 12 patients were negative for B27.

References

1. Morris R, Metzger AL, Bluestone R, Terasaki PI: HL-A W27-A clue to the diagnosis and pathogenesis of Reiter's syndrome. N Engl J Med 290:554-556, 1974
2. Wagner LP, Fessel WJ: HL-A27 (W27) absent in gonococcal arthritis. Lancet i:1094-1095, 1975

Psoriatic Arthropathy (Unspecified)

Population Association

Based on a combined analysis of the frequency data from the studies given in Table 6.14, B13, BW16, B27, and BW38 antigens were significantly increased in the patients. It should be noted that B13, B16, and B17 were also associated with psoriasis.

Disease Heterogeneity

In the 75 psoriatic arthropathy and 157 psoriatic patients studied by Eastmond and Woodrow,[1] there was no significant antigen difference with respect to family history (positive or negative) of psoriasis.

Lambert et al[2] and Metzger et al.[3] compared B27-positive and -negative patients with respect to sex ratio, age at onset of psoriasis and arthritis, and mean duration of arthritis and psoriasis. The 2 groups of patients did not differ significantly. Lambert et al.[2] obtained similar results for severity of arthritis, severity of skin psoriasis, prevalence of nail changes, iritis, sacroiliitis, and ankylosing spondylitis.

Family Data

See ref. 4.

See also refs. 5-17.

TABLE 6.14. Psoriatic Arthropathy (Unspecified)

	Patients		Controls				
Country/Population	n	%+	n	%+	RR	χ^2	Ref.
HLA-A1							
China	10	50	100	10	8.62	10.66	18
HLA-B13							
Canada	28	7	160	8	1.03	0.00	19
U.S.A.	52	12	126	4	3.19	4.05	20
Yugoslavia	60	18	302	7	2.96	7.66	21
England	82	7	1000	4	1.93	2.31	1
Denmark	44	9	2103	4	2.63	3.91	22
	266	11	3691	4	2.35	15.54	
	Heterogeneity χ^2 (4 df)					2.39	
HLA-BW16							
Canada	34	12	200	1	11.95	10.85	23
U.S.A.	52	25	800	5	6.42	28.30	24
Yugoslavia	60	7	302	5	1.54	0.67	21
Denmark	44	11	2103	5	2.55	4.24	22
Sweden	25	12	100	5	2.70	2.10	25
	215	14	3505	5	3.87	37.60	
	Heterogeneity χ^2 (4 df)					8.55	
HLA-B17							
Canada	28	21	160	11	2.23	2.57	19
U.S.A.	52	19	800	9	2.45	6.15	24
U.S.A.	52	17	126	8	2.35	3.29	20
	104	18	926	9	2.41	9.43	
	Heterogeneity χ^2 (1 df)					0.00	
Yugoslavia	60	25	302	8	3.85	14.22	21
England	82	20	1000	6	3.97	21.17	1
Denmark	44	25	2103	8	3.94	15.76	22
Sweden	25	20	100	5	4.66	6.05	25
	343	21	4591	8	3.32	66.26	
	Heterogeneity χ^2 (6 df)					2.95	
HLA-B27							
China	10	40	100	4	14.85	13.16	18
Canada	28	21	160	9	2.77	3.97	19
Canada	48	21	573	9	2.76	7.53	26
	76	21	733	9	2.76	11.51	
	Heterogeneity χ^2 (1 df)					0.00	
U.S.A.	4	25	91	7	5.31	3.11	27
U.S.A.	52	25	800	8	3.90	16.38	24
	56	25	891	8	4.04	19.40	
	Heterogeneity χ^2 (1 df)					0.09	

TABLE 6.14. *(continued)*

Country/Population	Patients n	Patients %+	Controls n	Controls %+	RR	χ^2	Ref.
HLA-B27							
Yugoslavia	60	27	302	12	2.73	9.09	21
England	82	28	1000	8	4.51	31.55	1
Denmark	44	30	2103	8	5.02	24.04	22
Sweden	25	48	100	14	5.52	12.89	25
	343	27	5129	8	3.84	104.60	
	Heterogeneity χ^2 (7 df)					3.98	
HLA-BW38							
Canada	28	36	160	7	7.33	17.12	19
U.S.A.	52	17	800	2	10.17	29.18	24
U.S.A.	52	23	126	4	6.74	13.22	20
	104	20	926	2	8.62	42.04	
	Heterogeneity χ^2 (1 df)					0.37	
	132	23	1086	3	8.18	59.08	
	Heterogeneity χ^2 (2 df)					0.45	

References

1. Eastmond CJ, Woodrow JC: The HLA system and the arthropathies associated with psoriasis. Ann Rheum Dis 36:112-120, 1977
2. Lambert JR, Wright V, Rajah SM, Moll JMH: Histocompatibility antigens in psoriatic arthritis. Ann Rheum Dis 35:526-530, 1976
3. Metzger AL, Morris RI, Bluestone R, Terasaki: HLA in psoriatic arthropathy. Arthritis Rheum 18:111-115, 1975
4. Guilhou JJ, Meynadier J, Seignalet J, Guilhou E: Les antigenes d'histocompatibilite dans le psoriasis-correlation avec l'arthropathie psoriasique; etudes familiales. Dermatologica 148:129-134, 1974
5. Dequeker J, Decock T, Walravens M, Van De Putte I: A systematic survey of the HLA B27 prevalence in inflammatory rheumatic diseases. J Rheumatol 5:452-459, 1978
6. Gunther VW, Richter KV: Haufigbeitsverteilung von histokompatibilitatsantigenen (HLA) bei dermatologischen erkranbungen. Dermatol Monatsschr 161:402-404, 1975
7. Schumacher TM, Genant HK, Kellet MJ, Mall JC, Fye KH: HLA-B27 associated arthropathies. Radiology 126:289-297, 1978
8. Moll JMH, Wright V: Familial occurrence of psoriatic arthritis. Ann Rheum Dis 32:181-201, 1973
9. Brewerton DA, James DCO: The histocompatibility antigen (HL-A 27) and disease. Semin Arthritis Rheum 4:191-207, 1975
10. McClusky OE, Lordon RE, Arnett FC Jr: HL-A 27 in Reiter's syndrome and psoriatic arthritis: A genetic factor in disease susceptibility and expression. J Rheumatol 1:263-268, 1974
11. Kozin F, Duquesnoy R, Rodey GE, Lightfoot RW, Ryan LM Jr: High prevalence of HLA-CW1 and CW2 antigens in spondylarthritis. Arthritis Rheum 21:889-895, 1978
12. Seignalet J, Sany J, Serre H: Systeme HL-A, spondylarthrite ankylosante rhumatisme psoriasique. Nouv Presse Med 3:1958, 1974
13. Lauter SA, Vasey FB, Espinoza LR, Bombardier C, Osterland CK: Homozygosity for HLA-B27 in psoriatic arthritis and spondylitis. Arthritis Rheum 20:1569-1570, 1977
14. Molin L: Psoriatic arthritis. Ann Clin Res 8:305-311, 1976
15. Sagredo JP, Eguren TT, Valverde VR: Anti gene d'histocompatibilite HLA-B27 dans les arthrites seronegatives et les lombalgies idiopathiqus. Rev Rhum 47:409-413, 1980
16. Sach JA: HLA systems and rheumatic diseases. Curr Top Pathol 71:235-262, 1982
17. Cazalis P, Dryll A, Ryckewaert A: Complexes HLA et rhumatisme psoriasique. Rev Rhum 47:529-534, 1980
18. Song FJ: HLA antigens and psoriasis. Natl Med J China 62:239-242, 1982
19. Espinoza LR, Vasey FB, Oh JH, Wilkinson R, Osterland CK: Association between HLA-BW38 and peripheral psoriatic arthritis. Arthritis Rheum 21:72-75, 1978
20. Murray C, Mann DL, Gerber LN, Barth W, Perlmann S, Decker JL, et al.: Histocompatibility alloantigens in psoriasis and psoriatic arthritis. J Clin

Invest 66:670-675, 1980
21. Jajic I, Kastelan A, Brnobic A, Kerhin V, Brkljacic L: HLA antigens in psoriatic arthritis and psoriasis. Arch Dermatol 113:1724-1725, 1977
22. Zachariae H, Hjortshoj A, Kissmeyer-Nielsen F, Svejgaard A, Svejgaard E, Zachariae E: HL-A antigens and psoriatic arthritis. Acta Derm Venereol (Stockh) 54:443-447, 1974
23. Buchanan R, Kraag G, Rosenthal D, Singal DP: HLA antigens and psoriatic arthritis. Transplant Proc 9:1873-1875, 1977
24. Arnett FC, Bias WB: HLA-BW38 and BW39 in psoriatic arthritis: Relationships and implications for peripheral and axial involvement. Arthritis Rheum 23:649-650, 1980
25. Marcusson J, Moller E, Thyresson N: HL-A antigens (17, 27, UPS) in psoriasis with special reference to patients with arthritic lesions. Acta Derm Venereol (Stockh) 55:297-300, 1975
26. Barraclough D, Russell AS, Percy JS: Psoriatic spondylitis: A clinical, radiological, and scintiscan survey. J Rheumatol 4:282-287, 1977
27. Nasrallah NS, Masi AT, Chandler RW, Feigenbaum SL, Kaplan SB: HLA-B27 antigen and rheumatoid factor negative (seronegative) peripheral arthritis: Studies in younger patients with early-diagnosed arthritis. Am J Med 63:379-386, 1977

Psoriatic Arthropathy (Central)

Population Association

Frequency data from studies given in Table 6.15 show that B13, BW16, B17, B27, and BW38 were significantly increased in this group of patients. It should be noted that BW16 was not increased in the peripheral form of this disease. B13, BW16, and B17 were also associated with psoriasis.

Disease Heterogeneity

Metzger et al.[1] studied the frequency of B27 in subgroups of patients based on sex, age at onset of psoriasis and arthritis, and mean duration of psoriasis and arthritis. There was no significant difference between B27-positive and B27-negative patients.

See also refs. 2–4.

References

1. Metzger AL, Morris RI, Bluestone R, Terasaki PI: HL-A W27 in psoriatic arthropathy. Arthritis Rheum 18:111-115, 1975
2. Sany J, Serre H, Seignalet J, Roux H, Maestraeci D, Recordier AM, et al: Relation enter rhumatisme psoriasique et systeme HL-A. Nouv Presse Med 4:3142-3143, 1975
3. Seignalet J, Sany J, Serre H: Interet pratique des groupes HL-A en rhumatologie. Semin Hop Paris 51:993-1000, 1975
4. Medsger TA Jr, Rodnan GP, Rabin B, Birnbaum N, Porter P: HL-A antigen 27 and psoriatic spondylitis. Arthritis Rheum 17:323, 1974
5. Jajic I, Kastelan A, Brnobic A, Kerhin V, Brkljacic L: HLA antigens in psoriatic arthritis and psoriasis. Arch Dermatol 113:1724-1725, 1977
6. Roux H, Mercier P, Maestracci D, Serratrice G, Sany J, Seignalet J, et al: Psoriatic arthritis and HLA antigens. J Rheumatol 4 (Suppl 3):64-65, 1977
7. Sany J, Seignalet JJ, Guilhou JJ, Serre H: HL-A et rhumatisme psoriasique. Rev Rhum Mal Osteoartic 42:451-460, 1975
8. Feldman JL, Hors J, Amor B, Cazalis P, Dryll A, Hacquart B: Antigenes HLA chez les malades atteints de rhumatisme psoriasique. Nouv Presse Med 5:477-480, 1976
9. Arnett FC, Bias WB: HLA-BW38 and BW39 in psoriatic arthritis: Relationships and implications for peripheral and axial involvement. Arthritis Rheum 23:649-650, 1980
10. Espinoza LR, Vasey FB, Oh JH, Wilkinson R, Osterland CK: Association between HLA-BW38 and peripheral psoriatic arthritis. Arthritis Rheum 21:72-75, 1978
11. Lambert JR, Wright V, Rajah SM, Moll JMH: Histocompatibility antigens in psoriatic arthritis. Ann Rheum Dis 35:526-530, 1976

Psoriatic Arthropathy (Peripheral)

Population Association

A combined analysis of all available data in Table 6.16 shows that B13, BW16, B17, B27, and BW38 are significantly increased in the patients. B13 and B17 are also associated with psoriasis.

Disease Heterogeneity

In the study by Metzger et al.,[1] patients were grouped on the basis of sex, age at onset of psoriasis and arthritis, and mean duration of psoriasis and arthritis. There were no significant differences between B27-positive and B27-negative groups.

Family Data

See refs. 2 and 3.

See also refs. 4–7.

References

1. Metzger AL, Morris RI, Bluestone R, Terasaki PI: HL-A W27 in psoriatic arthropathy. Arthritis Rheum 18:111-115, 1975
2. Marcusson J, Moller E, Rosenthal L, Lindwall N, Thyresson N: Psoriasis and arthritic lesions in relation to the inheritance of HLA genotypes: A family study. Acta Derm Venereol 58:511-520, 1978
3. Marcusson J, Elman A, Moller E, Thyresson N: Psoriasis, sacroiliitis and peripheral arthritis occur in patients with same HLA haplotype: Preliminary family report and hypothetical explanation of interaction between MHS products. Tissue Antigens 8:131-138, 1976
4. Sany J, Serre H, Seignalet J, Roux H, Maestraeci D, Recordier AM, et al: Relation enter rhumatisme psoriasique et systeme HL-A. Nouv Presse Med 4:3142-3143, 1975
5. Seignalet J, Sany J, Serre H: Interet pratique des groupes HL-A en rhumatologie. Semin Hop Paris 51:993-1000, 1975
6. Esdaile JM, Dwosh IL, Urowitz MB, Smythe HA, Falk J: HLA B27 in rheumatoid factor-negative polyarthritis. Ann Intern Med 86:699-702, 1977
7. Bluestone R, Morris RI, Metzger AL, Terasaki PI: (HLA) W27 and the spondylitis of chronic inflammatory bowel disease and psoriasis. Ann Rheum Dis 34:31-32, 1975
8. Lambert JR, Wright V J, Rajah SM, Moll JMH: Histocompatibility antigens in psoriatic arthritis. Ann Rheum Dis 35:526-530, 1976
9. Roux H, Mercier P, Maestracci D, Serratrice G, Sany J, Seignalet J, et al: Psoriatic arthritis and HLA antigens. J Rheumatol 4 (Suppl 3):64-65, 1977
10. Sany J, Seignalet JJ, Guilhou JJ, Serre H: HL-A et rhumatisme psoriasique. Rev Rhum Mal Osteoartic 42:451-460, 1975
11. Feldman JL, Hors J, Amor B, Cazalis P, Dryll A, Hacquart B: Antigenes HLA chez les malades atteints de rhumatisme psoriasique. Nouv Presse Med 5:477-480, 1976
12. Karvonen J, Lassus A, Sievers U, Tiilikainen A: HL-A antigens in psoriatic arthritis. Ann Clin Res 6:304-307, 1974
13. Arnett FC, Bias WB: HLA-BW38 and BW39 in psoriatic arthritis: Relationships and implications for peripheral and axial involvement. Arthritis Rheum 23:649-650, 1980
14. Eastmond CJ, Woodrow JC: The HLA system and the arthropathies associated with psoriasis. Ann Rheum Dis 36:112-120, 1977
15. Espinoza LR, Vasey FB, Oh JH, Wilkinson R, Osterland CK: Association between HLA-BW38 and peripheral psoriatic arthritis. Arthritis Rheum 21:72-75, 1978
16. Brewerton DA, Caffrey M, Nicholls AN, Walters D, James DCO: HL-A27 and arthropathies associated with ulcerative colitis and psoriasis. Lancet i: 956-957, 1974

Psoriatic Arthropathy (Peripheral and Sacroiliitis)

Population Association

In a small sample of 22 French patients, a significant association with BW38 was reported by Roux et al.[1] (Table 6.17). Also, in the combined data of Lambert et al.,[2] Roux et al.,[1] and Karvonen et al.,[3] there was a marginally significant increase of B17 in the patients (Table 6.17).

TABLE 6.15. Psoriatic Arthropathy (Central)

	Patients		Controls				
Country/Population	n	%+	n	%+	RR	χ^2	Ref.
HLA-B13							
U.S.A.	23	9	254	4	2.75	2.20	1
Yugoslavia	19	16	302	7	2.80	2.98	5
France	18	18	264	5	4.50	6.05	6
France	9	22	264	5	6.05	6.06	7
France	26	19	152	5	4.51	6.74	8
	53	19	680	5	4.85	18.73	
	Heterogeneity χ^2 (2 df)					0.12	
	95	16	1236	5	3.88	22.97	
	Heterogeneity χ^2 (4 df)					1.05	

TABLE 6.15. *(continued)*

Country/Population	Patients n	Patients %+	Controls n	Controls %+	RR	χ^2	Ref.
HLA-BW16							
U.S.A.	23	39	800	5	12.24	32.58	9
Yugoslavia	19	11	302	5	2.74	2.28	5
	42	26	1102	5	7.79	31.35	
	Heterogeneity χ^2 (1 df)					3.51	
HLA-B17							
U.S.A.	23	17	800	9	2.26	2.48	9
U.S.A.	23	13	254	9	1.69	0.79	1
	46	15	1054	9	1.99	3.14	
	Heterogeneity χ^2 (1 df)					0.14	
Yugoslavia	19	16	302	8	2.43	2.25	5
France	26	12	152	6	2.31	1.79	8
France	18	11	264	4	3.45	3.16	6
France	9	0	264	4	1.21	0.03	7
	53	10	680	4	2.43	4.31	
	Heterogeneity χ^2 (2 df)					0.67	
	118	13	2036	7	2.22	9.55	
	Heterogeneity χ^2 (5 df)					0.96	
HLA-B27							
Canada	6	83	160	9	35.35	17.32	10
U.S.A.	23	35	254	6	8.41	18.98	1
U.S.A.	23	35	254	6	8.41	18.98	1
U.S.A.	23	48	800	8	10.58	31.44	9
	69	39	1308	7	9.22	69.22	
	Heterogeneity χ^2 (2 df)					0.18	
Yugoslavia	19	47	302	12	6.47	15.72	5
England	28	60	1000	8	16.91	52.75	11
France	9	22	264	9	3.27	2.78	7
France	26	50	152	4	22.25	33.09	8
France	18	50	264	9	9.92	21.54	6
	53	45	680	8	10.55	52.76	
	Heterogeneity χ^2 (2 df)					4.64	
	175	47	3450	8	10.75	202.99	
	Heterogeneity χ^2 (8 df)					9.60	
HLA-BW38							
Canada	6	0	160	7	0.98	0.00	10
U.S.A.	23	30	800	2	21.19	38.04	9
France	18	14	264	3	5.76	6.65	6
France	26	27	152	3	11.29	16.26	8
	44	22	416	3	8.40	22.36	
	Heterogeneity χ^2 (1 df)					0.55	
	73	23	1376	3	10.33	53.58	
	Heterogeneity χ^2 (3 df)					7.37	

TABLE 6.16. Psoriatic Arthropathy (Peripheral)

	Patients		Controls				
Country/Population	n	%+	n	%+	RR	χ^2	Ref.
HLA-B13							
U.S.A.	17	6	254	4	2.11	0.87	1
England	54	11	1000	4	3.15	6.91	8
France	68	16	264	5	3.62	9.43	9
France	43	12	264	5	2.71	3.78	10
France	44	9	162	5	1.98	1.35	11
	155	13	690	5	2.87	13.83	
	Heterogeneity χ^2 (2 df)					0.73	
Finland	17	12	326	24	0.52	1.06	12
	243	12	2270	7	2.37	16.11	
	Heterogeneity χ^2 (5 df)					7.30	
HLA-BW16							
U.S.A.	29	14	800	5	3.37	5.62	13
U.S.A.	17	12	254	6	2.50	1.83	1
	46	13	1054	5	3.02	7.33	
	Heterogeneity χ^2 (1 df)					0.12	
Finland	17	0	326	12	0.21	2.29	12
	63	10	1380	7	2.11	3.88	
	Heterogeneity χ^2 (2 df)					5.86	
HLA-B17							
U.S.A.	17	35	254	9	5.54	10.73	1
U.S.A.	29	21	800	9	2.83	5.46	13
	46	26	1054	9	3.75	15.23	
	Heterogeneity χ^2 (1 df)					0.96	
England	40	30	433	8	4.98	18.15	14
England	54	24	1000	6	5.04	23.16	8
	94	27	1433	7	5.01	41.31	
	Heterogeneity χ^2 (1 df)					0.00	
France	44	23	152	6	4.60	10.39	11
France	68	26	264	4	8.21	27.13	9
France	43	30	264	4	10.05	27.38	12
	155	26	680	4	7.45	63.35	
	Heterogeneity χ^2 (2 df)					1.55	
Finland	17	6	326	11	0.74	0.16	15
	312	25	3493	7	5.06	110.57	
	Heterogeneity χ^2 (7 df)					11.99	
HLA-B27							
Canada	22	5	160	9	0.73	0.16	15
Canada	8	25	171	5	6.93	6.38	6
	30	10	331	7	2.27	2.27	
	Heterogeneity χ^2 (1 df)					4.27	

TABLE 6.16. *(continued)*

Country/Population	Patients n	Patients %+	Controls n	Controls %+	RR	χ^2	Ref.
U.S.A.	17	18	254	6	3.75	4.61	1
U.S.A.	29	7	800	8	1.05	0.01	13
	46	11	1054	8	1.99	2.49	
	Heterogeneity χ^2 (1 df)					2.12	
England	54	9	1000	8	1.23	0.22	8
England	40	33	433	8	5.70	22.10	14
	94	19	1433	8	3.08	15.46	
	Heterogeneity χ^2 (1 df)					6.86	
France	68	7	264	9	0.82	0.17	9
France	43	12	264	9	1.46	0.63	10
France	44	7	162	4	1.93	1.06	11
	155	8	690	8	1.24	0.52	
	Heterogeneity χ^2 (2 df)					1.34	
West Germany	41	24	300	7	4.25	12.13	16
Finland	17	24	326	43	0.45	2.24	12
	383	14	4134	10	1.98	19.14	
	Heterogeneity χ^2 (10 df)					30.56	
HLA-BW38							
Canada	22	46	160	7	10.95	22.35	15
U.S.A.	29	7	800	2	4.38	5.12	13
France	44	18	152	3	6.73	11.16	11
France	68	6	264	3	2.17	1.82	9
	112	11	416	3	3.83	11.02	
	Heterogeneity χ^2 (1 df)					1.96	
	163	15	1376	3	5.47	35.71	
	Heterogeneity χ^2 (3 df)					4.74	

TABLE 6.17. Psoriatic Arthropathy (Peripheral and Sacroiliitis)

Country/Population	Patients n	Patients %+	Controls n	Controls %+	RR	χ^2	Ref.
HLA-B17							
England	17	14	1000	6	2.96	3.12	2
France	22	14	264	4	4.23	5.40	1
Finland	19	11	326	11	1.19	0.07	3
	58	13	1590	7	2.50	6.45	
	Heterogeneity χ^2 (2 df)					2.14	
HLA-BW38							
France	22	17	264	3	6.89	9.83	1

Family Data

See ref. 4.
See also ref. 5.

References

1. Roux H, Mercier P, Maestracci D, Serratrice G, Sany J, Seignalet J, et al: Psoriatic arthritis and HLA antigens. J Rheumatol 4 (Suppl 3):64-65, 1977
2. Lambert JR, Wright V, Rajah SM, Moll JMH: Histocompatibility antigens in psoriatic arthritis. Ann Rheum Dis 35:526-530, 1976
3. Karvonen J, Lassus A, Sievers U, Tiilikainen A: HL-A antigens in psoriatic arthritis. Ann Clin Res 6:304-307, 1974
4. Marcusson J, Moller E, Rosenthal L, Lindwall N, Thyresson N: Psoriasis and arthritic lesions in relation to the inheritance of HLA genotypes: A family study. Acta Derm Venereol 58:511-520, 1978
5. Bluestone R, Morris RI, Metzger AL, Terasaki PI: (HLA) W27 and the spondylitis of chronic inflammatory bowel disease and psoriasis. Ann Rheum Dis 34:31-32, 1975

Post-*Yersinia* Arthritis

Population Association

The first reports from Finland by Aho et al.[1-3] showed a significant increase of B27 in arthritis patients who had *Yersinia* infection prior to the onset of arthritis. In 2 subsequent reports the data from Finland[4-7] and Denmark[1,5,6] showed similar results (Table 6.18).

In another study from Belgium,[8,11] B27 was present in 56% of the 25 patients[11] compared with only 6.6% in the controls (the number of controls is unknown). Thus, the existing data show a strong association of B27 with the arthritis developed after *Yersinia* infection.

Disease Heterogeneity

In the sample of 49 patients studied by Aho et al.[2] only 6 were B27-negative. Four of these B27-negative patients had monoarthritis of short duration (less than 1 month). Only 5 of the 43 B27-positive patients had this type of monoarthritis. B27-negative patients also had mild or somewhat atypical disease.

In the B27-positive group of patients studied by Leirisalo et al.[6] inflammatory urologic symptoms, ocular inflammation, and back pain during the acute disease were significantly more common than in B27-negative patients. Also, the duration of the disease was longer, and erythrocyte sedimentation rate, white blood cell count, and agglutinin titers for *Yersinia* organism were significantly higher in B27-positive patients.

Leirisalo et al.[9,10] studied chemotaxis, chemokinesis, and spontaneous locomotion of polymorphonuclear leukocytes of patients and healthy controls. B27-positive individuals (both patients and controls) showed a significantly higher response to chemotactic stimulus than B27-negative individuals. On the basis of these experiments the authors have suggested that these high responder polymorphonuclear leukocytes may contribute to the more severe inflammatory symptoms in *Yersinia* arthritis patients.

See also ref. 11.

References

1. Aho K, Ahvonen P, Alkio P, Sairanen E, Sievars K, Tiilikainen A: HL-A27 in reactive arthritis following infection. Ann Rheum Dis 34:29-30, 1975

TABLE 6.18. Post-*Yersinia* Arthritis

Country/Population	Patients n	Patients %+	Controls n	Controls %+	RR	χ^2	Ref.
HLA-B27							
Denmark	41	54	1967	9	11.79	61.05	6
Finland	103	81	900	14	25.60	151.03	6
Finland	49	88	326	14	41.62	72.03	2
	152	83	1226	14	29.12	222.16	
	Heterogeneity χ^2 (1 df)					0.90	
	193	77	3193	11	21.44	277.79	
	Heterogeneity χ^2 (2 df)					6.31	

TABLE 6.19. Postgonorrhoic Arthritis

Country/Population	Patients n	Patients %+	Controls n	Controls %+	RR	χ^2	Ref.
HLA-B27							
Denmark	19	47	1541	8	10.22	27.05	1

2. Aho K, Ahvonen P, Lassus A, Sievers K, Tiilikainen A: HL-A27 in reactive arthritis: A study of Yersinia arthritis and Reiter's disease. Arthritis Rheum 17:521-526, 1974
3. Aho K, Ahvonen P, Lassus A, Sievers K, Tiilikainen A: Genetic background of reactive arthritis. Duodecim 90:824-831, 1974
4. Leirisalo M, Laitinen O, and Tiilikainen A: HLA phenotypes in patients with rheumatic fever, rheumatic heart disease, and Yersinia arthritis. J Rheumatol 4 (Suppl 3):78-83, 1977
5. Laitinen O, Leirisalo M, Skylv G: Relation between HLA-B27 and clinical features in patients with Yersinia arthritis. Arthritis Rheum 20:1121-1124, 1977
6. Leirisalo M, Skylv G, Kousa M, Voipio-Pulkki LM, Suoranta H, Nissila M, et al: Followup study on patients with Reiter's disease and reactive arthritis, with special reference to HLA-B27. Arthritis Rheum 25:249-259, 1982
7. Leirisalo M, Skylv G, Kousa M, Voipio-Pulkki LM, Suoranta H, Nissila M, et al: HLA-B27 and clinical characteristics of reactive arthritis. Scand J Rheumatol 42:9, 1982
8. Dequeker J, Decock T, Walravens M, Van De Putte I: A systematic survey of the HLA B27 prevalence in inflammatory rheumatic diseases. J Rheumatol 5:452-459, 1978
9. Leirisalo M, Repo H, Tiilikanen A, Kosunen TU, Laitinen O: Chemotaxis in Yersinia arthritis: HLA-B27 positive neutrophils show high stimulated motility in vitro. Arthritis Rheum 23:1036-1044, 1980
10. Repo H, Leirisalo M, Tiilikainen A, Laitinen O: Chemotaxis in Yersinia arthritis: In vitro stimulation of neutrophil migration by HLA-B27 positive and negative sera. Arthritis Rheum 25:655-661, 1982
11. Dequeker J, Jamar R, Walravens M: HLA-B27, arthritis and Yersinia entertocolitica infection. J Rheumatol 7:706-710, 1980

Postgonorrhoic Arthritis

Population Association

In 19 Danish patients suffering from arthritis preceded by gonococcal infection (*Neisseria gonorrhoeae*), 9 were B27-positive.[1] This frequency was significantly different from controls (Table 6.19).

Reference

1. Friis J: HL-A27 in Neisseria infected patients with arthritis (abstract). Scand J Rheumatol Suppl 8, 1975

Postshigellosis Arthritis

Population Association

Aho et al.[1] showed a very high frequency of B27 in patients who, after a *Shigella flexneri*-induced dysentery, had contracted Reiter's disease (Table 6.20).

Reference

1. Aho K, Ahvonen P, Alkio P, Sairanen E, Sievars K, Tiilikainen A: HL-A27 in reactive arthritis following infection. Ann Rheum Dis 34:29-30, 1975

TABLE 6.20. Postshigellosis Arthritis

Country/Population	Patients n	Patients %+	Controls n	Controls %+	RR	χ^2	Ref.
HLA-B27							
Finland	13	85	323	14	28.69	25.20	1

Postmeningococcal Arthritis

Population Association

Friis[1] reported the B27 frequency in 14 Danish patients with meningococcal meningitis who also developed arthritis. Only 1 patient was B27-positive (7%). The frequency of B27 in 1541 healthy Danes was 8.1% (125/1541); thus, there was no significant difference between the patients and the controls.

In all patients the symptoms subsided in a few weeks and no joint symptoms were present at followup.

Reference

1. Friis J: HL-A27 in Neisseria infected patients with arthritis (abstract). Scand J Rheumatol (Suppl 8), 1975

Postrubella Vaccination Arthropathy

Population Association

Robitaille et al.[1] reported no association with A and B loci antigens, especially B27, in 23 patients from London. A diagnosis of presumed rubella arthropathy was made in the presence of an arthropathy that developed during a clinical attack of rubella. The diagnosis was supported whenever possible by a rising titer to rubella or, when unavailable, by a history of contact with another known case of rubella. However, in many of these patients, the rise in antibody titer was not detected because they were examined too late. Thus, the authors have used the term "presumed arthropathy." The frequency of B27 was 13% (3/23) compared with 8% (48/600) in controls.

A more specific study was done by Griffiths et al.[2] Thirty-four American Caucasian patients selected for the study had received HPV-77 DK-12 rubella vaccine and subsequently experienced recurrent attacks of pain and stiffness of the knees. (Two patients were siblings and thus there were only 33 unrelated patients.) The antigen frequencies were compared with frequencies in a control population of 646 persons. Although B12 and B14 were increased in the patients, the difference was not significant after correction was made for 21 antigens compared in the study.

There were 18 male and 15 female patients and separate analysis of these 2 groups did not show any association.

References

1. Robitaille A, Cockburn C, James DCO, Ansell BM: HLA frequencies in less common arthropathies. Ann Rheum Dis 35:271-273, 1976
2. Griffiths MM, Spruance SL, Ogra PL, Thompson GR, Dewitt CW: HLA and recurrent episodic arthropathy associated with rubella vaccination. Arthritis Rheum 20:1192-1197, 1977

Post-*Salmonella* Arthritis

Population Association

Available data from Denmark,[1,2] Sweden,[3,4] Finland,[5] and England[6] clearly showed that in patients who had *Salmonella* infection and later developed arthritis, the frequency of B27 was significantly increased (Table 6.21). The results of the 5 studies were similar and there was no evidence of heterogeneity in the data.

See also ref. 7.

References

1. Friis J, Svejgaard A: Salmonella arthritis and HL-A27. Lancet i:1350, 1974
2. Leirisalo M, Skylv G, Kousa M, Voipio-Pulkki LM, Suoranta H, Nissila M, et al: Followup study on patients with Reiter's disease and reactive arthritis, with special reference to HLA-B27. Arthritis Rheum 25:249-259, 1982
3. Hakansson U, Eitrem R, Low B, Winblad S: HLA-antigen B27 in cases with joint affections in an outbreak of salmonellosis. Scand J Infect Dis 8:245-248, 1976
4. Hakansson U, Low B, Eitrem R, and Winblad S: HL-A27 reactive arthritis in an outbreak of salmonellosis. Tissue Antigens 6:366-367, 1975
5. Aho K, Ahvonen P, Alkio P, Sairanen E, Sievars K, Tiilikainen A: HL-A27 in reactive arthritis following infection. Ann Rheum Dis 34:29-30, 1975
6. Robitaille A, Cockburn C, James DCO, Ansell BM: HLA frequencies in less common arthropathies. Ann Rheum Dis 35:271-273, 1976
7. Hamza M, Ayed K, Gueddiche M, Zaiem A, Boujnah A, Ben Ayed H: Arthrite a Salmonella enteritidis chez un sujet HLA-B27. Nouv Presse Med 10:3321-3322, 1981

Septic Arthritis Due to *Klebsiella*

Population Association

Cox[1] reported a case of a woman from England with seronegative polyarthritis who had a septic knee due

TABLE 6.21. Post-*Salmonella* Arthritis

	Patients		Controls				
Country/Population	n	%+	n	%+	RR	χ^2	Ref.
HLA-B27							
England	13	92	600	8	92.17	34.71	6
Denmark	5	60	1541	8	16.04	13.01	1
Finland	16	94	323	14	64.78	29.10	8
Finland	6	100	900	14	79.59	16.63	2
	22	96	1223	14	69.50	45.71	
	Heterogeneity χ^2 (1 df)					0.02	
Sweden	13	69	446	10	18.63	26.44	4
	53	85	3810	10	35.46	114.82	
	Heterogeneity χ^2 (4 df)					5.07	

to *Klebsiella*. She was positive for B27. The author suggested that impaired immune response to *Klebsiella* may have contributed to the spread and persistence of low-grade infection in this patient (see also Ankylosing spondylitis).

Reference

1. Cox NI: Septic arthritis due to Klebsiella in a B27-positve patient. Lancet i:720, 1979

Reactive Arthritis After *Campylobacter jejuni* Enteritis

Population Association

Kosunen et al.[1] reported 7 cases of reactive arthritis among the 340 patients diagnosed as having *Campylobacter jejuni* enteritis. Five of the 7 patients were B27-positive, a significant increase compared with healthy controls (Table 6.22).

Reference

1. Kosunen TU, Kauranen O, Martio J, Pitkanen T, Ponka A, Hortling L, et al: Reactive arthritis after campylobacter jejuni enteritis in patients with HLA-B27. Lancet i:1312-1313, 1980

Reactive Arthritis After *Mycoplasma pneumoniae* Infection

Population Association

There was no significant deviation of any of the A, B, or C antigens in 12 patients from Finland reported by Ponka et al.[1]

Reference

1. Ponka A, Ponka T, Koskimies S: HLA antigens and arthritis to mycoplasma pneumoniae. Tissue Antigens 17:445-446, 1981

Sexually Acquired Reactive Arthritis

Population Association

Keat et al.[1] studied prospectively inflammatory arthritis, tendinitis, and fasciitis after nonspecific urethritis ("sexually acquired reactive arthritis") in 531 British men with nonspecific urethritis. The authors

TABLE 6.22. Reactive Arthritis after *Campylobacter jejuni* Enteritis

	Patients		Controls				
Country/Population	n	%+	n	%+	RR	χ^2	Ref.
HLA-B27							
Finland	7	71	323	14	13.16	12.71	1

TABLE 6.23. Sexually Acquired Reactive Arthritis

Country/Population	Patients n	Patients %+	Controls n	Controls %+	RR	χ^2	Ref.
HLA-B27							
England	54	67	280	7	25.99	80.15	2

defined arthritis after a proved or putative infection of the genital tract as sexually acquired reactive arthritis, the arthritis (referred to as "reactive") being a sterile inflammation of the synovial membrane, tendon, and fascia. Thus, this definition included patients with sexually acquired Reiter's syndrome.

Fifteen of the 531 men developed arthritis and had a new sexual contact before their joint symptoms started. Six of these 15 patients (40%) were B27-positive compared with 30 of 482 (6.2%) typed in the total sample. Nine of the 452 (2%) B27-negative patients (in the total sample) developed arthritis as compared with 6 of the 30 B27 positive (20%) patients ($p < 0.001$).

Chlamydia trachomatis was also isolated from the patients' cultures. Satisfactory cultures were obtained from 20 B27-positive patients and 9 (45%) were positive for *C. trachomatis*, a value not significantly different from 36.5% (140/384) in the total sample. Thus, there was no association between B27 and carriers of *C. trachomatis*.

In a second report by the same group of authors[2], 54 patients with arthritis associated with nongonococcal infection were typed for HLA-A and -B loci antigens. B27 was increased in the patients (Table 6.23).

Disease Heterogeneity

The group of 54 patients in the British study[2] consisted of 30 patients who presented directly to a rheumatology unit and 24 who initially attended a venereology clinic. The frequency of B27 was 83% in the first group (25/30) and 46% (11/24) in the second group. The authors report that patients in the second subgroup tended to have milder disease. Thus, B27-positive patients appeared to have significantly longer duration of disease symptoms and a higher frequency of extraarticular manifestations than those negative for B27.

References

1. Keat AC, Maini RN, Nkwazi GC, Pegrum GD, Ridgway GL, Scott JT: Role of Chlamydia trachomatis and HLA-B27 in sexually acquired reactive arthritis. Br Med J 1:605-607, 1978
2. Keat AC, Maini RN, Pegrum GD, Scott JT: The clinical features and HLA associations of reactive arthritis associated with non-gonococcal urethritis. Q J Med 48:323-342, 1979

Pseudopolyarthritis of the Spine

Population Association

Sany et al.[1] studied A and B loci antigens in 50 French patients with pseudopolyarthritis of the spine. These patients did not have temporal arthritis. B5 and BW38 were increased in the patient group (Table 6.24).

Reference

1. Sany J, Seignalet J, Serre H, Lapinski H: Systeme HLA et pseudo-polyarthrite rhizomelique. Semin Hop Paris 53:1689-1691, 1977

TABLE 6.24. Pseudopolyarthritis of the Spine

Country/Population	Patients n	Patients %+	Controls n	Controls %+	RR	χ^2	Ref.
HLA-B5							
France	50	24	300	13	2.15	4.46	1
HLA-BW38							
France	50	18	300	5	4.22	10.91	1

Ankylosing Spondylitis

Population Association

HLA-A and -B Loci Antigens

The 2 landmark papers by Schlosstein et al.[1] and Brewerton et al.[2] simultaneously published in April 1973 reported a spectacular association of B27 with ankylosing spondylitis (AS). In patients, the frequency of B27 ranged from 88% to 96% as compared with 4% to 8% in the controls (Table 6.25). These results, as the data in the table show, have been confirmed in many studies of patients with various racial backgrounds.

The frequency of B27 in American Black patients was not as high as that in Caucasians.[1,3–8] Hamza et al.[9] observed similar data in 40 patients from Tunisia (Table 6.25). Chalmers et al.[10] have reported 3 cases of AS in Zulu men from South Africa who were all positive for B27 (also see ref. 11).

In American Indian patients[12] B27 was as high as in Caucasian groups but because of its higher frequency in the general Indian population the relative risk was low (Table 6.25). Furthermore, Russell et al.[13] studied 138 adult (ages 20-42 years) American Cree Indian volunteers from Canada. Fourteen were positive for B27, 2 had radiologic evidence of sacroiliitis but none had definite AS.

B27 is very rare in the Japanese population but its frequency in AS patients is as high as in Caucasian populations (Table 6.25).

The data from Iran,[14] Iraq,[15] Israel,[16] India,[17–19] Mexico,[20] and Chile[21] were similar to those of other Caucasian populations from Europe and North America (Table 6.25).

Although precise data are not available, the prevalence of AS in Polynesians is rare and the frequency of B27 in these populations was also very low (0–2.6%) (see 22 and refs. therein).

Cleland et al.[23] have studied 118 aboriginies in an isolated community at Yuendumu, Central Australia. No individual was positive for B27. The authors also note that AS is not known to occur in the Australian aboriginie.

Female Caucasian AS patients have been HLA typed by Hill et al.,[24] Levitin et al.,[25] Jeannet et al.,[26] and Safwenberg et al.[27] The association with B27 in females was as strong as in males. Swezey et al.[28] reported data on 7 American Black female patients. Three of the 7 (42.86%) were positive for B27. This small sample contrasts with an 80% frequency of B27 in American Black male patients.[28].

HLA-C Locus Antigens

C locus antigen frequencies in AS patients have been studied by Bela et al.,[29] Van Den Berg-Loonen et al.,[30] Contu et al.,[31] Moller et al.,[32] and Safwenberg et al.[27] As the data in Table 6.25 show there were significant associations with CW1 and CW2 antigens. However, the relative risks were much lower than that with B27; the associations were most probably due to the linkage disequilibrium between B27 and these 2 antigens.

HLA-D/DR Locus Antigens

Dejelo et al.[33] reported 7 DR antigen frequencies (DR1-DR7) in 28 Caucasian and 8 American Black patients. When compared with 64 Caucasian and 12 Black controls no significant deviations were found. Similar results were also obtained by Raffoux et al.[34,35] in 50 French patients and by Braun et al.[36] in 16 American Caucasian and 6 American Black patients.

Kemple et al.[37] studied 8 D locus antigens in 44 patients and 45 normal Caucasians by the 1-way mixed leukocyte culture technique. The antigen frequencies did not differ between patients and controls (also see 38).

Bf Locus

Arnason et al.[39] typed 19 Icelandic patients with AS and 46 individuals without AS. All 19 patients were B27- and Bf^S positive. In 46 controls half had B27 and Bf^S and the other half had B27 and Bf^F. Thus, there was an increase of the B27-Bf^S haplotype in the patients. However, another report by Wells et al.[40] did not find such an increase in the data from Italy and England.

B7-Cross-Reactive Group

McLain et al.[41,42] reported a 100% frequency of B7-cross-reactive group (CREG) antigens (B7, BW22, B40, BW42) in 12 American Caucasian patients. In a control group of 36 healthy individuals the B7-CREG frequency was only 44%. In the data of Arnett et al.[43] 25 of the 27 AS patients had B27 but the remaining 2 B27-negative patients did not have any B7-CREG antigens.

Khan et al.[44] have also presented data on 10 B27-negative American Caucasian patients. Four (40%) had BW16 as compared with only 3.1% of 444 B27 negative healthy controls ($\chi^2 = 25.87$). The same group of authors[45] studied 34 American Black patients with AS. Of the 18 B27 negative group 10 were positive (55.6%) for B7. The frequency of B7

TABLE 6.25. Ankylosing Spondylitis

Country/Population	Patients n	Patients %+	Controls n	Controls %+	RR	χ^2	Ref.
HLA-B27							
U.S.A.—Black	23	48	60	2	32.31	19.13	3
U.S.A.—Black	10	80	914	4	80.54	40.79	1
	33	58	974	4	54.49	59.16	
	Heterogeneity χ^2 (1 df)					0.76	
Haida—A.I. (Canada)	17	100	222	50	35.00	11.78	12
Bella Coola—A.I. (Canada)	3	100	129	25	20.79	7.14	12
Singapore—Chinese	29	97	238	7	270.16	49.74	187
Japan	36	92	89	2	382.69	53.75	84
Japan	41	74	181	0	1003.13	42.52	188
Japan	58	86	130	2	241.13	72.53	189
Japan	27	67	78	0	310.16	28.23	190
	162	81	478	1	354.43	195.68	
	Heterogeneity χ^2 (3 df)					1.35	
	211	85	1067	15	207.90	255.54	
	Heterogeneity χ^2 (6 df)					10.14	
Iran	25	92	400	3	292.15	70.92	14
Iraq	25	84	95	2	186.33	45.48	15
Tunisia	40	70	80	5	38.76	41.24	9
Jews (unspecified)	38	79	456	3	112.39	104.21	16
	128	80	1031	3	109.16	255.92	
	Heterogeneity χ^2 (3 df)					5.92	
India	17	94	60	3	276.71	34.07	17
India	40	83	118	2	187.47	59.08	19
	57	86	178	2	213.43	93.04	
	Heterogeneity χ^2 (1 df)					0.11	
Mexico	83	72	33	3	55.38	27.29	191
Mexico	51	69	305	6	33.43	86.48	20
	134	71	338	6	36.87	113.42	
	Heterogeneity χ^2 (1 df)					0.35	
Chile	16	81	132	5	67.42	38.66	21
	150	72	470	6	41.61	151.45	
	Heterogeneity χ^2 (2 df)					0.98	
Canada	12	92	200	9	77.97	29.14	192
Canada	50	90	295	9	82.25	85.14	58
	62	90	495	9	81.12	114.27	
	Heterogeneity χ^2 (1 df)					0.00	
U.S.A.	40	88	906	8	76.98	87.81	1
U.S.A.	5	100	1863	8	126.11	19.93	193
U.S.A.	27	96	540	9	167.52	48.56	194
U.S.A.	8	88	104	4	111.20	26.48	195
U.S.A.	50	94	485	8	154.26	85.14	3
U.S.A.	29	83	306	9	45.02	58.64	196
	159	91	4204	8	89.81	322.67	
	Heterogeneity χ^2 (5 df)					3.89	

TABLE 6.25. *(continued)*

Country/Population	Patients n	Patients %+	Controls n	Controls %+	RR	χ^2	Ref.
HLA-B27							
Australia	47	92	306	8	115.92	82.00	86
Australia	44	87	26	7	66.32	30.94	197
	91	90	332	8	96.61	112.58	
	Heterogeneity χ^2 (1 df)					0.37	
Czechoslovakia	134	93	84	27	33.77	76.20	198
East Germany	134	88	300	12	51.76	159.33	199
Hungary	55	93	352	13	78.73	76.25	29
Yugoslavia	134	93	158	13	83.04	123.65	98
BENELUX	108	81	250	8	47.06	135.20	200
BENELUX	118	81	778	10	37.51	195.60	30
BENELUX	31	90	200	9	77.82	56.33	201
BENELUX	62	97	1000	7	339.14	89.06	202
	319	85	2228	8	52.61	464.81	
	Heterogeneity χ^2 (3 df)					11.38	
England	145	88	451	9	71.57	205.85	62
England	67	94	174	10	123.26	84.12	203
England	75	96	75	4	429.08	69.67	2
England	35	100	89	14	422.06	32.78	204
England	39	69	433	8	24.71	72.04	24
England	17	82	597	9	40.67	41.19	77
England	28	64	433	8	19.76	51.26	76
	406	88	2252	9	53.73	531.27	
	Heterogeneity χ^2 (6 df)					25.64	
France	27	96	270	9	166.00	46.54	205
France	53	81	152	4	91.43	78.08	206
	80	86	422	7	110.49	124.19	
	Heterogeneity χ^2 (1 df)					0.43	
Italy	22	68	320	5	37.84	52.99	207
Italy	21	90	1428	4	177.59	68.65	97
Italy	26	77	398	5	58.77	68.76	208
	69	78	2146	4	64.90	186.60	
	Heterogeneity χ^2 (2 df)					3.80	
Spain	50	94	700	6	210.28	96.77	209
Switzerland	95	93	56	8	129.81	68.95	210
Switzerland	31	87	500	7	79.52	72.40	26
	126	92	556	7	98.41	140.95	
	Heterogeneity χ^2 (1 df)					0.39	
Sardinia	38	82	494	5	80.41	96.39	31
Finland	7	86	326	14	26.82	16.09	211
Norway	52	96	788	11	157.32	71.64	212
Norway	122	92	788	10	98.34	181.96	32
	174	93	1576	11	110.32	253.13	
	Heterogeneity χ^2 (1 df)					0.47	

TABLE 6.25. *(continued)*

Country/Population	Patients n	Patients %+	Controls n	Controls %+	RR	χ^2	Ref.
HLA-B27							
Sweden	26	92	500	11	75.98	48.72	27
Sweden	50	94	692	17	66.04	62.48	213
Sweden	66	100	100	12	941.64	42.51	214
	142	96	1292	14	97.79	148.35	
	Heterogeneity χ^2 (2 df)					5.36	
	2180	89	17917	9	69.11	3021.93	
	Heterogeneity χ^2 (39 df)					73.32	
HLA-CW1							
BENELUX	118	29	778	7	5.43	48.00	30
Sardinia	12	25	57	4	7.32	5.89	31
Sweden	26	46	500	7	11.24	33.72	27
	156	32	1335	7	6.58	85.32	
	Heterogeneity χ^2 (2 df)					2.29	
HLA-CW2							
Hungary	55	58	352	14	8.36	47.44	29
BENELUX	118	46	778	9	8.57	94.12	30
Sardinia	12	58	57	25	3.95	4.97	31
Norway	122	41	788	10	6.24	70.94	32
Sweden	26	42	500	9	7.34	23.36	27
	333	46	2475	10	7.27	238.60	
	Heterogeneity χ^2 (4 df)					2.23	

in 59 B27 negative Black controls was 23.7% ($p <$ 0.025).

In view of these inconsistent data the significance of association with other antigens in the B27 negative group remains unclear.

B27 Positivity and the Prevalence of AS

Epidemiologic studies (46 and refs. in 47 and 48) have estimated that the population prevalence of AS is 0.25 to 2.2 per 1,000. Recent epidemiologic studies of Calin and Fries,[48-50] using the B27 test, have shown that the actual prevalence of AS is much higher. Seventy-eight (30 males and 48 females) B27-positive blood donors selected from a group of apparently healthy subjects were evaluated by postal questionnaires and pelvic radiography. Fourteen individuals (6 males [20%] and 8 females [16.7%]) satisfied the criteria for definite AS. Thus, for a B27-positive person of either sex there is a 20% probability that AS will develop. These data suggest a population prevalence of 10-15 per 1,000. A similar study by Cohen et al.[51] found approximately 25% B27-positive men at risk for AS (6 AS in 24 B27-positives). Epidemiologic studies of AS in the Hungarian population by Gomor et al.[52] have also revealed that among males with B27 the frequency of AS was 2.9% and in B27-positive females was 0.58%. Similar data are also available in 2 French studies by Thorel et al.[53] and Alcalay et al.[54].

These high estimates of prevalence were not observed in an Australian study by Christiansen et al.[47,55]. When studying the population of Bussetlon, Western Australia, they found 168 of 2745 people (6.1%) were B27-positive. Questionnaire and clinical assessments of 139 B27 positive individuals did not show a single case of AS. Radiographs, available from 22% of the B27 positive individuals, were also reviewed. These authors[55] stated that they used questionnaires similar to that of Calin and Fries[48] and obtained sacroiliac radiographs in a higher percentage of the study group. In the data from this study a maximum prevalence of AS was 0.04% in the general population and 0.7% in B27-positive individuals. Thus, these estimates were similar to those found in the earlier epidemiologic surveys (also see 56).

Disease Heterogeneity

Radiological Data
Radiologic features of B27-positive and -negative AS patients have been evaluated in several studies. Only the studies of Russell et al.[57,58] and Namey et al.[59] found radiologic evidence of more severe disease in a B27-positive group as compared with the group as a whole or a subgroup matched for age, sex, and duration of disease.In the report of Namey et al.[59] 23 of the 34 patients were positive for B27 and they had a mean index of 2.09 by quantitative sacroiliac scintigraphy. Only 5 of these B27-positive patients had early radiographic sacroiliitis. The 11 B27 negative patients had a mean index of 1.52 and none had radiographic sacroiliitis. However, the data from 8 other reports[16,60–66] did not show any difference between B27-positive and -negative patients. Thus, the data from other reports did not support the conclusions of Russell et al.[57,58] and Namey et al.[59]

Age at Onset
In a report by Woodrow and Eastmond[62] age at onset data were available on 137 patients. The age of clinical onset in B27-negative patients was higher overall than that in B27-positive patients ($p = 0.012$). Brautbar et al.[16] also noted that B27-negative patients had a relatively later age at onset. On the other hand, the data of Khan et al.[66] and Van Der Linden et al.[64] did not reveal any difference between the 2 groups.

Duration of the Disease
There was no significant difference between B27-positive and -negative patients.[60,61,67]

Acute Anterior Uveitis
Khan et al.[66,68] and Nahir et al.[60] and Scharf et al.[69] compared the frequency of acute anterior uveitis in B27-positive and B27-negative patients. In both studies acute anterior uveitis was found to be associated with AS present in B27 positive individuals.

Peripheral Joints
Khan et al.[66] found no difference in the frequency of peripheral joint involvement between 63 B27-positive and 15 B27-negative patients. In the data of Woodrow and Eastmond[62] 5 patients had evidence of a seronegative peripheral arthritis resembling peripheral psoriatic arthritis and 3 of these were negative for B27.

Sex
In a report by Van Der Linden et al.[64] on 187 patients the male/female ratio in the group with B27 did not differ from that in the group without B27.

Clinical Difference
Gerber et al.[63] reported no clinical differences between 88 B27-positive and 7 B27-negative patients from Germany.

Prognosis of AS
No correlation was found between B27 and prognosis of the disease.[67]

Hygienic Conditions
Doury et al.[67] subdivided their AS patients into groups living under poor hygienic conditions and those living under normal hygienic conditions. There was no significant difference in the B27 frequency between the 2 groups.

Severity of the Disease
No significant difference between B27-positive and -negative groups was found.[6,67]

Antibody Titers to Streptokinase/Streptodornase
Christiansen et al.[70] have reported significantly higher titers in the B27-positive individuals, with or without AS, than in their B27-negative relatives.

Spondylodiscitis
Modena et al.[71] have reported that in a group of 64 patients with AS, 9 had a peculiar type of spondylodiscitis characterized by quite diffuse and marked sclerosis of multiple vertebral bodies with only minimal erosions of the adjacent vertebral plates whereas classic syndesmophytosis was absent. These patients also had bilateral sacroiliitis. B27 was present in only 1 of these 9 patients.

Pain
No difference was found between B27-positive and -negative groups.[66]

Degree of Deformity
No difference was found between B27-positive and -negative groups.[66]

Functional Ability
No difference was found between B27-positive and -negative patients.[66]

Reconstructive Surgery
The number of patients who needed reconstructive surgery was not significantly different in B27-positive and -negative groups.[66]

Homozygosity for B27
Khan et al.[72] calculated the frequency of apparent homozygotes for B27 as 15.5% in 58 B27-positive Caucasian patients. This frequency was significantly ($p < 0.0005$) greater than the estimated expected frequency of 4.2%. The authors suggested that B27 homozygotes are more susceptible to developing AS than are B27 heterozygotes. Clinical features of AS, however, showed no difference between heterozygotes and apparent homozygotes.

Family Data

Families with 2 or more AS patients were studied in several reports.[19,29,73–98] From these data it was clear that within a family the disease did not always segregate with the marker haplotype and there were members with the marker haplotype but without the disease. Thus, several authors have proposed the hypotheses of 1 major HLA-linked gene with reduced penetrance or 2 or more genes responsible for AS. In most of the aforementioned family studies data were available on only a few small pedigrees (generally 2 or 3) and no formal genetic or linkage analyses are available.

Based on an analysis of 27 families from Japan, Shirakura et al.[84] have proposed 2 genes for AS—1 an autosomal dominant gene linked with HLA and the other an X-linked recessive gene.

In the pedigree data of Sturrock et al.,[89,90] Dick et al.,[88] Cross et al.,[86] Van Der Linden et al.,[91,93] and De Bruyere et al.[92] there was also evidence of more than 1 gene responsible for the development of AS.

The genetic analyses of pedigrees by Kidd et al.[96] and Daneo et al.[97] have shown that susceptibility to AS is inherited as an autosomal dominant gene with incomplete penetrance. This incomplete penetrance may be due to environmental factors or interaction with an allele at another locus.

Strosberg et al.[87] studied a pedigree of 66 members covering 4 generations. There were 7 cases of AS, and 4 of these were in a single sibship of 13. Nine markers (ABO, Rh, P, Kell, MN, Gm, HLA, HP, and AcP) were tested on all individuals and lod scores were calculated for all 9 markers. Lod scores for all the markers (including HLA) except AcP (acid phosphatase) were negative (> -2.0) for recombination values of 0.0–0.30. The scores for AcP were all positive. The maximum was 0.873 at 0.0% recombination. It should be noted that a lod score of $+3.0$ is generally considered as evidence in favor of linkage and a score of -2.0 is regarded as evidence against linkage (also see 99).

B27 Test in the Diagnosis of Ankylosing Spondylitis

The extraordinary high association of B27 with AS has stimulated considerable interest in this test as a diagnostic tool in rheumatologic diseases. The data from several reports[55,100–103] have shown that the B27 test was useful in the diagnosis of AS and other B27-associated diseases. Calin et al.,[104–107] however, have argued that this test is of limited value in the clinical diagnosis (for details see the above reports and refs. therein; also see 108-110).

Khan and Khan,[111] using probability calculations based on Bayes' theorem (for details see chapter on Statistical Methods), have argued that the usefulness of the B27 test is dependent on the pretest likelihood (probability) of the disease. The test is most useful when the pretest probability of AS in a given patient is near 50%. Thus, a highly experienced physician may be able to decide on the diagnosis of AS after clinical history and radiographic examinations of the patient. The B27 test will not be very useful for him/her. On the other hand, physicians with less experience in this disease (and consequently less pretest probability of diagnosis) may find the test very useful in some patients.

It should be noted that some of the current research is being focused on monoclonal antibodies that will recognize B27 antigens of only AS patients and not of healthy individuals.[112–115] The discovery of such an antibody will obviously significantly enhance the usefulness of this test.

In an interesting study by Sany et al.[116] 23 patients (15 men and 8 women), ages 17-64 years, with unclassified B27 inflammatory rheumatic disease were followed during a mean period of 28 months. None of the patients had psoriasis, colopathy, or features of Reiter's syndrome. Using New York or Rome criteria AS was not diagnosed in a single patient. After a 28-month period using clinical and radiographic data the diagnosis of AS was established in 7 patients on the basis of the Rome criteria. With New York criteria AS was definite in 6 and probable in 1 patient. Thus, 7 of the 23 B27-positive patients

(30.43%) who initially had unclassified rheumatism developed AS. The authors have suggested the usefulness of the B27 test in unclassified inflammatory arthritides that could be related to AS.

Cross-Reactivity Between B27 and *Klebsiella*

Experiments by Ebringer et al.[117–120] using immunodiffusion, bacterial agglutination ($p < 0.025$), hemaagglutination ($p < 0.001$), and radioimmunoassays ($p < 0.001$), have shown that sera from rabbits immunized with B27 lymphocytes had increased activity against *Klebsiella* and enterobacter antigens. Rabbit anti-*Klebsiella* sera had lymphocytotoxic activity against B27 lymphocytes obtained from AS patients ($p < 0.001$). Immunoprecipitin lines were also produced by the antilymphocyte sera against extracts from *Yersinia enterocolitica* and *Shigella sonnci* microorganisms.

The same group of authors[119] also showed that human monospecific B27 typing sera had increased binding activity for *Klebsiella* extracts by hemagglutination ($p < 0.0001$), radiobinding assay ($p < 0.025$), and radiolabeled antigen completion assay ($p < 0.002$).

Similar results were also reported independently by Geczy et al.[121–130] These investigators showed that an antiserum raised in rabbits against an isolate of *Klebsiella pneumoniae* lysed the lymphocytes of B27-positive AS patients. The lymphocytes of B27-positive and B27-negative healthy controls did not react with this antiserum. Furthermore, the lymphocytotoxic activity of these anti-*Klebsiella* sera can be absorbed by B27-positive AS lymphocytes but not by B27-positive and B27-negative healthy lymphocytes. The lymphocytes of B27-negative AS patients were also not lysed by anti-*Klebsiella* sera. These data suggest that some *Klebsiella* antigens cross-react with a gene product closely associated with B27 or "modified B27" in patients with AS. Thus, B27 appears to be an essential component of a hypothetical "alloantigen-*Klebsiella* complex" with which some *Klebsiella* antigens may cross-react.

Furthermore, there are several interesting conclusions that have emerged from these studies and are summarized in a review paper by Geczy et al.[130]

1. The antibodies produced against *Klebsiella* K43 and K21 specifically lyse the B27-positive lymphocytes of about 80% of AS patients, 60% of those with Reiter's syndrome or B27-positive asymmetrical peripheral arthritis, and 20% of patients with B27-positive uveitis without an arthropathy. The lymphocytes of the clinically normal B27-positive individuals were not lysed.

2. *Klebsiella* isolates that cross-react with an HLA-B27-associated structure on the lymphocytes of AS patients do not share capsular serotypes or bacteriophage types.

3. The modification of B27, or of a closely related structure, in AS patients was not a direct genetic effect. The lymphocytes from the first-degree relatives who share the B27-contained haplotype with the affected individual do not undergo lysis or exposure to anti-*Kebsiella* serum.

4. The modification of a B27-associated structure was present on lymphoid cells, fibroblasts, and platelets but not on spermatozoa or erythrocytes.[129] Epstein-Barr virus-induced lymphoblastoid cell lines and skin fibroblasts (derived from B27-positive AS patients) after 10-20 generations in culture were lysed by the anti-*Klebsiella* serum. Thus, apparently repeated exposure of the B27 antigen to *Klebsiella* product was not necessary for the continued expression of the cell-surface modification.

Geczy et al.[122,130] have done experiments to show that B27 lymphocytes from healthy individuals, which are not lysed by an antiserum against *Klebsiella* K43, can be rendered susceptible to lysing after incubation in the culture filtrate of *Klebsiella* K43. These data suggest a specific modification by a *Klebsiella* K43-derived soluble factor of a B27-associated lymphoid cell component. The capacity of this factor to convert lymphocytes of B27-positive healthy individuals could be specifically absorbed by B27-positive healthy lymphocytes, but not by B27-positive AS, B27-negative AS, or by B27-negative healthy lymphocytes. These results suggest that B27-positive healthy cells carry a hypothetical receptor that can specifically bind a *Klebsiella* K43 antigenic determinant.

Druery et al.[126] have performed experiments to identify the cross-reactive component of the *Klebsiella* and its relationship to the factor present in *Klebsiella* culture filtrates. Polyacrylamide gel electrophoresis of cell wall material of *Klebsiella* K43 showed the presence of 4 major protein bands. Antisera were raised in rabbits for each of these and were tested for their cytotoxic effects on the lymphocytes of B27-positive AS patients. An antiserum to 1 component only, of 40,000–52,000 daltons molecular weight, reproduced the activity of the whole serum.

Further studies[126] on the K43 filtrate indicated that the modifying factor appeared to reside in a 25,000–

50,000-dalton component. Immunoelectrophoresis of anti-K43 serum showed overlapping bands in the culture filtrate and in the 40,000–52,000-dalton cell wall fraction and these appeared to be identical on immunodiffusion. Antibody to the cell wall component removed both the modifying activity and the appropriate protein band from the filtrate. These data suggest that a 40,000–52,000-dalton component of the *Klebsiella* K43 cell wall is cross-reactive with a determinant on the lymphocytes of B27-positive AS patients. It is similar to or identical to a modifying factor in a K43 culture filtrate that renders the lymphocytes of B27-positive healthy individuals susceptible to lysis by anti-*Klebsiella* antiserum.

In a later report[130] the molecular weight, based on Biogel P-100 chromatography, of the B27-related modifying factor was estimated to be 26–30,000 daltons (as compared with the earlier estimate of 40–52,000 daltons.[126] The authors have noted that the newer estimate is probably more accurate.

It is interesting to note a study by Archer[131] in which cross-reactivity between B27 and *Klebsiella pneumoniae* MX100 was also investigated. No evidence of cross-reaction was found.

It should be added that Dilley et al.[132] have also studied the cell surface susceptibility of human skin fibroblasts from patients with AS, Reiter's disease, and also from normal volunteers. *In vitro* cell damage studies showed that susceptibilities to *Yersinia enterocolitica, Salmonella minnesota, cytomegalovirus, herpes simplex* virus, *Ureaplasma urealyticum, Mycoplasma hominis,* and *Chlamydia trachomatis* were the same in both B27-positive and -negative individuals.

Pease et al.[133] have reported some data on the cytotoxic activities of sera raised in rabbits to 3 strains of *Yersinia enterocolitica*. No cytotoxic activity against the lymphocytes of B27-positive AS patients, B27-positive healthy individuals, or B27-negative individuals was found. The activity of the B27 antigen was also not absorbed out by any of the *Yersinia* antigens.

Molecular Structure of the B27 Antigen

Recent studies have been directed toward elucidating the biochemical structure of the B27 antigen. Grumet et al.[113] and Trapani et al.[115] have reported monoclonal antibodies for detecting the B27 antigen. Although these antibodies are better reagents for B27 typing they were not able to detect any difference between healthy and AS B27 antigens. In a second report Grumet et al.[114] described another monoclonal antibody (B27M2) that reacted with only 87% of the healthy B27-positive individuals. However, no difference between the B27 present in healthy and AS patients was found. Kaneoka et al.[112] have studied the molecular properties of the two variants of B27 recognized by B27M2. They were found to have different isoelectric points and could be distinguished from each other and from a different (BW44) control antigen.

Molders et al.[134] have done biochemical analyses of B27 antigens from individuals that were HLA-ABC identical by serology but distinct in cell-mediated lympholysis typing. B27 exists in two types: W type and K type. HLA-B27 K type was reported to have a more basic isoelectric point than W type.

In another study by Karr et al.[135] biosynthetically radiolabeled B27 molecules from AS patients and healthy individuals were compared by two-dimensional gel electrophoresis and tryptic peptide mapping with high-pressure liquid chromatography. The authors did not find any structural difference, as detected by electrophoresis, in the B27 molecule from an AS patient and a normal individual.

The research in the area of monoclonal antibodies and molecular characteristics of HLA antigens is progressing rapidly. In the near future this may lead to a better understanding of the mechanisms of HLA and disease associations in general and the nature of B27 and AS association in particular.

See also refs. 136–186 and 215–232.

References

1. Schlosstein L, Terasaki PI, Bluestone R, Pearson CM: High association of an HL-A antigen, W27, with ankylosing spondylitis. N Engl J Med 288:704-706, 1973
2. Brewerton DA, Caffrey M, Hart FD, James DCO, Nicholls A, Sturrock RD: Ankylosing spondylitis and HL-A 27. Lancet i:904-907, 1973
3. Khan MA, Braun WE, Kushner I, Gracek DE, Muir WA, Steinberg AG: HLA B27 in ankylosing spondylitis: Differences in frequency and relative risk in American blacks and Caucasians. J Rheumatol 4(Suppl 3):39-43, 1977
4. Khan M, Kushner I, Braun W: Low incidence of HLA-B27 in American blacks with spondyloarthropathies. Lancet i:483, 1976
5. Good AE, Kawanishi H, Schultz JS: HLA B27 in blacks with ankylosing spondylitis or Reiter's disease. N Engl J Med 294:166-167, 1976
6. Khan MA, Braun WE, Kushner I: Low frequency of HLA-B27 in American blacks with ankylosing spondylitis (AS). Clin Res 24:331a, 1976
7. Khan MA, Kushner I, Braun WE, Schacter BZ, Steinberg AG: HLA-B7 and ankylosing spondylitis

in American blacks. N Engl J Med 297:513, 1977
8. Ruderman RJ and Ward FE: HLA-B27 in black patients with ankylosing spondylitis: Lancet i:610, 1977
9. Hamza M, Ayed HB, Akyed K: HLA-B27 et spondylarthrite ankylosante en tunise. Nouv Presse Med 9:1171-1172, 1980
10. Chalmers IM, Seedat YK, Mudaliar MY: Ankylosing spondylitis in three Zulu men negative for the HLA B27 antigen. S Afr Med J 52:567-569, 1977
11. Klemp P, Meyers OL, Du Toit ED: HLA-B27 and ankylosing spondylitis in African blacks. Arthritis Rheum 25:716-717, 1982
12. Gofton JP, Chalmers A, Price GE, Reeve CE: HL-A 27 and ankylosing spondylitis in B.C. Indians. J Rheumatol 2:314-318, 1975
13. Russell AS, Davis P, Schlaut J: Prevalence of ankylosing spondylitis and HLA-B27 in a North American Indian population: A pilot study. Can Med Assoc J 116:148-149, 1977
14. Davatchi F, Nikbin B, Ala F: Histocompatibility antigens (HLA) in rheumatic disases in Iran. J Rheumatol 4 (Suppl 3):36-38, 1977
15. Al-Rawi ZS, Al-Shakarchi HA, Hasan F, Thewaini AJ: Ankylosing spondylitis and its association with the histocompatibility antigen HL-A B27: An epidemiological and clinical study. Rheumatol Rehab 17:72-75, 1978
16. Brautbar C, Porat S, Nelken D, Gabriel KR, Cohen T: HLA B27 and ankylosing spondylitis in the Israeli population. J Rheumatol 4 (Suppl 3):24-32, 1977
17. Sengupta S, Sehgal S, Aikat BK, Deodhar SD, James DCO: HLA B27 in ankylosing spondylitis in India. Lancet i:1209-1210, 1977
18. Malaviya AN, Mehra NK, Adhar G, Jindal K, Bhargawa S, Batta RK, et al: HLA B27 in patients with seronegative spondarthritides. J Rheumatol 6:413-416, 1979
19. Bale UM, Mehta MM, Contractor NM, Bhatia HM, Tilve GH: HLA antigens in ankylosing spondylitis: The association of HLA-B27. Indian J Med Res 71:96-103, 1980
20. Fraga A, Gorodezky C, Lavalle C, Castro-Escobar LE, Magana L, Escobar-Gutierrez A: HLA-B27 in Mexican patients with ankylosing spondylitis. Arthritis Rheum 22:302, 1979
21. Macera C, Losada M, Melendez M, Fuentes C, Mauritz M: HLA-B27 antigen in ankylosing spondylitis and other forms of rheumatism. Rev Med Chil 105:90-92, 1977
22. Caughey DE, Gow J: Ankylosing spondylitis in Polynesian races. NZ Med J 81:268, 1975
23. Cleland LG, Hay JAR, Milazzo SC: Absence of HL-A 27 and of ankylosing spondylitis in Central Australian aboriginals. Scand J Rheumatol (Suppl 8), Abstr 30-05, 1975
24. Hill HFH, Hill AGS, Bodmer JG: Clinical diagnosis of ankylosing spondylitis in women and relation to presence of HLA-B27. Ann Rheum Dis 35:267-270, 1976
25. Levitin PM, Gough WW, Davis JS: HLA-B27 antigen in women with ankylosing spondylitis. JAMA 235:2621-2622, 1976
26. Jeannet M, Saudan Y, Bitter T: HL-A27 in female patients with ankylosing spondylitis. Tissue Antigens 6:262-264, 1975
27. Safwenberg J, Domeij-Nyberg B, Kjallman M: HLA antigens in females with ankylosing spondylitis and other forms of seronegative rheumatic diseases. Scand J Rheumatol 7:177-182, 1978
28. Swezey RL, Zucker LM, Terasaki PI: Reduced prevalence of HL-A antigen W27 in black females with ankylosing spondylitis. J Rheumatol 1:260-262, 1974
29. Bela G, Eva GK: HLA-B27 antigen spondylitis ankylopoeticaban (Bechterew-betegsegben). Orv Hetil 118: 616-619, 1977
30. Van Den Berg-Loonen EM, Dekker-Saeys BJ, Meuwissen SGM, Nijenhuis LE, Engelfriet CP: Histocompatibility antigens and other genetic markers in ankylosing spondylitis and inflammatory bowel diseases. J Immunogenet 4:167-175, 1977
31. Contu L, Capelli P, Sale S: HLA B27 and ankylosing spondylitis: A population and family study in Sardinia. J Rheumatol 4 (Suppl 3):18-23, 1977
32. Moller P, Vinje O, Berg K: HLA antigens, psoriasis and acute anterior uveitis in Bechterew's syndrome (ankylosing spondylitis). Clin Genet 21:215-221, 1982
33. Dejelo CL, Braun WE, Khan MA, Clough JD: HLA-DR antigens and ankylosing spondylitis. Transplant Proc 10:971-972, 1978
34. Raffoux C, Faure G, Netter P, Streiff F, Pourel J,Gaucher A: No association of known DRW antigens with ankylosing spondylitis. Arthritis Rheum 21:997, 1978
35. Gaucher A, Raffoux C, Netter P, Faure G, Pourel J, Streiff F: HLA DRW dans la spondylarthrite ankylosante. Rev Rhum Mal Osteoartic 45:335-338, 1978
36. Braun WE, Dejelo CL, Clough JD, Beck KA, Schacter BZ, Khan MA: No association of known DR antigens with ankylosing spondylitis. N Engl J Med 298:744-745, 1978
37. Kemple K, Gatti RA, Leibold W, Klinenberg J, Bluestone R: HLA-D locus typing in ankylosing spondylitis and Reiter's syndrome. Arthritis Rheum 22:371-375, 1979
38. Roy R, Hebert J, Latulippe L, Latulippe L: Possible association between HLA-D locus and ankylosing spondylitis. Arthritis Rheum 22:94-95, 1979
39. Arnason A, Thorsteinson J, Sigurbergsson K: An-

kylosing spondylitis, HLA-B27 and BF. Lancet i:339-340, 1978
40. Wells LJ, Edwards JH, Webley M, James DCO, Brewerton DA, Mackintosh P, et al: Ankylosing spondylitis, HLA, and BF. Lancet i:104-105, 1979
41. McLain DA, Luehrman LK, Rodey GE, Schwartz BD: An HLA public antigen is more common than HLA-B27 in patients with ankylosing spondylitis. Arthritis Rheum 23:718, 1980
42. Schwartz BD, Luehrman LK: An HLA public antigen can act as a target antigen in cell mediated lympholysis. Arthritis Rheum 23:743, 1980
43. Arnett FC, Hochberg MC, Bias W: Cross-reactive HLA antigens in B27-negative Reiter's syndrome and sacroiliitis. Johns Hopkins Med J 141:193-197, 1977
44. Khan MA, Kushner I, Braun WE: B27-negative HLA-BW16 in ankylosing spondylitis. Lancet i:1370-1371, 1978
45. Khan MA, Kushner I, Braun WE: A subgroup of ankylosing spondylitis associated with HLA-B7 in American blacks. Arthritis Rheum 21:528-530, 1978
46. Cater ET, McKenna CH, Brian DD, Kurland LT: Epidemiology of ankylosing spondylitis in Rochester, Minnesota, 1935-1973. Arthritis Rheum 22:365-370, 1979
47. Christiansen FT, Hawkins BR, Dawkins RL, Owen ET, Potter RM: The prevalence of ankylosing spondylitis among B27 positive normal individuals- a reassessment. J Rheumatol 6:713-718, 1979
48. Calin A, Fries JF: Striking prevalence of ankylosing spondylitis in "healthy" W27 positive males and females. N Engl J Med 293:835-839, 1975
49. Calin A, Fries JF: Ankylosing spondylitis and epidemic Reiter's syndrome: Genetics and environment. Ann Rheum Dis 35:287, 1976
50. Calin A, Fries JF, Payne R: HL-A antigens and ankylosing spondylitis. Br Med J 3:650, 1975
51. Cohen LM, Mittal KK, Schmid FR, Rogers LF, Cohen KL: Increased risk for spondylitis stigmata in apparently healthy HL-AW27 men. Ann Intern Med 84:1-7, 1976
52. Gomor B, Gyodi E, Bakos L: Distribution of HLA B27 and ankylosing spondylitis in the Hungarian population. J Rheumatol 4(Suppl 3):33-35, 1977
53. Thorel JB, Cavelier B, Bonneav JC, Simonin JL, et al: Etude d'une population porteuse de l'antigene HLA B27 comparee a celle d'une population temoin non B27 a la recherche de la spondylarthrite ankylosante. Rev Rhum Mal Osteoartic 45:275-282, 1978
54. Alcalay M, Amor B, Haider F, Alcalay D, Orfila J, Tanzer J, et al: Ankylosing spondylitis and chlamydial infection in apparently healthy HLA B27 blood donors. J Rheumatol 6:439-446, 1979
55. Christiansen F, Zilko P, Dawkins RL: Ankylosing spondylitis in HLA-B27-positive individuals: Use in diagnosis. Br Med J 1:125, 1979
56. Whitfield AGW: Ankylosing spondylitis. J R Coll Physicians Lond 11:107-120, 1976
57. Russell AS, Lentle BC, Schlaut J: Radiologic and scintiscan findings in HLA-B27 negative patients with ankylosing spondylitis. J Rheumatol 3:321-323, 1976
58. Russell AS, Schlaut J, Percy JS, Dossetor JB: HL-A (transplantation) antigens in ankylosing spondylitis and Crohn's disease. J Rheumatol 1:203-209, 1974
59. Namey TC, Mcintyre J, Buse M, Leroy EC: Nucleographic studies of axial spondarthritides. I. Quantitative sacroiliac scintigraphy in early HLA B27-associated sacroiliitis. Arthritis Rheum 20:1058-1064, 1977
60. Nahir M, Scharf Y, Brik R, Scharfy Y, Gidasi O, Barzilai A: The influence of HL-A B27 on the clinical picture of ankylosing spondylitis. Rheumatol Rehab 18:10-12, 1979
61. Spencer DG, Park WM, Dick HM, Papazoglou SN, Buchanan WW: Radiological manifestations in 200 patients with ankylosing spondylitis: Correlation with clincal features and HLA B27. J Rheumatol 6:305-315, 1979
62. Woodrow JC, Eastmond CJ: HLA B27 and the genetics of ankylosing spondylitis. Ann Rheum Dis 37:504-509, 1978
63. Gerber N, Ambrosini GC, Boni A, Fehr K, Wagenhauser FJ: Spondylitis ankylosans (Bechterew) und gewebsantigen HLA-B27: Z Rheumatol 36:224-229, 1977
64. Van Der Linden JMJP, De Ceulaer K, Van Romunde LKJ, Cats A: Ankylosing spondylitis without HLA B27. J Rheumatol 4(Suppl 3):54-56, 1977
65. Bandilla K, Berg D, Semmler H, Pfannenstiel P: HLA B27 typing in combination with bone scanning for differential diagnosis of back pain. J Rheumatol 4 (Suppl 3):114, 1977 (Abstr)
66. Khan MA, Kushner I, Braun WE: Comparison of clinical features in HLA-B27 positive and negative patients with ankylosing spondylitis. Arthritis Rheum 20:909-912, 1977
67. Doury P, Pattin S, Roue R, Hainaut J: HLA-B27 antigen in ankylosing spondylitis and Reiter's disease. J Rheumatol 4 (Suppl 3):110, 1977 (Abstr)
68. Khan MA, Kushner I, Braun WE: Association of HLA-A2 with uveitis in HLA-B27 positive patients with ankylosing spondylitis. Arthritis Rheum 23:703, 1980
69. Scharf J, Nahir M, Scharf J, Briek R, Gidoni O, Brazilai A, et al: Anterior uveitis in ankylosing

spondylitis: A histocompatibility study. Ann Ophthalmol 11:1061-1062, 1979
70. Christiansen FT, Hawkins BR, Dawkins RL: Immune function in ankylosing spondylitics and their relatives: Influence of disease and HLA B27. Clin Exp Immunol 33:270 275, 1978
71. Modena V, Migone N, Daneo V, Carbonara AO, Di Vittorio S, Viara M: Spondylodiscitis and ankylosing spondylitis: HLA typing and nosological implications. Ann Rheum Dis 37:510-512, 1978
72. Khan MA, Kushner I, Braun WE, Zachary AA, Steinberg AG: HLA-B27 homozygosity in ankylosing spondylitis: Relationship to risk and severity. Tissue Antigens 11:434-438, 1978
73. Espinoza L, Oh JH, Kinsella TD, Stacey CH, Osterland CK, Dove FB: Ankylosing spondylitis: Family studies and HL-A 27 antigen distribution. J Rheumatol 1:254-259, 1974
74. Scharf J, Miller B, Zonis S, Scharf J, Nahir M, Gidoni O, et al: HL-A27 antigen associated with uveitis and ankylosing spondylitis in a family. Am J Ophthalmol 82:139-140, 1976
75. Lockshin MD, Fotino M, Gough WW, Litwin SD: Ankylosing spondylitis and HL-A. Am J Med 58:695-703, 1975
76. Eastmond CJ, Woodrow JC: The HLA system and the arthropathies associated with psoriasis. Ann Rheum Dis 36:112-120, 1977
77. Dick HM, Sturrock RD, Goel GK, Henderson N, Canesi B, Rooney PJ, et al: The association between HL-A antigens, ankylosing spondylitis and sacro-iliitis. Tissue Antigens 5:26-32, 1975
78. James DCO: Ankylosing spondylitis and HL-A 27. Ann Rheum Dis 34:1-3, 1975
79. Spencer DG, Dick HM, Ferguson-Smith MA, El-Ghobarey, Dick WC: Genotypic and phenotyic family studies of individuals homozygous and heterozygous for HLA-B27, with and without ankylosing spondylitis. Scott Med J 23:312-313, 1978
80. Falace P, Ruderman RJ, Ward FE, Swift M: Histocompatibility typing and the counseling of families with ankylosing spondylitis. Clin Genet 13:380-383, 1978
81. Arnett FC Jr, Schacter BZ, Hochberg MC, Hsu S, Bias WB: Homozygosity for HLA-B27: Impact on rheumatic disease expression in two families. Arthritis Rheum 20:797-804, 1977
82. Hochberg MC, Bias WB, Arnett FC: Family studies in HLA-B27 associated arthritis. Medicine 57:463-475, 1978
83. Gerber N, Von Felten A, Boni A, Wagenhauser F: Spondylitis ankylosans (Bechterew) und gewebsantigen HLA-B 27: Erblichbeit der spondylitis ankylosans (Bechterew). Z Rheumatol 36:230-238, 1977
84. Shirakura R, Mori T, Shichikawa, Tsujimoto M, Manabe H: Genetic significance of HLA B27 in ankylosing spondylitis. A study of 27 families. J Rheumatol 4 (Suppl 3):110, 1977 (Abstr)
85. Scholz S, Schattenkirchner M, Harms K, Steinbauer-Rosenthal I, Albert ED: Family studies in HL-A associated diseases. Z Immun Forsch 148:387-388, 1975
86. Cross RA, Rigby R, Dawkins RL: The significance of HL-A W27 in ankylosing spondylitis and Reiter's syndrome with three family studies. Aust NZ J Med 5:108-111, 1975
87. Strosberg JM, Allen FH Jr, Calabro JJ, Harris ED JR: Ankylosing spondylitis in a large kindred: Clinical and genetic studies. Tissue Antigens 5:205-212, 1975
88. Dick HM, Dick WC, Sturrock RD, Dick WC, Buchanan WW: Inheritance of ankylosing spondylitis and HL-A W27. Lancet ii:24-25, 1974
89. Sturrock RD, Dick HM, Henderson N, Dick WC: Family studies in ankylosing spondylitis. Ann Rheum Dis 34:39-41, 1975
90. Sturrock RD, Dick HM, Henderson N, Goel GK, Lee P, Dick WC, et al: Association of HL-A27 and AJ in juvenile rheumatoid arthritis and ankylosing spondylitis. J Rheumatol 1:269-273, 1974
91. Van Der Linden JMJP, Cats A, Keuning JJ, Van Rood JJ, Wuisman JHC: HL-A27 and ankylosing spondylitis. Ann Rheum Dis 34 (Suppl):53-54, 1975
92. De Bruyere M, De Deuxchaisnes CHN: Segregation of HL-A27 and ankylosing spondylitis in an informative kindred. Tissue Antigens 7:15-22, 1976
93. Van Der Linden JMJP, Keuning JJ, Wuisman JHC, Cats A, Van Rood JJ: HL-A27 and ankylosing spongylitis. Lancet i:520, 1975
94. Christiansen FT, Owen ET, Dawkins RL, Hanrahan P: Symptoms and signs among relatives of patients with HLA B27 ankylosing spondylitis. J Rheumatol 4 (Suppl 3):11-17, 1977
95. Cohen T: Are homozygotes for HLA B27 more susceptible to ankylosing spondylitis?. N Engl J Med 295:342-343, 1976
96. Kidd KK, et al: Genetic analysis of HLA-associated diseases: The illness-susceptible gene frequency and sex ratio in ankylosing spondylitis. In Dausset J, Svejgaard A (eds): HLA and Disease, pp 72-79, Munskgaard, Copenhagen, 1977
97. Daneo V, Migone N, Modena V, Bianchi SD, Alfieri G, Diotallevi P, et al: Family studies and HLA typing in ankylosing spondylitis and sacroiliitis. J Rheumatol 4 (Suppl 3):5-10, 1977
98. Kastelan A, Durinovic-Bello I, Jajic I: The HLA genes and haplotypes in ankylosing spondylitis. Periodicum Biologrum 82:57-63, 1980
99. Hersh AH, Stecher RM, Solomon WM, Wolpaw R, Hauser H: Heredity in ankylosing spondylitis:

A study of 50 families. Am J Hum Genet 391-408, 1951
100. Bingham WF: The role of HLA B27 in the diagnosis and management of low-back pain and sciatica. J Neurosurg 47:561-566, 1977
101. Golding DN, Jenkins WJ: Histocompatibility testing in doubtful cases of ankylosing spondylitis. Lancet ii:522-523, 1974
102. Smith DL, Regan MG: HLA-B27 typing: Letter. Ann Intern Med 92:872, 1980
103. Kaplan H: HLA-B27 typing: Letter. Ann Intern Med 92: 871-872, 1980
104. Calin A: HLA-B27: To type or not to type?. Ann Intern Med 92:208-211, 1980
105. Calin A, Porta J, Fries JF, Schurman DJ: The clinical history as a screening test for ankylosing spondylitis. J Rheumatol 4 (Suppl 3):111, 1977 (Abstr)
106. Calin A: HLA-B27 typing: Comment. Ann Intern Med 92:872, 1980
107. Editorial: HLA-B27 in 1982: Reappraisal of a clinical test. Ann Intern Med 96:114-115, 1982
108. Curtis DL, Epstein WV: Implications of W27 screening. N Engl J Med 294:226, 1976
109. Middleton D: Do clinicians really want to know about HLA-B27? Lancet ii:877, 1982
110. Calin A, Fries JF, Schurman D, Payne R: The close correlation between symptoms and disease expression in HLA B27 positive individuals. J Rheumatol 4:277-281, 1977
111. Khan MA, Khan MK: Diagnostic value of HLA-B27 testing in ankylosing spondylitis and Reiter's syndrome. Ann Intern Med 96:70-76, 1982
112. Kaneoka H, Engleman EG, Grumet FC: Immunochemical variants of HLA-B27. J Immunol 130:1288-1292, 1983
113. Grumet FC, Fendly BM, Engleman EG: Monoclonal anti-HLA-B27 antibody: Production and lack of detectable typing difference between patients with ankylosing spondylitis, Reiter' syndrome, and normal controls. Lancet ii:174, 1981
114. Grumet FC, Fendly BM, Fish L, Foung S, Engleman EG: Monoclonal antibody (B27M2) subdividing HLA-B27. Hum Immunol 5:61-72, 1982
115. Trapani JA, Vaughan HA, Sparrow RL, Tait BD, McKenzie IFC: Description of a mouse monoclonal anti-HLA-B27 antibody HLA-ABC-m3. Hum Immunol 7:205-216, 1983
116. Sany J, Rosenberg F, Panis G, Serre H, Seignalet J: Unclassified HLA-B27 inflammatory rheumatic diseases: Followup of X3 patients. Arthritis Rheum 23:258-259, 1980
117. Ebringer A, Avakian H, Cowling P, Welsh J, Wooley P, Panayi G, et al: Ankylosing spondylitis, HLA B27, and *Klebsiella*: Cross reactivity studies with rabbit anti-lymphocyte sera and human tissue typing sera. Ann Rheum Dis 39:194, 1980
118. Welsh J, Avakian H, Cowling P, Ebringer A, Wooley P, Panayi G, et al: Ankylosing spondylitis, HLA-B27 and Klebsiella: 1. Cross reactivity studies with rabbit antisera. Br J Exp Pathol 61:85-91, 1980
119. Avakian H, Welsh J, Ebringer A, Entwistle CC: Ankylosing spondylitis, HLA-B27 and *Klebsiella*. II. Cross-reactivity studies with human tissue typing sera. Br J Exp Pathol 61:92-96, 1980
120. Ebringer A: Ankylosing spondylitis, immune-response-genes and molecular mimicry. Lancet i:1186, 1979
121. Geczy AF, Alexander K, Bashir HV: A factor(s) in Klebsiella culture filtrates specifically modifies an HLA-B27-associated cell-surface component. Nature 283:782-784, 1980
122. Geczy AF, Alexander K, Bashir HV, Edmonds JP: Characterization of a factor(s) present in Klebsiella culture filtrates that specifically modifies an HLA-B27 associated cell surface components. J Exp Med 152:331s-340s, 1980
123. Seager K, Bashir HV, Geczy AF, Edmonds J, De Vere-Tyndall A: Evidence for a specific B27-associated cell surface marker on lymphocytes of patients with ankylosing spondylitis. Nature 277:68-70, 1979
124. Geczy AF, Yap J: HLA-B27, *Klebsiella*, and ankylosing spondylitis. Lancet i:719-720, 1979
125. Geczy AF, Bashir HV, Alexander K, Edmonds JP: Cross-reactivity between environmental agents and HLA-B27. Lancet i:50, 1980
126. Druery C, Bashir H, Geczy AF, Alexander K, Edmonds J: Search for Klebsiella cell wall components cross-reactive with lymphocytes of B27+ AS+ individuals. Hum Immunol 1:151-160, 1980
127. Seager K, Bashir HV, Geczy AF, Edmonds J, De Vere-Tyndall A: Evidence for a specific B27-associated cell surface marker on lymphocytes of patients with ankylosing spondylitis. Nature 277:68-70, 1979
128. Geczy AF, Seager K, Bashir HV, De Vere-Tyndall A, Edmonds J: The role of *Klebsiella* in the pathogenesis of AS: II. Evidence for a specific B27-associated marker on the lymphocytes of patients with AS. J Clin Lab Immunol 3:23-28, 1980
129. Alexander K, Edwards C, Misko IS, Geczy AF, Bashir HV, Edmonds JP: The distribution of a specific HLA-B27-associated cell surface component on the tissues of patients with ankylosing spondylitis. Clin Exp Immunol 45:158-164, 1981
130. Geczy AF, Alexander K, Bashir HV, Edmonds JP, Upfold L, Sullivan J: HLA-B27, Klebsiella and ankylosing spondylitis: Biological and chemical studies. Immunol Rev 70:23-50, 1983

131. Archer JR: Search for cross-reactivity between HLA B27 and Klebsiella pneumoniae. Ann Rheum Dis 40:400-403, 1981
132. Dilley D, Fan PT, Bluestone R: Absence of cytotoxic effect of selected pathogens on HLA B27 positive fibroblasts. Proc Soc Exp Biol Med 159:184-186, 1978
133. Pease P, England G, Tyler R, Mackintosh P: HLA B27, Yersinia enterocolitica, and ankylosing spondylitis. Ann Rheum Dis 39:415-416, 1980
134. Molders HH, Breuning MH, Ivanyi P, Ploegh HL: Biochemical analysis of variant HLA-B27 antigens. Hum Immunol 6:111-117, 1983
135. Karr RW, Hahn Y, Schwartz BD: Structural identity of human histocompatibility leukocyte antigen-B27 molecules from patients with ankylosing spondylitis and normal individuals. J Clin Invest 69:443-450, 1982
136. Hoshino K, Inouye H, Unokuchi T, Ito M, Tamaoki N, Tsuji K: HLA and disease in Japanese. In Dausset J, Svejgaard A (eds): HLA and Disease, p 249, De L'institut National De La Sante Et De La Recherche Medicale, Paris, 1976
137. Percy JS, Russell AS: Prevalence of ankylosing spondylitis and its association with HL-A27. J Rheumatol 2:351-354, 1975
138. Goldenberg DL, Gibbons RB: Ankylosing spondylitis: A case positive for rheumatoid factor and HL-A27 (W27). JAMA 235:284-285, 1976
139. Dequeker J, Decock T, Walravens M, Van De Putte I: A systematic survey of the HLA B27 prevalence in inflammatory rheumatic diseases. J Rheumatol 5:452-459, 1978
140. Saari KM: Family studies on uveitis and ankylosing spondylitis. Am J Ophthalmol 83:424-425, 1977
141. Sikora K, Webster S, Sachs J, Festenstein H: Associated clinical syndromes in a patient homozygous for HLA B27. Br Med J 1:1184-1186, 1978
142. Sonozaki H Mitsui H: Rheumatism and HL-A antigens. Nippon Rinsho 36:3159-3163, 1978
143. Editorial: Enterobacter, B27, and ankylosing spondylitis. Lancet i:1242, 1978
144. Canoso JJ, Saini M, Hermos JA: Whipple's disease and ankylosing spondylitis simultaneous occurrence in HLA-B27 positive male. J Rheumatol 5:79-84, 1978
145. Rose BS: Familial reactive arthritis of Reiter's and ankylosing spondylitis types in the HLA B7 geno type. NZ Med J 83:107-109, 1976
146. Truog P, Steiger U, Loewi G, Neuhaus K: HL-A B27 associated rheumatic disease. Schweiz Med Wochenschr 105:1733-1735, 1975
147. Editorial: HL-A W27 and ankylosing spondylitis. Med J Aust 1:287-288, 1976
148. Bluestone R, Pearson CM: Ankylosing spondylitis and Reiter's syndrome: Their interrelationship and association with HLA B27. Adv Intern Med 22:1-19, 1977
149. Doury P, Pattin S, Thevenot J, Wahl D: L'association antigene HLA W27-spondylarthrite ankylosante. Nouv Presse Med 5:90, 1976
150. Doury P, Pattin S, Thevenot J, Wahl D: Antigene HLA W27 et spondylarthrite ankylosante. Semin Hop Paris 52:1551-1553, 1976
151. Seignalet J, Sany J, Serre H: Interet pratique des groupes HL-A en rhumatologie. Sem Hop Paris 51:993-1000, 1975
152. Schumacher TM, Genant HK, Kellet MJ, Mall JC, Fye KH: HLA-B27 associated arthropathies. Radiology 126:289-297, 1978
153. Neumuller J, Partsch G, Tausch G, Prohaska E, Eberl R: Prevalence of HLA B27 in ankylosing spondylitis. J Rheumatol 4 (Suppl 3):109, 1977 (Abstr)
154. Bluestone R, Goldberg LS, Weisbart RH, Morris RI, Holber OW: Aberrant immunity in (HL-A) W27-positive rheumatic disease. Ann Rheum Dis 34:46-48, 1975
155. Sachs JA, Brewerton DA: HLA, ankylosing spondylitis and rheumatoid arthritis. Br Med Bull 34:275-278, 1978
156. Delage JM, Bergeron P, Simard J, Lehner-Netsch G, Prochazka E: Hereditary C7 deficiency: Diagnosis and HLA studies in a French-Candian family. J Clin Invest 60:1061-1069, 1977
157. Myers BW , Cheatum DE: Ankylosing spondylitis in a black woman: Association with HL-A W27. JAMA 231:278-279, 1975
158. Marcolongo R, Contu L: Les antigenes HL-A dans la polyarthrite chronique rhumatismale et la spondylarthrite ankylosante en sardaigne. Nouv Presse Med 3: 2023, 1974
159. Arnett FC, Hochberg MC, Bias WB: HLA-C locus antigens in HLA-B27 associated arthritis. Arthritis Rheum 21:885-888, 1978
160. Kozin F, Duquesnoy R, Rodey GE, Lightfoot RW, Ryan LM JR: High prevalence of HLA-CW1 and CW2 antigens in spondylarthritis. Arthritis Rheum 21:889-895, 1978
161. Spielmann W: Das HLA-blutgruppen-system und seine beziehungen zu den erkrankungen des bewegungsapparates. Z Orthop 116:546-548, 1978
162. Editorial: *Klebsiella* and ankylosing spondylitis—molecular mimicry. Lancet i:1012-1013, 1979
163. Spencer DG: Spondylitis and related syndromes: Scottish symposium on rheumatic diseases. Scott Med J 23:81-84, 1978
164. Kentala E, Repo UK, Lehtipuu AL, Vuornos T: HLA-antigens and pulmonary upper lobe fibrocystic changes with and without ankylosing spondylitis. Scand J Respir Dis 59:8-12, 1978

165. Mitsui H, Juji T, Sonozaki H, Watanabe N: Distribution of HLA-B27 in patients with juvenile rheumatoid arthritis. Pediatrics 60:562, 1977
166. Shankar PS, Scott JH, Anderson CL: Pulmonary disease in ankylosing spondylitis positive for rheumatoid factor and HLA-B 27. Indian J Chest Dis Allied Sci 19:27-31, 1977
167. Macurova H, Truhlar P, Ivaskova E, Bavorova H, Ivanyi P: Asociace HL-A antigenu W27 s ankylozujici spondylartritidou. Cas Lek Cesk 113:799-800, 1974
168. Caffrey MFP, James DCO: Human lymphocyte antigen association in ankylosing spondylitis. Nature 242:121, 1973
169. Seignalet J, Sany J, Serre H: Systeme HL-A, spondylarthrite ankylosante rhumatisme psoriasique. Nouv Presse Med 3:1958, 1974
170. Amor B, Feldmann JL, Delbarre F, Hors J, Beaujan MM, Dausset J: L'antigene HL-A W27 sa frequence dans la spondylarthrite ankylosante et le syndrome de fiessinger-leroy-reiter. Nouv Presse Med 3:1373-1374, 1974
171. Le Goff P, Le Menn G, Youinou P, Clavier J, Baret M, Saleun JP: L'antigene HLA-B27 chez les sujets atteints de proliferation osseuse. Nouv Presse Med 7:120-121, 1978
172. Hudgins WR: Ankylosing spondylitis and sciatica. J Neurosurg 48:668-669, 1978
173. Bigar F, Gerber N, Von Felten A: Acute iridocyclitis, ankylosing spondylitis (Bechterew) and congenital tissue antigens. Klin Monatsbl Augenheilkd 172:597-601, 1978
174. Vischer TL, Jeannet M, Boussina I: HL-A27 diagnosis of rheumatic diseases. Lancet i:1001, 1974
175. Schattenkirchner M, Schurer W, Scholz S, Steinbauer-Rosenthal I, Albert ED: Spondylitis ankylosans (sp. a.) und histokompatibilitatsantigen HL-A27. Munch Med Wochenschr 116:1109, 1974
176. Brewerton DA: HL-A27 and disease. J Bone Joint Surg 57B:247, 1975
177. Amor B, Kahan A, Georgiadis AE: Transient loss of HLA B27. Lancet i:284, 1978
178. Van Den Berg-Loonen PM, Dekker-Saeys AJ, Meuwissen SGM, Nijenhuis LE: Histocompatibility antigens and other markers in ankylosing spondylitis and inflammatory bowel disease. J Rheumatol 4 (Suppl 3):57-59, 1977
179. Khan MA: Race-related differences in HLA association with ankylosing spondylitis and Reiter's disease in American blacks and whites. J Natl Med Assoc 70:41-42, 1978
180. Veys EM, Coigne E, Mielants H, Verbruggen A: HLA et polyarthrite chronique juvenile. Rev Rhum Mal Osteoartic 43:491-495, 1976
181. Keat AC, Barnes RMR: HL-A27-associated arthritis. Rheumatol Rehab 15:87-91, 1976
182. Ott H: Interet de la recherche de l'antigene HLA-B27 dans le diagnostic des arthropathies inflammatoires seronegatives. Rev Med Suisse Romande 98:111-117, 1978
183. Laroche CL, Cremer GA, Patri B, Remy JM, Letellier PH: Associattion de maladie de Behcet et de pelvispondylite chez un sujet ne presentant pas l'antigene HLA W27. Semin Hop Paris 51:2501-2508, 1975
184. Libich M, Majsky A, Bartsch D: HLA-B 27 (W27) antigen and other immunological factors in ankylosing spondylarthritis. Cas Lek Cesk 114:1521-1523, 1975
185. Welfling J: Spondylarthrite ankylosante et antigene HL-A 27. Nouv Presse Med 3:891-892, 1974
186. Doury P: Antigene HLA-B27 et spondylarthrite ankylosante. Nouv Presse Med 9:2160-2161, 1980
187. Chan SH, Satkunananthan K, Wee GB, Srinivasan N, Chacha P: HLA-B27 and Chinese ankylosing spondylitis. Singapore Med J 21:710-712, 1980
188. Mitsui H, Juji T, Sonozaki H: Juvenile ankylosing spondylitis, its clinical features and HLA-B27. Arch Orthop Unfallchir 87:31-37, 1977
189. Tsujimoto M, Okabe N: HLA and orthopedic disease. Nippon Rinsho 36:2346-2347, 1978
190. Sonozaki H, Seki H, Chang S, Okuyama M, Juji T: Human lymphocyte antigen, HL-A27, in Japanese patients with ankylosing spondylitis. Tissue Antigens 5:131-136, 1975
191. Orozco-Medina JH, Vazquez-Escobosa C: HLA antigens in ankylosing spondylitis. Rev Invest Clin 33:369-372, 1981
192. Singal DP, De Bosset P, Gordon DA, Smythe HA, Urowitz MB, Koehler BE: HLA antigens in osteitis condensans ilii and ankylosing spondylitis. J Rheumatol 4 (Suppl 3):105-108, 1977
193. Schaller JG, Ochs HD, Thomas ED, Nisperos B, Feigl P, Wedgwood RJ: Histocompatibility antigens in childhood-onset arthritis. J Pediatr 88:926-930, 1976
194. Mills DM, Arai Y, Gupta RC: HL-A antigens and sacroiliitis. JAMA 231:268-270, 1975
195. McClusky OE, Lordon RE, Arnett FC Jr: HL-A 27 in Reiter's syndrome and psoriatic arthritis: A genetic factor in disease susceptibility and expression. J Rheumatol 1:263-268, 1974
196. Duquesnoy RJ, Kozin F, Rodey GE: High prevalence of HLA-B27, CW1 and CW2 in patients with seronegative spondyloarthritis. Tissue Antigens 12:58-62, 1978
197. Zilko PJ, Thevathasan M, Dawkins RL: Immune function in ankylosing spondylitis: Apparent relationship between steptococcal responses and HLA B27. J Rheumatol 4 (Suppl 3):49-53, 1977
198. Kuthan F, Streda A, Parma R, Krepelkova M, Hill Z, Valnickova Z: Diagnostic importance of

the incidence of tissue antigen HLA-B27 in some rheumatic diseases. Vnitr Lek 25:578-583, 1979
199. Wegener VS, Mach J: Zur assoziation von ankyosierender spondylitis (Morbus Bechterew) und HLA system. Z Arztl Fortbild (Jena) 74:895-898, 1980
200. Huaux J, Fiasse R, De Bruyere M, De Deuxchaisnes CN: HLA B27 in regional enteritis with and without ankylosing spondylitis or sacroiliitis. J Rheumatol 4 (Suppl 3):60-63, 1977
201. De Deuxchaisnes CN, Huaux JP, Fiasse R, De Bruyere M: Ankylosing spondylitis, sacroiliitis, regional enteritis, and HL-A27. Lancet i:1238-1239, 1974
202. Veys EM, Coigne E, Mielants H, Verbruggen A: HLA and juvenile chronic polyarthritis. Tissue Antigens 8:61-65, 1976
203. Sachs JA, Sterioff S, Robinette M, Wolf E, Curry MLF, Festenstein H: Ankylosing spondylitis and the major histocompatibility system. Tissue Antigens 5:120-127, 1975
204. Calin A, Grahame R, Tudor M, Kennedy L: "Ankylosing rheumatoid arthritis," ankylosing spondylitis and HL-A antigens. Lancet i:874-875, 1974
205. Sany J, Serre H, Seignalet J: Antigene HL-A et pelvispondylites rhumatismales atypiques. Rev Rhum Mal Osteoartic 43:97-103, 1976
206. Amor B, Feldmann JL, Delbarre F, Hors J, Beaujan MM, Dausset J: HL-A antigen W27- A genetic link between ankylosing spondylitis and Reiter's syndrome? N Engl J Med 290:572, 1974
207. Ferri S, Conighi C, Buzzanca G, Albertazzi R, Mattiuz PL: Contribution to the study of the prevalence of HLA-B27 antigen in ankylosing spondylitis in Italy. Rev Rhum Mal Osteoartic 49:355-358, 1982
208. Marcolongo R, Contu L: HL-A antigens associated with rheumatoid arthritis and ankylosing spondylitis in an ethnic homogeneous population. Biomedicine 23:88-91, 1975
209. Ercilla MG, Brancos MA, Breysse Y, Alonso G, Vives J, Castillo R, et al: HLA antigens in Forestier's disease, ankylosing spondylitis, and polyarthrosis of the hands. J Rheumatol 4 (Suppl 3):89-93, 1977
210. Gerber N, Ambrosini GC, Boni A, Ossola A, Wagenhauser FJ, Fehr K, et al: Spondylitis ankylosans (Bechterew) and gewebsantigen HLA-B27. Z Rheumatol 36:219-223, 1977
211. Isomaki H, Koota K, Martio J, Nissila M, Tiilikainen A: HL-A27 and arthritis. Ann Clin Res 7:138-145, 1975
212. Reiten T, Skavdal KO, Solheim BG: HLA B27 in ankylosing spondylitis. J Rheumatol 4 (Suppl 3):109, 1977 (Abstr)
213. Bjelle A, Cedergren B, Dahlqvist SR: HLA B27 in the population of northern Sweden. Scand J Rheumatol 11:23-26, 1982
214. Moller E, Olhagen B: Studies on the major histocompatibility system in patients with ankylosing spondylitis. Tissue Antigens 6:237-246, 1975
215. Grahame R, Kennedy L, Wood PHN: HL-A27 and the diagnosis of back problems. Rheumatol Rehab 14:168-172, 1975
216. Rudge SR, Treadwell BLJ: HLA B27 negative ankylosing spondylitis-A rare condition. Aust NZ J Med 10:227-229, 1980
217. Vital Durand D, Rouhier D, Brette R: Could the HLA-B27 antigen be a predisposing factor in the development of fibrotic changes? J Urol 124:162, 1980
218. Edelman J and Walters D: HLA B27 negative ankylosing spondylitis with unusually severe and generalized peripheral arthritis. Med J Aust 2:730, 1980
219. Kuberski T: Histocompatibility antigens and the sexually transmitted diseases. Am Vener Dis Assoc 7:203-205, 1980
220. Rosenbaum JT: Why HLA-B27: An analysis based on two animal models. Ann Intern Med 94:261-263, 1981
221. Moller E, Link H, Matell G, Olhagen B, Stendahl L: LD alleles in ankylosing spondylitis, myasthenia gravis, multiple sclerosis and neuritis. In Kissmeyer-Nielsen F (ed): Histocompatiblity Testing 1975, pp 778-781, Munksgaard, Copenhagen, 1975
222. Calin A, Fries JF: On the reassesssment of the prevalence of AS among B27 positive normal individuals. J Rheumatol 7:577-578, 1980
223. Rate RG, Morse HG, Bonnel MD, Kuberski TT: "Navajo arthritis" reconsidered: Relationship to HLA-B27. Arthritis Rheum 23:1299-1302, 1980
224. Faure G, Raffoux C, Netter P, Pourel J, Streiff F, Gaucher A: Spondylarthrites ankylosants sans antigene HLA B27. Nouv Presse Med 9:51,1982
225. Nashel DJ, Leonard A, Mann DL, Guccion JG, Katz AL, Sliwinski AJ: Ankylosing spondylitis and systemic lupus erythematosus. Arch Intern Med 142:1227-1228, 1982
226. Calin A: Epidemiology of the rheumatic diseases, with a focus on HLA. Curr Ther Res 30:S15-S23, 1981
227. Ebringer RW: HLA-B27 and the link with rheumatic diseases: Recent developments. Clin Sci 59:405-410, 1980
228. Sach JA: HLA systems and rheumatic diseases. Curr Top Pathol 71:235-262, 1982
229. Veys EM, Verbruggen G, Hermanns P, Mielants H, Van Bruwaene P, De Brabanter G, et al: Peripheral blood T lymphocytes subpopulations in HLA-B27 related rheumatic diseases:Ankylosing

spondylitis and reactive synovitis. J Rheumatol 10:140-143, 1983

230. Dawkins RL, Christiansen FT, Kay PH, Garlepp M, McCluskey J, Hollingsworth PN, et al.: Disease associations with complotypes, supratypes and haplotypes. Immunol Rev 70:5-22, 1983
231. Coughlan RJ, Molony J, Bresnihan B: Ankylosing spondylitis: A two year experience. Irish Med J 74:190-191, 1981
232. Jacobs JC, Berdon WE, Johnston AD: HLA-B27-associated spondyloarthritis and enthesopathy in childhood: Clinical, pathologic, and radiographic observations in 58 patients. J Pediatr 100:521-528, 1982

Ankylosing Spondylitis in Inflammatory Bowel Disease

Population Association

Available data from the United States[1] and The Netherlands[2,3] showed a significant increase of B27 in patients with this disease (Table 6.26). In 20 patients with inflammatory bowel disease and spondylitis and/or peripheral arthritis from Belgium[4] the frequency of B27 was 40% compared with 6.6% in a normal population of unknown size. Dekker-Saeys et al.[2] summarized 8 studies in which small numbers of patients with ankylosing spondylitis and inflammatory bowel disease were typed for B27. In each study the frequency of B27 was higher in the patients (range 14%–91%) as compared with 6%–10% found in healthy Caucasian populations.

Disease Heterogeneity

In the study by Hyla et al.[1] there were 11 patients with inflammatory bowel disease and radiographic sacroiliitis and only 1 (9.1%) was positive for B27. The frequency of this antigen in 91 controls was 6.6%.

References

1. Hyla JF, Franck WA, Davis JS: Lack of association 4 of HLA B27 with radiographic sacroiliitis in inflammatory bowel disease. J Rheumatol 3:196-200, 1976
2. Dekker-Saeys BJ, Meuwissen SGM, Van Den Berg-Loonen EM, DE Hass WHD, Meijers AF, Tytgat GNJ: Clinical characteristic of histocompatibility typing (HLA B27) in 50 patients with both ankylosing spondylitis and inflammatory bowel disease. Ann Rheum Dis 37:36-41, 1978
3. Van Den Berg-Loonen EM, Dekker-Saeys BJ, Meuwissen SGM, Nijenhuis LE, Engelfriet CP: Histocompatibility antigens and other genetic markers in ankylosing spondylitis and inflammatory bowel diseases. J Immunogenet 4: 167-175, 1977
4. Dequeker J, Decock T, Walravens M, Van De Putte I: A systematic survey of the HLA B27 prevalence in inflammatory rheumatic diseases. J Rheumatol 5:452-459, 1978

Seronegative "Spondylitic Variant" Syndrome

Population Association

In a mixed group of 25 patients from Canada,[1] B27 was significantly increased (Table 6.27). The sample included 7 patients with Reiter's syndrome, 5 with incomplete Reiter's syndrome, 8 with psoriatic peripheral arthritis, and 5 with inflammatory bowel disease and peripheral arthritis. In the last subgroup, 3 had Crohn's disease and 2 had ulcerative colitis.

TABLE 6.26. Ankylosing Spondylitis in Inflammatory Bowel Disease

	Patients		Controls				
Country/Population	n	%+	n	%+	RR	χ^2	Ref.
HLA-B27							
U.S.A.	4	75	91	7	28.91	12.61	1
BENELUX	39	50	778	10	8.95	43.01	3
	43	52	869	10	10.19	54.26	
	Heterogeneity χ^2 (1 df)					1.36	

TABLE 6.27. Seronegative "Spondylitic Variant" Syndrome

	Patients		Controls				
Country/Population	n	%+	n	%+	RR	χ^2	Ref.
HLA-B27							
Canada	25	44	171	5	14.28	27.10	1

Reference

1. Esdaile JM, Dwosh IL, Urowitz MB, Smythe HA, and Falk J: HLA B27 in rheumatoid factor-negative polyarthritis. Ann Intern Med 86:699-702, 1977

Vertebral Ankylosing Hyperostosis (Forestier's Disease)

Population Association

Shapiro et al.[1] found a highly significant increase of B27 in 47 American Caucasian patients (Table 6.28). Similar results were also reported from Czechoslovakia by Svec et al.[2] However, as the data in Table 6.28 show, 4 other studies by Perry et al.,[3] Brigode and Francois.[4] Ercilla et al.[5] and Rosenthal et al.[6,7] could not confirm this association. The significant increase of B27 in the combined data is due primarily to the results of Shapiro et al.[1] and Svec et al.[2]

Similar inconsistent results were found in the case of B8. Rosenthal et al.[6,7] observed a significant association with B8 that was not confirmed in 3 other studies given in Table 6.28.

In the data of Brigode and Francois.[4] on 50 Belgian patients (Table 6.28) CW4 was found to be increased.

Disease Heterogeneity

Shapiro et al.[1] found no difference between B27-positive and -negative patients with respect to roentgenograms of the spine and peripheral joints.

See also refs. 8–10.

TABLE 6.28. Vertebral Ankylosing Hyperostosis (Forestier's Disease)

	Patients		Controls				
Country/Population	n	%+	n	%+	RR	χ^2	Ref.
HLA-B8							
U.S.A.	27	30	1205	21	1.67	1.57	1
BENELUX	50	14	466	21	0.65	1.19	4
Spain	50	10	700	10	1.08	0.03	5
Switzerland	50	42	1244	18	3.31	17.05	6
	177	23	3615	18	1.67	7.72	
	Heterogeneity χ^2 (3 df)					12.12	
HLA-B27							
Jews (unspecified)	18	6	60	7	1.09	0.01	3
U.S.A.	47	34	1205	8	5.98	31.60	1
Czechoslovakia	43	33	760	9	5.03	22.67	2
BENELUX	50	6	466	7	0.97	0.00	4
Spain	50	4	700	6	0.80	0.13	5
Switzerland	50	8	1244	7	1.28	0.26	6
	240	16	4375	7	3.04	35.66	
	Heterogeneity χ^2 (4 df)					19.01	
HLA-CW4							
BENELUX	50	4	466	26	0.15	10.13	4

TABLE 6.29. Sacroiliitis

Country/Population	Patients n	Patients %+	Controls n	Controls %+	RR	χ^2	Ref.
HLA-B27							
Pima—A.I.	38	26	400	18	1.64	1.73	6
Italy	39	44	1428	4	18.81	73.74	3
Italy	17	71	320	5	42.72	45.88	5
	56	52	1748	4	23.58	118.04	
	Heterogeneity χ^2 (1 df)					1.59	
Sweden	60	70	100	12	16.26	47.42	1
Sweden	14	71	500	11	18.38	27.41	2
	74	70	600	11	16.97	74.80	
	Heterogeneity χ^2 (1 df)					0.03	
	130	62	2348	6	20.39	192.28	
	Heterogeneity χ^2 (3 df)					2.18	
HLA-CW1							
Sweden	14	57	500	7	17.05	28.36	2

References

1. Shapiro RF, Utsinger PD, Wiesner KB, Resnik D, Bryan BL, Castles JJ: The association of HLA-B27 with Forestier's disease (vertebral ankylosing hyperostosis). J Rheumatol 3:4 8, 1976
2. Svec V, Nyulassy S, Zlnay D, Buc M, Schultz P: HLA B27 antigen in ankylosing vertebral hyperostosis. Cas Lek Cesk 118:527-529, 1979
3. Perry JD, Wolf H, Festenstein H, Storey GO: Ankylosing hyperostosis: A study of HLA A, B, and C antigens. Ann Rheum Dis 38:72-73, 1979
4. Brigode M, Francois RJ: Histocompatibility antigens in vertebral ankylosing hyperostosis. J Rheumatol 4:429-434, 1977
5. Ercilla MG, Brancos MA, Breysse Y, Alonso G, Vives J, Castillo R, et al: HLA antigens in Forestier's disease, ankylosing spondylitis, and polyarthrosis of the hands. J Rheumatol 4 (Suppl 3):89-93, 1977
6. Rosenthal M, Bahous I, Muller W: Increased freqency of HLA B8 in hyperostotic spondylosis. J Rheumatol 4 (Suppl 3):94-96, 1977
7. Rosenthal M, Bahous I, Muller W: HL-A B27 and modified bone formation. Lancet i:543, 1976
8. Querol JR, Gonzalez GE: HLA-B27 and modified bone formation. Lancet i:482-483, 1976
9. Schumacher TM, Genant HK, Kellet MJ, Mall JC, Fye KH: HLA-B27 associated arthropathies. Radiology 126:289-297, 1978
10. Shapiro RF, Wiesner KB, Bryan BL, Utsinger PD, Resnick D, Castles JJ: HLA-B27 and modified bone formation. Lancet i:230-231, 1976

Sacroiliitis

Population Association

Studies of Moller et al.[1] and Safwenberg et al.[2] from Sweden and of Migone et al.[3,4] and Ferri et al.[5] from Italy reported a highly significant association with B27 (Table 6.29). However, the increase of B27 was not as high as in ankylosing spondylitis. In the report of Safwenberg et al.,[2] CW1 was also increased in the patients (Table 6.29).

Calin et al.[6] reported B27 frequencies in 38 Pima Indian patients in the United States (Table 6.29). In the total sample, the B27 increase was not significant. However, 8 of 16 male patients were positive (50%) for B27. In 22 female patients, only 2 were positive for B27. Thus, in the subgroup of male patients, the association with B27 was significant (also see 7).

Searles et al.[8] reported some data on Zuni Indians (United States) in which 4 of 7 B27-positive males had either X-ray evidence of sacroiliitis or positive physical findings on back examination. None of the 5 B27-positive females had X-ray evidence of sacroiliitis.

Kuberski et al.[9] have surveyed the frequencies of B27 and sacroiliitis in 100 Navajo and 100 Hopi Indians (United States). Although the data on control groups were not given there were significant associations between the presence of B27 and sacroilliitis in 2 populations.

Moller and Olhagen[1] also did MLC typings on Swedish patients. No association was found.

Disease Heterogeneity

In the data of Migone et al.[3] and of Safwenberg et al.,[2] there was a higher percentage of male B27-positive patients. In addition, Migone et al.[3] found the onset of the first osteoarticular complaints at an earlier age in B27-positive individuals. The severity of sacroiliitis (expressed as bilateral vs. unilateral involvement) was also significantly greater among B27-positive patients ($p = 0.028$).

Family Data

Migone et al.[3,4] found a higher frequency (20%) of sacroiliitis in the families of B27-positive probands as compared with only 3.7% in the families of B27-negative probands. (See also 10.)

See also refs. 1, and 11-13.

References

1. Moller E, Olhagen B: Studies on the major histocompatibility system in patients with ankylosing spondylitis. Tissue Antigens 6:237-246, 1975
2. Safwenberg J, Domeij-Nyberg B, Kjallman M: HLA antigens in females with ankylosing spondylitis and other forms of seronegative rheumatic diseases. Scand J Rheumatol 7:177-182, 1978
3. Migone N, Modena V, Daneo V, Carbonara AO, Ceppellini R: Sacroiliitis and HLA: A clinical and genetical study. Ann Rheum Dis 37:513-517, 1978
4. Daneo V, Migone N, Modena V, Bianchi SD, Alfieri G, Diotallevi P, et al: Family studies and HLA typing in ankylosing spondylitis and sacroiliitis. J Rheumatol 4 (Suppl 3):5-10, 1977
5. Ferri S, Conighi C, Buzzanca G, Albertazzi R, Mattiuz PL: Contribution to the study of the prevalence of HLA-B27 antigen in ankylosing spondylitis in Italy. Rev Rhum Mal Osteoartic 49:355-358, 1982
6. Calin A, Bennett PH, Jupiter J, Terasaki PI: HLA-B27 and sacroiliitis in Pima Indians - association in males only. J Rheumatol 4 (Suppl 3):44-48, 1977
7. Lisse JR, Kuberski TT, Bennett PH, Knowler WC, Gofton JP, Calin A, et al.: High risk of sacroiliitis in HLA-B27-positive Pima Indian men. Arthritis Rheum 25:236-237, 1982
8. Searles RP, Voyles WF, Billowitz E, Thouk GM, Messner RP: Prevalence of HLA-B27 and sacroiliitis in a prospective study of Zuni Indians. Tissue Antigens 14:174-176, 1979
9. Kuberski TT, Morse HG, Rate RG, Bonnell MD, Wood JG Jr, Bennett PH: A hospital-based survey of radiological sacroiliitis and HLA-B27 and Cw2 in Navajo and Hopi Indians. Hum Immunol 3:77-83, 1981
10. Arnett FC, Enlow RW, Bias WB: Sacroiliitis in the old order Amish. Am J Med Genet 12:333-342, 1982
11. Marcusson J, Elman A, Moller E, Thyresson N: Psoriasis, sacroiliitis and peripheral arthritis occur in patients with same HLA haplotype: Preliminary family report and hypothetical explanation of interaction between MHS products. Tissue Antigens 8:131-138, 1976
12. Hochberg MC, Bias WB, Arnett FC: Family studies in HLA-B27 associated arthritis. Medicine 57:463-475, 1978
13. De Deuxchaisnes CN, Huaux JP, Fiasse R, De Bruyere M: Ankylosing spondylitis, sacroiliitis, regional enteritis, and HL-A27. Lancet i:1238-1239, 1974

Polyarthrosis of Hands

Population Association

There has been no association with A and B loci antigens in 50 patients (and 700 normal controls) from Spain[1]. Gomez et al.[2] reported similar results.

References

1. Ercilla MG, Brancos MA, Breysse Y, Alonso G, Vives J, Castillo R, et al: HLA antigens in Forestier's disease, ankylosing spondylitis, and polyarthrosis of the hands. J Rheumatol 4 (Suppl 3):89-93, 1977
2. Gomez JM, Cunilla MAB, Goncales GE: Histocompatibility antigens in polyarthrosis in the hand. Ann Rheum Dis 35:287, 1976

Mechanical Disorders of Spine

Population Association

When comparing 21 Iranian patients with 400 healthy controls, Davatchi et al.[1] found no significant deviations in A and B loci antigens, especially B27.

Reference

1. Davatchi F, Nikbin B, Ala F: Histocompatibility antigens (HLA) in rheumatic disases in Iran. J Rheumatol 4 (Suppl 3):36-38, 1977

Osteoarthritis

Population Association

Six Ashkenazi and 12 nonAshkenazi Jewish patients from Israel were typed for A and B loci antigens by Brautbar et al.[1] There was no significant deviation in any of the antigen frequencies. Mattingly and Mowat.[2] have also reported no HLA associations in a group of 16 English osteoarthritic patients with ectopic ossification after total hip replacement.

See also ref. 3.

References

1. Brautbar C, Porat S, Nelken D, Gabriel KR, Cohen T: HLA B27 and ankylosing spondylitis in the Israeli population. J Rheumatol 4 (Suppl 3):24-32, 1977
2. Mattingly PC, Mowat AG: HLA antigens in patients with ectopic ossification after total hip replacement. J Rheumatol 7:582, 1980
3. Poulter LW, Duke O, Hobbs S, Janossy G, Panayi G: Histochemical discrimination of HLA-DR positive cell populations in the normal and arthritic synovial lining. Clin Exp Immunol 48:381-388, 1982

Osteitis Condensans Ilii

Osteitis condensans ilii is a radiologic diagnosis defined as a unilateral or bilateral triangular bony sclerosis of the lower ilium, sparing the sacral portion of the sacroiliac joint.

Population Association

Twenty-five Caucasian female patients from Canada[1] were typed for A and B loci antigens. No significant association, when compared with 200 controls, was found.

Reference

1. Singal DP, De Bosset P, Gordon DA, Smythe HA, Urowitz MB, Koehler BE: HLA antigens in osteitis condensans ilii and ankylosing spondylitis. J Rheumatol 4 (Suppl 3):105-108, 1977

Juvenile Dermatomyositis

Population Association

In a small sample of American Caucasian patients a significant association with B8 was reported by Pachman et al.[1,2] In a later study the same group of authors[3] concluded that DR3 was also increased. Table 6.30 shows the B8 and DR3 antigen frequency data from 2 subsequent reports[4,5] by the authors on a larger sample that included the patients studied in the previous reports.

Disease Heterogeneity

Pachman et al.[3] also measured autoantibodies to thyroid microsomes, smooth muscle, immunoglobulin, mitochondria, nuclei, DNA, ENA, RNP, Sm, or PM-I in B8- and/or -DR3 positive and -negative patients. There was no difference between these groups.

In 7 American Caucasian and 9 American Black patients with adult dermatomyositis, no association with DR locus antigens was reported by Hirsch et al.[6].

References

1. Pachman LM, Jonasson O, Cannon RA, Friedman JM: HLA-B8 in juvenile dermatomyositis. Lancet ii:567-568, 1977
2. Pachman LM, Jonasson O, Cannon RA, Friedman JM: Increased frequency of HLA-B8 in juvenile dermatomyositis. Lancet ii:1238, 1977

TABLE 6.30. Juvenile Dermatomyositis

	Patients		Controls				
Country/Population	n	%+	n	%+	RR	χ^2	Ref.
HLA-B8							
U.S.A.	67	37	867	18	2.69	14.06	5
HLA-DR3							
U.S.A.—Black	6	83	168	28	9.21	7.13	4
Mexico	9	78	88	16	15.48	13.90	4
U.S.A.	36	53	979	23	3.76	15.73	4

TABLE 6.31. Caplan's Syndrome

	Patients		Controls				
Country/Population	n	%+	n	%+	RR	χ^2	Ref.
HLA-BW45							
England	56	11	250	1	10.94	12.74	1

3. Pachman LM, Maryjowski MC, Friedman JM, Jonasson O, Radvany RM, Sharp GC, et al: Immunogenetic studies of juvenile dermatomyositis: Increased occurrence of HLA-B8, DRW3, and their relation to PM-I and other autoantibodies. Arthritis Rheum 23:728, 1980
4. Friedman JM, Pachman LM, Maryjowski ML, Radvany RM, Crowe WE, Hanson V, et al: Immunogenetic studies of juvenile dermatomyositis: HLA-DR antigen frequencies. Arthritis Rheum 26:214-216, 1983
5. Friedman JM, Pachman LM, Maryjowski ML, Jonasson O, Battles ND, Crowe WE, et al: Immunogenetic studies of juvenile dermatomyositis. HLA antigens in patients and their families. Tissue Antigens 21:45-49, 1983
6. Hirsch TJ, Enlow RW, Bias WB, Arnett FC: HLA-D related (DR) antigens in polymyositis: Evidence for clinical and immunogenetic heterogeneity. Arthritis Rheum 23:689, 1980

Caplan's Syndrome

Patients with this syndrome have rheumatoid arthritis associated with pneumoconiosis.

Population Association

Wagner and Darke[1] studied the A and B loci antigens in 56 Welsh coal workers with Caplan's syndrome. When compared with frequencies in 250 people living in the Cardiff area and occupationally not exposed to coal dust BW45 was significantly increased in the patients (Table 6.31). The frequency of BW45 was 4.5% in 135 normal coal workers.

Disease Heterogeneity

In the British study[1] 50 patients tested for rheumatoid factor (RF) were divided into 2 groups: 31 positive and 19 negative. In 31 patients with RF the frequency of BW45 was 16%, compared with 0% in 19 negative patients. In comparisons of BW45 in the RF-positive group with that in the nonexposed healthy population (0.8% in 250 individuals) BW45 also showed a significant difference (corrected $p = 0.0064$).

Reference

1. Wagner MMF, Darke C: HLA-A and B antigen frequencies in Welsh coalworkers with pneumoconiosis and Caplan's syndrome. Tissue Antigens 14:165-168, 1979

Neurogenic Paraosteoarthropathy

Population Association

Minaire et al.[1] first reported a significant association with B18 in 43 French patients with spinal cord injury with paraosteoarthropathies (ossifications of the paraarticular soft tissues but no change in the joints). Later the same group of authors[2] extended the study to a larger sample size. In the second report on 66 patients (43 with spinal cord injury and 23 with severe head injury) they observed that B18 was significantly increased (Table 6.32). The frequency of B18 from 2 other French studies[3,4] and a combined analysis of all the data are given in Table 6.32.

In a small sample of 28 patients Betuel et al.[4] also reported a significant increase of antigen DR7.

Weiss et al.[5] also reported A and B loci antigen frequencies in 20 Israeli patients (12 with severe craniocerebral injury and 8 with spinal cord injury). Common to all those patients was radiologically proven periarticular new bone formation. Hip, shoulder, elbow, and knee joints were the most frequently involved. When compared with 631 controls, no significant frequency deviations were observed. Antigen B18 was slightly increased in the patients but not significantly (Table 6.32).

Disease Heterogeneity

In the French study[2] there were 34 patients without paraosteoarthropathies (25 with spinal cord injury and 9 with severe head injury). The frequency of

TABLE 6.32. Neurogenic Paraosteoarthropathy

	Patients		Controls				
Country/Population	n	%+	n	%+	RR	χ^2	Ref.
HLA-B18							
Jews (unspecified)	20	10	631	7	1.78	0.81	5
France	58	19	300	12	1.76	2.36	3
France	31	23	100	10	2.70	3.72	4
France	66	26	341	8	4.05	17.20	2
	155	23	741	10	2.75	20.48	
	Heterogeneity χ^2 (2 df)					2.80	
HLA-DR7							
France	28	57	100	17	6.26	16.57	4

B18 in that group was 0% but not significantly different from that of the group with paraosteoarthropathies (if probability of 0.001 is corrected for 26 antigens tested in this study). The frequency of B18 was the same in spinal cord injury (25.6%) and head injury (25.7%) patients.

References

1. Minaire P, Betuel H, Pilonchery G: System HLA chez les blesses medullaires atteints de para-osteo-arthropathies neurogenes. Nouv Presse Med 7:3044, 1978
2. Minaire P, Betuel H, Girard R, Pilonchery G: Neurologic injuries, paraosteoarthropathies, and human leukocyte antigens. Arch Phys Med Rehab 61:214-215, 1980
3. Seignalet J, Moulin M, Pelissier J, Romain M, Bouffeard-Vercelli M, Lapinski H, et al: HLA and neurogenic paraosteoarthropathies. Tissue Antigens 21:268-269, 1983
4. Betuel H, Minaire P, Gebuhrer L, Girard R, Bertrand J, Lacroix B: Neurogenic paraosteoarthropathies (POA). In Terašaki PI (ed): Histocompatibility Testing 1980, pp 715-716. UCLA Tissue Typing Laboratory, Los Angeles, 1981
5. Weiss S, Grosswasser Z, Ohri A, Mizrachi Y, Orgad S, Efter T, et al: Histocompatibility (HLA) antigens in heterotopic ossification associated with neurological injury. J Rheumatol 6:88-91, 1979

Spondylarthritis in Chronic Brucellosis

Population Association

Hodinka et al.[1] reported a significant increase of B27 in 27 Hungarian patients (Table 6.33) with chronic brucellosis. In addition, they had a history of exudative arthritis, severe back pain, or clinical signs of arthritis or painful and limited spine movements with a tenderness of the dorsolumbar vertebrae and sacroiliac joints on physical examination. Radiologic evidence of sacroiliitis or osteochondritis of the dorsal vertebrae was also present.

Reference

1. Hodinka L, Gomor B, Meretey K, Zahumansky Z, Geher P, Telegdy L, et al: HLA-B27-associated spondylarthritis in chronic brucellosis. Lancet i:499, 1978

TABLE 6.33. Spondylarthritis in Chronic Brucellosis

	Patients		Controls				
Country/Population	n	%+	n	%+	RR	χ^2	Ref.
HLA-B27							
Hungary	27	44	352	13	5.26	16.76	1

Amyloidosis in Rheumatoid Arthritis

Population Association

The HLA frequency data are available in only 1 study on 26 Finnish patients with rheumatoid arthritis and secondary amyloidosis[1]. The frequency of B27 was significantly increased in the patient group (Table 6.34).

Reference

1. Pasternack A, Tiilikainen A: HLA-B27 in rheumatoid arthritis and amyloidosis. Tissue Antigens 9:80-89, 1977

Gout

Population Association

Sixty-six American Caucasian patients and 906 controls were typed for A and B loci antigens by Schlosstein et al.[1] No association was observed with any of the antigens.

Reference

1. Schlosstein L, Terasaki PI, Bluestone R, Pearson CM: High association of an HL-A antigen, W27, with ankylosing spondylitis. N Engl J Med 288:704-706, 1973

Reiter's Disease

Population Association

The initial reports by Brewerton et al.[1] and Morris et al.[2] showed a strong disease association with B27. This was confirmed in several subsequent reports on various Caucasian groups. The frequency data from these studies are given in Table 6.35. The reports with mixed ethnic groups and without information on controls are listed only in the bibliography.

Good et al.[3] reported only 1 (14.29%) B27 positive in a sample of 7 American Black patients. Khan et al.[4,5] also studied 19 American Black patients and found 7 (36.84%) positive for B27. The B27 phenotype frequency in the American Black population is about 2.30%.

In a report from India by Malaviya et al.[6] 18 of the 20 patients (90%) were reported to be positive for B27. The gene frequency of B27 in that population (of unknown size) was 4.26%.

C locus typing has been done by Kozin et al.[7] and Kemple et al.[8] in American Caucasian and American Black patients with no significant association found.

HLA-D locus typing of 31 patients by Kemple et al.[8] also did not show any association with these antigens.

Arnett et al.[9] reported that, of the 10 patients (from a total of 44) with Reiter's disease who were B27-negative, 7 (70%) had another B locus antigen that was immunologically cross-reactive with B27 (B7, BW22, and BW42). On the basis of this result the authors hypothesized a direct role of HLA antigens in the pathogenesis of the disease. This increase of B7 cross-reacting groups in B27 negative patients was not observed in 23 B27-negative patients studied by Khan et al.[4] In this study, the frequency of these cross-reactive antigens was not significantly different from that in the control population.

Disease Heterogeneity

The patients studied by McClusky et al.[10] were subdivided into groups based on the course of the disease and the presence or absence of uveitis. Fifteen of the 17 B27-positive patients had chronic or relapsing course as compared with only 2 in 11 B27-negative patients ($p < 0.001$). Similarly, uveitis and the presence of high fever and severe weight loss were more frequent in B27-positive patients compared with B27-negative patients. Aho et al.[11] reported that B27-negative Finnish patients usually had a mild or somewhat atypical disease. In an analysis of 160 patients

TABLE 6.34. Amyloidosis in Rheumatoid Arthritis

	Patients		Controls				
Country/Population	n	%+	n	%+	RR	χ^2	Ref.
HLA-B27							
Finland	26	62	120	16	8.23	21.20	1

TABLE 6.35. Reiter's Disease

Country/Population	Patients n	Patients %+	Controls n	Controls %+	RR	χ^2	Ref.
HLA-B27							
Navajo —A.I.	16	88	100	36	10.65	12.40	52
Canada	12	75	171	5	48.87	32.82	53
U.S.A.	99	77	202	8	36.88	109.70	13
U.S.A.	14	79	306	9	33.43	32.81	54
U.S.A.	30	63	104	4	36.01	38.16	10
U.S.A.	24	96	1863	8	184.85	48.73	2
U.S.A.	23	74	540	9	27.09	49.26	55
U.S.A.	30	80	65	8	39.87	37.67	19
U.S.A.	16	88	906	8	68.85	42.28	56
	236	78	3986	8	41.23	352.89	
	Heterogeneity χ^2 (6 df)					5.72	
Australia	6	100	306	8	146.77	20.99	57
New Zealand	38	82	514	7	56.58	86.73	58
England	63	75	33	6	37.35	29.31	59
England	20	65	150	8	19.94	31.93	60
England	50	68	194	8	23.36	64.68	21
England	33	76	33	6	38.61	25.81	1
	166	72	410	8	25.88	150.81	
	Heterogeneity χ^2 (3 df)					0.92	
France	46	80	152	4	85.57	72.64	61
West Germany	21	86	413	7	70.55	52.93	62
Denmark	48	65	2103	8	21.02	99.01	63
Denmark	26	77	1967	9	31.94	60.90	12
Denmark	9	89	562	8	65.02	27.35	64
	83	71	4632	8	26.32	185.25	
	Heterogeneity χ^2 (2 df)					2.01	
Finland	40	90	326	14	49.37	60.33	11
Finland	61	92	323	14	64.06	81.32	65
Finland	18	83	326	14	26.40	32.08	66
Finland	134	82	900	14	27.45	189.19	12
Finland	25	92	326	14	57.22	40.94	67
	278	86	2201	14	35.45	399.82	
	Heterogeneity χ^2 (4 df)					4.04	
Sweden	20	95	692	17	63.26	30.70	68
	906	80	13477	9	37.13	1374.35	
	Heterogeneity χ^2 (24 df)					23.93	

(134 Finnish and 30 Danish) Leirisalo et al.[12] found more severe acute disease (more frequent back pain, urologic symptoms, mucocutaneous manifestations, and a longer duration of the disease) and more frequent chronic back pain and sacroiliitis in patients with B27. A similar increase in disease severity has also been reported by Schultz et al.[13]. The sample in this study consisted of 86 Caucasians and 13 American Black patients. See also comments in reference 14.

Doury et al.[15] grouped their 46 French patients on the basis of living conditions. B27 was present in 57.9% of the patients living under poor hygienic conditions as compared with 81.8% in those living under normal hygienic conditions. The difference between the 2 groups was not significant. However, the frequency of B27 was found to be significantly increased ($p < 0.01$) in patients with long duration ($\geqslant 6$ months) of the disease (19/22 vs. 8/18 in group with disease of $\leqslant 5$ months duration).

In a followup study, Calin and Fries[16] reported data on an epidemic of post-*Shigella* Reiter's syndrome. Five of the original 10 patients were traced, HLA-typed, and clinically evaluated 13 years after the initial episode. Four patients had a chronic course, had persistent active disease, and were B27-positive. One had minimal disease, was without any symptons, and was also B27-negative.

In an interesting experiment, Dilley et al.[17] studied the susceptibility of B27-positive and -negative fibroblasts to *Chlamydia trachomatis, Ureaplasma, Urealyticum, Salmonella,* and *Yersinia*. There was no evidence for differential susceptibility related to the presence or absence of B27 antigen.

Family Data

Families with one or more affected individuals have been studied in several reports.[18–22] Linkage analysis is not available in any of these reports. There are very few families with 2 or more patients.[20,21,23] In these families, there are affected siblings with different haplotypes and healthy siblings who frequently carry the haplotype with the "disease gene."

See also refs. 24–48.

Diagnostic Value of HLA-B27 Test

In an interesting paper on the analysis of the predictive value of the HLA-B27 test, Khan and Khan,[49] using Bayes' theorem on some illustrative cases, have concluded that the B27 test has an overall greater clinical usefulness than the pelvic radiograph as an aid to diagnosis of Reiter's syndrome. This conclusion, however, has been argued in an accompanying editorial by Calin[50] and also in a subsequent comment by Merz.[51] Thus there is no general agreement on the clinical utility of the B27 test for this disease.

See also refs. 69—76.

References

1. Brewerton DA, Caffrey M, Nicholls A, Walters D, Oates JK, James DCO: Reiter's disease and HL-A27. Lancet ii:996-997, 1973
2. Morris R, Metzger AL, Bluestone R, Terasaki PI: HL-A W27- A clue to the diagnosis and pathogenesis of Reiter's syndrome. N Engl J Med 290:554-556, 1974
3. Good AE, Kawanishi H, Schultz JS: HLA B27 in blacks with ankylosing spondylitis or Reiter's disease. N Engl J Med 294:166-167, 1976
4. Khan MA, Askari AD, Braun WE, Aponte CJ: Low association of HLA-B27 with Reiter's syndrome in blacks. Ann Intern Med 90:202-203, 1979
5. Khan MA: Race-related differences in HLA association with ankylosing spondylitis and Reiter's disease in American blacks and whites. J Natl Med Assoc 70:41-42, 1978
6. Malaviya AN, Mehra NK, Adhar G, Jindal K, Bhargawa S, Batta RK, et al: HLA B27 in patients with seronegative spondarthritides. J Rheumatol 6:413-416, 1979
7. Kozin F, Duquesnoy R, Rodey GE, Lightfoot RW, Ryan LM Jr: High prevalence of HLA-CW1 and CW2 antigens in spondylarthritis. Arthritis Rheum 21:889-895, 1978
8. Kemple K, Gatti RA, Leibold W, Klinenberg J, Bluestone R: HLA-D locus typing in ankylosing spondylitis and Reiter's syndrome. Arthritis Rheum 22:371-375, 1979
9. Arnett FC, Hochberg MC, Bias W: Cross-reactive HLA antigens in B27-negative Reiter's syndrome and sacroiliitis. Johns Hopkins Med J 141:193-197, 1977
10. McClusky OE, Lordon RE, Arnett FC: HL-A 27 in Reiter's syndrome and psoriatic arthritis: A genetic factor in disease susceptibility and expression. J Rheumatol 1: 263-268, 1974
11. Aho K, Ahvonen P, Lassus A, Sievers K, Tiilikainen A: HL-A27 in reactive arthritis: A study of Yersinia arthritis and Reiter's disease. Arthritis Rheum 17:521-526, 1974
12. Leirisalo M, Skylv G, Kousa M, Voipio-Pulkki LM, Suoranta H, Nissila M, et al.: Followup study on patients with Reiter's disease and reactive arthritis, with special reference to HLA-B27. Arthritis Rheum 25:249-259, 1982
13. Schultz JS, Good AE, Sing CF, Kapur JJ: HLA profile and Reiter's syndrome. Clin Genet 19:159-167, 1981
14. Calin A, Marks SH: Reactive arthritis. Br Med J 281:311-312, 1980
15. Doury P, Pattin S, Roue R, Hainaut J: HLA-B27 antigen in ankylosing spondylitis and Reiter's disease. J Rheumatol (Suppl 3):110, 1977 (Abstr)
16. Calin A, Fries JF: An "experimental" epidemic of Reiter's syndrome revisited: Follow-up evidence on genetic and environmental factors. Ann Intern Med 84:564-566, 1976
17. Dilley D, Fan PT, Bluestone R: Absence of cytotoxic effect of selected pathogens on HLA B27 positive fibroblasts. Proc Soc Exp Biol Med 159:184-186, 1978

18. Arnett FC Jr, Schacter BZ, Hochberg MC Hsu S, Bias WB: Homozygosity for HLA-B27: Impact on rheumatic disease expression in two families. Arthritis Rheum 200:797-804, 1977
19. McCarthy MK, Gibbons RB, Jennings PB, Fariss BL, Goldenberg DL: Familial studies in HLA-B27 positive Reiter's syndrome. Milit Med 142:674-677, 1977
20. Kousa M, Lassus A, Karvonen J, Tillikainen A, Aho K: Family study of Reiter's disease and HLA B27 distribution. J Rheumatol 4:95-102, 1977
21. Woodrow JC, Treanor B, Usher N: The HL-A system in Reiter's syndrome. Tissue Antigens 4:533-540, 1974
22. Hochberg MC, Bias WB, Arnett FC: Family studies in HLA-B27 associated arthritis. Medicine 57:463-475, 1978
23. Yunus M, Calabro JJ, Miller KA, Masi AT: Family studies with HLA typing in Reiter's syndrome. Am J Med 70:1210-1214, 1981
24. Dequeker J, Decock T, Walravens M, Van De Putte I: A systematic survey of the HLA B27 prevalence in inflammatory rheumatic diseases. J Rheumatol 5:452-459, 1978
25. Brewerton DA: HL-A27 in Reiter's disease and psoriatic arthropathy. Int J Dermatol 14:39-40, 1975
26. Arnett FC, McClusky OE, Schacter BZ, Lordon RE: Incomplete Reiter's syndrome: Discriminating features and HL-A W27 in diagnosis. Ann Intern Med 84:8-12, 1976
27. Pajarre R, Kero M. Nail changes as the first manifestations of the HLA-B27 inheritance. Dermatologica 154:350-354, 1977
28. Khan M, Kushner I, Braun W: Low incidence of HLA-B27 in American blacks with spondyloarthropathies. Lancet i:483, 1976
29. Rose BS: Familial reactive arthritis of Reiter's and ankylosing spondylitis types in the HLA-B7 genotype. NZ Med J 83:107-109, 1976
30. Bluestone R, Pearson CM: Ankylosing spondylitis and Reiter's syndrome: Their interrelationship and association with HLA B27. Adv Intern Med 22: 1-19, 1977
31. Seignalet J, Sany J, Serre H: Interet pratique des groupes HL-A en rhumatologie. Semin Hop Paris 51:993-1000, 1975
32. Schumacher TM, Genant HK, Kellet MJ, Mall JC, Fye KH: HLA-B27 associated arthropathies. Radiology 126:289-297, 1978
33. Bluestone R, Goldberg LS, Weisbart RH, Morris RI, Holber OW: Aberrant immunity in (HL-A) W27-positive rheumatic disease. Ann Rheum Dis 34:46-48, 1975
34. Calin A: HLA-B27: To type or not to type? Ann Int Med 92:208-211, 1980
35. Kuthan F, Streda A, Parma R, Krepelkova M, Hill Z, Valnickova Z: Diagnostic importance of the incidence of tissue antigen HLA-B27 in some rheumatic diseases. Vnitr Lek 25:578-583, 1979
36. Arnett FC, Hochberg MC, Bias WB: HLA-C locus antigens in HLA-B27 associated arthritis. Arthritis Rheum 21:885-888, 1978
37. Jones MB, Smith PW, Olnhausen RW: Reiter's syndrome after salmonella infection: Occurrence in HLA-B27 positive brothers. Arthritis Rheum 22:1141, 1979
38. Alcalay M, Amor B, Haider F, Alcalay D, Orfila J, Tanzer J, et al: Ankylosing spondylitis and chlamydial infection in apparently healthy HLA B27 blood donors. J Rheumatol 6:439-446, 1979
39. Doury P, Pattin S, Roue R, Hainaut J: Relation entre antigene HLA B27 et pronostic a court terme du syndrome de fiessinger leroy reiter. Nouv Presse Med 5:2635-2636, 1976
40. Aho K, Ahvonen P, Lassus A, Sievers K, Tiilikainen A: Genetic background of reactive arthritis. Duodecim 90:824-831, 1974
41. Amor B, Feldmann JL, Delbarre F, Hors J, Beaujan MM, Dausset J: L'antigene HL-A W27 sa frequence dans la spondylarthrite ankylosante et le syndrome de fiessinger-leroy-reiter. Nouv Presse Med 3:1373-1374, 1974
42. Schulman P: Salicylate hepatotoxicity and HL-A W27. Ann Intern Med 84:754-755, 1976
43. Nasrallah NS, Masi AT, Chandler RW, Feigenbaum SL, Kaplan SB: HLA-B27 antigen and rheumatoid factor negative (seronegative) peripheral arthritis: Studies in younger patients with early-diagnosed arthritis. Am J Med 63:379-386, 1977
44. Vischer TL, Jeannet M, Boussina I: HL-A27 diagnosis of rheumatic diseases. Lancet i:1001, 1974
45. Calin A, Fries JF: Ankylosing spondylitis and epidemic Reiter's syndrome: Genetics and environment. Ann Rheum Dis 35:287, 1976
46. Keat AC, Barnes RMR: HL-A27-associated arthritis. Rheumatol Rehabil 15:87-91, 1976
47. Rosenthal M, Thiel G: Reitersche krankheit nach salmonella-infektion bei einem HLA-B27-trager. Schweiz Med Wochenschr 110:920-922, 1980
48. Calin AC, Barnett M: HLA 27 positive, negative, or both? N Engl J Med 302:1366-1367, 1980
49. Khan MA, Khan MK: Diagnostic value of HLA-B27 testing in ankylosing spondylitis and Reiter's syndrome. Ann Intern Med 96:70-76, 1982
50. Editorial: HLA-B27 in 1982: Reappraisal of a clinical test. Ann Intern Med 96:114-115, 1982
51. Merz D: Non-utility of the HLA-B27 test. Ann Intern Med 96:383-384, 1982
52. Morse HG, Rate RG, Bonnell MD, Kuberski T: High frequency of HLA-B27 and Reiter's syndrome in Navajo Indians. J Rheumatol 7:900-902, 1980

53. Esdaile JM, Dwosh IL, Urowitz MB, Smythe HA, Falk J: HLA B27 in rheumatoid factor-negative polyarthritis. Ann Intern Med 86:699-702, 1977
54. Duquesnoy RJ, Kozin F, Rodey GE: High prevalence of HLA-B27, CW1 and CW2 in patients with seronegative spondyloarthritis. Tissue Antigens 12:58-62, 1978
55. Mills DM, Arai Y, Gupta RC: HL-A antigens and sacroiliitis. JAMA 231:268-270, 1975
56. McGlamory JC: HL-A27 in Reiter's syndrome. Milit Med 141:95-96, 1976
57. Cross RA, Rigby R, Dawkins RL: The significance of HL-A W27 in ankylosing spondylitis and Reiter's syndrome with three family studies. Aust NZ J Med 5:108-111, 1975
58. Caughey DE, Hawkes JG, Mills KR, Douglas R: Reiter's disease and HL-A27. Curr Med Res Opin 2:17-22, 1974
59. Nicholls A: Reiter's disease and HL-A27. Ann Rheum Dis 34:27-28, 1975
60. Woodrow JC: HL-A27 and Reiter's syndrome. Lancet ii:671-672, 1973
61. Amor B, Feldmann JL, Delbarre F, Hors J, Beaujan MM, Dausset J: HL-A antigen W27- A genetic link between ankylosing spondylitis and Reiter's syndrome? N Engl J Med 290:572, 1974
62. Lange CE, Muller N: HLA-B27 bei morbus reiter unter besonderer berucksichtigung oligosymptomatischer verlaufsformen. Z Hautkr 52:1153-1159, 1977
63. Zachariae H, Friis J, Graudal H, Hjorthoj A, Kissmeyer-Nielsen F, Svejgaard A, et al.: Reiter's disease and the histocompatibility antigen, HL-A27. Scand J Rheumatol 4:13-15, 1975
64. Zachariae H, Hjortshoj A, Kissmeyer-Nielsen F: Reiter's disease and HL-A27. Lancet ii:565-566, 1973
65. Aho K, Ahvonen P, Alkio P, Sairanen E, Sievars K, Tiilikainen A: HL-A27 in reactive arthritis following infection. Ann Rheum Dis 34:29-30, 1975
66. Isomaki H, Koota K, Martio J, Nissila M, Tiilikainen A: HL-A27 and arthritis. Ann Clin Res 7:138-145, 1975
67. Kousa M, Tiilikainen A, Karvonen J, Lassus A: Psoriatic arthritis and Reiter's disease: HLA antigens in mixed cases. Ann Clin Res 8:312-316, 1976
68. Bjelle A, Cedergren B, Dahlqvist SR: HLA B27 in the population of northern Sweden. Scand J Rheumatol 11:23-26, 1982
69. Kuberski T: Histocompatibility antigens and the sexually transmitted diseases. Am Vener Dis Assoc 7:203-205, 1980
70. Rosenbaum JT: Why HLA-B27: An analysis based on two animal models. Ann Intern Med 94:261-263, 1981
71. Friis J: Reiter's disease with childhood onset having special reference to HLA B27. Scand J Rheumatol 9:250-252, 1980
72. Rate RG, Morse HG, Bonnel MD, Kuberski TT: "Navajo arthritis" reconsidered: Relationship to HLA-B27. Arthritis Rheum 23:1299-1302, 1980
73. Hodinka L, Geher P, Meretey K, Gyodi EK, Petranyi GG, Bozsoky S: Lavamisole-induced neutropenia and agranulocytosis: Association of HLA B27 leukocyte agglutinating and lymphocytotoxic antibodies. Int Arch Allergy Appl Immunol 65:460-464, 1981
74. Sach JA: HLA systems and rheumatic diseases. Curr Top Pathol 71:235-262, 1982
75. Leirisalo M, Skylv G, Kousa M, Voipio-Pulkki LM, Suoranta H, Nissila M, et al.: HLA-B27 and clinical characteristics of reactive arthritis. Scand J Rheumatol 42:9, 1982
76. Seedat YK, Duminiet H: Reiter's syndrome in a Black patient. S Afr Med J 61:289, 1982

CHAPTER 7

Dermatology

Psoriasis Vulgaris

Population Association

HLA-A and -B Loci

The association of psoriasis with HLA-B13 and -B17 in American Caucasian populations was first reported by Russell et al.[1] and White et al.[2] in 1972. Since then, several investigators have observed these associations in Caucasian patients from the United States, Canada, and various European and Asian countries (Table 7.1). However, the association with B13 is not consistent in all of the studies. This discrepancy cannot be attributed to the differences between the populations or the sample size. Other studies on the same populations with smaller sample size reported a significant increase in the frequency of B13. This type of discrepancy was probably the result of serologic and/or technical problems associated with typing some of the HLA specificities. Data on the frequency of B17 in various Caucasian groups are more consistent; all of the studies reported a significant increase in frequency. The combined estimate of relative risk for all the Caucasian groups is 5.30 (Table 7.1). In later studies, B37 was also significantly increased in psoriasis patients.

The pooled analyses of all the Caucasian groups also showed that the frequencies of B7, B8, and B12 were significantly decreased in the patient groups. However, as is apparent from the data in Table 7.1, a significant decrease was not observed in all the studies.

The frequencies of B13 and B17 were also increased, though not significantly, in Ashkenazi Jewish patients studied during the Seventh International Histocompatibility Workshop[3] and by Gazit et al.[4] A significant increase in the frequency of B37 was observed in both studies.

Tsuji et al.[5] and Hawkins et al.[6] did not find any difference in the frequencies of B13 and B17 in Japanese patients. In the Seventh Histocompatibility Workshop data,[3] however, a significant increase of B13 was observed. There was a significant heterogeneity between these 2 data sets. The antigen B37 was significantly associated with psoriasis in Japanese.

HLA-C Locus

Ryder and Svejgaard[7] indicated in 1977 that antigen T7 (now called CW6) showed an association stronger than that with HLA-B13 and -B17 in a Danish population. Data collected during the Seventh Histocompatibility Workshop (ref. 3; see also Scandinavian Regional Report in the same book) showed for the first time that psoriasis was more frequently associated with CW6 than with B13, B17, or B37. This was further confirmed by the data from several studies given in Table 7.1. The association of CW6 with psoriasis also seemed to be stronger than that of B locus antigens in Japanese patients.

HLA-D/DR Locus

Grosse-Wilde et al.[8] first reported that a locally defined specificity, HLA-D EI (DW11), was significantly increased in a sample of 72 German patients. The relative risk of 5.35 for EI was higher than that with B13 or B17. Another locally defined specificity, DMA, was shown by McMichael et al.[9] to be greatly increased, with a relative risk of 10.85 in 38 American Caucasian patients.

Raffoux et al.[10] first reported an association of DR7 with psoriasis in a group of 40 French patients (Table 7.1). Since then this association has been confirmed in several studies on Caucasian and Japanese patients (Table 7.1). It should be noted that the combined estimate of relative risk for DR7 in Caucasians is less than that for B13, B17, B37, and CW6.

Nature of the Primary Association

On the basis of the higher relative risk associated with CW6 and the existence of linkage disequilibrium between CW6 and B13 and between CW6 and B17, it can be concluded that the association of psoriasis with either B13 or B17 is secondary to that with CW6. The relative risk values for CW6 are also higher than for DR7 in Caucasian and Japanese patients (Table 7.1), and there is a significant linkage disequilibrium between CW6 and DR7. Furthermore, a significant linkage disequilibrium also exists between DR7 and B13 and between DR7 and B17. Thus, at present it seems (on the basis of relative risk) that the primary association of psoriasis is with CW6. It should also be noted that psoriasis is the only disease showing a strong association with an antigen of the C locus.

Disease Heterogeneity

Age at Onset

In the original papers of Russell et al.[1] and White et al.[2], it was observed that the age at onset was significantly lower (< 35 years) in patients with B13 and B17. This correlation was confirmed in subsequent reports by several investigators (e.g., refs. 6, 11). Brenner et al.[12] reported that the patients with onset between 10 and 20 years showed a significantly higher frequency of CW6 than patients with onset between 35 and 45 years. In the data of Tiwari et al.[13] and Hawkins et al.[6] DR7 was also found to be significantly increased in patients with age at onset < 35 years.

However, in 112 Japanese patients studied during the Eighth International Histocompatibility Workshop,[6] B37, BW39, and CW6 were found to be significantly increased in all 3 groups: total sample, age at onset < 35 years, and those with age at onset ⩾ 35 years.

Relatives

A significant correlation between B17 and the presence of psoriasis in close relatives was also observed by White et al.[2] The frequency of the disease among close relatives of B17 patients was 16.3%, as compared with only 5.4%, 1.5%, and 8.1% for B13, B12, and "all others," respectively. Similar results were also reported by Svejgaard et al.,[14] Gunn et al.,[15] Woodrow et al.,[16] Moller et al.,[11] and Krulig et al.[17] However, in a sample of 1054 German patients,[18] no correlation with family history was observed.

Body Surface

Krulig et al.[17] reported that B16 and/or B17 were associated with psoriasis that involved > 50% of the body surface as well as nails.

Streptococcal Infection

An association between B13 and a history of antecedent severe streptococcal infection was observed by Krain et al.[19] A study by Gross et al.[20] of antistreptolysin-O titers in 110 German patients showed that the mean value of the titer was significantly lower in B13- positive patients, and it was hypothesized that this may have been the reason for the correlation between streptococcal infection and B13 positivity reported by Krain et al.[19] In a study of cellular immune responses in 28 hospitalized patients,[20] specific cell-mediated immunity to A-streptococcal cell wall and cell membrane antigen occurred significantly more often in patients than in controls. However, no significant correlation between HLA (B13 and B17) and cellular immune reactivity to A-streptococcal antigen or clinical course was found. The frequency of a history of antecedent streptococcal infection was also studied by Svejgaard et al.[14] They found no difference among B13-positive, B17-positive, B13-negative, and B17-negative patients. The frequency of various HLA antigens in the patients with high (or low) antistreptolysin-O titer was the same. Thus, these 2 reports contradicted the results of Krain et al.[19] and Bertrams et al.[21]

Clinical Status

Turowski et al.[22] subgrouped 136 Polish patients on the basis of their clinical status. The skin lesions of the patients in the first subgroup were stationary for a long period of time. The second subgroup consisted of patients with peripheral spreading of skin lesions. The patients in the third subgroup were characterized by "very rapid occurrence of small papules and their high aptitude to disseminate."[22] No significant difference between the subgroups was found.

Extent of Skin Lesions

Turowski et al.[22] reported a higher frequency of B17 (66.67%) in 42 patients who had lesions on > 50%

> 50% of the skin as compared with only 28.72% in 94 patients with lesions on < 50% of the skin.

Family History
In the report of Tiwari et al.[13] 10 of the 17 patients (58.82%) with a positive family history of psoriasis were positive for DR7 as compared with 16 of 39 patients (41.03%) without a family history (p = 0.0002).

Presence of Arthritis
DR7 was also found to be increased (52.50%) in 40 patients with arthritis reported by Tiwari et al.[13] Its frequency in 24 patients without arthritis was 33.33% (p = 0.0001).

Thalassotherapy
In a study by Zlatkov et al.[23] 192 Bulgarian patients were evaluated after 4 weeks of thalassotherapy. Fifty (26.04%) were in full clinical remission, 116 (60.42%) showed great or moderate improvement, and 26 patients (13.54%) did not show any improvement. B13 and B17 frequencies did not differ significantly among the 3 groups of patients.

Case Rate
An interesting analysis of the correlation between HLA antigen frequency and psoriasis case rate (percentage of psoriasis cases reported from a dermatologic clinic or a special survey) has been made by Thomas.[24] The case rate was significantly correlated (RR = 0.8242) with B17 but not with B13. It was indicated that this may be the result of "two genotypes for the etiology of psoriasis." However, if the primary association of psoriasis is with CW6 or DR7, then any analysis in terms of B13 and B17 may not provide useful information.

Family Data

Psoriasis is an inherited disease, but the actual mode of inheritance is not well established. Genetic hypotheses—including the occurrence of irregular dominant gene, incomplete sex-limited gene, 2 pairs of autosomal recessive genes, and polygenes—have been proposed by various workers to explain the pedigree data (see refs. 25-28, as well as the studies cited in these papers). After reviewing the data of many authors, Kimberling and Dobson[27] concluded that an autosomal dominant pattern of inheritance seems most consistent with the available data. In McKusick's[29] catalog of "Mendelian Inheritance in Man" psoriasis is listed under the category of dominantly inherited disorders with an additional notation to indicate "inheritance proved (in the judgment of the author)."

Many investigators have studied the segregation of HLA antigens in families with at least 2 affected individuals.[1,2,14–17,30–39] It is clear from their data that the disease can develop in the absence of B13, B17, and other associated antigens, and frequently within a family the "psoriasis gene" does not segregate with the "marker haplotype." Pietrzyk et al.[39] analyzed 39 Polish families with 7 pairs of siblings affected with psoriasis. In this sib pair test the authors could not find significant evidence of linkage with HLA. The observed number of sib pairs were also found to be consistent with the distribution expected for a recessive as well as the dominant mode of inheritance for the disease gene. In another study of multiple-case families (number unknown) Svejgaard et al.[14] calculated a recombination frequency of 13% between a hypothetical psoriasis locus and HLA.

It should be noted that in the aforementioned studies complete pedigree data for all of the families and the methods of ascertainment are not available. Thus, it is difficult to perform any appropriate genetic analysis on the pooled data.

However, family data with complete pedigree diagrams have been reported by Karvonen et al.[31] (all of the families were selected for the presence of B13 or B17), Civatte et al.,[32] and Espinoza et al.[37] Thirteen families with at least 2 affected individuals were also studied during the Eighth International Histocompatibility Workshop. A linkage analysis using the lod score method was done on these pedigrees, excluding those of Karvonen et al.[31]; the total lod score data are given in Table 7.2. Assuming a dominant mode of inheritance of the "psoriasis gene," there is significant evidence of tight linkage (lod score 3.54) at the penetrance values of 10%-25%. Strong evidence of linkage also exists at penetrance values ranging from 25% to 50% (Table 7.2). However, at these levels of penetrance the linkage is quite loose. This indication of loose linkage may be the consequence of genetic heterogeneity of the disease or problems associated with the mode of inheritance of the disease gene specified in the statistical model. It should be pointed out that similar patterns of lod scores have been observed in diseases such as diabetes and multiple sclerosis.

See also refs. 40–70 and 91–97.

TABLE 7.1. Psoriasis Vulgaris

Country/Population	Patients n	Patients %+	Controls n	Controls %+	RR	χ^2	Ref.
HLA-A1							
Singapore—Chinese	70	6	330	0	46.86	12.23	71
China	60	35	100	10	4.69	13.86	72
	130	19	430	2	6.25	22.26	
	Heterogeneity χ^2 (1 df)					3.83	
HLA-B7							
Canada	24	16	200	17	1.01	0.00	73
Canada	32	22	160	14	1.79	1.58	74
	56	19	360	16	1.40	0.94	
	Heterogeneity χ^2 (1 df)					0.64	
U.S.A.	101	14	113	32	0.35	9.23	17
U.S.A.	60	8	126	31	0.21	10.73	75
U.S.A.	156	13	386	22	0.54	5.53	2
U.S.A.	44	18	89	20	0.90	0.05	1
	361	13	714	25	0.46	19.68	
	Heterogeneity χ^2 (3 df)					5.85	
Bulgaria	192	9	1085	10	0.91	0.13	23
Czechoslovakia	45	6	231	26	0.21	7.64	76
Hungary	80	15	450	20	0.73	0.97	77
Yugoslavia	65	8	302	18	0.43	3.61	78
England	61	16	204	33	0.40	6.23	15
England	125	15	233	32	0.38	11.66	16
	186	15	437	32	0.39	17.88	
	Heterogeneity χ^2 (1 df)					0.01	
France	31	13	591	19	0.70	0.52	32
France	110	6	231	18	0.31	8.14	79
	141	8	822	19	0.43	7.04	
	Heterogeneity χ^2 (1 df)					1.62	
West Germany	90	10	353	20	0.46	4.55	80
West Germany	104	16	442	28	0.50	6.06	18
West Germany	72	22	5046	27	0.78	0.80	8
	266	16	5841	27	0.58	9.62	
	Heterogeneity χ^2 (2 df)					1.78	
Denmark	76	11	562	35	0.24	15.65	14
Denmark	80	15	1541	27	0.49	5.28	14
	156	13	2103	29	0.36	18.65	
	Heterogeneity χ^2 (1 df)					2.28	
Finland	45	20	326	29	0.64	1.45	81
Finland	37	11	900	24	0.43	3.02	82
Finland	10	10	326	29	0.39	1.48	83
Finland	125	18	326	29	0.55	5.50	84
	217	17	1878	27	0.54	10.87	
	Heterogeneity χ^2 (3 df)					0.58	

TABLE 7.1. *(continued)*

Country/Population	Patients n	Patients %+	Controls n	Controls %+	RR	χ^2	Ref.
HLA-B7							
Norway	50	12	788	30	0.34	6.79	11
Sweden	51	26	93	28	0.91	0.05	85
Sweden	50	14	100	29	0.42	3.91	86
Sweden	87	24	198	41	0.46	7.38	87
	188	22	391	35	0.55	8.82	
	Heterogeneity χ^2 (2 df)					2.52	
	2003	14	15402	25	0.52	89.88	
	Heterogeneity χ^2 (26 df)					38.06	
HLA-B8							
Canada	32	16	160	21	0.76	0.31	74
Canada	24	21	200	24	0.90	0.05	73
	56	18	360	23	0.83	0.31	
	Heterogeneity χ^2 (1 df)					0.05	
U.S.A.	44	14	89	20	0.68	0.64	1
U.S.A.	156	10	386	16	0.60	3.10	2
U.S.A.	101	16	113	22	0.68	1.22	17
	301	13	588	18	0.64	4.85	
	Heterogeneity χ^2 (2 df)					0.11	
Bulgaria	192	8	1085	13	0.60	3.55	23
Czechoslovakia	45	12	231	19	0.62	1.08	76
Hungary	80	4	450	19	0.20	9.58	77
Yugoslavia	65	17	302	14	1.29	0.51	78
England	125	17	233	32	0.44	9.02	16
England	61	18	204	28	0.58	2.32	15
	186	17	437	30	0.49	10.96	
	Heterogeneity χ^2 (1 df)					0.37	
France	31	6	591	17	0.39	2.28	32
France	110	12	231	16	0.73	0.87	79
	141	11	822	17	0.64	2.36	
	Heterogeneity χ^2 (1 df)					0.80	
West Germany	104	13	442	19	0.65	1.91	18
West Germany	72	15	5046	19	0.78	0.60	8
West Germany	90	10	353	20	0.46	4.55	80
	266	13	5841	19	0.63	5.88	
	Heterogeneity χ^2 (2 df)					1.19	
Denmark	76	17	562	23	0.70	1.26	14
Denmark	80	10	1541	24	0.37	7.66	14
	156	13	2103	24	0.53	7.10	
	Heterogeneity χ^2 (1 df)					1.82	

TABLE 7.1. *(continued)*

Country/Population	Patients n	Patients %+	Controls n	Controls %+	RR	χ^2	Ref.
HLA-B8							
Finland	45	4	326	18	0.24	5.14	81
Finland	37	5	900	20	0.26	4.62	82
Finland	10	0	326	18	0.22	2.12	83
Finland	125	7	326	18	0.36	8.00	84
	217	6	1878	19	0.30	19.37	
	Heterogeneity χ^2 (3 df)					0.52	
Norway	50	22	788	25	0.87	0.16	11
Sweden	51	18	93	28	0.58	1.70	85
Sweden	50	18	100	16	1.17	0.13	86
Sweden	87	15	198	25	0.54	3.37	87
	188	17	391	23	0.68	3.07	
	Heterogeneity χ^2 (2 df)					2.13	
	1943	12	15276	20	0.59	49.73	
	Heterogeneity χ^2 (25 df)					26.02	
HLA-B12							
Canada	32	19	160	24	0.78	0.29	74
Canada	24	16	200	31	0.47	2.11	73
	56	18	360	28	0.62	1.85	
	Heterogeneity χ^2 (1 df)					0.55	
U.S.A.	156	10	386	23	0.38	11.38	2
U.S.A.	44	23	89	25	0.91	0.05	1
U.S.A.	101	16	113	22	0.68	1.22	17
	301	14	588	23	0.55	9.16	
	Heterogeneity χ^2 (2 df)					3.49	
Bulgaria	192	11	1085	18	0.57	5.40	23
Czechoslovakia	45	16	231	27	0.54	2.23	76
Hungary	80	9	450	23	0.35	7.43	77
Yugoslavia	65	15	302	18	0.83	0.26	78
England	61	33	204	36	0.88	0.17	15
England	125	38	233	27	1.66	4.63	16
	186	36	437	31	1.31	2.12	
	Heterogeneity χ^2 (1 df)					2.68	
France	31	13	591	29	0.40	3.40	32
France	110	26	231	34	0.69	2.16	79
	141	23	822	30	0.61	4.63	
	Heterogeneity χ^2 (1 df)					0.93	
West Germany	90	16	353	19	0.83	0.36	80
West Germany	104	13	442	24	0.49	5.64	18
West Germany	72	15	5046	23	0.61	2.35	8
	266	15	5841	23	0.63	6.83	
	Heterogeneity χ^2 (2 df)					1.52	

TABLE 7.1. *(continued)*

Country/Population	Patients n	Patients %+	Controls n	Controls %+	RR	χ^2	Ref.
HLA-B12							
Denmark	76	26	562	22	1.26	0.71	14
Denmark	80	18	1541	26	0.64	2.37	14
	156	22	2103	25	0.91	0.20	
	Heterogeneity χ^2 (1 df)					2.88	
Finland	45	13	326	15	0.90	0.06	81
Finland	125	12	326	15	0.79	0.60	84
Finland	10	20	326	15	1.65	0.54	83
Finland	37	8	900	15	0.57	1.12	82
	217	12	1878	15	0.83	0.73	
	Heterogeneity χ^2 (3 df)					1.58	
Norway	50	14	788	29	0.42	4.85	11
Sweden	50	14	100	15	0.95	0.01	86
Sweden	87	26	198	29	0.87	0.24	87
	137	22	298	24	0.89	0.23	
	Heterogeneity χ^2 (1 df)					0.03	
	1892	18	15183	23	0.73	22.90	
	Heterogeneity χ^2 (24 df)					36.67	
HLA-B13							
Singapore—Chinese	70	37	330	19	2.51	10.73	71
China	60	62	100	18	7.22	29.39	72
Japan	54	7	66	6	1.18	0.06	5
Japan	40	17	123	1	15.31	12.12	3
Japan	112	6	805	3	2.16	3.31	6
	206	8	994	3	2.63	8.80	
	Heterogeneity χ^2 (2 df)					6.69	
	336	24	1424	8	3.33	42.88	
	Heterogeneity χ^2 (4 df)					12.74	
Jews—Ashkenazi	29	14	384	6	2.75	3.65	3
Jews (unspecified)	46	15	368	7	2.44	4.14	4
	75	15	752	6	2.56	7.77	
	Heterogeneity χ^2 (1 df)					0.03	
Caucasians (unspecified)	63	6	1506	6	1.12	0.05	6
Canada	32	13	160	8	1.83	1.18	74
Canada	24	16	200	5	3.81	5.11	73
Canada	25	20	384	6	4.12	7.75	3
	81	16	744	6	3.09	12.70	
	Heterogeneity χ^2 (2 df)					1.34	
U.S.A.	101	9	113	7	1.30	0.30	17
U.S.A.	44	27	89	3	10.40	13.99	1
U.S.A.	156	15	386	5	3.33	14.41	2
U.S.A.	66	17	558	4	4.98	17.84	13
U.S.A.	60	15	126	4	4.04	6.66	75
	427	15	1272	5	3.62	45.04	
	Heterogeneity χ^2 (4 df)					8.17	

TABLE 7.1. *(continued)*

Country/Population	Patients n	Patients %+	Controls n	Controls %+	RR	χ^2	Ref.
HLA-B13							
Bulgaria	192	20	1085	7	3.33	31.63	23
Czechoslovakia	45	51	231	9	10.29	40.03	76
Hungary	80	35	450	9	5.43	35.82	77
Poland	136	30	240	14	2.62	13.62	22
Yugoslavia	65	22	302	7	3.76	13.14	78
England	126	7	233	5	1.45	0.70	16
England	61	20	204	3	7.72	17.31	15
	187	11	437	4	3.05	11.56	
	Heterogeneity χ^2 (1 df)					6.45	
France	31	10	591	3	3.99	5.74	32
France	83	13	264	5	2.85	6.34	88
France	110	13	231	4	3.51	8.87	79
France	40	18	340	5	4.27	10.04	10
	264	13	1426	4	3.53	30.50	
	Heterogeneity χ^2 (3 df)					0.49	
West Germany	104	23	442	8	3.44	18.53	18
West Germany	72	19	5046	6	3.77	19.91	8
West Germany	90	33	353	7	6.48	38.44	80
	266	25	5841	6	4.34	74.23	
	Heterogeneity χ^2 (2 df)					2.64	
Austria	77	30	450	5	8.07	41.70	12
Denmark	80	15	1541	4	4.35	19.98	14
Denmark	76	21	562	3	8.55	34.56	14
Denmark	45	7	1967	4	2.06	1.87	89
	201	15	4070	4	4.88	51.24	
	Heterogeneity χ^2 (2 df)					5.18	
Finland	125	24	326	8	3.61	19.87	84
Finland	10	24	326	8	4.05	4.34	83
Finland	37	35	900	6	8.51	35.01	82
Finland	40	40	384	6	10.34	38.12	3
Finland	45	24	326	8	3.68	11.07	81
	257	28	2262	7	5.40	100.77	
	Heterogeneity χ^2 (4 df)					7.63	
Norway	50	8	788	2	4.60	8.25	11
Sweden	51	8	93	4	2.05	1.18	85
Sweden	50	4	100	2	2.03	0.72	86
Sweden	87	7	198	1	6.41	6.99	87
	188	6	391	2	3.06	7.18	
	Heterogeneity χ^2 (2 df)					1.71	
	2579	19	21495	5	4.13	488.39	
	Heterogeneity χ^2 (35 df)					62.68	

TABLE 7.1. *(continued)*

Country/Population	Patients n	Patients %+	Controls n	Controls %+	RR	χ^2	Ref.
HLA-BW16							
Canada	24	13	200	1	13.44	10.77	73
U.S.A.	101	22	113	5	5.03	12.11	17
Bulgaria	192	7	1085	8	0.89	0.15	23
Yugoslavia	65	3	302	5	0.71	0.28	78
England	61	7	204	3	2.50	2.38	15
France	31	10	591	7	1.67	0.86	32
West Germany	72	13	5046	3	5.03	21.94	8
West Germany	104	11	442	3	4.00	11.76	18
	176	12	5488	3	4.57	33.52	
	Heterogeneity χ^2 (1 df)					0.19	
Denmark	80	9	1541	5	1.98	3.15	14
Denmark	76	9	562	5	1.97	2.58	14
	156	9	2103	5	1.98	5.73	
	Heterogeneity χ^2 (1 df)					0.00	
Finland	45	13	326	12	1.16	0.11	81
Finland	125	12	326	12	1.02	0.00	84
Finland	37	19	900	9	2.48	4.87	82
Finland	10	20	326	12	2.13	1.21	83
	217	14	1878	11	1.41	2.69	
	Heterogeneity χ^2 (3 df)					3.50	
Sweden	50	8	100	5	1.68	0.68	86
	1073	11	12064	5	1.97	36.31	
	Heterogeneity χ^2 (14 df)					36.55	
HLA-B17							
Singapore—Chinese	70	14	330	14	1.03	0.01	71
China	60	27	100	6	5.48	12.38	72
Japan	40	2	123	1	2.31	0.68	3
Japan	54	2	66	0	3.93	1.24	5
	94	2	189	1	2.87	1.81	
	Heterogeneity χ^2 (1 df)					0.11	
	224	12	619	9	1.99	6.37	
	Heterogeneity χ^2 (3 df)					7.93	
Jews—Ashkenazi	29	14	384	5	3.32	5.00	3
Jews (unspecified)	46	24	368	15	1.83	2.77	4
	75	20	752	10	2.21	6.93	
	Heterogeneity χ^2 (1 df)					0.85	
Canada	25	28	384	5	7.52	17.70	3
Canada	24	21	200	6	4.29	7.13	73
Canada	32	28	160	11	3.17	6.58	74
	81	26	744	7	4.63	29.66	
	Heterogeneity χ^2 (2 df)					1.75	

TABLE 7.1. *(continued)*

Country/Population	Patients n	Patients %+	Controls n	Controls %+	RR	χ^2	Ref.
HLA-B17							
U.S.A.	101	31	113	6	6.64	19.60	17
U.S.A.	66	21	558	9	2.73	9.40	13
U.S.A.	156	26	386	8	4.01	28.90	2
U.S.A.	44	23	89	9	2.96	4.86	1
U.S.A.	60	38	126	8	6.80	22.01	75
	427	28	1272	8	4.12	79.99	
	Heterogeneity χ^2 (4 df)					4.78	
Bulgaria	192	24	1085	6	4.95	57.91	23
Czechoslovakia	45	20	231	9	2.58	5.04	76
Hungary	80	31	450	10	4.05	24.21	77
Poland	136	40	240	11	5.32	39.20	22
Yugoslavia	65	34	302	8	5.88	28.67	78
England	61	46	204	10	7.52	35.10	15
England	125	50	233	6	15.16	71.90	16
	186	49	437	8	10.91	104.76	
	Heterogeneity χ^2 (1 df)					2.24	
France	31	58	591	7	17.96	55.82	32
France	40	25	300	6	5.26	15.36	10
France	110	22	231	4	6.53	22.96	79
France	83	27	264	4	8.61	31.03	88
	264	28	1386	6	8.73	119.70	
	Heterogeneity χ^2 (3 df)					5.47	
West Germany	104	22	442	8	3.25	16.56	18
West Germany	90	33	353	11	3.97	24.67	80
West Germany	72	25	5046	8	3.90	25.19	8
	266	27	5841	8	3.71	66.12	
	Heterogeneity χ^2 (2 df)					0.30	
Austria	77	35	450	8	6.17	39.02	12
Denmark	80	36	1541	8	6.49	56.94	14
Denmark	76	28	562	8	4.49	26.07	14
Denmark	45	29	1967	8	4.79	22.63	89
	201	31	4070	8	5.36	104.56	
	Heterogeneity χ^2 (2 df)					1.08	
Finland	125	18	326	4	5.17	21.31	84
Finland	40	16	384	5	3.75	8.08	3
Finland	45	29	326	4	9.67	29.26	81
Finland	37	19	900	4	5.85	16.88	82
Finland	10	60	326	4	33.44	29.52	83
	257	21	2262	4	6.82	95.92	
	Heterogeneity χ^2 (4 df)					9.13	

TABLE 7.1. *(continued)*

Country/Population	Patients n	Patients %+	Controls n	Controls %+	RR	χ^2	Ref.
HLA-B17							
Norway	50	20	788	6	4.02	14.10	11
Sweden	51	28	93	7	4.93	10.75	85
Sweden	87	10	198	1	9.25	10.85	87
Sweden	50	22	100	5	5.06	9.20	86
	188	18	391	3	5.71	30.15	
	Heterogeneity χ^2 (2 df)					0.65	
	2515	29	19949	7	5.30	808.88	
	Heterogeneity χ^2 (34 df)					55.54	
HLA-B37							
Japan	54	20	66	5	4.30	5.98	5
Japan	112	14	805	2	7.95	33.06	6
Japan	40	35	123	2	22.37	24.09	3
	206	20	994	2	8.49	59.46	
	Heterogeneity χ^2 (2 df)					3.68	
Jews—Ashkenazi	29	10	384	2	5.89	7.64	3
Jews (unspecified)	46	7	368	2	3.95	4.94	4
	75	8	752	2	4.79	12.38	
	Heterogeneity χ^2 (1 df)					0.20	
Caucasians (unspecified)	63	11	1506	3	4.20	12.42	6
Canada	25	4	384	2	2.82	1.63	3
Canada	32	6	160	2	3.36	2.38	74
	57	5	544	2	3.09	3.99	
	Heterogeneity χ^2 (1 df)					0.02	
England	61	2	204	0	11.67	4.10	15
France	31	0	591	2	0.75	0.08	32
West Germany	72	4	5046	2	2.37	2.63	8
Austria	77	9	450	2	4.89	10.40	12
Denmark	45	16	424	1	17.83	24.34	89
Finland	125	6	505	1	6.11	11.17	84
Finland	40	2	384	2	1.51	0.24	3
Finland	45	9	505	1	9.90	13.50	81
Finland	37	3	900	2	2.11	1.01	82
	247	5	2294	2	4.57	21.27	
	Heterogeneity χ^2 (3 df)					4.66	
Norway	50	4	788	2	2.45	1.94	11
Sweden	51	12	93	5	2.52	2.43	85
Sweden	50	6	100	3	2.05	0.97	86
	101	9	193	4	2.32	3.36	
	Heterogeneity χ^2 (1 df)					0.05	
	804	7	12040	2	3.95	71.14	
	Heterogeneity χ^2 (14 df)					18.10	
HLA-BW57							
Caucasians (unspecified)	63	19	1506	7	3.20	12.72	6

TABLE 7.1. *(continued)*

Country/Population	Patients n	Patients %+	Controls n	Controls %+	RR	χ^2	Ref.
HLA-CW6							
Singapore—Chinese	70	4	88	6	0.70	0.28	71
Japan	112	23	805	3	9.60	56.90	6
Japan	40	55	40	5	18.73	18.87	90
Japan	40	53	123	7	14.18	33.76	3
	192	36	968	4	11.54	108.43	
	Heterogeneity χ^2 (2 df)					1.10	
	262	27	1056	4	8.50	93.16	
	Heterogeneity χ^2 (3 df)					16.65	
Jews—Ashkenazi	29	34	384	23	1.76	2.04	3
Jews (unspecified)	46	48	98	15	5.10	16.68	4
	75	43	482	21	2.98	15.13	
	Heterogeneity χ^2 (1 df)					3.59	
Caucasians (unspecified)	63	51	1506	18	4.73	36.58	6
Canada	25	64	384	23	5.79	17.79	3
U.S.A.	60	50	126	13	6.52	26.83	75
Austria	77	74	125	26	7.89	40.51	12
Finland	37	46	462	7	11.21	43.10	82
Finland	40	50	405	7	13.07	50.07	3
	77	48	867	7	12.12	93.09	
	Heterogeneity χ^2 (1 df)					0.09	
Sweden	51	48	93	7	11.47	27.04	85
	353	56	3101	15	7.51	233.81	
	Heterogeneity χ^2 (6 df)					8.12	
HLA-DMA							
U.S.A.	38	42	142	6	10.85	26.45	9
HLA-DW-EI							
West Germany	72	22	394	5	5.35	22.00	8
HLA-DR7							
Japan	108	6	792	1	6.38	13.36	6
Japan	40	20	33	0	17.52	7.00	90
	148	10	825	1	7.65	19.65	
	Heterogeneity χ^2 (1 df)					0.72	
Caucasians (unspecified)	76	43	1385	23	2.53	15.33	6
U.S.A.	69	45	218	22	2.89	13.52	13
U.S.A.	60	58	126	24	4.30	19.63	75
	129	51	344	23	3.43	32.32	
	Heterogeneity χ^2 (1 df)					0.83	
France	40	60	166	21	5.53	21.77	10
Sweden	51	41	93	18	3.12	8.78	85
	296	48	1988	23	3.27	74.92	
	Heterogeneity χ^2 (4 df)					4.11	

TABLE 7.2. Total Lod Scores of 35 Families with Psoriasis. Dominant Psoriasis Gene with Different Levels of Penetrance

Penetrance of the Psoriasis Gene	Recombination Fraction, Θ										Maximum lod score	Θ at the Maximum lod score	Heterogeneity χ^2 34 df
	0.00	0.05	0.10	0.15	0.20	0.25	0.30	0.35	0.40	0.45			
0.10	3.54	3.41	3.04	2.56	2.05	1.55	1.08	0.68	0.35	0.13	3.54	0.00	8.53
0.30	1.74	2.90	2.90	2.57	2.10	1.60	1.11	0.68	0.34	0.11	2.90	0.05	15.43
0.50	−0.86	1.93	2.33	2.21	1.89	1.48	1.06	0.66	0.33	0.10	2.33	0.10	20.13
0.70	−5.67	0.00	1.05	1.39	1.40	1.25	0.98	0.66	0.34	0.10	1.40	0.20	26.70
0.90	−19.47	−5.69	−2.56	−0.83	0.16	0.61	0.71	0.58	0.34	0.10	0.71	0.30	30.93

χ^2 for heterogeneity among pedigrees is not significant.

References

1. Russell TJ, Schultes LM, Kuban DJ: Histocompatibility (HL-A) antigens associated with psoriasis. N Engl J Med 287:738-740, 1972
2. White SH, Newcomer VD, Mickey MR, Terasaki PI: Disturbance of HL-A antigen frequency in psoriasis. N Engl J Med 287:740-743, 1972
3. Batchelor JR, Morris PJ: Psoriasis: Joint report. In Bodmer W, et al. (eds): Histocompatibility Testing 1977. Munksgaard, Copenhagen, 1977, pp 230-231
4. Gazit E, Brenner S, Efter T, Orgad S, Mizrachi Y, Krawowski A: HLA antigens in patients with psoriasis. Tissue Antigens 12:195-199, 1978
5. Tsuji K, Nose Y, Ito M, Ozawa A, Matsuo I, Niizuma K, et al: HLA antigens and susceptibility to psoriasis vulgaris in a non-Caucasian population. Tissue Antigens 8:29-33, 1976
6. Hawkins BR, Tiwari JL, Lowe N, Wolfish P, Pollock CA, Cho YW, et al: HLA and psoriasis. In Terasaki PI (ed): Histocompatibility Testing 1980. UCLA Tissue Typing Laboratory, Los Angeles, 1981, pp 711-714
7. Ryder LP , Svejgaard A: Histocompatibility associated diseases. In Loor F, Roelants E (eds): B and T cells in Immune Recognition. John Wiley and Sons, New York, 1977, pp 437-456
8. Grosse-Wilde H, Wustner H, Albert ED, Kuntz B, Scholz S, Braun-Falco O: HLA-D typing in 72 psoriasis vulgaris patients: Distribution of seven HLA-D alleles. Tissue Antigens 11:427-433, 1978
9. McMichael AJ, Morhenn V, Payne R, Saszuki T, Farber EM: HLA C and D antigens associated with psoriasis. Br J Dermatol 98:287-292, 1978
10. Raffoux C, Streiff F, Blum F, Weber M, Beurey J: Groupage HLA-DRW chez 40 patients atteints de psoriasis. C R Soc Biol (Paris) 174:28-32, 1980
11. Moller P, Berg K, Vinje O: HLA phenotypes and joint affection in psoriasis, acute anterior uveitis and chronic prostatitis. Clin Genet 19:266-270, 1981
12. Brenner W, Gschnait F, Mayr WR: HLA, B13, B17, B37 and CW6 in psoriasis vulgaris: Association with the age of onset. Arch Dermatol Res 262:337-339, 1978
13. Tiwari JL, Lowe NJ, Abramovits W, Hawkins BR, Park MS: Association of psoriasis with HLA-DR7. Br J Dermatol 106:227-230, 1982
14. Svejgaard A, Stahl-Nielsen L, Svejgaard E, Kissmeyer-Nielsen F, Mjortshoj A, Zachariae H: HL-A in psoriasis vulgaris and in pustular psoriasis: Population and family studies. Br J Dermatol 91:145-153, 1974
15. Gunn I, Leheny W, Lakshmipathi T, Lamont MA, Fade M: HLA antigens in a Scottish psoriatic population. Tissue Antigens 14:157-164, 1979
16. Woodrow JC, Dave VK, Usher N, Anderson J: The HL-A system and psoriasis. Br J Dermatol 92:427-436, 1975
17. Krulig L, Farber EM, Grumet FC, Payne RO: Histocompatibility (HL-A) antigens in psoriasis. Arch Dermatol 111:857-860, 1975
18. Schoefinius HH, Braun-Falco O, Scholz S, Steinbauer-Rosenthal I, Wank R, Albert ED: Histokompatibilita tsantigene (HL-A) bei psoriasis. Dtsch Med Wochenschr 99:440-444, 1974
19. Krain LS, Newcomer VD, Terasaki PI: HL-A antigen in psoriasis. N Engl J Med 288:1245, 1973
20. Gross WL, Packhauser U, Hahn G, Westphal E, Christopher SE: Lymphocyte activation by streptococcal antigens in psoriasis. Br J Dermatol 97:529-536, 1977
21. Bertrams J, Lattke CL, Kuwert E: Correlation of antistreptolysin-O-titer to HL-A13 in psoriasis. N Engl J Med 291:631, 1974
22. Turowski G, Pietrzyk JJ, Kapinska-Mrowka M: Locus B HLA antigens in psoriatic patients. Population and family studies and clinical relationship. Arch Dermatol Res 271:315-324, 1981

23. Zlatkov NB, Minev M, Dourmishev AL, Martinova F: HLA system and therapy in psoriasis. Dermatologica 166:156-160, 1983
24. Thomas RJ: Psoriasis: Case rate-HL-A antigen frequency correlations. Dermatologica 154:23-31, 1977
25. Watson W, Cann HM, Faber EM, Nall ML: The genetics of psoriasis. Arch Dermatol 105:197-207, 1972
26. Lomholt G: Environment and genetics in psoriasis. Ann Clin Res 8:290-297, 1976
27. Kimberling W, Dobson RL: The inheritance of psoriasis. J Invest Dermatol 60:538-540, 1973
28. Pietrzyk JJ, Turowski G, Kapinska-Mrowka M, Rozanski B: Family studies in psoriasis. I. Complex segregation analysis. Arch Dermatol Res 273:287-294, 1982
29. McKusick VA: Mendelian Inheritance in Man: Catalogs of Autosomal Dominant, Autosomal Recessive, and X-linked Phenotypes, 6th edit. The Johns Hopkins University Press, 1983
30. Marcusson J, Moller E, Rosenthal L, Lindwall N, Thyresson N: Psoriasis and arthritic lesions in relation to the inheritance of HLA genotypes: A family study. Acta Dermatol Venereol 58:511-520, 1978
31. Karvonen J, Tiilikainen A, Lassus A: HLA antigens in psoriasis: A family study. Ann Clin Res 8:298-304, 1976
32. Civatte J, Lazarovici C, Ganas P, Leon S, Hors J, Contu L, et al: Le systeme HL-A dans le psoriasis: etude de 31 familles. Ann Dermatol Venereol 104:525-532, 1977
33. Marcusson J, Elman A, Moller E, Thyresson N: Psoriasis, sacroiliitis and peripheral arthritis occur in patients with same HLA haplotype: Preliminary family report and hypothetical explanation of interaction between MHS products. Tissue Antigens 8:131-138, 1976
34. Marcusson J, Moller E, Thyresson N: Penetration of HLA-linked psoriasis-predisposing gene(s): A family investigation. Acta Dermatol Venereol 56:453-463, 1976
35. Schoefinius HH, Braun-Falco O, Scholz S, Steinbauer-Rosenthal I, Wank R, Albert ED: HL-A antigens and psoriasis. N Engl J Med 291:51, 1974
36. Marcusson J, Moller E: HLA antigens in a psoriasis family: Comparative studies with MLC, HTC, PLT and serological HLA-DR determinants. Tissue Antigens 14:279-295, 1979
37. Espinoza LR, Bombardier C, Gaylord SW, Lauter S, Vasey FB, Osterland CK: Histocompatibility studies in psoriasis vulgaris: Family studies. J Rheumatol 7:445-452, 1980
38. Turowski G, Pietrzyk JJ, Turowska B, Kapinska-Mrowka M: Immunogenetic aspects of psoriasis in the light of population and family studies. Acta Med Pol 21:269-275, 1980
39. Pietrzyk JJ, Turowski G, Kapinska-Mrowka M: Family studies in psoriasis. II. Inheritance of HLA genotypes. Arch Dermatol Res 273:295-300, 1982
40. Hoshino K, Inouye H, Unokuchi T, Ito M, Tamaoki N, Tsuji K: HLA and disease in Japanese. In Dausset J, Svejgaard A (eds): HLA and Disease. De L'institut National De La Sante Et De La Recherche Medicale, Paris 1976, p 249
41. Roux H, Mercier P, Maestracci D, Serratrice G, Sany J, Seignalet J, et al: Psoriatic arthritis and HLA antigens. J Rheumatol 4 (Suppl 3):64-65, 1977
42. Morhenn V, Engleman E, Farber EM: Significance of HLA antigens and the mixed lymphocyte reaction in psoriasis. Acta Dermatol Venereol (Suppl) 87:12-14, 1979
43. Rimbaud PP, Meynadier J, Guilhou JJ, Clot J, Seignalet J, Guilhou E: Troubles immunitaires et antigenes d'histocompatiabilite dans le psoriasis. Ann Dermatol Venereol 101:359-374, 1974
44. Stancl I, Nyulassy S: Konjugale psoriasis und ihre beziehung zu den histokompatibilitatsantigenen. Hautarzt 28:407-408, 1977
45. Angelini G, Vena GA, Lomuto M, Meneghini CL: On cell-mediated immune response in psoriatic patients. Acta Dermatol Venereol (Suppl) 87:29-30, 1979
46. Gunther VW, Richter KV: Haufigbeitsverteilung von histokompatibilitatsantigenen (HLA) bei dermatologischen erkranbungen. Dermatol Monatsschr 161:402-404, 1975
47. Wood C: The pathogenesis of HLA-associated psoriasis. Med Hypotheses 4:111-122, 1978
48. Ozawa A: Histocompatibility antigens in psoriasis vulgaris. Jpn J Dermatol 86:205-216, 1976
49. Walter H, Brachtel R, Eckes L, Hilling M: Psoriasis vulgaris and genetic markers. Hum Genet 37:169-181, 1977
50. Stancl I, Sinka L, Bohunska S, Cervenkova D: Niektore aspekty genetiky psoriazy. Bratisl Lek Listy 63:366-369, 1975
51. Guilhou JJ, Meynadier J, Clot J: Pathogenie du psoriasis: Realites et hypotheses. Nouv Presse Med 7:1291-1295, 1978
52. Scandinavian Regional Report. In Bodmer W, et al. (eds): Histocompatibility Testing 1977. Munksgaard, Copenhagen, 1978, pp 499-511
53. Beckman L, Bergdahl K, Cedergren B, Damber MG, Linden S, Von Schoultz B, et al: Increased serum levels of the pregnancy zone protein in psoriasis. Acta Dermatol Venereol 57:403-406, 1977
54. Clot J, Guilhou JJ, Meynadier J, Paradis B, Andary M: Immunological aspects of psoriasis. Br J Dermatol 99:25-30, 1978
55. Beckman L, Bergdahl K, Cedergren B, Liden S: Genetic markers in psoriasis. Acta Dermatol Venereol 57:247-251, 1977

56. Svejgaard A, Svejgaard E, Nielsen LS, Jacobsen B: Some speculations on the associations between HL-A and disease based on studies of psoriasis patients and their families. Transplant Proc 5:1797-1798, 1973
57. Zachariae H, Kragballe K, Thestrup-Pedersen K, Kissmeyer-Nielsen F: HLA antigens in methrotrexate-induced liver cirrhosis. Acta Dermatol Venereol 60:165-166, 1980
58. Sany J, Seignalet JJ, Guilhou JJ, Serre H: HL-A et rhumatisme psoriasique. Rev Rhum Mal Osteoartic 42:451-460, 1975
59. Majsky A, Novotny F: HLA antigens in psoriasis vulgaris and patients' siblings. Tissue Antigens 9:131, 1977
60. Moll JMH, Wright V: Familial occurrence of psoriatic arthritis. Ann Rheum Dis 32:181-201, 1973
61. Mayr WR, Gschnait F, Brenner W: HLA B13, B17 und CW6 bei psoriasis vulgaris beziehung zum alter des patienten bei der erstmanifestation. Wien Klin Wochenschr 91:164-166, 1979
62. Marcusson J, Moller E, Thyresson N: Genetic problems concerning psoriasis. Acta Dermatol Venereol (Suppl) 87:28, 1979
63. Rogers RS: Genetics of psoriasis. Minn Med 58:326-327, 1975
64. Krain LS: Histocompatibility antigens: A laboratory and epidemiologic tool. J Invest Dermatol 62:67-73, 1974
65. Lattke CL, Heitmann HJ, Bertrams J, Kuwert E: Generische faktoren bei der psoriasis vulgaris: Histocompatibilitats (HL-A)-antigene. Hautarzt 25:39, 1974
66. Seignalet J, Sany J, Serre H: HL-A antigens and arthropathies in psoriasis. Lancet i:1350, 1974
67. Raffoux C, Streiff F, Blum F, Weber M, Beurey J: HLA-DRW7 dans le psoriasis vulgaire. C R Acad Sci Paris 290:883-884, 1980
68. Editorial: Histocompatibility (HL-A) antigens and psoriasis (letter by resident's journal club). Arch Dermatol 112:1030, 1976
69. Grumet CF, Krulig L, Farber EM, Payne RO: Histocompatibility (HL-A) antigens and psoriasis. Arch Dermatol 112:1030, 1976
70. Raffoux C, Streiff F, Jacobi C, Blum F, Ducommun F, Beurey J: Groupage HLA-DRW chez 40 patients atteints de psoriasis. Nouv Presse Med 9:1038, 1980
71. Chan SH, Tan T, Wee GB, Kamarudin A, Rajan VS: HLA and psoriasis in Chinese. Dermatologica 163:348-352, 1981
72. Song FJ: HLA antigens and psoriasis. Natl Med China 62:239-242, 1982
73. Buchanan R, Kraag G, Rosenthal D, Singal DP: HLA antigens and psoriatic arthritis. Transplant Proc 9:1873-1875, 1977
74. Espinoza LR, Vasey FB, Oh JH, Wilkinson R, Osterland CK: Association between HLA-BW38 and peripheral psoriatic arthritis. Arthritis Rheum 21:72-75, 1978
75. Murray C, Mann DL, Gerber LN, Barth W, Perlmann S, Decker JL, et al: Histocompatibility alloantigens in psoriasis and psoriatic arthritis. J Clin Invest 66:670-675, 1980
76. Novotny F, Majsky A: HLA antigens in psoriatics and their family members. Cesk Dermatol 52:222-226, 1977
77. Stenszky V, Nagy E, Szerze P, Ladanyi E: HL-A antigens and lymphocytotoxic antibodies in psoriasis vulgaris. Dermatol Monatschr 162:35-38, 1976
78. Jajic I, Kastelan A, Brnobic A, Kerhin V, Brkljacic L: HLA antigens in psoriatic arthritis and psoriasis. Arch Dermatol 113:1724-1725, 1977
79. Seignalet J, Clot J, Guilhou JJ, Duntze F, Meynadier J, Robinet-Levy M: HL-A antigens and some immunological parameters in psoriasis. Tissue Antigens 4:59-68, 1974
80. Schunter F, Schieferstein G: HL-A antigene bei psoriasis vulgaris. Hautarzt 25:82-83, 1974
81. Karvonen J, Tiilikainen A, Lassus A: HL-A antigens in patients with persistent palmoplantar pustulosis and pustular psoriasis. Ann Clin Res 7:112-115, 1975
82. Tilikainen A, Lassus A, Karvonen J, Vartiainen P, Julin M: Psoriasis and HLA-CW6. Br J Dermatol 102:179-184, 1980
83. Karvonen J, Lassus A, Sievers U, Tiilikainen A: HL-A antigens in psoriatic arthritis. Ann Clin Res 6:304 307, 1974
84. Karvonen J: HL-A antigens in psoriasis with special reference to the clinical type, age of onset, exacerbations after respiratory infections and occurrence of arthritis. Ann Clin Res 7:301-311, 1975
85. Marcusson JA, Johannesson A, Moller E: HLA-A, B, C and DR antigens in psoriasis. Tissue antigens 17:525-529, 1981
86. Marcusson J, Moller E, Thyresson N: HL-A antigens (17, 27, UPS) in psoriasis with special reference to patients with arthritic lesions. Acta Dermatol Venereol 55:297-300, 1975
87. Beckman L, Bronnestam R, Cedergrem B, Liden S: HL-A antigens, blood groups, serum groups and red cell enzyme types in psoriasis. Hum Hered 24:496-506, 1974
88. Sany J, Serre H, Seignalet J, Roux H, Maestraeci D, Recordier AM, et al: Relation enter rhumatisme psoriasique et systeme HL-A. Nouv Press Med 4:3142-3143, 1975
89. Nyfors A, Svejgaard A: The relation of HL-A antigens to liver histology in methotrexate-treated psoriatics. Acta Dermatol Venereol 56:235-238, 1976
90. Tsuji K, Inouye H, Nose Y, Sasazuki T, Ozawa A, Ohkido M: Further study on HLA-A, B, C, D, DR and haplotype antigen frequencies in psoriasis vulgaris. Acta Dermatol Venereol 87:107-108, 1979

91. Voorhees JJ: Pathophysiology of psoriasis. Ann Rev Med 28:467-473, 1977
92. Itakura K, Moriuchi J, Wakisaka A, Nakai Y, Kano T, and Aizawa M: Psoriasis vulgaris and HLA in Japanese. In Terasaki PI (ed): Histocompatibility Testing 1980. UCLA Tissue Typing Laboratory, Los Angeles, 1981, p 950
93. Karvonen J, Reunala T, Lokki J, Tiilikainen A, Lassus A: Theoretical considerations on HLA-associated illness-susceptibility genes in dermatitis herpetiformis and psoriasis. Tissue Antigens 14:331-335, 1979
94. Morhenn VB, Abel EA, Mahrle G: Expression of HLA-DR antigen in skin from patients with psoriasis. J Invest Dermatol 78:165-168, 1982
95. Moller P, Vinje O, Berg K: HLA antigens, psoriasis and acute anterior uveitis in Bechterew's syndrome (ankylosing spondylitis). Clin Genet 21:215-221, 1982
96. Sprenger-Klasen I, Franz HE, Rodermund OE: Besserun der psoriasis durch hamoldialyse: Beziehung zu eirner bestimmten HLA-antigen-konstellation? Dtsch Med Wochenschr 105:925-928, 1980
97. Cazalis P, Dryll A, Ryckewaert A: Complexes HLA et rhumatisme psoriasique. Rev Rhum 47:529-534, 1980

Pustular Psoriasis

Population Association

In 97 Danish[1] and 15 Finnish[2,3] patients, the frequency of B27 was increased (Table 7.3). The total sample in the Danish study consisted of 30 patients with localized pustular psoriasis of palms and soles, 14 with typical acrodermatitis continua, 35 with persistent palmoplantar pustulosis, also known as pustulosis palmaris et plantaris, and 18 patients with generalized pustular psoriasis. In the Finnish study, all of the patients were classified as generalized psoriasis cases.

The antigens B13 and B17 were not increased in pustular psoriasis. Thus, these 2 types of psoriasis may be genetically distinct etiologic entities.

See also ref. 4.

References

1. Zachariae H, Peterson HO, Kissmeyer-Nielsen F, Lamm L: HL-A antigens in pustular psoriasis. Dermatologica 154:73-77, 1977
2. Karvonen J: HL-A antigens in psoriasis with special reference to the clinical type, age of onset, exacerbations after respiratory infections and occurrence of arthritis. Ann Clin Res 7:301-311, 1975
3. Karvonen J, Tiilikainen A, Lassus A: HL-A antigens in patients with persistent palmoplantar pustulosis and pustular psoriasis. Ann Clin Res 7:112-115, 1975
4. Svejgaard A, Stahl-Nielsen L, Svejgaard E, Kissmeyer-Nielsen F, Mjortshoj A, Zachariae H: HL-A in psoriasis vulgaris and in pustular psoriasis: Population and family studies. Br J Dermatol 91:145-153, 1974

Guttate Psoriasis

Population Association

Like psoriasis vulgaris, guttate psoriasis also shows association with B13, B17, and CW6 (Table 7.4). The relative risks, although based on only 2 studies, are somewhat higher than those for psoriasis vulgaris.

See also ref. 1.

TABLE 7.3. Pustular Psoriasis

Country/Population	Patients n	Patients %+	Controls n	Controls %+	RR	χ^2	Ref.
HLA-B27							
Denmark	97	18	562	8	2.55	9.74	1
Finland	15	53	326	14	6.81	14.11	3
Finland	16	56	326	14	7.64	16.55	2
	31	55	652	14	7.22	30.63	
	Heterogeneity χ^2 (1 df)					0.03	
	128	27	1214	11	3.93	35.42	
	Heterogeneity χ^2 (2 df)					4.98	

Table 7.4. Guttate Psoriasis

	Patients		Controls				
Country/Population	n	%+	n	%+	RR	χ^2	Ref.
HLA-B13							
England	62	13	1036	4	3.73	11.32	2
Finland	22	41	900	6	10.97	30.08	3
	84	20	1936	5	6.03	38.02	
	Heterogeneity χ^2 (1 df)					3.38	
HLA-B17							
England	62	48	1036	8	10.57	73.59	2
Finland	22	23	900	4	7.55	16.42	3
	84	41	1936	6	9.77	89.66	
	Heterogeneity χ^2 (1 df)					0.35	
HLA-CW6							
Finland	22	73	462	7	33.68	52.63	3

References

1. Raznatovsky IM, Domeseva TV: On the morphology and immunology of parapsoriasis gutta. Vestn Dermatol Venereol 616:17-20, 1978
2. Williams RC, Mckenzie AW, Roger JH, Joysey VC: HL-A antigens in patients with guttate psoriasis. Br J Dermatol 95:163-167, 1976
3. Tiilikainen A, Lassus A, Karvonen J, Vartiainen P, Julin M: Psoriasis and HLA-CW6. Br J Dermatol 102:179-184, 1980

Erythrodermic Psoriasis

Population Association

In 16 Finnish patients,[1] A28, B13, and B17 were significantly increased (Table 7.5).

Reference

1. Karvonen J: HL-A antigens in psoriasis with special reference to the clinical type, age of onset, exacerbations after respiratory infections and occurrence of arthritis. Ann Clin Res 7:301-311, 1975

Persistent Palmoplantar Pustulosis (Pustulosis Palmaris et Plantaris)

Population Association

The results of 5 independent studies on Caucasian populations are not consistent (Table 7.6).

Antigen B8 was significantly increased in the British study but not in Finnish, German, and Danish samples. In the combined analysis, this association was marginally significant with some evidence of heterogeneity in the data. In 2 reports from Denmark[1]

Table 7.5. Erythrodermic Psoriasis

	Patients		Controls				
Country/Population	n	%+	n	%+	RR	χ^2	Ref.
HLA-A28							
Finland	16	38	326	12	4.58	8.87	1
HLA-B13							
Finland	16	31	326	8	5.35	9.66	1
HLA-B17							
Finland	16	25	326	4	8.33	12.80	1

TABLE 7.6. Persistent Palmoplantar Pustulosis (Pustulosis Palmaris et Plantaris)

	Patients		Controls				
Country/Population	n	%+	n	%+	RR	χ^2	Ref.
HLA-B8							
England	93	39	280	19	2.72	14.94	4
West Germany	70	27	500	25	1.12	0.17	5
West Germany	20	15	32	13	1.22	0.07	6
	90	24	532	24	1.14	0.23	
	Heterogeneity χ^2 (1 df)					0.01	
Finland	22	9	326	18	0.55	0.90	2
	205	29	1138	21	1.62	7.35	
	Heterogeneity χ^2 (3 df)					8.74	
HLA-B13							
England	93	0	280	6	0.08	5.87	4
West Germany	20	10	32	16	0.66	0.30	6
West Germany	70	0	500	2	0.33	1.10	5
	90	2	532	3	0.52	1.12	
	Heterogeneity χ^2 (1 df)					0.28	
Denmark	35	0	562	3	0.44	0.61	1
Finland	22	5	326	8	0.85	0.05	2
	240	1	1700	4	0.44	4.17	
	Heterogeneity χ^2 (4 df)					3.76	
HLA-BW35							
England	93	15	280	13	1.20	0.31	4
West Germany	70	13	500	13	1.04	0.01	5
West Germany	20	10	32	19	0.54	0.66	6
	90	12	532	13	0.92	0.07	
	Heterogeneity χ^2 (1 df)					0.61	
Denmark	35	34	562	13	3.50	11.64	1
Finland	22	41	326	19	2.99	6.29	2
	240	19	1700	14	1.67	8.16	
	Heterogeneity χ^2 (4 df)					10.75	

and Finland[2] BW35 was also increased in the patients. However, in the pooled sample this was only marginally significant (Table 7.6). All interesting frequency data are given in Table 7.6.

No association was observed in 35 Japanese patients studied by Tsuji et al.[3]

References

1. Zachariae H, Peterson HO, Kissmeyer-Nielsen F, Lamm L: HL-A antigens in pustular psoriasis. Dermatologica 154:73-77, 1977
2. Karvonen J, Tiilikainen A, Lassus A: HL-A antigens in patients with persistent palmoplantar pustulosis and pustular psoriasis. Ann Clin Res 7:112-115, 1975
3. Tsuji K, Nose Y, Ito M, Ozawa A, Matsuo I, Niizuma K, et al: HLA antigens and susceptibility to psoriasis vulgaris in a non-Caucasian population. Tissue Antigens 8:29-33, 1976
4. Ward JM, Barnes RMR: HLA antigens in persistent palmoplantar pustulosis and its relationship to psoriasis. Br J Dermatol 99:477-483, 1978

5. Rosen K, Lindholm A, Mobacken H, Sandberg L: HLA antigens associated with pustulosis palmoplantaris. Dermatol Monatsschr 168:182-185, 1982
6. Djawari D, Deinlein E: Zur immunologie des Bakterid Andrews. II. HLA-typisierung. Dermatol Monatsschr 166:305-308, 1980

Flexural Psoriasis (Psoriasis Inversus, Intertriginous Psoriasis)

This form of psoriasis affects the groin, axilla, submammary areas, and other body folds. It is estimated that in 3-6% of the patients, flexural or genital areas alone are affected.

Population Association

Karvonen[1] studied A and B loci in 12 cases of flexural psoriasis and 326 normal controls from Finland. There was no difference in the frequencies between patients and controls.

Reference

1. Karvonen J: HL-A antigens in psoriasis with special reference to the clinical type, age of onset, exacerbations after respiratory infections and occurrence of arthritis. Ann Clin Res 7:301-311, 1975

Pemphigus Vulgaris

Population Association

HLA-A and B Loci

The first report, published by Katz et al.[1] in 1973, on the association of HLA with pemphigus showed a significant increase of B13 in American Caucasian patients. However, this was not confirmed in any of the later studies, probably because the sample consisted of a mixture of Jews and others representing "a wide spectrum of cultural and ethnic backgrounds." During the same year, another paper by Krain et al.[2] showed a significant association of A10 with this disease (Table 7.7) in American Jewish patients. This association was later confirmed in 2 independent studies on American Jews by Park et al.[3] and Israeli Jews by Brautbar et al.[4] and David et al.[5] In these studies, BW38 and only the A26 split of A10 (not A25) were found to be increased in the patient groups.

In a group of 43 Japanese patients studied by Hashimoto et al.,[6] A26 was also found to be associated with this disease (Table 7.7).

Chan and Tan[7] typed 40 Chinese patients from Singapore for A and B loci antigens. Unlike in Japanese patients no antigen was found to be increased or decreased in this population. The frequency of

TABLE 7.7. Pemphigus Vulgaris

	Patients		Controls				
Country/Population	n	%+	n	%+	RR	χ^2	Ref.
HLA-A10							
Singapore—Chinese	40	5	330	6	0.99	0.00	7
Jews—Ashkenazi	28	61	94	20	6.04	15.94	2
U.S.A.	15	20	870	11	2.26	1.95	2
U.S.A.	18	22	251	16	1.59	0.73	1
	33	21	1121	12	1.87	2.50	
	Heterogeneity χ^2 (1 df)					0.19	
HLA-A26							
Japan	43	42	60	17	3.43	7.60	6
Jews—Ashkenazi	30	70	52	25	6.62	14.77	4
Jews—Ashkenazi	45	69	50	28	5.50	15.14	5
	75	69	102	26	5.97	29.83	
	Heterogeneity χ^2 (1 df)					0.08	
Jews—Non-Ashkenazi	11	64	40	13	10.47	10.71	5
Jews—Non-Ashkenazi	9	22	38	13	2.03	0.77	4
	20	45	78	13	5.10	9.18	
	Heterogeneity χ^2 (1 df)					2.29	

TABLE 7.7. *(continued)*

Country/Population	Patients n	Patients %+	Controls n	Controls %+	RR	χ^2	Ref.
HLA-A26							
Jews (unspecified)	22	41	72	19	2.93	4.51	3
	117	60	252	20	4.89	42.12	
	Heterogeneity χ^2 (4 df)					3.77	
HLA-B7							
U.S.A.	15	7	870	25	0.32	2.30	2
Greece	20	40	280	13	4.50	10.33	8
	35	26	1150	22	2.14	3.70	
	Heterogeneity χ^2 (1 df)					8.93	
HLA-BW22							
U.S.A.	15	7	870	5	2.02	0.85	2
Greece	20	35	231	5	10.14	19.12	8
	35	23	1101	5	5.98	16.93	
	Heterogeneity χ^2 (1 df)					3.04	
HLA-BW38							
Jews—Ashkenazi	30	70	52	27	5.99	13.48	4
Jews—Ashkenazi	45	71	50	28	6.03	16.53	5
	75	71	102	27	6.01	30.01	
	Heterogeneity χ^2 (1 df)					0.00	
Jews—Non-Ashkenazi	11	9	40	9	1.28	0.07	5
Jews—Non-Ashkenazi	9	33	38	10	4.29	3.36	4
	20	20	78	9	2.55	2.43	
	Heterogeneity χ^2 (1 df)					1.00	
Jews (unspecified)	22	55	72	24	3.76	7.29	3
	117	59	252	21	4.60	37.93	
	Heterogeneity χ^2 (4 df)					2.81	
HLA-DR2							
Japan	20	0	73	37	0.04	9.21	10
Japan	17	0	144	39	0.04	8.93	9
	37	0	217	38	0.04	18.13	
	Heterogeneity χ^2 (1 df)					0.00	
HLA-DR4							
Japan	17	41	144	33	1.43	0.52	9
Japan	20	55	73	30	2.79	4.27	10
	37	49	217	32	2.00	3.90	
	Heterogeneity χ^2 (1 df)					0.90	
Jews—Ashkenazi	30	97	52	46	24.74	16.24	4
Jews—Non-Ashkenazi	9	67	38	26	5.19	5.21	4
Jews (unspecified)	23	91	72	25	24.56	23.18	3
	62	90	162	32	14.65	41.52	
	Heterogeneity χ^2 (2 df)					3.11	

A10 in this sample is given in Table 7.7 for comparison.

In the original paper by Krain et al.,[2] no HLA association was observed in American Caucasian patients. However, in a later report on 20 Greek Caucasian patients,[8] BW22 was reported to be significantly associated with pemphigus. This association is also significant in the combined analysis of American and Greek patients (Table 7.7).

HLA-DR Locus

In the paper by Park et al.,[3] a very strong association of DR4 was reported in Jewish patients. The frequency of DR4 was 91% in patients as compared with 25% in controls. Similar data on Israeli Ashkenazi patients were reported by Brautbar et al.[4] In a small sample (n = 9) of non-Ashkenazi Jews, the association with DR4 was only marginally significant (uncorrected $p = 0.045$).[4] This strong association of pemphigus vulgaris with DR4 is very similar to that of ankylosing spondylitis with B27 and of narcolepsy with DR2. These are the only 3 diseases where almost all the patients have the associated antigens.

In 2 reports from Japan[9,10] there is no evidence of a significant association with DR4. However, in both of these studies DR2 was not present in any of the patients, thus showing a highly significant negative association with the disease (Table 7.7)

In view of a strong linkage disequilibrium between A26-BW38, A26-DR4, and BW38-DR4 and a much stronger association with DR4, it can be concluded that the primary association of the disease in Jewish patients is with HLA-DR4.

See also refs. 11–13.

References

1. Katz SI, Dahal MV, Penneys N, Trapani RJ, Rogentine N: HL-A antigens in pemphigus. Arch Dermatol 108:53-55, 1973
2. Krain LS, Terasaki PI, Newcomer VD, Mickey MR: Increased frequency of HL-A10 in pemphigus vulgaris. Arch Dermatol 108:803-805, 1973
3. Park MS, Terasaki PI, Ahmed AR, Tiwari JL: HLA-DRW4 in 91% of Jewish pemphigus vulgaris patients. Lancet ii:441-442, 1979
4. Brautbar C, Moscovitz M, Livshits T, Haim S, Hacham-Zadeh S, Cohen HA, et al: HLA-DRW4 in pemphigus vulgaris patients in Israel. Tissue Antigens 16:238-243, 1985
5. David M, Zamir R, Segal R, Gazit E, Feuerman EJ: HLA antigens in Jews with pemphigus vulgaris. Dermatologica 163:326-330, 1981
6. Hashimoto K, Yoshiharu M, Nakata S, Matsuyama M: HLA-A10 in pemphigus among Japanese. Arch Dermatol 113:1518-1519, 1977
7. Chan SH, Tan T: HLA and pemphigus in Chinese. Dermatologica 163:205-206, 1981
8. Zervas J, Tosca A, Apostolakis I, Varelzidis A: HLA and pemphigus. Br J Dermatol 101:357-358, 1979
9. Sakural M, Takigawa M, Terasaki PI, Imamura S, Sakurami T, Ueno Y, et al: Absence of HLA-DRW2 in Japanese pemphigus vulgaris. J Invest Dermatol 76:70-71, 1981
10. Masamichi M, Hashimoto K, Yamasaki Y, Shirakura R, Higuchi R, Miyajima T, et al: HLA-DR antigens in pemphigus among Japanese. Tissue Antigens 17:236-238, 1981
11. Hashimoto T, Nishikawa T, Kurihara S, Hatano H: Complement-fixing pemphigus antibodies. Arch Dermatol 114:1191-1192, 1978
12. Hoshino K, Inouye H, Unokuchi T, Ito M, Tamaoki N, Tsuji K: HLA and disease in Japanese. In Dausset J, Svejgaard A (eds): HLA and Disease. De L'institut National De La Sante Et De La Recherche Medicale, Paris 1976, p 249
13. Sakurami T, Ueno Y, Iwaki Y, Park MS, Terasaki PI, Saji H: HLA-DR specificities among Japanese with several autoimmune disease. Tissue Antigens 19:129-133, 1982

Pemphigus Foliaceus

Population Association

The association of pemphigus foliaceus with HLA has been studied in Japanese patients by Hashimoto et al.[1] As in pemphigus vulgaris, the frequency of A26 was significantly increased in a group of 25 patients (Table 7.8). It is important to note that some patients with pemphigus erythematosus (Senear-Usher syndrome) were also included in the sample, for there was no clear-cut separation of the clinical features between the 2 diseases.

In a later report by the same group of authors[2] a significant association with DR4 was also observed (Table 7.8).

References

1. Hashimoto K, Yoshiharu M, Nakata S, Matsuyama M: HLA-A10 in pemphigus among Japanese. Arch Dermatol 133:1518-1519, 1977

TABLE 7.8. Pemphigus Foliaceus

Country/Population	Patients n	Patients %+	Controls n	Controls %+	RR	χ^2	Ref.
HLA-A26							
Japan	25	48	60	17	4.35	8.41	1
HLA-DR4							
Japan	17	71	73	30	5.33	9.10	2

2. Masamichi M, Hashimoto K, Yamasaki Y, Shirakura R, Iguchi R, Miyajima T, et al.: HLA-DR antigens in pemphigus among Japanese. Tissue Antigens 17:238-239, 1981

Bullous Pemphigoid

Population Association

In a study of 19 American Caucasian patients typed for A and B loci antigens in 1977, no statistically significant difference was observed.[1] Similar results were obtained by Hashimoto et al.[2] in a sample of 41 Japanese patients.

However, a later report by Lohrisch et al.[3] showed a significant increase of AW24 in 11 German patients (Table 7.9). In the data of Ahmed et al.[1] on 19 American Caucasian patients the frequency of A9 (AW23 and AW24 are splits of A9) was 16% as compared with 23% in 60 controls. These patients were not typed for AW24.

References

1. Ahmed AR, Cohen E, Blumenson LE, Provost TT: HLA in bullous pemphigoid. Arch Dermatol 113:1121, 1977
2. Hashimoto K, Miki Y, Nakata S, Matsuyama M, Takashi M: HLA antigens in bullous pemphigoid among Japanese. Arch Dermatol 115:96-97, 1979
3. Lohrisch VI, Freistedt B, Haustein UF: HLA-merkmale beim parapemphigus. Dermatol Monatsschr 166:247-248, 1980

Benign Mucosal Pemphigoid (Cicatrical Pemphigoid, Ocular Pemphigus)

Population Association

Mondino et al.[1] studied A and B loci antigens in 20 American Caucasian patients and 245 controls. The frequency of B12 was 45% in patients as compared with 19.6% in controls (uncorrected Fisher's exact $p = 0.02$).

Reference

1. Mondino BJ, Brown SI, Rabin BS: HLA antigens in ocular cicatricial pemphigoid. Br J Ophthalmol 62:265-267, 1978

Benign Familial Pemphigus (Hailey-Hailey's Disease)

This disease is rare and is inherited as a dominant gene. The family history, however, is observed in only about 70% of the patients.

Population Association

The only data available are from a small sample of Finnish patients studied by Karvonen and Tiilikainen.[1] HLA-A and -B loci were typed in 9 unrelated patients and the results compared with 326 normal controls. The frequency of B8 was 44% in patients and 17% in controls. Similarly, the frequencies of

TABLE 7.9. Bullous Pemphigoid

Country/Population	Patients n	Patients %+	Controls n	Controls %+	RR	χ^2	Ref.
HLA-AW24							
West Germany	11	63	500	21	6.09	9.74	3

TABLE 7.10. Subacute Cutaneous Lupus Erythematosus

	Patients		Controls				
Country/Population	n	%+	n	%+	RR	χ^2	Ref.
HLA-B8							
U.S.A.	26	65	100	23	5.98	15.27	3
HLA-DR3							
U.S.A.	26	77	100	22	11.05	23.37	3

B5 (33% vs. 13%) and BW40 (33% vs. 15%) were also increased in the patient group. None of these, however, was statistically significant.

Reference

1. Karvonen J, Tiilikainen A: HLA antigens in Hailey-Hailey's disease. Tissue Antigens 8:277-278, 1976

Subacute Cutaneous Lupus Erythematosus

Population Association

HLA-A, -B, -C, and -DR antigens were studied in 26 American Caucasian patients by Stastny and Gilliam.[1-3] The frequencies of B8 and DR3 were significantly increased in the patients (Table 7.10). This, when compared with the absence of HLA association in the patients with chronic lupus erythematosus, has led these authors to propose that subacute cutaneous lupus erythematosus is a separate clinical entity.

Disease Heterogeneity

The 26 patients studied in the aforementioned study[3] were subdivided into annular type (n = 15) and papulosquamous type. DR3 was significantly increased in both groups.

References

1. Stastny P, Gilliam JN: HLA-A1, B8, DRW3 in patients with a distinct form of lupus erythematosus. Transplant Proc 11:1869-1870, 1979
2. Sontheimer RD, Stastny P, Maddison P, Reichlin M, Gilliam JN: Anti-RO and LA antibodies and further HLA associations in subacute cutaneous lupus erythematosus. Arthritis Rheum 23:750, 1980
3. Sontheimer RD, Stastny P, Gilliam JN: Human histocompatibility antigen associations in subacute cutaneous lupus erythematosus. J Clin Invest 67:312-316, 1981

Discoid Lupus Erythematosus

Population Association

The existing data do not show any consistency in the nature of HLA association for discoid lupus erythematosus. The first report in 1975 by Stenszky et al.[1] on 33 patients from Hungary showed a significant increase in the frequency of B5 and BW22 (uncorrected probabilities were 0.0106 and 0.0237, respectively). During the same year, in 60 German patients,[2] A1 and B8 were found to be increased (no frequency data are given). No significant difference was observed in American Caucasian patients studied by Prystowsky and Gilliam[3] and Stastny and Gilliam.[4]

No significant change in any antigen was observed in a group of 69 patients from England.[5] However, when the patients were dichotomized according to their age at onset, B7 was significantly increased in young men and women (15–39 years). In women with age at onset > 40 years, the frequency of B8 was increased. The authors have used these results to argue for the existence of genetic heterogeneity in this disease.

No HLA association was observed in 36 American Black patients studied by Prystowsky and Gilliam.[3]

References

1. Stenszky V, Nagy E, Szerze P: Examination of HL-A antigens and lymphocytotoxic antibodies in discoid lupus erythematosus. Acta Dermatol Venereol 55:131-133, 1975
2. Gunther VW, Richter KV: Haufigbeitsverteilung von histokompatibilitatsantigenen (HLA) bei dermatologischen erkranbungen. Dermatol Monatsschr 161:402-404, 1975
3. Prystowsky SD, Gilliam JN: Discoid lupus erythematosus as part of a larger disease spectrum. Arch Dermatol 111:1448-1452, 1975
4. Stastny P, Gilliam JN: HLA-A1, B8, DRW3 in patients with a distinct form of lupus erythematosus. Transplant Proc 11:1869-1870, 1979

5. Millard LG, Rowell NR, Rajah SM: Histocompatibility antigens in discoid and systemic lupus erythematosus. Br J Dermatol 96:139-144, 1977

Atopic Dermatitis

Population Association

The first report on 45 American Caucasian patients and 870 controls by Krain and Terasaki[1] showed increased frequencies of A3 (33% vs. 19% in controls) and A9 (33% vs. 21% in controls) in patients. This, however, was not confirmed in 27 French patients[2] or in 103 German patients.[3,4] In the French study,[2] a significant association with BW35 was reported (Table 7.11). The frequency data from other reports are not available and thus this association with BW35 cannot be evaluated in the combined sample.

Ohkido et al.[5] studied 100 unrelated Japanese patients and found no association with A and B loci antigens (also see ref.6).

Disease Heterogeneity

The Japanese patients[5] were divided into 4 subgroups: with and without allergic rhinitis and with and without bronchial asthma. There was no significant difference in the antigen frequencies between the groups.

Family Data

HLA typing of families with more than one affected member has been done in several studies. In 23 French,[2] 17 English,[7] and 35 Japanese[5] families, there was no evidence of disease segregation with specific haplotypes. Thus, in these 3 studies, data did not support linkage between atopic dermatitis and HLA. On the other hand, Scholz et al.[3,4] studied 19 families with more than one patient. Their analysis showed that the observed distribution of atopic dermatitis and HLA haplotypes was not random and thus there was evidence that the disease segregated with HLA haplotypes ($p = 0.00028$). In another study of one Danish family,[8] all affected members had the A2-BW35-CW4 haplotype.

Complete pedigree data are available in only 2 studies.[7,8]

References

1. Krain LS, Terasaki PI: HL-A types in atopic dermatitis. Lancet i:1059-1060, 1973
2. Goudemand J, Defrenne C, Desmons F: HLA antigens and atopic dermatitis. Monogr Allergy 11:24-29, 1977
3. Scholz S, Ziegler E, Wustner H, Braun-Falco O, Albert ED: HLA family studies in patients with atopic dermatitis. Monogr Allergy 11:44, 1977
4. Scholz S, Ziegler E, Schoeffinius H, Braun-Falco O, Kuntz B, Schiessl B, et al: HLA family studies in patients with atopic dermatitis. Z Immunitaetsforsch 152:313-315, 1976
5. Ohkido M, Ozawa A, Matsuo I, Miizuma K, Nakano M, Tsuji K, et al: HLA antigens and suceptibility to atopic dermatitis. Monogr Allergy 11:36-43, 1977
6. Hoshino K, Inouye H, Unokuchi T, Ito M, Tamaoki N, Tsuji K: HLA and disease in Japanese. In Dausset J, Svejgaard A (eds): HLA and Disease. De L'institut National De La Sante Et De La Recherche Medicale, Paris 1976, p 249
7. Mackie RM, Dick HM: A study of HLA antigen distribution in families with atopic dermatitis. Allergy 34:19-23, 1979
8. Larsen FS, Grunnet N, Vase P: HLA antigens in atopic dermatitis: A family study. Dermatologica 160:17-20, 1979

Atopy (Unspecified, Includes Eczema)

Population Association

The data of Escobar-Gutierrez et al.[1] on 100 Mexican Mestizo atopic patients showed a significant association with B7 (Table 7.12).

De Vries et al.[2] found no association with A, B, and C loci antigens in 80 healthy sailors from the Netherlands. These sailors were not given vaccine to vaccinia virus due to infantile eczema. In these

TABLE 7.11. Atopic Dermatitis

Country/Population	Patients n	Patients %+	Controls n	Controls %+	RR	χ^2	Ref.
HLA-BW35							
France	27	37	326	12	4.35	12.34	2

TABLE 7.12. Atopy (Unspecified, Includes Eczema)

	Patients		Controls				
Country/Population	n	%+	n	%+	RR	χ^2	Ref.
HLA-BW4							
BENELUX	80	41	6215	60	0.47	11.47	2
HLA-B7							
Mexico	100	36	200	16	2.93	14.73	1

patients the frequency of BW4 was significantly increased (Table 7.12).

Turner et al.[3] studied 40 British Caucasian patients with atopic eczema and another sample of 40 patients with hay fever. When compared with 1036 controls, none of the A and B loci antigens were found to be associated with these conditions.

Family Data

Geerts et al.[4] reported a family of 17 individuals, "of whom 7 had an atopic history, at least bronchial asthma and/or hay fever, inherited from the maternal grandfather of the proband." Six descendants had inherited the haplotype A11-B27 from the grandfather and 3 nonatopics did not have this haplotype.

See also refs. 5–7.

References

1. Escobar-Gutierrez A, Gorodezky C, Salazar-Mallen M: Distribution of some of the HL-A system lymphocyte antigens in Mexicans. Vox Sang 25:151-155, 1973
2. De Vries RRP, Van Rood JJ, Lange PC: HLA-W4 and W6 antigens and allergic disorders. Lancet i:151, 1977
3. Turner MW, Brostoff J, Wells RS, Stokes CR, Soothill JF: HLA in eczema and hay fever. Clin Exp Immunol 27:43-47, 1977
4. Geerts SJ, Pottgens H, Limburg M, Van Rood JJ: Predisposition for atopy or allergy linked to HL-A. Lancet i:461, 1975
5. Gunther VW, Richter KV: Haufigbeitsverteilung von histokompatibilitatsantigenen (HLA) bei dermatologischen erkranbungen. Dermatol Monatsschr 161:402-404, 1975
6. Ozawa A: Atopic diseases and HL-A antigens. Nippon Rinsho 36:3176-3180, 1978
7. Turner MW, Brostoff J, Wells RS, Soothill JF: Histocompatibility antigens in atopy with special reference to eczema and hay fever. Monogr Allergy 11:19-23, 1977

Dermatitis Herpetiformis

Population Association

Data are available only for Caucasian populations from Europe, the United States, and Australia (Table 7.13). In all of these populations, A1 and B8 were significantly associated with dermatitis herpetiformis (DH). It is also clear from Table 7.13 that the association with A1 was not as strong as that with B8.

Studies of D locus antigens by Solheim et al.[1] and Thomsen et al.[2] indicated that DW3 showed a much stronger association with this disease (RR = 21.81). Similar results have been obtained for DR3 in 3 independent studies from Italy,[3] Austria,[4] and Norway[5] (Table 7.13). Mann et al.[6] also reported 2 antisera (B-1 and W-1) that reacted with B lymphocytes from 78.96% (15/19) and 100% (15/15), respectively, of the DH patients.

Thus, based on these high relative risks and the fact that highly significant linkage disequilibria exist between A1-B8 and B8-DR3, it can be concluded that the primary association of DH is most probably with DW3/DR3.

Park et al.[7] have found a highly significant association with the antigen Te24 in American Caucasian patients (Table 7.13). The Te24 antigen is associated with DR3 and DR7 and is an allele of the postulated second DR locus.

Disease Heterogeneity

A high proportion of the patients with DH have abnormalities of the jejunal mucosa similar to the typical symptoms in gluten-sensitive enteropathy (celiac disease). These jejunal abnormalities in DH patients also respond to gluten-free diet. Thus the frequencies of A1 and B8 have been investigated in patients with and without jejunal abnormalities.

Gebhard et al.[8] first reported that 84% of patients with associated villous atrophy (determined by small intestinal biopsy) had B8, a figure similar to that

TABLE 7.13. Dermatitis Herpetiformis

Country/Population	Patients n	Patients %+	Controls n	Controls %+	RR	χ^2	Ref.
HLA-Te 24							
U.S.A.	44	93	174	26	32.70	40.77	7
HLA-A1							
U.S.A.	26	62	251	29	3.90	10.95	23
U.S.A.	33	76	92	28	7.72	20.61	24
	59	70	343	29	5.33	30.31	
	Heterogeneity χ^2 (1 df)					1.25	
England	38	61	180	32	3.27	10.82	10
England	35	54	175	35	2.16	4.45	11
	73	58	355	33	2.67	14.62	
	Heterogeneity χ^2 (1 df)					0.65	
Austria	21	62	3000	27	4.31	11.57	4
Finland	61	64	326	17	8.53	51.11	9
	214	63	4024	27	4.58	98.60	
	Heterogeneity χ^2 (5 df)					10.92	
HLA-B8							
U.S.A.	33	85	92	18	23.32	36.39	24
U.S.A.	55	64	174	17	8.47	39.61	7
U.S.A.	49	88	184	24	21.48	47.70	13
U.S.A.	28	68	42	17	9.56	16.93	8
U.S.A.	26	58	251	24	4.30	12.68	23
	191	74	743	21	10.13	143.21	
	Heterogeneity χ^2 (4 df)					10.09	
Australia	14	71	700	24	7.24	13.19	25
England	40	85	1967	24	16.80	45.68	2
England	38	79	180	26	10.17	31.29	10
England	35	60	175	33	3.00	8.76	11
	113	75	2322	25	7.40	75.35	
	Heterogeneity χ^2 (2 df)					10.38	
Italy	32	50	431	14	6.10	23.93	3
Austria	21	67	3000	18	8.93	24.61	4
Finland	61	87	326	17	30.81	77.36	9
Norway	34	79	1628	25	10.73	34.77	1
Norway	32	84	1628	25	14.60	35.50	5
	66	81	3256	25	12.31	70.01	
	Heterogeneity χ^2 (1 df)					0.26	
	498	75	10778	22	9.89	414.94	
	Heterogeneity χ^2 (13 df)					33.46	
HLA-DW3							
England	40	93	157	20	45.16	44.25	2
Norway	20	75	136	19	11.84	22.18	1
	60	87	293	20	21.81	63.46	
	Heterogeneity χ^2 (1 df)					2.97	

TABLE 7.13 *(continued)*

Country/Population	Patients n	Patients %+	Controls n	Controls %+	RR	χ^2	Ref.
HLA-DW7							
England	40	25	157	8	3.82	8.82	2
HLA-DR3							
U.S.A.	44	80	174	19	16.18	46.66	7
Italy	32	69	125	16	11.15	30.30	3
Austria	21	86	160	20	21.33	27.20	4
Norway	29	97	120	25	62.01	27.82	5
	126	82	579	20	17.30	128.16	
	Heterogeneity χ^2 (3 df)					3.82	

reported for gluten-sensitive enteropathy. Only 33% of the patients without gastrointestinal disease had B8, and thus there was no significant difference between this and the normal control group. The authors concluded that B8 in DH is associated mainly in those patients who have gastrointestinal abnormalities.

In later studies by several authors,[9–12] the frequency of B8 did not differ significantly in patients with and without abnormal biopsies. The results of Gebhard et al.[8] were probably the result of the less restricted criteria of diagnosing DH.

Rate of Acetylation of Dapsone

Dapsone (widely used to control the rash in DH) is acetylated by patients at various rates, and hence they can be classified into slow and rapid acetylators. In 61 Finnish patients studied by Reunala et al.,[9] B8 occurred in 81% of 28 slow acetylators and in 77% of 22 rapid acetylators. Thus, there was no significant difference in the frequency of B8 (and also A1) between the 2 groups.

Pattern of Immunoglobulin Deposition in Skin

It has been reported by several authors that there is a small subgroup of DH patients in whom the bound IgA occurs in a linear band along the basement membrane zone of skin instead of the more usual granular IgA deposits in the dermal papillae. Lawley et al.[13] studied 10 patients with linear IgA deposits and 49 with granular deposits. HLA-B8 was found in 30% of the patients with linear deposits and in 88% of those with granular deposits. The former was not significantly different from that of the control population. On the basis of these results, the authors concluded that the patients with linear IgA deposits have a disease that is pathophysiologically different from that of patients with granular IgA deposits. More data are needed to verify this interesting observation.

Family Data

Gebhard et al.[8] described 2 small DH families (a total of 9 members in both) with HLA typing. In each family affected individuals shared one haplotype.

Karvonen et al.[14] using Finnish data on the observed number of patients homozygous for B8, estimated the frequency of the B8-associated DH susceptibility gene to be 0.0005. In this analysis DH susceptibility gene appeared to be dominant.

See also refs. 15–22, 26, and 27.

References

1. Solheim BG, Ek J, Thune PO, Bablien K, Bratlie A, Rankin B, et al: HLA antigens in dermatitis herpetiformis and coeliac disease. Tissue Antigens 7:57-59, 1976
2. Thomsen M, Platz P, Marks J, Ryder LP, Shuster S, Svejgaard A, et al: Association of LD-8A and LD-12A with dermatitis herpetiformis. Tissue Antigens 7:60-62, 1976
3. Richiardi P, Borell I, Malavasi F, Curtoni ES, Berti E, Gianotti F, et al: HLA antigens in juvenile dermatitis herpetiformis. Acta Dermatol Venereol 61:241-244, 1981
4. Pehamberger H, Holubar K, Mayer WR: HLA-DR3

in dermatitis herpetiformis. Br J Dermatol 104: 321-324, 1981
5. Solheim BG, Albrechtsen D, Thorsby E, Thune P: Strong association between an HLA-DW3 associated B cell alloantigen and dermatitis herpetiformis. Tissue Antigens 10:114-118, 1977
6. Mann DL, Nelson DL, Katz SI, Nelson DL, Abelson LD, Strober W: Specific B-cell antigens associated with gluten-sensitive enteropathy and dermatitis herpetiformis. Lancet i:110-111, 1976
7. Park MS, Terasaki PI, Ahmed AR, Zone J: The 90% incidence of HLA antigen (Te24) in dermatitis herpetiformis. Tissue Antigens 22:263-266, 1983
8. Gebhard RL, Katz SI, Marks J, Shuster S, Trapani RJ, Rogentine GN, et al: HL-A antigen type and small-intestine disease in dermatitis herpetiformis. Lancet ii:760-762, 1973
9. Reunala T, Salo OP, Tiilikainen A, Mattila MJ: Histocompatibility antigens and dermatitis herpetiformis with special reference to jejunal abnormalities and acetylator phenotype. Br J Dermatol 94:139-143, 1976
10. Seah PP, Fry L, Kearney JW, Campbell E, Mowlray JF, Stewart JS, et al: A comparison of histocompatibility antigens in dermatitis herpetiformis and adult coeliac disease. Br J Dermatol 94:131-138, 1976
11. White AG, Barnetson RSTC, Da Costa JAG, McClelland DBL: The incidence of HL-A antigens in dermatitis herpetiformis. Br J Dermatol 89:133-136, 1973
12. Barnetson RSC, Heading RC, White AG: HL-A8 and dermatitis herpetiformis. Lancet ii:1027, 1973
13. Lawley TJ, Strober W, Yaoita H, Katz SI: Small intestinal biopsies and HLA types in dermatitis herpetiformis patients with granular and linear IgA skin deposits. J Invest Dermatol 74:9-12, 1980
14. Karvonen J, Reunala T, Lokki J, Tiilikainen A, Lassus A: Theoretical considerations on HLA-associated illness-susceptibility genes in dermatitis herpetiformis and psoriasis. Tissue Antigens 14:331-335, 1979
15. Marks JM: HLA-DW3 in dermatitis herpetiformis. Lancet i:750, 1976
16. Scott BB, Young S, Rajah SM, Marks J, Losowsky MS: The incidence of coeliac disease and HL-A8 in dermatitis herpetiformis. Gut 16:845, 1975
17. Diaz LA, Lamkin BC, Dubin HV: Juvenile dermatitis herpetiformis. Arch Dermatol 115:584-586, 1979
18. Davies MG, Davies PG: Dermatitis herpetiformis, glomerulonephritis, and HLA-DRW3. Lancet ii:911, 1979
19. Gebhard RL, Falchuk ZM, Katz SI, Sessoms C, Rogentine GN, Strober W: Immunologic concomitants of small intestinal disease and relationship to histocompatibility antigen HL-A8. J Clin Invest 54:98-103, 1974
20. White AG, Barnetson RSTC, Da Costa JAG, McClelland DBL: HL-A and disordered immunity. Lancet i:108, 1973
21. Grenier R, Rostas A, Wilkinson RD: Dermatitis herpetiformis and leiomyomas with HLA-B8, a marker of immune diseases. Can Med Assoc J 115:882-884, 1976
22. Scott BB, Losowsky MS, Rajah SM: HL-A8 and HL-A12 in coeliac disease. Lancet ii:171, 1974
23. Katz SI, Falchuk ZM, Dahl MV, Rogentine GN, Strober W: HL-A8: A genetic link between dermatitis herpetiformis and gluten-sensitive enteropathy. J Clin Invest 51:2977-2980, 1972
24. Katz SI, Hertz KC, Rogentine GN, Strober W: HLA-B8 and dermatitis herpetiformis in patients with IgA deposits in skin. Arch Dermatol 113:155-156, 1977
25. Morris PJ, Vaughan H, Tait BD, Mackay IR: Histocompatibility antigens (HLA): Association with immunopathic diseases and with response to microbial antigens. Aust NZ J Med 7:616-624, 1977
26. Scott H, Brandtzaeg P, Solheim BG, Thorsby E: Relation between HLA-DR like antigens and secretory component (SC) in jejunal epithelium of patients with coeliac disease or dermatitis herpetiformis. Clin Exp Immunol 44:233-238, 1981
27. Lawley TJ, Hall RP, Fauci AS, Katz SI, Hamburger MI, Frank MM: Defective Fc-receptor functions associated with the HLA-B8/DRw3 haplotype: Studies in patients with dermatitis herpetiformis and normal subjects. N Engl J Med 304:185-192, 1981

Psoriasiform Napkin Dermatitis

Psoriasiform napkin dermatitis is a characteristic eruption in infants predominantly in the napkin (diaper) area. This disease has many features of psoriasis and some investigators have called this true psoriasis. Others have classified this as a special seborrheic eczema due to napkin irritation (for details, see references in 1).

Population Association

Skoven and Hjortshoj[1] typed 14 Danish patients for A and B antigens and compared the results with 1967 controls. The frequencies of B13, B17, and B37 (antigens associated with psoriasis, see Psoriasis) were not significantly different from controls. However, they were significantly lower than those in a population of 220 psoriatics. If these results are confirmed in other studies, they may suggest that psoriasis and psoriasiform napkin dermatitis have different etiologic entities.

TABLE 7.14. Seborrheic Dermatitis

	Patients		Controls				
Country/Population	n	%+	n	%+	RR	χ^2	Ref.
HLA-B12							
Japan	17	47	66	11	6.82	10.56	1

Reference

1. Skoven IG, Hjortshoj A: HLA-antigens and psoriasiform napkin dermatitis. Dermatologica 157:225-228, 1978

Seborrheic Dermatitis

Population Association

Population data based on a small (n = 17) sample of Japanese patients typed for A and B antigens[1] showed a significant association with B12 (Table 7.14). In this study, the frequency of AW30 and 31 was also increased (29.41% in patients vs. 3.02% in 66 controls).

Reference

1. Tsuji K, Nose Y, Ito M, Ozawa A, Matsuo I, Niizuma K, et al: HLA antigens and susceptibility to psoriasis vulgaris in a non-Caucasian population. Tissue Antigens 8:29-33, 1976

Epidermolysis Bullosa

Population Association

Gedde-Dahl and Thorsby[1] have presented data on 24 Norwegian patients with 4 types of recessive epidermolysis bullosa (EB) (see below). The frequencies were reported to be close to the expected frequencies in a Norwegian control population.

Disease Heterogeneity

The 24 patients studied by Gedde-Dahl and Thorsby[1] were a mixture of 4 types of recessive EB: Hallopeau-Siemens (dermolytic), inversa (dermolytic), progressive, and acquisita. There was no HLA difference between these 4 types of EB. Also, linkage analysis of several types of EB did not reveal linkage with HLA (see below).

Family Data

Gedde-Dahl and Thorsby[1] also reported lod score calculations on 16 families with different types of EB: 2 families with dominant EB simplex-Ogna type, 2 with dominant EB simplex-Weber-Cockayne type, 1 with dominant EB simplex-mottled pigment type, 2 with dominant EB dystrophica-Cockayne-Touraine type, 2 with dominant EB dystrophica-Pasini type, 1 with recessive EB dystrophica-Hallopeau-Siemens type, 3 with recessive EB dystrophica-inversa type, and 3 with recessive EB dystrophica-progressive type. In this data there was no evidence of close linkage with HLA (negative lod scores).

Ozawa et al.[2] also published data on 1 large Japanese pedigree (27 members) with 11 patients with dominant EB dystrophica-Cockayne-Touraine type. Although no lod scores were calculated, the apparent segregation of the disease with haplotypes did not show evidence of close linkage. Only 5 of the 7 HLA-typed patients had a common haplotype (AW24-B5).

References

1. Gedde-Dahl T JR, Thorsby E: HLA and epidermolysis bullosa. Arch Dermatol 113:1722-1723, 1977
2. Ozawa A, Matsuo I, Niizuma K, Ohkido M, Nose Y, Tsuji K: HLA antigens and dominant dystrophic epidermolysis bullosa in a family study. Tissue Antigens 12:233-235, 1978

Vitiligo

Population Association

An increased frequency of B13 in 28 German patients was reported by Gunther and Richter.[1] However, in 90 French patients, no significant difference was observed by Retornaz et al.[2]

Foley et al.[3] found a marginally significant in-

TABLE 7.15. Vitiligo

Country/Population	Patients n	Patients %+	Controls n	Controls %+	RR	χ^2	Ref.
HLA-A1							
U.S.A.—Black	48	38	107	15	3.42	9.83	5
HLA-A2							
U.S.A.—Black	48	48	107	24	2.89	8.68	5
HLA-A10							
U.S.A.—Black	48	8	107	27	0.26	6.60	5
HLA-AW31							
U.S.A.—Black	48	17	107	5	3.75	5.80	5
HLA-DR4							
U.S.A.	48	48	979	28	2.37	8.78	3

crease of DR4 in a sample of 48 American Caucasian patients (Table 7.15).

In 48 American Black patients, the frequencies of A1, A2, and AW31 were increased and that of A10 was decreased.[5] None of this, however, would be significant if the probabilities were corrected for multiple comparisons.

Nonsignificant results were also obtained by Metzker et al.[4] in 77 Jewish patients from Israel. When the patients were subdivided according to their ethnic origin, a high frequency of B13 was found in Moroccan Jews (n = 18).

Disease Heterogeneity

In the data of Retornaz et al.,[2] no association was observed even when patients were grouped according to sex, age at onset, extent of skin lesions, involvement of the pigmentary system of hair follicles, and provocation by an external cause. However, when the patients were subdivided into those with and without antithyroid antibodies, B13 was significantly increased in the patients with the antibodies (n = 13).

In the Israeli Jewish patients, the subdivision according to ethnic origin and age at onset showed a relatively high frequency of B13 in young (< 20 years) Moroccans, with a relative risk of 9.3 (p = 0.002). In young Yemenites, there was a significant increase in BW35 (RR = 13.89).

Family Data

In a 3-generation family, 4 of the 5 members with vitiligo were typed for HLA and no haplotype was found to be associated with the disease.[2]

References

1. Gunther VW, Richter KV: Haufigbeitsverteilung von histokompatibilitatsantigenen (HLA) bei dermatologischen erkranbungen. Dermatol Monatsschr 161:402-404, 1975
2. Retornaz G, Betuel H, Ortonne JP, Thivolet J: HL-A antigens and vitiligo. Br J Dermatol 95:173-175, 1976
3. Foley LM, Lowe NJ, Misheloff E, Tiwari JL: Association of HLA-DR4 with vitiligo. J Am Acad Dermatol 8:39-40, 1983
4. Metzker A, Zamir R, Gazit E, David M, Feuerman EJ: Vitiligo and the HLA system. Dermatologica 160:100-105, 1980
5. Kachru RB, Telischi RB, Mittal KK: HLA antigens and vitiligo in an American black population. Tissue Antigens 12:396-397, 1978

Urticaria

Population Association

In a report from Belgium by Van Nesle and Bouillenne,[1] BW35 was associated with the acute form (total duration of the symptoms less than 2 months) of urticaria (Table 7.16).

Disease Heterogeneity

The Belgian study[1] also contained data on 27 patients with chronic urticaria (total duration of the symptoms longer than 2 months). The frequency of BW35 in this group (26%) was not significantly different from controls. It should also be noted that there was no significant difference (χ^2 = 2.805) in the frequency of BW35 between acute and chronic forms of the

TABLE 7.16. Urticaria

	Patients		Controls				
Country/Population	n	%+	n	%+	RR	χ^2	Ref.
HLA-BW35							
BENELUX	27	52	1517	24	3.42	10.66	1

disease. Thus, additional data from independent studies would be necessary to confirm the association of BW35 with this disease.

Subgrouping of patients on the basis of age at onset and history of previous atopic respiratory disease did not show significant deviations in the frequencies of BW35 or any other A and B loci antigens.

Reference

1. Van Neste D, Bouillenne C: HLA antigens and urticaria. Arch Dermatol Res 261:213-215, 1978

Acne Conglobata

Population Association

A study of 65 German patients from the Munich area[1] showed no significant deviations in A and B loci antigen frequencies when compared with 1142 controls.

Reference

1. Schackert K, Scholz S, Steinbauer-Rosenthal I, Albert ED, Wahk R, Plewig G: HL-A antigens in acne conglobata: A negative study. Arch Dermatol 110:468, 1974

Alopecia Areata

Population Association

In 47 Finnish patients,[1] a highly significant association with B12 was observed (Table 7.17). At the same time, data on 70 German patients did not show any clear association with HLA. The frequency of A9 in this material was increased, though not significantly so, after correction for the multiple comparisons. A third study from France[2] did not find any significant association. However, in the combined analysis (Table 7.17), the associations with these 2 antigens are highly significant.

In the Jewish patients from Israel[3] the disease appeared to be associated with B18.

Disease Heterogeneity

In the Finnish sample,[1] there were 29 patients with patchy alopecia areata (patchy alopecia of the scalp) and the association with B12 was even stronger in this subgroup (RR = 5.41, χ^2 = 20.80). In the 14 patients with alopecia totalis (total hair loss of the scalp), B12 was increased but not significantly. There were 4 patients with alopecia universalis (hair loss of the entire body) and none had B12.

Van Neste et al.[2] classified the patients according to their response to a single immunizing dose of 2 mg of 1-chloro-2,4-dinitrobenzene. In 19 "high responders" the frequency of A3 was 15.8% as compared with 63.6% in 11 "low responders" ($p < 0.025$, corrected p not significant).

In the Israeli study [3] the association with B18 was not influenced by sex, age at onset, or by the type of alopecia.

Family Data

The report by Hacham-Zadeh et al.[3] included information on 2 small families. One patient had an affected mother and both of them carried B18. In the second family parents and both children were affected. No member of this family was positive for either B12 or B18.

References

1. Kianto U, Reunala T, Karvonen J, Lassus A, Tiilikainen A: HLA-B12 in alopecia areata. Arch Dermatol 113:1716, 1977
2. Van Neste D, Szapiro E, Breuillard F, Goudemand J: A study of HLA antigens and immune response to DNCB in alopecia areata. Clin Exp Dermatol 5:389-394, 1980
3. Hacham-Zadeh S, Brautbar C, Cohen CA, Cohen T: HLA and alopecia areata in Jerusalem. Tissue Antigens 18:71-74, 1981

TABLE 7.17. Alopecia Areata

Country/Population	Patients n	Patients %+	Controls n	Controls %+	RR	χ^2	Ref.
HLA-A9							
France	30	30	326	21	1.65	1.54	2
West Germany	70	33	1142	19	2.12	8.29	4
Finland	47	32	326	18	2.17	5.28	1
	147	32	1794	19	2.03	14.79	
	Heterogeneity χ^2 (2 df)					0.32	
HLA-B12							
France	30	40	326	26	1.92	2.91	2
West Germany	70	27	1142	23	1.26	0.70	4
Finland	47	38	326	15	3.48	14.16	1
	147	33	1794	22	1.90	12.14	
	Heterogeneity χ^2 (2 df)					5.63	
HLA-B18							
Jews—Ashkenazi	14	21	453	8	3.38	4.05	3
Jews—Non-Ashkenazi	31	26	262	6	5.56	13.62	3
	45	24	715	7	4.62	17.24	
	Heterogeneity χ^2 (1 df)					0.42	

4. Kuntz BME, Selzle D, Braun-Falco O, Scholz S, Albert ED: HLA antigens in alopecia areata. Arch Dermatol 113:1717, 1977

2. Cohen IK, McCoy BJ, Mohanakumar T, Diegelmann RF: Immunoglobulin, complement, and histocompatibility antigen studies in keloid patients. Plast Reconstr Surg 63:689-695, 1979

Keloids and Hypertrophic Scars

Population Association

In a sample of 40 Italian patients with keloids and/or hypertrophic scars, B14 was significantly increased (Table 7.18).[1] In another study of 25 American Black patients, no HLA association was observed.[2]

References

1. Laurentaci G, Dioguardi D: HLA antigens in keloids and hypertrophic scars. Arch Dermatol 113:1726, 1977

Lichen Planus

Population Association

Data are available on 241 patients from England, Denmark, and Israel (Table 7.19). In the original report of Lowe et al.,[1] a significant increase in the frequency of A3 was observed. An increase in B5, though nonsignificant, was also noted. In French and Danish patients, no significant association with either A3 or B7 was found. However, these 2 antigens are significantly increased in the total sample and there

TABLE 7.18. Keloids and Hypertrophic Scars

Country/Population	Patients n	Patients %+	Controls n	Controls %+	RR	χ^2	Ref.
HLA-B14							
Italy	40	20	131	4	5.75	9.89	1

TABLE 7.19. Lichen Planus

Country/Population	Patients n	Patients %+	Controls n	Controls %+	RR	χ^2	Ref.
HLA-A3							
Jews (unspecified)	52	14	631	18	0.78	0.40	4
England	57	55	300	30	2.83	12.88	1
France	43	37	591	26	1.69	2.66	2
Denmark	89	33	1967	27	1.34	1.67	3
	189	41	2858	27	1.76	13.09	
	Heterogeneity χ^2 (2 df)					4.12	
HLA-A28							
Jews (unspecified)	52	23	631	8	3.50	12.81	4
Jews (unspecified)	22	36	631	8	6.58	17.79	4
	74	27	1262	8	4.45	29.37	
	Heterogeneity χ^2 (1 df)					1.23	
HLA-B5							
Jews (unspecified)	52	27	631	18	1.72	2.84	4
England	57	19	300	9	2.41	5.36	1
France	43	21	591	13	1.84	2.60	2
Denmark	89	14	1967	11	1.36	1.02	3
	189	17	2858	11	1.74	7.54	
	Heterogeneity χ^2 (2 df)					1.43	

is no evidence of heterogeneity in the data (Table 7.19).

In 52 Israeli Jewish patients, the frequency of A28 was increased but not significantly if the probability values are adjusted for the number of antigens compared in the sample.

Disease Heterogeneity

Subdivision of patients in terms of age at onset of skin lesions, extent of the lesions, sex, and presence or absence of mucosal lesions did not reveal any clinical subgroup of patients with a strong or no association.[1-3]

When 52 Israeli Jewish patients were divided into diabetic and nondiabetic (based on standard oral glucose tolerance test), the frequency of A28 in 22 nondiabetic patients was significantly increased (36% in patient vs. 8% in 631 controls). Only one of 13 diabetic patients was A28-positive, and this frequency of 7.7% was not different from that of the control group. Thus, in Jewish patients, there is some indication that there may be 2 forms of lichen planus: one associated with A28 but the other not associated with A28 and probably etiologically related to diabetes.[4]

References

1. Lowe NJ, Cudworth AG, Woodrow JC: HL-A antigens in lichen planus. Br J Dermatol 95:169-171, 1976
2. Saurat JH, Lemarchand F, Hors J, Nunez-Roldan A, Gluckman E, Dausset J: HLA markers and lymhocytotoxins in lichen planus. Arch Dermatol 113:1719-1720, 1977
3. Veien NK, Risum G, Paulli Jorgensen H, Svejgaard A: HLA antigens in patients with lichen planus. Acta Dermatol Venereol 59:205-209, 1979
4. Halevy S, Zamir R, Gazit E, Feuerman EJ: HLA system in relation to carbohydrate metabolism in lichen planus. Br J Dermatol 100:683-686, 1979

Lichen Sclerosus et Atrophicus

Population Association

Harrington and Gelsthorpe[1] studied 50 Caucasian females from England. Only A and B loci antigens

TABLE 7.20. Lichen Sclerosus et Atrophicus

	Patients		Controls				
Country/Population	n	%+	n	%+	RR	χ^2	Ref.
HLA-B40							
England	50	28	3000	13	2.66	9.87	1

were typed. The authors noted an increase of B40 antigen in the patient group (Table 7.20).

Reference

1. Harrington CI, Gelsthrope K: The associaton between lichen sclerosus et atrophicus and HLA-B40. Br J Dermatol 104:561-562, 1981

Pityriasis Rubra Pilaris

Population Association

Eleven Finnish patients were studied for A and B loci antigens by Niemi et al.,[1] and no significant difference in any of the frequencies was observed.

Reference

1. Niemi KM, Kousa M, Storgards K, Karvonen J: Pityriasis rubra pilaris. Dermatologica 152:109-118, 1976

Generalized Granuloma Annulare

Population Association

In 19 Israeli Jewish patients,[1] BW35 was significantly increased (Table 7.21). If the generalized form of granuloma annulare is truly associated with HLA, then this may be indicative of a different pathogenesis of the 2 forms of the disease.

Reference

1. Friedman-Birnbaum R, Haim S, Gideone O, Barzilai A: Histocompatibility antigens in granuloma annulare. Br J Dermatol 98:425-428, 1978

Localized Granuloma Annulare

Population Association

In 13 Israeli Jewish patients studied by Friedman-Birnbaum et al.,[1] no difference in the frequencies of A and B loci antigens was observed. Similar results were also observed for A, B, and C loci antigens in 46 Swedish patients.[2] However, an increased frequency of AW29 was noted in these patients (10.9% vs. 3.8%, Fisher's exact probability = 0.043).

References

1. Friedman-Birnbaum R, Haim S, Gideone O, Barzilai A: Histocompatibility antigens in granuloma annulare. Br J Dermatol 98:425-428, 1978
2. Mobacken H, Lindholm A, Sandberg L: HLA antigens in localized granuloma annulare. Acta Dermatol Venereol 59:76-77, 1978

Kawasaki's Disease (Mucocutaneous Lymph Node Syndrome)

Population Association

The report of Kato et al.[1] on 205 Japanese patients showed significant associations with BW22 and

TABLE 7.21. Granuloma Annulare

	Patients		Controls				
Country/Population	n	%+	n	%+	RR	χ^2	Ref.
HLA-BW35							
Jews (unspecified)	19	95	70	36	22.55	15.52	1

TABLE 7.22. Kawasaki's Disease

Country/Population	Patients n	Patients %+	Controls n	Controls %+	RR	χ^2	Ref.
HLA-BW22							
Japan	32	14	76	9	1.69	0.76	2
Japan	205	25	500	12	2.44	18.02	1
	237	24	576	12	2.35	18.44	
	Heterogeneity χ^2 (1 df)					0.34	
HLA-BW51							
Jews (unspecified)	12	58	90	7	16.67	18.00	5
U.S.A.	23	30	244	3	13.52	21.92	3
HLA-BW54							
Japan	205	23	500	9	3.01	23.85	1
Japan	32	21	76	13	1.80	1.25	2
	237	23	576	10	2.78	24.28	
	Heterogeneity χ^2 (1 df)					0.82	

BW54 (a split of BW22). In a second paper from Japan,[2] these antigen frequencies were also found to be increased in 32 patients. This increase, however, was not statistically significant (Table 7.22).

Highly significant associations with BW51 have been reported in American Caucasian patients by Krensky et al.,[3,4] and in Israeli Jews by Keren et al.[5] (Table 7.22).

The frequencies of DR locus antigens were also studied in 51 American Caucasian patients by Kerensky et al.[4] However, no significant deviation of any antigen was found in this report.

Disease Heterogeneity

Kato et al.[1] also grouped their patients based on the presence of coronary aneurysms. In 22 patients with coronary aneurysms the frequency of BW15 was found to be 27.3% compared with that of patients without aneurysms (12.7%) or healthy controls (6.8%). This difference was significant at $p < 0.02$ (corrected for the number of comparisons).

Krensky et al.[4] reported data on 23 American Caucasian patients studied during an epidemic in the Boston area. Ten patients were also HLA-typed prior to this epidemic. In these 10 patients the frequency of BW51 was 70% as compared with 3% in 246 controls. In the group studied during the epidemic no patient was positive for BW51. There was, however, an increase of BW44 (50% in the patients vs. 27% in 255 controls). There was no DR antigen difference between the 2 groups.

References

1. Kato S, Kimura M, Tsuji K, Kusakawa S, Asai T, Juji T, et al: HLA antigens in Kawasaki disease. Pediatrics 61:252-255, 1978
2. Matsuda I, Hattori S, Nagata N, Fruse A, Nambu H, Itakura K, Wakisaka A: HLA antigens in mucocutaneous lymph node syndrome. Am J Dis Child 131:1417-1418, 1977
3. Krensky AM, Berenberg W, Shanley K, Yunis EJ: HLA antigens in mucocutaneous lymph node syndrome in New England. Pediatrics 67:741-743, 1981
4. Krensky AM, Grady S, Shanley KM, Berenberg W, Yunis EJ: Epidemic and endemic HLA-B and DR associations in mucocutaneous lymph node syndrome. Hum Immunol 6:75-77, 1983
5. Keren G, Danon YL, Orgad S, Kalt R, Gazit E: HLA Bw51 is increased in mucocutaneous lymph node syndrome in Israeli patients. Tissue Antigens 20:144-146, 1982

Behçet's Disease

Population Association

In 1973 Ohno et al.[1] have showed that in 21 Japanese patients, the frequency of B5 was 71.4% as compared with 30.8% in 78 controls. This association with B5 was later confirmed in several studies in Japanese

TABLE 7.23. Behçet's Disease

Country/Population	Patients n	Patients % +	Controls n	Controls % +	RR	χ^2	Ref.
HLA-B5							
Japan	20	50	166	16	5.17	11.99	25
Japan	50	60	92	28	3.78	13.39	26
Japan	23	70	553	38	3.66	8.72	3
Japan	17	88	141	38	9.90	12.47	12
Japan	44	75	78	31	6.41	20.23	13
Japan	45	67	114	35	3.69	12.81	27
	199	67	1144	33	4.59	76.57	
	Heterogeneity χ^2 (5 df)					3.03	
Turkey	26	85	138	25	15.26	26.05	28
Turkey	19	84	150	27	12.47	18.75	29
	45	85	288	26	13.92	44.74	
	Heterogeneity χ^2 (1 df)					0.07	
Tunisia	31	54	80	24	3.63	8.88	30
Jews (unspecified)	22	59	615	22	5.01	14.36	14
Jews + Arabs (Israel)	21	71	24	13	13.81	14.00	6
	119	69	1007	23	7.17	75.09	
	Heterogeneity χ^2 (4 df)					6.95	
Mexico	10	70	105	31	4.73	5.77	31
U.S.A.	26	12	523	10	1.38	0.34	2
England	9	56	283	12	8.99	12.07	32
England	60	25	100	12	2.41	4.50	5
England	28	18	613	9	2.37	3.28	33
	97	26	996	10	3.11	16.32	
	Heterogeneity χ^2 (2 df)					3.52	
France	11	55	591	13	8.00	13.32	34
Greece	16	75	200	19	11.72	19.63	35
	150	31	2310	12	3.81	39.92	
	Heterogeneity χ^2 (5 df)					13.21	
HLA-BW51							
Japan	23	61	553	21	5.75	17.24	3
Turkey	22	82	52	23	13.53	19.07	4
England	14	21	34	12	1.98	0.82	4
HLA-DR7							
Turkey	19	16	49	22	0.74	0.22	4
England	12	8	28	18	0.54	0.49	4
England	51	39	70	17	3.05	7.16	5
	63	33	98	17	2.24	4.55	
	Heterogeneity χ^2 (1 df)					3.10	

and Caucasian populations (Table 7.23). The only nonsignificant difference was reported by O'Duffy et al.[2] in a sample of 26 American Caucasian patients (Table 7.23).

In a later paper, Ohno et al.[3] reported that BW51, one split of B5, was associated in Japanese patients (Table 7.23). BW52, the other split of B5, was less frequent in the Japanese population (approximately

14%) and there was no increase in the patients. Yazici et al.[4] also found similar results in Turkish patients (Table 7.23).

In Lehner's et al. study[5] DR7 was significantly associated with this disease. However, data from 2 other reports given in Table 7.23 do not confirm this association.

It is interesting to note that this disease has some features of Reiter's disease (e.g., ocular inflammation, synovitis, and mucosal ulceration). However, unlike in Reiter's disease, B27 is not increased in this disorder.

Disease Heterogeneity

In their first report, Ohno et al.[1] also measured complement-fixing antibody to *Chlamydia*. There was no difference in the frequency of B5 between the patients with and without chlamydial antibody.

O'Duffy et al.[2] classified their patients according to the system involvement and HLA types. No relationship was found. Similarily, no association between HLA and severity or type of lesion was found in the study of Haim et al.[6]

In the Turkish study by Yazici et al.[7] 41 of the 49 patients (84%) were positive for B5. Forty of the 49 (82%) B5-positive patients had a nonspecific skin hyperreactivity to needle prick (positive pathergy). No patient was reactive for B5 and the pathergy test. In another report by the same group of authors[8] subgrouping of 119 patients on the basis of age at onset, sex, incidence of ocular disease, arthritis, thrombophlebitis, and erythema nodosum did not show any specific relationship with any A and B loci antigens.

Lehner et al.[5] compared A, B, and DR loci antigens in 4 types of Behcet's disease: mucocutaneous (n = 16), arthritic (n = 14), neurologic (n = 10), and ocular (n = 11). B12 was found to be significantly increased in the total sample mucocutaneous subgroup and in the arthritic subgroups. There was a highly significant increase of B5 in the ocular subgroup. In another report by the same group of authors[9] the ratio of IgA:IgG in immune complexes was found to be low in patients with B12 but high in those with B5 or DR2. It should be noted that no other study has reported any association of this disease with B12.

Family Data

Families with 2 or more affected members have been studied by several authors.[10–15] These data showed that affected siblings in a family share at least 1 haplotype. No formal linkage analysis is available in any of these studies. However, inspection of the data shows some evidence of linkage with HLA.

See also refs. 16–24 and 36–38.

References

1. Ohno S, Aoki K, Sugiura S, Nakayama E, Itakura K, Aizawa M: HL-A5 and Behcet's disease. Lancet ii:1383-1384, 1973
2. O'Duffy JD, Taswell HF, Elveback LR: HL-A antigens in Behcet's disease. J Rheumatol 3:1-3, 1976
3. Ohno S, Asanuma T, Sugiura S, Wakisaka A, Aizawa M, Itakura K: HLA-BW51 and Behcet's disease. JAMA 240:529, 1978
4. Yazici H, Chamberlain MA, Schreuder I, D'Amaro J, Muftuooglu M: HLA antigens in Behcet's disease: A reappraisal by a comparative study of Turkish and British patients. Ann Rheum Dis 39:344-348, 1980
5. Lehner T, Welsh KI, Batchelor JR: The relationship of HLA-B and DR phenotypes to Behcet's syndrome, recurrent oral ulceration and the class of immune complexes. Immunology 47:581-587, 1982
6. Haim S, Gideoni O, Barzilai A: The histocompatibility antigens in patients with Behcet's disease. Acta Dermatol Venereol 57:243-245, 1977
7. Yazici H, Tuzun Y , Pazarli H, Yalcin B, Yurdakul S, Muftuoglu A: The combined use of HLA-B5 and pathergy test as diagnostic markers of Behcet's disease in Turkey. J Rheumatol 7:206-210, 1980
8. Muftuoglu AU, Yazici H, Yurdakul S, Pazarli H, Ozyazgan Y, Tuzun Y, et al: Behcet's disease: Lack of correlation of clinical manifestations with HLA antigens. Tissue Antigens 17:226-230, 1981
9. Lehner T, Welsh KL, Batchelor JR: Relationship of HLA phenotype to immunoglobulin present in immune complexes from patients with Behcet's syndrome. Tissue Antigens 17:357-361, 1981
10. Ohno S, Aoki K, Sugiura S, Nakayama E, Itakura K: Immunohematological studies on Behcet's disease histocompatibility (HL-A) antigens and I blood group system. Nippon Ganka Gakkai Zasshi 77:1452-1460, 1973
11. Nahir M, Scharf Y, Gidoni O, Barzilai A, Friedman-Birnbaum R, Haim S: HL-A antigens in Behcet's disease. Dermatologica 156:205-208, 1978
12. Takano M, Miyajima T, Kiuchi M, Ohmori K, Amemiya H, Yokoyama T, et al: Behcet's disease and the HLA system. Tissue Antigens 8:95-99, 1976
13. Ohno S, Nakayama E, Sugiura S, Itakura K, Aoki K, Aizawa M: Specific histocompatibility antigens associated with Behcet's disease. Am J Ophthalmol 80:636-641, 1975

14. Brautbar C, Chajek T, Ben-Tuvia S, Lamm L, Cohen T: A genetic study of Behcet disease in Israel. Tissue Antigens 11:113-120, 1978
15. Goolamali SK, Comaish JS, Hassanyeh F, Stephens A: Familial Behcet's syndrome. Br J Dermatol 95:637-642, 1976
16. Hoshino K, Inouye H, Unokuchi T, Ito M, Tamaoki N, Tsuji K: HLA and disease in Japanese. In Dausset J, and Svejgaard A (eds): HLA and Disease. De L'institut National De La Sante Et De La Recherche Medicale, Paris 1976, p 249
17. Miyajima T, Omori K, Aoki M, Yokoyama T, Hashizumo T: Bechet's disease and HL-A antigens. Nippon Rinsho 36:3147-3150, 1978
18. Sugiura S, Sanefuji M, Ohno S: Immunological studies on Behcet's and Harada's diseases. Mod Prob Ophthalmol 16:267-278, 1976
19. Rosselet E, Saudan Y, Jeannet M: Recherche des antigenes HL-A dans la maladie de Behcet. Ophthalmologica 172:116-119, 1976
20. Chamberlain MA: Behcet's disease. Br Med J 2:1369-1370, 1978
21. Vadot E, Betuel H: Interet du groupage HLA dans la maladie de behcet. Bull Soc Ophtalmol Fr 77:257-259, 1977
22. Ohno S: Study on HL-A antigens in Behcet disease. Nippon Ganka Gakkai Zasshi Acta 78:1158-1163, 1974
23. Laroche CL, Cremer GA, Patri B, Remy JM, Letellier PH: Associattion de maladie de Behcet et de pelvispondylite chez un sujet ne presentant pas l'antigene HLA W27. Semin Hop Paris 51:2501-2508, 1975
24. Schwartz BD, Luehrman LK, Lee J, Rodey GE: A public antigenic determinant in the HLA-B5 cross reacting group-A basis for cross-reactivity and a possible link with Behcet's disease. Hum Immunol 1:37-54, 1980
25. Ono A, Kurita K, Tsuchiya M, Yamanaka I, Tsuji K: HLA antigens of intrathymic and peripheral lymphocytes in autoimmune disease. Keio J Med 24:367-376, 1975
26. Ohno S, Sugiura S: HLA antigens and Behcet's disease. Nippon Ganka Gakkai Zasshi 82:95-98, 1978
27. Okinami S, Hayashi M, Uyama M, Nakagawa J, Ikehara Y: HLA antigens in the patients with Behcet's disease, sarcoid-uveitis, and endogenous uveitis. Nippon Ganka Gakkai Zasshi 81:43-47, 1977
28. Ersoy F, Berkel I, Firat T, Kazokoglu H: HLA antigens associated with Behcet's disease. Arch Dermatol 113:1720-1721, 1977
29. Yazici H, Akokan G, Yalcin B, Muftuoglu A: The high prevalence of HLA-B5 in Behcet's disease. Clin Exp Immunol 30:259-261, 1977
30. Hamza M, Ben Ayed HB, Sohier R, Betuel H: Frequence de l'antigene HLA-B5 au cours de la maladie de Behcet. Nouv Press Med 7:3263, 1978
31. Lavalle C, Alarcon-Segovia D, Giudice-Knipping JAD, Fraga A: Association of Behcet's syndrome with HLA-B5 in the Mexican Mestizo population. J Rheumatol 8:325-327, 1981
32. Crews SJ, Mackintosh P, Barry DR, Willshaw HE: HLA antigens and certain types of uveitis. Trans Ophthalmol Soc UK 99:156-159, 1979
33. Chamberlain MA: Behcet's syndrome in 32 patients in Yorkshire. Ann Rheum Dis 36:491-499, 1977
34. Bloch-Michel E, Binaghi D, Campinchi R: Maladie de Behcet, uveites behcetoides et systeme HLA. Bull Soc Ophthalmol Fr 76:1081-1083, 1976
35. Psilas K, Polymenidis Z, Georgiades G: Le HLA-B5 antigene dans le syndrome d'adamantiades-behcet. J Fr Ophtalmol 2:701-704, 1979
36. Ohno S: Immunogenetic studies on various ocular diseases. Nippon Ganka Gakkai Zasshi 83:1875-1908, 1980
37. Hamza M, Ben Ayed H: Association agranulocytose par le levamisole et HLA B27 dans la maladie de Behcet. Nouv Presse Med 8:3167-3168, 1979
38. Jung RT, Chalmers TM, Joysey VC: HLA in Behcet's disease. Lancet i:694, 1976

Xeroderma Pigmentosum

Population Association

In a study of 16 Tunisian families (see below) when parents of the patients were compared with a control population, no difference in the HLA frequencies was observed.[1]

Family Data

A total of 37 patients and 108 relatives in 16 Tunisian families, were typed for A and B loci antigens.[1] Eleven families with at least 2 patients (in the same generation) provided data for linkage analysis. No evidence of linkage was observed in this data based on a sib-pair test outlined by the authors. (For some comments on this particular method see reference 2.) See also ref. 3.

References

1. Giraldo G, Degos L, Beth E, Gharbi RM, Day NK, Dastal H, et al: HLA antigens in 16 families with xeroderma pigmentosum. Tissue Antigens 9:167-170, 1977
2. Hodge SE, Berkel AI, Gatti RA, Boder E, Spence MA: Ataxia-telangiectasia and xeroderma pigmentosum: No evidence of linkage to HLA. Tissue Antigens 15:313-317, 1980

TABLE 7.24. Keratoacanthoma

	Patients		Controls				
Country/Population	n	%+	n	%+	RR	χ^2	Ref.
HLA-BW35							
France	25	36	200	13	3.79	8.81	1

3. Giraldo G, Degos L, Beth E, Sasportes M, Marelli A, Gharbi R, et al: C8 deficiency in a family with xeroderma pigmentosum: Lack of linkage to the HL-A region. Clin Immunol Immunopathol 8:377-384, 1977

Desquamative Erythroderma

Population Association

In a small sample of 10 French patients, Bost et al.[1] have not found any deviations in A or B loci antigens.

Reference

1. Bost M, Levy G, Arvieux J, Bensa J: Les antigenes d'histocompatibilite (HLA A et B) dans les erythrodermies desquamatives du nourisson: Maladie de Leiner-Moussous. Nouv Press Med 10:2751, 1981

Hutchinson-Guilford Progeria Syndrome

Population Association

Brown et al.[1] found no evidence of association with any of the A and B loci antigens in a single sample of 9 American Caucasian patients.

Reference

1. Brown WT, Darlington GJ, Arnold A, Fotino M: Detection of HLA antigens on progeria syndrome fibroblasts. Clin Genet 17:213-219, 1980

Werner's Syndrome

Family Data

Perez-Rojah et al.[1] published a 3-generation pedigree from Venezuela in which 5 individuals were affected by the disease. The two grandparents were first cousins. In this pedigree the disease was not segregating with any particular haplotype.

Reference

1. Perez-Rojas G, Marcano N, Gonzales L, Penchaszadeh G, Moya P, Bianco N, et al: HLA complex in Werner's disease. In Terasaki PI (eds): Histocompatibility Testing 1980. UCLA Tissue Typing Laboratory, Los Angeles, 1981, pp 945-946

Keratoacanthoma

Population Association

The frequencies of A, B, and C loci antigens in 25 French patients were compared with that in 200 controls by Gualde et al.[1] An increase of BW35 was observed (Table 7.24).

Reference

1. Gualde N, Bonnetblanc JM, Malinvaud G: HLA antigens and keratoacanthoma. Tissue Antigens 17:349-350, 1981

Felty's Syndrome

Population Association

In 22 patients from the Netherlands a significant increase of DR4 has been reported by Dinant et al.[1] (Table 7.25).

Reference

1. Dinant HJ, Muller WH, Van Den Berg-Loonen EM, Nijenhuis LE, Engelfriet CP: HLA-DRW4 in Felty's syndrome. Arthritis Rheum 23:1336, 1980

Goltz-Gorlin Syndrome (Dermal Hypoplasia)

Family Data

The HLA typings of a 3-generation pedigree with several affected members has been reported by Linss

TABLE 7.25. Felty's Syndrome

	Patients		Controls				
Country/Population	n	%+	n	%+	RR	χ^2	Ref.
HLA-DR4							
BENELUX	22	95	84	31	29.46	19.88	1

TABLE 7.26. Erythema Multiforme

	Patients		Controls				
Country/Population	n	%+	n	%+	RR	χ^2	Ref.
HLA-B15							
Ireland	29	24	200	5	6.00	12.12	1

et al.[1] In this pedigree the segregation of the haplotypes and the disease did not show strong evidence of linkage with the HLA complex.

Reference

1. Linss VG, Schielinsky Ch, Schmidt G: HLA-system und navobasaliomatose (Gorlin-Goltz-syndrome). Dermatol Monatsschr 167:377-379, 1981

Geographic Tongue

Population Association

Marks and Tait[1] studied A, B, and C loci antigens in 95 Australian patients with geographic tongue (benign migratory glossitis). When compared with 586 normal controls no significant deviations were observed.

Reference

1. Marks R, Tait B: HLA antigens in geographic tongue. Tissue Antigens 15:60-62, 1980

Erythema Multiforme

Population Association

A highly significant association with B15 in 29 Irish patients has been reported by Middleton et al.[1] (Table 7.26).

Reference

1. Middleton D, Hutchison TH, Lynd J: HLA antigen frequency in erythema multiforme and in recurrent herpes simplex. Tissue Antigens 21:264-267, 1983

CHAPTER 8

Neurology

Multiple Sclerosis

Population Association

A and B Loci

Relatively large numbers of studies have been done on the association of HLA antigens with multiple sclerosis (MS). As the data in Table 8.1 show, A3 and B7 were significantly increased in most of the studies on Caucasians from Europe and North America. A notable exception is the report by Poskanzer et al.[1] on patients from the Orkney Islands (a high-prevalence area) in which no association with the A, B, D, and DR loci antigens was found (Table 8.1). This association was not present in Italy, Iran, and India (all in a medium-to-low risk zone). In Indian patients an association with B12 has been reported.[2–4] In a sample of 71 Caucasians from South Africa and 40 from Zimbabwe (a low-risk-zone), no HLA association was observed (Table 8.1).

In Jewish patients from Israel, Brautbar et al.[5,6] found an increased frequency of B40. However,in two other reports from Israel on 45 patients and 47 controls Brautbar et al.[7,8] did not find any association with A, B, C, D, and DR loci antigens. In these reports the B40 frequency data were not given. B60 and B61 (splits of B40) were reported to be completely absent in patients as well as controls (see also ref. 9).

In Japan, where MS is very rare, increased frequencies of B8,[10] BW22,[11] and B40[12] have been reported. Eleven patients were also studied during the Eighth International Histocompatibility Workshop. No association was found[9]. In view of these inconsistent results it appears that MS in Japanese patients is not associated with HLA (see below).

In a study of 31 American Black patients, B40 was significantly increased[13]. No association was found in 11 South African Black patients[14].

Gyodi et al.[15] have noted that MS is almost completely absent (incidence = 0.004%) in the Gypsy population of Hungary (compared with the incidence of 0.06% in the entire Hungarian population). Only one Gypsy patient was observed, and he was positive for B7 and DR2.

HLA-D/DR Locus

MS patients have been typed for D/DR locus antigens by many investigators (Table 8.1) and the available results consistently showed a strong association with DW2/DR2 antigens. The combined estimates of RR for DW2 and DR2 in Caucasian patients were higher than those for A3 and B7 (Table 8.1). The association with DW2 was also evident in American Black patients.[13] No D and DR antigens were increased in the Japanese. Recent data from Brautbar et al.[7,8] showed that no D and DR loci antigens are significantly associated with MS in Israeli Jews. In 32 Arab patients (28 Jordanians [including 6 Bedouins], 2 Syrians, and 2 Lebanese), an association with DR4 (BT102) has also been reported by Kurdi et al.[16]

Thus, the existing data reveal that MS was strongly associated with the antigens of the D/DR locus in all the studied populations with the exception of Israeli Jews and Japanese. (In Iranians,[17] South Af-

TABLE 8.1. Multiple Sclerosis

Country/Population	Patients n	Patients %+	Controls n	Controls %+	RR	χ^2	Ref.
HLA-A2							
Iran	35	29	100	28	1.07	0.03	17
South Africa	71	41	71	39	1.09	0.06	14
Canada	100	42	143	49	0.76	1.15	104
Canada	224	44	253	47	0.89	0.43	27
	324	43	396	48	0.84	1.33	
	Heterogeneity χ^2 (1 df)					0.25	
U.S.A.	135	41	147	55	0.57	5.49	105
U.S.A.	94	36	871	51	0.54	7.47	106
U.S.A.	106	43	107	45	0.92	0.09	37
U.S.A.	56	41	100	49	0.73	0.92	107
	391	40	1225	51	0.65	11.27	
	Heterogeneity χ^2 (3 df)					2.69	
Australia	50	34	713	48	0.57	3.58	41
Australia	46	41	700	50	0.70	1.38	108
	96	37	1413	49	0.63	4.71	
	Heterogeneity χ^2 (1 df)					0.25	
Czechoslovakia	40	33	301	49	0.52	3.53	109
Hungary	88	51	60	48	1.13	0.13	110
England	51	45	96	52	0.76	0.65	1
France	261	37	356	52	0.54	13.53	32
France	82	44	358	50	0.79	0.96	111
	343	39	714	51	0.61	12.90	
	Heterogeneity χ^2 (1 df)					1.59	
West Germany	111	36	5046	52	0.52	10.81	112
West Germany	1000	43	1000	51	0.73	12.82	113
West Germany	393	49	255	55	0.79	2.22	114
	1504	44	6301	52	0.71	22.98	
	Heterogeneity χ^2 (2 df)					2.87	
Italy	17	41	149	42	0.98	0.00	115
Switzerland	60	35	176	43	0.72	1.15	116
Finland	60	32	116	60	0.32	12.00	39
	3045	42	11018	51	0.69	56.99	
	Heterogeneity χ^2 (19 df)					21.38	
HLA-A3							
Iran	35	43	100	18	3.39	8.53	17
India	18	0	144	13	0.18	2.70	2
Caucasians (unspecified)	66	33	959	23	1.67	3.62	9
South Africa	71	25	71	28	0.86	0.16	14
Canada	224	38	253	25	1.83	9.28	27
Canada	100	36	143	24	1.77	4.12	104
Canada	136	36	143	24	1.77	4.75	117
	460	37	539	24	1.80	18.14	
	Heterogeneity χ^2 (2 df)					0.01	

TABLE 8.1 *(continued)*

	Patients		Controls				
Country/Population	n	%+	n	%+	RR	χ^2	Ref.
HLA-A3							
U.S.A.	154	34	906	24	1.64	7.03	30
U.S.A.	106	25	107	22	1.18	0.27	37
U.S.A.	94	40	871	24	2.12	11.34	106
U.S.A.	135	27	147	24	1.17	0.34	105
U.S.A.	56	43	100	23	2.50	6.73	107
U.S.A.	330	29	136	29	1.00	0.00	118
	875	31	2267	24	1.49	16.20	
	Heterogeneity χ^2 (5 df)					9.51	
Australia	46	37	700	20	2.37	7.63	108
Australia	50	46	713	28	2.19	7.32	41
	96	42	1413	24	2.27	14.92	
	Heterogeneity χ^2 (1 df)					0.03	
Czechoslovakia	40	33	301	25	1.50	1.32	109
Hungary	88	37	60	20	2.29	4.75	110
West European (unspecified)	214	32	332	21	1.77	8.29	11
England	24	4	14	21	0.21	2.77	54
England	51	25	96	30	0.79	0.38	1
	75	18	110	29	0.65	1.43	
	Heterogeneity χ^2 (1 df)					1.72	
France	82	35	368	28	1.39	1.67	111
France	261	34	356	25	1.54	5.94	32
	343	34	724	27	1.49	7.50	
	Heterogeneity χ^2 (1 df)					0.11	
West Germany	160	34	165	28	1.32	1.37	119
West Germany	1000	36	1000	29	1.38	11.14	113
West Germany	111	27	5046	30	0.87	0.41	112
West Germany	393	36	255	27	1.52	5.66	114
	1664	35	6466	30	1.32	13.97	
	Heterogeneity χ^2 (3 df)					4.61	
Italy	176	23	245	18	1.36	1.62	9
Italy	17	18	149	17	1.19	0.08	115
	193	23	394	18	1.33	1.65	
	Heterogeneity χ^2 (1 df)					0.05	
Switzerland	60	43	176	28	1.94	4.68	116
Finland	60	38	116	45	0.75	0.78	39
Sweden	22	27	100	30	0.90	0.05	120
Sweden	105	39	135	30	1.49	2.14	22
	127	37	235	30	1.33	1.40	
	Heterogeneity χ^2 (1 df)					0.79	
	4432	34	14163	27	1.46	75.06	
	Heterogeneity χ^2 (29 df)					40.56	

TABLE 8.1 *(continued)*

Country/Population	Patients n	Patients %+	Controls n	Controls %+	RR	χ^2	Ref.
HLA-A11							
Iran	35	20	100	3	7.33	9.46	17
HLA-B7							
Iran	35	25	100	8	3.76	6.73	17
India	18	0	144	11	0.21	2.14	2
Caucasians (unspecified)	66	41	959	16	3.66	24.60	9
South Africa	71	42	71	31	1.60	1.84	14
Zimbabwe	40	38	705	26	1.76	2.98	18
Canada	136	44	143	24	2.47	12.21	117
Canada	100	46	143	24	2.68	12.59	104
Canada	224	41	253	22	2.45	19.64	27
Canada	26	50	294	20	3.97	11.62	11
	486	43	833	22	2.63	54.84	
	Heterogeneity χ^2 (3 df)					1.22	
U.S.A.	135	34	147	23	1.72	4.17	105
U.S.A.	330	35	136	29	1.31	1.52	108
U.S.A.	56	39	100	21	2.38	5.79	107
U.S.A.	94	28	871	24	1.24	0.83	106
U.S.A.	154	31	906	25	1.35	2.57	30
U.S.A.	106	27	107	19	1.56	1.91	37
	875	33	2267	24	1.45	13.68	
	Heterogeneity χ^2 (5 df)					3.11	
Australia	37	54	332	18	5.29	22.51	11
Australia	50	46	713	27	2.31	8.27	41
Australia	46	37	700	21	2.23	6.60	108
	133	45	1745	23	2.85	33.14	
	Heterogeneity χ^2 (2 df)					4.25	
Czechoslovakia	40	43	301	27	2.05	4.51	109
East Germany	100	36	1446	25	1.70	6.06	28
Hungary	133	32	717	15	2.67	21.60	15
Hungary	88	37	60	18	2.60	6.00	110
	221	34	777	15	2.66	27.60	
	Heterogeneity χ^2 (1 df)					0.00	
West European (unspecified)	214	35	332	18	2.44	19.76	11
BENELUX	46	41	503	23	2.34	7.43	26
BENELUX	46	37	49	37	1.00	0.00	24
	92	39	552	24	1.72	4.76	
	Heterogeneity χ^2 (1 df)					2.67	
England	51	35	96	36	0.96	0.01	1
England	28	58	14	21	4.59	4.91	54
	79	43	110	34	1.34	0.85	
	Heterogeneity χ^2 (1 df)					4.06	
France	261	44	356	26	2.23	21.53	32
France	82	45	368	26	2.33	11.48	111
	343	44	724	26	2.26	32.99	
	Heterogeneity χ^2 (1 df)					0.02	

TABLE 8.1 *(continued)*

Country/Population	Patients n	Patients %+	Controls n	Controls %+	RR	χ^2	Ref.
HLA-B7							
West Germany	1000	35	1000	26	1.53	19.00	113
West Germany	160	34	165	27	1.39	1.88	119
West Germany	100	36	1446	25	1.70	6.06	121
West Germany	111	45	5046	27	2.22	17.22	112
West Germany	393	36	255	31	1.25	1.70	114
	1764	36	7912	27	1.56	40.40	
	Heterogeneity χ^2 (4 df)					5.46	
Italy	176	16	245	11	1.54	2.28	9
Italy	17	18	149	12	1.77	0.86	115
	193	16	394	11	1.58	3.10	
	Heterogeneity χ^2 (1 df)					0.04	
Switzerland	60	37	176	22	2.08	5.31	116
Finland	60	33	116	31	1.10	0.08	39
Sweden	22	50	100	29	2.42	3.66	120
Sweden	105	49	135	29	2.34	9.91	22
	127	49	235	29	2.36	13.57	
	Heterogeneity χ^2 (1 df)					0.00	
	4964	37	19655	24	1.86	245.39	
	Heterogeneity χ^2 (37 df)					65.55	
HLA-B8							
Japan	41	5	213	0	27.60	8.11	10
HLA-B12							
Iran	35	11	100	10	1.18	0.08	17
India	18	78	144	14	19.62	27.40	2
India	18	78	756	7	42.94	49.07	4
	36	78	900	8	29.69	75.47	
	Heterogeneity χ^2 (1 df)					1.00	
South Africa	71	20	71	20	1.00	0.00	14
Canada	100	22	143	29	0.70	1.46	104
Canada	224	17	253	30	0.48	10.80	27
	324	19	396	30	0.55	11.28	
	Heterogeneity χ^2 (1 df)					0.99	
U.S.A.	135	15	147	27	0.48	5.92	105
U.S.A.	106	25	107	20	1.33	0.76	37
U.S.A.	94	19	871	23	0.80	0.68	106
U.S.A.	56	14	100	19	0.72	0.57	107
	391	19	1225	23	0.77	2.63	
	Heterogeneity χ^2 (3 df)					5.30	
Australia	50	22	707	31	0.65	1.65	41
Australia	46	17	700	26	0.61	1.66	108
	96	20	1407	29	0.63	3.29	
	Heterogeneity χ^2 (1 df)					0.01	

TABLE 8.1 *(continued)*

Country/Population	Patients n	Patients %+	Controls n	Controls %+	RR	χ^2	Ref.
HLA-B12							
Czechoslovakia	40	13	301	26	0.46	2.96	109
Hungary	88	16	60	25	0.58	1.87	110
West European (unspecified)	214	17	332	28	0.53	8.51	11
England	51	22	96	30	0.67	1.02	1
France	261	18	356	32	0.47	14.94	32
France	82	16	368	31	0.44	7.05	111
	343	18	724	31	0.46	21.96	
	Heterogeneity χ^2 (1 df)					0.04	
West Germany	111	14	5046	23	0.56	4.69	112
West Germany	393	15	255	25	0.53	9.98	114
West Germany	1000	16	1000	22	0.68	11.62	113
	1504	16	6301	23	0.63	24.98	
	Heterogeneity χ^2 (2 df)					1.30	
Italy	17	18	149	19	1.04	0.00	115
Switzerland	60	10	176	28	0.30	7.48	116
Finland	60	12	116	13	0.94	0.02	39
	3259	17	11354	25	0.61	73.85	
	Heterogeneity χ^2 (20 df)					19.80	
HLA-B15							
Iran	35	3	100	2	1.77	0.38	17
South Africa	71	10	71	4	2.43	1.90	14
Canada	100	6	143	12	0.49	2.32	104
Canada	224	8	253	9	0.88	0.15	27
	324	7	396	10	0.73	1.40	
	Heterogeneity χ^2 (1 df)					1.07	
U.S.A.	135	6	147	10	0.59	1.48	105
U.S.A.	56	2	100	2	1.15	0.02	107
U.S.A.	106	12	107	8	1.54	0.94	37
U.S.A.	94	3	871	8	0.41	2.70	106
	391	6	1225	8	0.79	0.82	
	Heterogeneity χ^2 (3 df)					4.32	
Australia	50	6	548	10	0.66	0.60	41
Czechoslovakia	40	5	301	13	0.43	1.84	109
Hungary	88	4	60	15	0.26	5.26	110
England	51	16	96	12	1.41	0.53	1
France	261	8	356	13	0.59	3.77	32
France	82	6	368	14	0.43	3.58	111
	343	8	724	14	0.54	6.97	
	Heterogeneity χ^2 (1 df)					0.38	
West Germany	393	5	255	8	0.61	2.45	114
West Germany	1000	9	1000	15	0.56	16.73	113
West Germany	111	14	5046	14	1.03	0.01	112
	1504	8	6301	14	0.64	15.24	
	Heterogeneity χ^2 (2 df)					3.96	

TABLE 8.1 *(continued)*

Country/Population	Patients n	Patients %+	Controls n	Controls %+	RR	χ^2	Ref.
HLA-B15							
Italy	17	12	149	6	2.45	1.60	115
Switzerland	60	20	176	16	1.33	0.60	116
Finland	60	20	116	20	1.01	0.00	39
	2999	8	10163	13	0.71	18.10	
	Heterogeneity χ^2 (18 df)					28.38	
HLA-BW22							
Japan	20	40	123	15	3.77	7.07	11
HLA-B40							
U.S.A.—Black	31	52	268	1	90.33	51.10	13
Japan	43	23	46	44	0.39	4.28	12
Jews—Ashkenazi	152	18	292	7	2.89	12.06	6
Jews—Non-Ashkenazi	46	22	167	11	2.31	3.99	6
Jews (unspecified)	41	22	171	8	3.26	6.83	5
	239	19	630	8	2.80	22.54	
	Heterogeneity χ^2 (2 df)					0.34	
HLA-DW2							
U.S.A.—Black	31	35	34	0	37.92	11.39	13
Canada	121	47	98	20	3.48	16.62	48
Canada	62	48	77	19	3.84	12.72	27
Canada	121	47	98	20	3.48	16.62	47
	304	47	273	20	3.57	45.90	
	Heterogeneity χ^2 (2 df)					0.05	
U.S.A.	330	52	136	18	4.86	41.49	118
U.S.A.	131	47	120	18	3.97	22.52	30
U.S.A.	44	49	109	23	3.18	9.74	23
	505	50	365	19	4.17	72.79	
	Heterogeneity χ^2 (2 df)					0.96	
Australia	40	63	34	18	7.20	14.09	41
West European (unspecified)	139	53	156	21	4.19	31.05	11
BENELUX	35	40	82	18	2.99	6.32	26
BENELUX	46	54	49	20	4.51	11.27	24
	81	48	131	19	3.65	17.16	
	Heterogeneity χ^2 (1 df)					0.43	
England	41	44	78	40	1.18	0.19	1
West Germany	111	54	5046	21	4.41	59.78	112
West Germany	160	43	165	21	2.81	17.59	119
	271	48	5211	21	3.72	75.30	
	Heterogeneity χ^2 (1 df)					2.07	
Finland	54	57	54	32	2.76	6.70	45
Sweden	11	45	132	18	3.73	4.82	122
Sweden	105	47	135	30	2.06	7.22	22
Sweden	22	59	45	27	3.73	6.27	120
	138	49	312	24	2.48	16.75	
	Heterogeneity χ^2 (2 df)					1.55	
	1573	50	6614	21	3.49	265.43	
	Heterogeneity χ^2 (16 df)					19.56	

TABLE 8.1 *(continued)*

Country/Population	Patients n	Patients %+	Controls n	Controls %+	RR	χ^2	Ref.
HLA-DR2							
Caucasians (unspecified)	66	56	959	26	3.60	25.28	9
Canada	22	50	294	28	2.56	4.83	11
U.S.A.	44	56	109	30	2.93	8.83	23
U.S.A.	56	84	72	33	10.10	29.39	123
U.S.A.	94	49	90	26	2.70	10.11	37
	194	61	271	29	3.78	41.36	
	Heterogeneity χ^2 (2 df)					6.97	
Australia	28	52	332	22	3.81	11.87	11
Hungary	177	43	84	19	3.15	13.65	15
West European (unspecified)	134	41	332	22	2.46	16.96	11
England	41	55	78	50	1.22	0.27	1
England	59	83	30	33	9.31	19.92	124
	100	72	108	45	2.56	9.67	
	Heterogeneity χ^2 (1 df)					10.52	
France	94	53	113	35	2.08	6.71	32
Italy	176	37	245	23	1.96	9.69	9
Switzerland	60	60	100	34	2.87	10.07	116
	1051	51	2838	27	2.78	141.91	
	Heterogeneity χ^2 (12 df)					25.65	
HLA-DR4							
Arabs (Non-Magrebian)	32	88	43	35	12.08	18.38	16
HLA-DRW6							
Japan	11	55	123	18	5.38	7.80	11

rican Caucasian and Black patients,[14] and Caucasians from Zimbabwe[18] D/DR typing was not done.) As mentioned earlier MS is very rare in Japan and it may be associated with yet undefined antigens of the D/DR locus, as was recently found in the case of Italian patients.[9]

Bf and GLO Loci

Stewart et al.[19] have reported an increased frequency of Bfs in 162 MS patients compared with 470 controls. However, this increase was a result of the strong linkage disequilibrium between Bfs and DW2 in patients as well as normal controls. In the same study[19] no association of MS with any of the GLO alleles was found.

In an interesting paper Comings[20] reported an association of Pc 1 Duarte, a common polymorphism of a human brain protein, with MS. Pc 1 Duarte was present in 52.5% (21/40) of the patients compared with 31% (48/152) of the controls, giving a relative risk value of 2.4.

Disease Heterogeneity

Progression of MS

Jersild et al.[21] first reported that patients negative for DW2 (LD-7a) had a significantly slower progression than those positive for DW2. Similar results, albeit statistically nonsignificant, were also obtained by Stendahl-Brodin et al.[22] In this study when the patients were divided into 2 groups—malignant course (persistent moderate-severe disability within 5 years after onset) and benign course (slight to no disability after 10 years)—the highest frequency of DW2 was observed in 17 patients of the first group (59% vs. 41% in 44 patients with benign course). In 19 patients with the most benign course (slight to no disability after 20 years), the frequency of DW2 was 37%. In Walker et al.'s data[23] patients with DR2 were found to have a higher progression coefficient, suggesting more severe disease.

Studies by van den Berg-Loonen and Lucas,[24] Moller et al.,[25] Reekers et al.,[26] Paty et al.,[27] Poskanzer et al.,[1] Meyer-Rienecker et al.,[28] Poser et al.,[29] and Myers et al.[30] on a large sample of patients did not show any association between DW2 (or B7) and progression of MS.

Clinical course, as measured by the rate of progression, and its relationship with B7 was analyzed in 396 German patients by Bertrams et al.[31]. B7 was significantly increased in 152 patients with a progressive course with bouts ($p = 0.0429$) and also in 117 patients with the progressive form without bouts ($p = 0.0299$). No significant increase was noted in patients with a remittant and progressive course with bouts.

It has been reported by van den Berg-Loonen and Lucas[24] that 45% of the patients with the chronic progressive form of MS were positive for DR2. The frequency of DW2 was higher in the patients with bouts as compared with the patients with the chronic progressive form. Similar results were reported by Reekers et al.[26]

Madigand et al.[32] have compared A3, B7, and DR2 frequencies in remitting and progressive subgroups of patients. A1 was found to be significantly increased in progressive type of patients. When compared with controls the frequency of DR2 was significantly increased only in the remitting subgroup. In this report patients were also subdivided on the basis of "benign MS" and "severe MS." No significant HLA difference was found between these 2 subgroups.

Oligoclonal Immunoglobulin G in Cerebrospinal Fluid

In the cerebrospinal fluids (CSF) of approximately 75-90% of the MS patients increased concentrations of oligoclonal immunoglobulin G (IgG) have been reported by many investigators. Eighty-eight of the 105 patients studied by Stendahl-Brodin[22] showed oligoclonal IgG on agarose gel electrophoresis. The frequencies of B7 and DW2 in this group, although increased, were not significantly different from those in the group without oligoclonal IgG. Similar results were observed by Reekers et al.[26] and van den Berg-Loonen and Lucas.[24] Only the results of Moller et al.[25] have shown an association between the occurrence of oligoclonal IgG in CSF and a higher frequency of DR2. Thus the bulk of data does not support any correlation between the presence of oligoclonal IgG in CSF and HLA-DW2/DR2.

Age at Onset

No association between age at onset and HLA-DW2 has been observed.[22,26,27]

Hypersensitive Response to Brain Antigen

HLA-B7 has been determined to be significantly less common in patients showing a hypersensitive response to brain antigen (16% in 19 patients positive for the leukocyte migration test vs. 55% in 20 patients negative for this test[33]).

Improvement After Immunosuppressive Therapy

No correlation was observed in 32 patients between clinical response to immunosuppressive treatment with prednisone and cyclophosphamide and DR2.[26]

Hypocomplementemic MS

Approximately 30% of the MS patients showed persistent or fluctuating low C3 levels.[34] Trouillas and Betuel et al.[34,35] have reported that B18 and B7 were strongly associated with hypocomplementemic and normocomplementemic groups of patients, respectively. A significant correlation between A3 and a hypocomplementemic group has also been reported in 58 Italian patients.[36]

Since B18 is not associated with MS, the significance of this observation in terms of disease heterogeneity is not clear.

Antimeasles Antibody Titer

There are 18 different reports on various Caucasian populations in which measles antibody titer in MS patients and its association with HLA was studied (Table 8.2). It is clear from Table 8.2 that the results are inconsistent. In most of these studies HLA antigens were not associated with the antibody titer. Furthermore, the results of the studies showing association are also variable. For example, Walker et al.[23] reported an association with B40. In 106 patients of Visscher et al.[37] low antibody titer was found to be associated with DW2. In another report by the same group of authors[38] measles antibody titers were significantly lower in siblings sharing no haplotypes with the patients. Thus, most of the data on Caucasians provides only negative results. Also, in 19 Black patients from South Africa[14] no difference between patients and controls and no HLA association was noticed.

Antirubella Antibody

No associations with any HLA antigens were observed in 5 different studies.[39–43] Only Eldridge et al.[44] observed higher antibody titer in B7 or DW2 patients. However, the sample size was small. Also, Ilonen et al.[45] reported high antibody titers in patients as compared with controls.

TABLE 8.2. Measles Antibody Titer and HLA Associations

Country	No. of Patients	Antibody Titer Patients vs. Controls	Antibody Titer Association with HLA	Ref.
Finland	60	No difference	No	39
USA	19	No difference	No	44
Sweden	95	No difference	No	22
Australia	50	No difference	No	41
England	51	No difference	No	43
England	24	No difference	No	54
Germany	941	No difference	No	101
USA	48	—	No	107
Norway	37	—	No	42
South Africa	73	High	No	14
Finland	54	High	—	45
USA	105	High	No	105
USA	15	High	—	40
USA	107	High	A3	30
USA	106	High	DW2 (low titer assoc w/DW2)	37
Canada	224	—	A3, B7, BW18, DW2	27
Denmark	57	—	A3, B7, BW18	84
USA	44	—	B40	23

Antibody to Herpes Simplex Type 1
Data of Visscher et al.,[37,38] Stewart et al.,[41] Poskanzer et al.,[43] and Ilonen et al.,[38] showed no difference between patients and controls and no association of antibody titer with HLA. Lehrich et al.[46] also found no difference between patients and controls. However, the same data showed that individuals (both patients and controls) with A3 and B7 had a high antibody titer but it was significant only in the patient group. Walker et al.[23] reported that DW7/DR7 antigens were associated with high titers. An association of antibody titer with DW2 was also reported by Paty et al.[47,48] Thus, there is no consistency in the results and no definite conclusion can be made.

Antibody to Herpes Simplex Type 2
In this case, the available data are also inconsistent. Lehrich et al.,[46] Poskanzer et al.,[43] and Visscher et al.[37,38] did not find any difference between patients and controls. However, as in the case of herpes simplex type 1, Lehrich et al.[46] reported an association between high titer and A3 and B7 in both patients and controls. This association was significant only in patients. A significant association with DW2 has also been observed by Paty et al.[48]

Antibody to Cytomegalovirus
No difference between patients and controls and no association with HLA was observed.[37,38,41,43]

Antibody to Epstein-Barr Capsid Antigen
A weak association with antibody titer and DW2 was found in patients but not in controls.[49]

Antibody to Parainfluenza Type 1
No difference between patients and controls and no association with HLA was observed.[40,43]

Antibody to Parainfluenza 3
No difference between patients and controls and no association with HLA was observed.[41]

Antibody to Mumps Virus
No difference between patients and controls and no association with HLA was observed.[41,43,45]

Antibody to Herpes Zoster
No association with HLA was observed.[47]

Antibody to Varicella
No association with HLA was observed.[43]

Mitogen Responsiveness
No response to phytohemagglutinin, concanavalin A, and pokeweed mitogen and no association with HLA was observed.[27,47,50]

Age at Onset of MS
In Walker et al.'s[23] study on 44 American Caucasian patients the age at onset of MS was significantly later

in the group with DR2 than in those without DR2 (mean 32.5 vs. 25.0 years, $p < 0.05$).

CSF C2

Delasnerie-Laupretre et al.[51] have measured C2 hemolytic activity in serum and CSF of 67 French patients. The average level of fluid C2 was found to be significantly reduced in B18 and B18 + DR2-positive patients.

Interferon Production

Salonen et al.[52,53] studied interferon production after stimulation of lymphocytes of stable MS patients with purified protein derivatives, pokeweed mitogen, phytohemagglutinin, and some viral antigens. There was some evidence of an association between low interferon production and DW2 antigen in these patients. Similar results were also observed by Gyodi et al.[15]

In another experiment Gyodi et al.[15] measured the responsiveness of natural killer cells to interferon activation. No association between high/low cytotoxic response and HLA antigens was found.

NK and K Cell Activity

Gyodi et al.[15] reported a significant association of low NK and K cell activity with B7 and DR2 antigens.

Lymphocyte Transformation Response to Viral Antigens

No significant difference between DR2/DW2-positive and -negative patients was observed.[23,45]

Leukocyte Migration Inhibition

No significant difference between A3/B7-positive or -negative patients was observed.[54]

Lymphocytotoxic Antibodies

Walker et al.[23] observed an association of B40 and DR7/DW7 with a decreased occurrence of lymphocytotoxic antibodies.

Effect of Azathioprine

In the study of Madigand et al.[32] 58 patients showed worsening of their condition during treatment with Imuran for more than 5 years. Another group of 62 patients did not show any deterioration of their condition. When compared with controls B7 was significantly increased in both groups. DR2 was significantly increased only in the group showing worsening of their condition.

Family Data

Many authors have studied the joint segregation of HLA and MS in families with 2 or more affected individuals.[9,35,41,44,55–65] Thus, published data are available on more than 125 pedigrees with at least 2 affected individuals in each pedigree. It is clear from these data that within a family MS does not always segregate with the marker haplotype, and there are many families in which MS has developed in the absence of B7 or DW2.

The results of the aforementioned studies are variable and inconsistent. Whereas some found evidence of linkage between HLA and MS, others have observed independent segregation of HLA haplotypes and MS in the families. Tiwari et al.[66] analyzed the published data on 72 pedigrees by the method of maximum likelihood. Since the mode of inheritance of MS is not clearly established, the data were analyzed for both the dominant and recessive models of inheritance and for penetrance values ranging from 5% to 95%. These results showed strong evidence of linkage (lod score > 3.0) even at the 95% penetrance level, although linkage was looser at higher penetrance values. The lod scores were similar in both dominant and recessive models of inheritance (dominant and recessive). Very similar results were also observed for 53 MS families studied during the 1980 Histocompatibility Workshop.[9] Thus, there was strong evidence in favor of linkage between HLA and an MS susceptibility gene (MSSG). The estimate of distance between HLA and MSSG was 15-20% recombination units. This anomalous result was not consistent with the idea that a population association between HLA (B7 or DW2) and MS was due to the linkage disequilibrium between MSSG and DW2. For such a linkage disequilibrium cannot exist unless the distance between HLA-D and MSSG is < 1% recombination unit. This high estimate of recombination may have been the result of the heterogeneity of the disease or of the method of linkage analysis in which linkage disequilibrium between DW2 (or B7) and MSSG has not been considered.

A more refined linkage analysis of published MS pedigree data has been published by Ho et al.[63] and also by Haile et al.[65] In these analyses the effect of linkage disequilibrium was considered. The results showed that a dominant MS susceptibility gene on chromosome 6 is tighly linked to the HLA system and that another gene for susceptibility to MS recombined freely with the HLA locus. Evidence of loose linkage observed in previous studies (e.g., ref. 66) is an abstract of this duality. The analysis of the sib pair data by Stewart et al.[64] has also favored a dominant gene hypothesis.

Weitkamp[67] and Suarez et al.[68] have proposed methods of analyzing sib pair data. The results of these methods also show that more than one gene may contribute to the susceptibillity to MS (see also ref. 69).

It is important to note that in standard Lod score analysis higher estimates of recombination (10–20%) have been obtained in other HLA-associated diseases, such as diabetes (see Diabetes) and psoriasis (see Psoriasis).

See also refs. 70–103 and 125–134.

References

1. Poskanzer DC, Terasaki PI, Prenney LB, Sheridan JL, Park MS: Multiple sclerosis in the Orkney and Shetland islands. III: Histocompatibility determinants. J Epidemiol Commun Health 34:253-257, 1980
2. Wadia NH, Trikannad VS, Krishnaswamy PR: Association of HLA-B12 with multiple sclerosis in India. Tissue Antigens 15:90-93, 1980
3. Wadia NH, Trikannad VS, Krishnaswamy PR: HLA antigens in multiple sclerosis amongst Indians. J Neurol Neurosurg Psychiatry 44:849-851, 1981
4. Trikannad VS, Wadia NH, Krishnaswamy PR: Multiple sclerosis and HLA-B12 in Parsi and non-Parsi Indians. A clarification. Tissue Antigens 19:155-157, 1982
5. Brautbar C, Cohen I, Kahana E, Alter M, Jorgensen F, Lamm L: Histocompatibility determinants in Israeli Jewish patients with multiple sclerosis. Tissue Antigens 10:291-302, 1977
6. Brautbar C, Alter M, and Kahana E: HLA antigens in multiple sclerosis. Neurology 6:50-53, 1976
7. Brautbar C, Amar A, Cohen I, Kahana E, Cohen T, Bloch D, et al: Histocompatibility (HLA) antigens and multiple sclerosis in Israelis. Isr J Med Sci 18:631-634, 1982
8. Brautbar C, Amar A, Cohen N, Oksenberg J, Cohen I, Kahana E, et al: HLA-D typing in multiple sclerosis: Israelis tested with European homozygous typing cells. Tissue Antigens 19:189-197, 1982
9. Tiwari JL, Morton NE, Lalouel JM, Terasaki PI, Zander H, Hawkins BR, et al: Multiple sclerosis. In Terasaki PI (ed): Histocompatibility Testing 1980. UCLA Tissue Typing Laboratory, Los Angeles, 1981, pp 687-692
10. Saito S, Naito S, Kawanami S, Kuroiwa Y: HLA studies on multiple sclerosis in Japan. Neurology 6:49, 1976
11. Batchelor JR, Morris PJ: Multiple sclerosis (MS): Joint report. In Bodmer W, et al. (eds): Histocompatibility Testing 1977. Munksgaard, Copenhagen, 1978, pp 207-211
12. Naito S, Kuroiwa Y, Itoyama T, Tsubaki T, Horikawa A, Sasazuki T, et al: HLA and Japanese MS. Tissue Antigens 12:19-24, 1978
13. Dupont B, Lisak RP, Jersild C, Hansen JA, Silberberg DH, Whitseti C, et al: HLA antigens in black American patients with multiple sclerosis. Transplant Proc 9:181-185, 1977
14. Fewster ME, Ames FR, Botha MC: Measles antibodies and histocompatibility types in multiple sclerosis. J Neurol Sci 43:19-26, 1979
15. Gyodi E, Benczur M, Palffy Gy, Talas M, Petranyi Gy, Foldes I, et al: Association between HLA B7,DR2 and dysfunction of natural- and antibody-mediated cytotoxicity without connection with the deficient interferon production in multiple sclerosis. Hum Immunol 4:209-217, 1982
16. Kurdi A, Ayesh I, Abdallat A, Maayta V, McDonald WS, Combston DAS, et al: Different B lymphocyte alloantigens associated with multiple sclerosis in Arabs and north Europeans. Lancet i:1123-1125, 1977
17. Lotfi J, Nikbin B, Derakhshan I, Aghai Z, Ala F: Histocompatibility antigens (HLA) in multiple sclerosis in Iran. J Neurol Neurosurg Psychiatry 41:699-701, 1978
18. Lowe RF, Moore HH, Briggs BR: The histocompatibility (HLA) antigen distribution in multiple sclerosis patients in Zimbabwe. Cent Afr J Med 26:234-236, 1980
19. Stewart GJ, Basten A, Kirk RL: Strong linkage disequilibrium between HLA-DW2 and Bfs in multiple sclerosis and in the normal population. Tissue Antigens 14:86-97, 1979
20. Comings DE: PC 1 Duarte, a common polymorphism of a human brain protein, and its relationship to depressive disease and multiple sclerosis. Nature 277:28-32, 1979
21. Jersild C, Fog T, Hansen GS, Thomsen M, Svejgaard A, Dupont B: Histocompatibility determinants in multiple sclerosis, with special reference to clinical course. Lancet ii:1221-1225, 1973
22. Stendahl-Brodin L, Link H, Moller E, Norrby E: Genetic basis of multiple sclerosis: HLA antigens, disease progression, and oligoclonal IGG in CSF. Acta Neurol Scand 59:297-308, 1979
23. Walker JE, Cook JD, Harrison P, Stastny P: HLA and the response of lymphocytes to viral antigens in patients with multiple sclerosis. Hum Immunol 4:71-78, 1982
24. van den Berg-Loonen EM, Lucas KJ: LD7a typing in 46 patients with multiple sclerosis. In Kissmeyer-Nielsen F (ed): Histocompatibility Testing 1975, Munksgaard, Copenhagen, 1975

25. Moller E, Link H, Matell G, Olhagen B, Stendahl L: LD alleles in ankylosing, myasthenia gravis, multiple sclerosis and neuritis. In Kissmeyer-Nielsen F (ed): Histocompatiblity Testing 1975. Munksgaard, Copenhagen, 1975, pp 778-781
26. Reekers P, Hommes OR, Creemers-Molenaar J, Wijnings J, Kunst VAJM, Van Rood JJ: HLA-typing and lymphocyte population studies in patients with multiple sclerosis. J Neurol Sci 33:143-153, 1977
27. Paty DW, Dossetor JB, Stiller CR, Cousin HK, Marchuk L, Furesz J, et al.: HLA in multiple sclerosis. J Neurol Sci 32:371-379, 1977
28. Meyer-Rienecker HJ, Wegener S, Hitzschke B, Richter KV: Multiple sclerosis - relation between HLA haplotype A25,B18 and disease progression. Acta Neurol Scand 66:709-712, 1982
29. Poser S, Ritter G, Bauer HJ, Grosse-Wilde H, Kuwert EK, Raun NE: HLA-antigens and the prognosis of multiple sclerosis. J Neurol 225:219-221, 1981
30. Myers LW, Ellison GW, Fewster ME, Terasaki PI, Opelz G: HLA and the immune response to measles in multiple sclerosis. Neurology 6:54-55, 1976
31. Bertrams J, Hoher PG, Kuwert E: HL-A antigens in multiple sclerosis. Lancet i:1287, 1974
32. Madigand M, Oger J, Fauchet R, Sabouraud O, Genetet B: HLA profiles in multiple sclerosis suggest two forms of disease and the existence of protective haplotypes. J Neurol Sci 53:519-529, 1982
33. Finkelstein S, Walford RL, Myers LW, Ellison GW: HL-A antigens and hypersensitivity to brain tissue in multiple sclerosis. Lancet i:736, 1974
34. Trouillas P, Berthoux F, Betuel H, Boisson D, Aimard G, Devic M: Hypocomplementaemic multiple sclerosis: Heterozygous C2 deficiency linked to HLA A10, B18. Lancet ii:1023, 1976
35. Trouillas P, Betuel H: Hypocomplementaemic and normocomplementaemic multiple sclerosis. J Neurol Sci 32:425-435, 1977
36. Caputo D, Bisaccia G, Sabbadini MG, Zibetti A: HLA-A3 linked C3 deficiency in multiple sclerosis. Boll Ist Sieroter Milan 56:260-263, 1977
37. Visscher BR, Myers LW, Ellison GW, Malmgren RM, Detels R, Lucia MV, et al: HLA types and immunity in multiple sclerosis. Neurology 29:1561-1565, 1979
38. Visscher BR, Sullivan CB, Detels R, Madden DL, Sever JL, Terasaki PI, et al: Measles antibody titers in multiple sclerosis patients and HLA-matched and unmatched siblings. Neurology (NY) 31:1142-1145, 1981
39. Ilonen J, Herva E, Reunanen M, Panelius M, Meurman O, Arstila A, et al: HLA antigens and antibody responses to measles and rubella viruses in multiple sclerosis. Acta Neurol Scand 55:299-309, 1977
40. Utermohlen V, Zabriskie JB: A suppression of cellular immunity in patients with multiple sclerosis. J Exp Med 138:1591-1595, 1973
41. Stewart GJ, Basten A, Guinan J, Bashir HV, Cameron J, Mcleod JG: HLA-DW2, viral immunity and family studies in multiple sclerosis. J Neurol Sci 32:153-167, 1977
42. Thorsby E, Helgesen A, Solheim BG, Vandvik B: HLA antigens in multiple sclerosis. J Neurol Sci 32:187-193, 1977
43. Poskanzer DC, Sever JL, Terasaki PI, Prenney LB, Sheridan JL, Park MS: Multiple sclerosis in the Orkney and Shetland Islands. V. The effect on viral titres of histocompatibility determinants. J Epidemiol Commun Health 34:265-270, 1980
44. Eldridge R, McFarland H, Sever J, Sadowsky D, Krebs H: Familial multiple sclerosis: Clinical, histocompatibility, and viral serological studies. Ann Neurol 3:72-80, 1978
45. Ilonen J, Reunanen M, Salmi A, Tiilikainen A: Lymphocyte blast transformation responses and viral antibodies in relation to HLA antigens in multiple sclerosis. J Neurol Sci 49:117-133, 1981
46. Lehrich JR, Arnason BGW: Histocompatibility types and viral antibodies. Arch Neurol 33:404-405, 1976
47. Paty DW, Cousin HK, Stiller CR, Boucher DW, Furesz J, Warren KG, et al: HLA-D typing, association of DW2 and absent immune responses towards herpes simplex (type 1) antigen in multiple sclerosis. Transplant Proc 9:1845-1848, 1977
48. Patty DW, Cousin HK, Stiller CR, Boucher DW, Warren K, Dossetor JB: HLA-DW2-related hyporesponsiveness to herpes simplex antigen in multiple sclerosis. Trans Am Neurol Assoc 102:49-51, 1977
49. Ellison GW, Myers LW, Sumaya CV, Terasaki PI, Opelz G, Holevoet MI: Epstein-Barr virus antibodies and histocompatibility type in multiple sclerosis. Trans Am Neurol Assoc 102:59-60, 1977
50. Paty DW, Cousin HK, Stiller CR: HLA antigens and mitogen responsiveness in multiple sclerosis. Transplant Proc 9:187-189, 1977
51. Delasnerie-Laupretre N, Suet-Hubert C, Marcelli-Barge A: Cerebrospinal fluid C2 and HLA system in multiple sclerosis. Tissue Antigens 19:79-84, 1982
52. Salonen R, Ilonen J, Reunanen M, Nikoskelainen J, Salmi A: PPD-, PWM-, and PHA-induced interferon in stable multiple sclerosis: Association with HLA-Dw2 antigen and clinical variables. Ann Neurol 11:279-284, 1982
53. Salonen R, Ilonen J, Reunanen M, Salmi A: Defective production of interferon-alpha associated

with HLA-DW2 antigen in stable multiple sclerosis. J Neurol Sci 55:197-206, 1982
54. Robertson P, Ward P, Brostff J, Pack S, Festenstein H, Sacks J, et al: Immunogenetic studies of multiple sclerosis patients in Caithness County, Scotland. Neuropathol Appl Neurobiol 6:299-305, 1980
55. Bertrams J, Kuwert E: HLA antigen segregation analysis in multiple sclerosis (MS) families. Z Immunitaets Forsch 152:201-208, 1976
56. Drachman DA, Davison WC, Mittal KK: Histocompatibility (HL-A) factors in familial multiple sclerosis. Arch Neurol 33:406-413, 1976
57. Alter M, Harshe M, Anderson VE, Emme L, Yunis EJ: Genetic association of multiple sclerosis and HL-A determinants. Neurology 26:31-36, 1976
58. Hens L, Carton H: HL-A determinants and familial multiple sclerosis: HL-A typing of 13 families with at least two affected members. Tissue Antigens 11:75-80, 1978
59. Visscher BR, Detels R, Dudley J, Haile RW, Malmgren RM, Terasaki PI, et al: Genetic susceptibility to multiple sclerosis. Neurology 29:1354-1360, 1979
60. Bird TD: Apparent familial multiple sclerosis in three generations: Report of a family with histocompatibility antigen typing. Arch Neurol 32:414-416, 1975
61. Zander H, Scholz S, Kuntz B, Albert ED: A sib-pair double-case study of the genetics of multiple sclerosis: An interim report on 34 pairs of affected siblings. In Bauer HJ, et al. (ed): Progress in Multiple Sclerosis. Springer-Verlag, 1980, pp 376-379
62. Zander H, Scholz S, Albert ED: Multiple sclerosis disease study: HLA-A,B,C and DRW haploytypes in 13 sib-pair double case families from West Germany. In Terasaki PI (ed): Histocompatibility Testing 1980. UCLA Tissue Typing Laboratory, Los Angeles, California, 1980, pp 947
63. Ho Z, Tiwari JL, Haile RW, Terasaki PI, Morton NE: HLA-linked and unlinked determinants of multiple sclerosis. Immunogenetics 15:509-517, 1982
64. Stewart GJ, McLeod JG, Basten A, Bashir HV: HLA family studies and multiple sclerosis: A common gene, dominantly expressed. Hum Immunol 3:13-29, 1981
65. Haile RW, Iselius L, Hodge SE, Morton NE, Detels R: Segregation and linkage analysis of 40 multiplex multiple sclerosis families. Hum Hered 31:252-258, 1981
66. Tiwari JL, Hodge SE, Terasaki PI, Spence MA: HLA and the inheritance of multiple sclerosis: Linkage analysis of 72 pedigrees. Am J Hum Genet 32:103-111, 1980
67. Weitkamp LR: HLA and disease: Predictions for HLA haplotype sharing in families. Am J Hum Genet 33:776-784, 1981
68. Suarez B, O'Rourke D, Van Eerdewegh P: Power of the affected-sib-pair method to detect disease susceptibility loci of small effect: An application to multiple sclerosis. Am J Med Genet 12:309-326, 1982
69. Spielman RS, Nathanson N: The genetics of susceptibility to multiple sclerosis. Epidemiol Rev 4:45-64, 1982
70. Olsson JE, Moller E, Link H: HLA haplotypes in families with high frequency of multiple sclerosis. Arch Neurol 33:808-812, 1976
71. Kuwert EK: Genetic aspects of multiple sclerosis with special regard to histocompatibility determinants. Acta Neurol Scand (Suppl) 55:23-42, 1977
72. Batchelor JR, Compston A, McDonald WI: The significance of the association between HLA and multiple sclerosis. Br Med Bull 34:279-284, 1978
73. Batchelor JR: Histocompatibility antigens and their relevance to multiple sclerosis. Br Med Bull 33:72-77, 1977
74. Compston DAS, Batchelor JR, Earl CJ, McDonald WI: Factors influencing the risk of multiple sclerosis developing in patients with optic neuritis. Brain 101:495-511, 1978
75. Santoli D, Trinchieri G, Zmijewski CM, Koprowski H: HLA-related control of spontaneous and antibody-dependent cell-mediated cytotoxic activity in humans. J Immunol 117:765-770, 1976
76. Terasaki PI, Mickey MR: A single mutation hypothesis for multiple sclerosis based on the HL A system. Neurology 26:56-58, 1976
77. Sachs JA: HLA antigens in multiple sclerosis. Proc R Soc Med 70:869-871, 1977
78. Poskanzer DC, Schapira K, Miller H: Epidemiology of multiple sclerosis in the counties of Northumberland and Durham. J Neurol Neurosurg Psychiatry 26:368-376, 1963
79. De Moerloose PH, Chardonnens X, Vassalli P, Jeannet M: Antigenes HLA-D des lymphocytes B et susceptibilite a certaines maladies. Schweiz Med Wochenschr 107:1461, 1977
80. Jersild C, Dupont J, Fog T, Hansen GS, Nielsen LS, Thomsen M, et al.: Histocompatibility-linked immune-response determinants in multiple sclerosis. Transplant Proc 5:1791-1796, 1973
81. Smeraldi E: Immunogenetica della sclerosi multipla: Relazione tra antigeni di istocompatibilita' e susceptibilita' alla malattia. Boll Ist Sieroter Milan 51:220-223, 1976
82. Jersild C, Svejgaard A, Fog T: HL-A antigens and multiple sclerosis. Lancet i: 1240-1241, 1972
83. Cazzullo CL, Smeraldi E: HL-A antigens and multiple sclerosis. Lancet ii:429-430, 1972
84. Jersild C, Ammitzboll T, Clausen J, Fog T: Asso-

ciation between HL-A antigens and measles antibody in multiple sclerosis. Lancet i:151-152, 1973
85. Hirsch MS: Virus markers in multiple sclerosis. N Engl J Med 294:1457-1458, 1976
86. Alter M, Quevedo J: Genetic segregation of multiple sclerosis and histocompatibility (HLA) haplotypes. J Neurol 222:67-74, 1979
87. Winchester RJ, Ebers G, Fu SM, Espinosa L, Zabriskie J, Kunkel HG: B-cell alloantigen AG 7A in multiple sclerosis. Lancet ii:814, 1975
88. Karis R: Segregation of HLA type in multiple sclerosis families. Ann Neurol 4:156-157, 1978
89. Paty DW, Cousin HK, Stiller CR, Dossetor JB: An HLA-D-linked low response to polyclonal B-cell activation in multiple sclerosis. Transplant Proc 10:973-975, 1978
90. Editorial: Multiple sclerosis and optic neuritis. Lancet i:85-86, 1979
91. Serjeantson S, Montagner A, Dry P, Stewart GJ: Absence of lymphocytotoxic antibodies in spouses of multiple-sclerosis patients. Lancet i:1347-1348, 1979
92. Kiessling WR, Pflughaupt KW: Antithyroid antibodies in multiple sclerosis. Lancet i:41, 1980
93. De Moerloose PPH, Jeannet M, Martins-Da-Silva B, Wener-Favre CH, Rohr J, Gauthier G: Antigenes HLA-DRW et la sclerose en plaques. Arch Suisses Neurol Neurochirurg Psychiatry 123:51-61, 1978
94. Alter M, Harshe M, Yunis EJ: Multiple sclerosis susceptibility and histocompatibility determinants. Neurology 25:489, 1975
95. Jersild C, Dupont B, Svejgaard A, Platz PJ, Ciongoli KA, Fog T: Genetic factors in multiple sclerosis: The major histocompatibility system (HL-A) and immunity. Neurology 25:488-489, 1975
96. Poskanzer DC, Schapira K, Brack RA, Miller H: Studies of blood groups, genetic linkage, trait association, and chromosomal pattern in multiple sclerosis. J Neurol Neurosurg Psychiatry 28:218-222, 1965
97. McFarlin DE, McFarland HF: Histocompatibility studies and multiple sclerosis. Arch Neurol 33:395-398, 1976
98. Kallen B, Low B, Nilsson O: Mixed leukocyte reaction and HL-A specificity at multiple sclerosis. Acta Neurol Scand 51:184-192, 1975
99. Strominger JL, Humphreys RE, Mccune JM, Parham P, Robb R, Springer T, et al: The immunoglobulin-like structure of human histocompatibility antigens. Fed Proc 35:1177-1182, 1976
100. Degos L, Dausset J: Histocompatibility determinants in multiple sclerosis. Lancet i:307-308, 1974
101. Bertrams J, Von Fisenne E, Hoher PG, Kuwert E: Lack of association between HL-A antigens and measles antibody in multiple sclerosis. Lancet ii:441, 1973
102. Editorial: Histocompatibility antigens and multiple sclerosis. Lancet ii:1286-1287, 1976
103. Rose AS, Ellison GW, Myers LW, Tourtellotte WW: Criteria for the clinical diagnosis of multiple sclerosis. Neurology 26:20-22, 1976
104. Paty DW, Mervart H, Campling B, Rand CG, Stiller CR: HL-A frequencies in patients with multiple sclerosis. Can J Neurol Sci 1:211-213, 1974
105. Fewster ME, Myers LW, Ellison GW, Walford RL: Histocompatibility types and measles antibodies in multiple sclerosis. J Neurol Sci 34:287-296, 1977
106. Naito S, Namerow N, Mickey MR, Terasaki PI: Multiple sclerosis: Association with HL-A3. Tissue Antigens 2:1-4, 1972
107. Arnason BGW, Fuller TC, Lehrich JR, Wray SH: Histocompatibility types and measles antibodies in multiple sclerosis and optic neuritis. J Neurol Sci 22:419-428, 1974
108. Morris PJ, Vaughan H, Tait BD, Mackay IR: Histocompatibility antigens (HLA): Association with immunopathic diseases and with response to microbial antigens. Aust NZ J Med 7:616-624, 1977
109. Vyumazal J, Krasenska J, Korinkova P, Majsky A: More experience of HLA antigen follow-up in patients with disseminated cerebrospinal sclerosis. Cesk Neurol Neurochir 43/76:284-289, 1980
110. Etelka H, Maria A, Gabor B: A HLA antigenek praedispositios jelentosege kulonbozo korkepekben es primaer immunhianyos allapotban. Orv Hetil 120:1747-1750, 1979
111. Oger J, Sabouraud O, Fauchet R, Genetet N, Menault F, Genetet B: Etude du systeme majeur d'histocompatibilite dans la sclerose en plaques. Rev Neurol 132:89-97, 1976
112. Grosse-Wilde H, Bertrams J, Schuppien W, Netzel B, Ruppelt W, Kuwert EK: HLA-D typing in 111 multiple sclerosis patients: Distribution of four HLA-D alleles. Immunogenetics 4:481-488, 1977
113. Bertrams HJ, Kuwert EK: Association of histocompatibility haplotype HLA-A3-B7 with multiple sclerosis. J Immunol 117:1906-1912, 1976
114. Bertrams J, Kuwert E, Liedtke U: HL-A antigens and multiple sclerosis. Tissue Antigens 2:405-408, 1972
115. Mazzilli MC, Baricordi O, Carolei A, Lulli P, Trabace S, Costanzi S: Distribuzione degli istoantigeni (HLA) nella sclerosi multipla. Boll Soc Ital Biol Sper 52:704-710, 1976
116. De Moerloose PH, Jeannet M, Martins-Da-Silva B, Werner-Favre CH, Rohr J, Cauthier G: Increased frequency of HLA-DRW2 and DRW3 in multiple sclerosis. Tissue Antigens 13:357-360, 1979
117. Paty DW, Furesz J, Boucher DW, Rand CG, Stiller CR: Measles antibodies as related to HL-A

types in multiple sclerosis. Neurology 26:651-655, 1976
118. Opelz G, Terasaki P, Myers L, Ellison G, Ebers G, Zabriskie J, et al: The association of HLA antigens A3, B7, and DW2 with 330 multiple sclerosis patients in the United States. Tissue Antigens 9:54-58, 1977
119. Poser S, Ritter G, Bauer HJ, Kuwert EK, Hoher PG, Grosse-Wilde H, et al: Histocompatibility patterns in multiple sclerosis. Findings of an epidemiological study. Nervenarzt 52:326-328, 1981
120. Stendahl-Brodin L, Link H, Moller E, Norrby E: Optic neuritis and distribution of genetic markers of the HLA system. Acta Neurol Scand 57:418-431, 1978
121. Meyer-Rienecker HJ, Wegener S, Hitzschke B, Richter KV: Multiple sclerosis - relation between HLA haplotype A25, B18 and disease progression. Acta Neurol Scand 66:709-712, 1982
122. Sandberg-Wollheim M, Platz P, Ryder LP, Nielsen LS, Thomsen M: HL-A histocompatibility antigens in optic neuritis. Acta Neurol Scand 52:161-166, 1975
123. Terasaki PI, Park MS, Opelz G, Ting A: Multiple sclerosis and high incidence of AB lymphocyte antigen. Science 193:1245-1247, 1976
124. Compston DAS, Batchelor JR, McDonald WI: B-lymphocyte alloantigens associated with multiple sclerosis. Lancet ii:1261-1265, 1976
125. Johnson KP: Multiple sclerosis and the immune system. Arch Neurol 37:535-536, 1980
126. Poskanzer DC, Prenney LB, Sheridan JL, Kondy JY: Multiple sclerosis in the Orkncy and Shetland islands. J Epidemiol Commun Health 34:229-239, 1980
127. Poskanzer DC, Sever JL, Sheridan JL, Prenney LB: Multiple sclerosis in the Orkney and Shetland islands. VI. Viral antibody titres and viral infections. J Epidemiol Cummun Health 34:258-264, 1980
128. Poskanzer DC, Sheriden JL, Prenney LB, Walker AM: Multiple sclerosis in the Orkney and Shetland Islands. II: The search for an exogenous aetiology. J Epidemiol Commun Health 34:240-252, 1980
129. Taylor R, Illsley R, Poskanzer DC: Multiple sclerosis in the Orkney and Shetland Islands. VI: The effects of migration and social structure. J Epidemiol Commun Health 34:271-276, 1980
130. Madigand M, Fauchet R, Oger J, Sabouraud O: Sclerose en plaques: Correlation possible entre formes cliniques et groupes HLA. Nouv Press Med 10:2349-2352, 1981
131. Stendahl-Brodin L: Studies on humoral immunity and HLA antigens in multiple sclerosis, optic neuritis and hereditary optic atrophy. Acta Ophthalmol Suppl 149:1-111, 1982
132. Ebers G: HLA typing in sibling pairs with multiple sclerosis. Lancet ii:1278, 1982
133. Compston A: Multiple sclerosis in the Orkneys. Lancet ii:98, 1981
134. Schroder R, Zander H, Andreas A, Mauff G: Multiple sclerosis: Immunogenetic analyses of sib-pair double case families. II. Studies on the association of MS with C2, C4, BF, C3, C6, and GLO polymorphisms. Immunobiology 164:160-170, 1983

Myasthenia Gravis

Population Association

HLA-A and -B locus frequency data on patients from Europe and the U.S.A. (Table 8.3) showed highly significant associations with A1 and B8 in the combined sample. The relative risk for B8 was higher (3.89) than that for A1 (2.41). The increased frequency of A1 in patients was most probably due to the linkage disequilibrium between this antigen and B8 (see ref. 1).

The studies of Kaakinen et al.[2] from Finland and of Moller et al.[3] from Sweden have shown that the association of DW3 in patients was not stronger than that with B8. Similar data are available in 3 reports (Table 8.3) on DR3. The increased frequency of this antigen in the combined sample was highly significant.

Yoshida et al.[4] reported a highly significant association with B12 in 63 Japanese patients. However, it is interesting to note that in an earlier report by the same authors[5] the frequency of B5 was 53% in 35 patients not typed for B12 as compared with 16% in 166 controls ($\chi^2 = 23.44$). In the later report[4] B5 was present in 36.5% of the patients and 40.6% of the controls and thus the difference between the 2 groups was not significant. In a sample of 59 Japanese and 17 Chinese patients tested during the 1980 Histocompatibility Workshop[6] no significant association was found.

One report on 37 patients from India[7] showed a marginally sgnificant increase of BW21 and BW35 in patients.

In an interesting study of Gm allotypes in 74 Japanese patients Nakao et al.[8] showed that Gm*1,2,21* was present in 40% of the patients as compared with 17.06% in 236 normal controls ($\chi^2 = 16.94$). In Caucasian patients an excess of phenotype 1,4,12 has been reported by Dawkins[6].

TABLE 8.3. Myasthenia Gravis

	Patients		Controls				
Country/Population	n	%+	n	%+	RR	χ^2	Ref.
HLA-A1							
Caucasians (unspecified)	67	43	3184	28	1.95	7.33	6
U.S.A.	71	21	90	24	0.85	0.19	10
U.S.A.	37	35	125	24	1.72	1.89	36
	108	26	215	24	1.18	0.39	
	Heterogeneity χ^2 (1 df)					1.69	
BENELUX	100	55	533	30	2.84	22.49	1
England	26	85	597	31	11.42	23.24	37
England	68	47	200	37	1.51	2.15	15
	94	58	797	33	2.43	13.11	
	Heterogeneity χ^2 (1 df)					12.27	
West Germany	54	41	600	23	2.34	8.68	11
Italy	60	35	172	23	1.81	3.41	6
Finland	159	35	326	17	2.62	19.09	12
Sweden	42	33	95	20	1.97	2.78	38
	684	41	5922	27	2.17	69.18	
	Heterogeneity χ^2 (9 df)					22.06	
HLA-B8							
India	37	24	118	12	2.33	3.40	7
Caucasians (unspecified)	67	34	3184	16	2.73	15.18	6
U.S.A.	28	40	855	18	3.07	8.63	17
U.S.A.	71	31	90	18	2.02	3.68	10
U.S.A.	28	29	200	16	2.19	3.18	14
	127	33	1145	18	2.40	14.82	
	Heterogeneity χ^2 (2 df)					0.68	
BENELUX	100	59	533	19	6.09	62.09	1
England	68	41	200	28	1.79	4.04	15
England	26	65	597	31	4.03	101.93	37
	94	48	797	30	2.35	13.29	
	Heterogeneity χ^2 (1 df)					2.69	
West Germany	54	43	600	17	3.69	20.16	11
Italy	60	25	172	13	2.24	4.85	6
Finland	159	48	326	18	4.18	45.09	12
Sweden	44	64	100	31	3.87	13.15	39
Sweden	42	47	95	19	3.71	10.99	38
	86	56	195	25	3.80	24.14	
	Heterogeneity χ^2 (1 df)					0.01	
	747	44	6952	18	3.35	185.13	
	Heterogeneity χ^2 (11 df)					17.85	

TABLE 8.3 *(continued)*

Country/Population	Patients n	Patients %+	Controls n	Controls %+	RR	χ^2	Ref.
HLA-B12							
Japan	63	40	271	17	3.25	15.49	4
HLA-BW21							
India	37	19	118	4	5.39	8.33	7
HLA-BW35							
India	37	24	118	7	4.12	7.95	7
HLA-DW3							
Sweden	44	36	100	19	2.38	4.84	39
HLA-DR3							
Caucasians (unspecified)	67	42	3184	21	2.74	16.52	6
U.S.A.	28	36	47	15	3.08	4.33	17
England	68	38	200	27	1.66	3.01	15
Italy	60	24	172	14	1.95	3.36	6
	223	35	3603	21	2.23	25.03	
	Heterogeneity χ^2 (3 df)					2.19	

Disease Heterogeneity

Sex

A1, B8, DW3, and DR3 antigen frequencies in male and female patients are available in some of the reports and they are given in Tables 8.4 and 8.5 (see also ref. 9). It is clear from these data that the association of B8 (and of A1) was significant only in female patients. The data in Table 8.3 are the sum of findings in males and females. In males these antigens were not associated with the disease. Yoshida et al.[4] reported similar results for B12 in Japanese patients.

In males DR3 and DW3 were also not associated with the disease (Table 8.4). The results of Moller et al.[3] and Kaakinen et al.[2] also did not associate DW3 in either sex. These 2 reports do not contain information about the sample size of controls and thus are not included in the tables.

Age at Onset

Several authors have reported a stronger association of B8 in patients with early onset of the disease.[2,10–14]. The early age at onset was defined by Pirskanen[12] as < 35 years and by Fritze et al.[10] as < 40 years. B12 was also strongly associated in female Japanese patients with age at onset < 30 years.[4].

As an example, in the data of Pirskanen[12] the frequency of B8 in 75 female Finnish patients with early onset was 72.0% as compared with 26.3% in 37 late onset patients and 17.5% in 326 controls.

The study of Safwenberg et al.[13] included only male patients. In 22 patients with age at onset < 35 years the frequency of B8 was 55% as compared with 16% in 32 patients with age at onset > 35 years and 19% in 500 controls. The results of Pirskanen[12] on male patients were similar. The studies of Gross et al.[11] and Fritze et al.[10] have shown a stronger association of B8 in all patients (males and females) with early onset. Compston et al.[15] have reported a lower mean age at onset in patients positive for A1, B8, and DR3 antigens.

Thymic Morphology

Fritze et al.[10] reported a highly significant increase of B8 in 21 patients with hyperplasia (57% in the patients with hyperplasia vs. 6% in 16 patients with thymoma and 18% in 90 controls). Similarly, in the 38 patients with hyperplastic thymus studied by Pirskanen[12] the frequency of B8 was 73.7% as compared with 14.29% in 7 patients with thymoma and 17.5% in 326 controls. In the Japanese study by Yoshida et al.[4] B12 was found in 44.6% of the 56 patients without thymoma and 0% in 7 patients with

TABLE 8.4. Myasthenia Gravis: Male

Country/Population	Patients n	Patients %+	Controls n	Controls %+	RR	χ^2	Ref.
HLA-A1							
U.S.A.	28	4	90	24	0.18	5.05	10
England	38	37	200	37	1.01	0.00	15
West Germany	21	23	600	23	1.07	0.02	11
Finland	47	19	326	17	1.19	0.20	12
Sweden	54	37	500	22	2.10	6.24	13
	188	26	1716	23	1.24	1.52	
	Heterogeneity χ^2 (4 df)					9.99	
HLA-B8							
Caucasians (unspecified)	31	19	3184	16	1.31	0.39	6
U.S.A.	12	33	855	18	2.37	2.33	17
U.S.A.	28	7	90	18	0.41	1.76	10
	40	15	945	18	1.14	0.10	
	Heterogeneity χ^2 (1 df)					4.00	
England	38	29	200	28	1.07	0.03	15
West Germany	21	23	600	23	1.07	0.02	11
Finland	47	26	326	18	1.63	1.93	12
Sweden	7	29	100	31	1.02	0.00	39
Sweden	54	31	500	19	1.94	4.59	13
	61	31	600	21	1.76	3.95	
	Heterogeneity χ^2 (1 df)					0.64	
	238	25	5855	18	1.39	4.53	
	Heterogeneity χ^2 (7 df)					6.53	
HLA-B12							
Japan	16	25	271	17	1.74	1.02	4
HLA-DW3							
Sweden	54	20	317	18	1.17	0.19	13
Sweden	7	14	100	19	0.95	0.00	39
	61	19	417	18	1.13	0.14	
	Heterogeneity χ^2 (1 df)					0.05	
HLA-DR3							
U.S.A.	12	25	47	15	1.97	0.93	17
England	38	32	200	27	1.29	0.47	15
	50	30	247	25	1.42	1.12	
	Heterogeneity χ^2 (1 df)					0.28	

thymoma. Thus, these data indicate stronger HLA associations in a subgroup of patients without thymoma (see also refs. 2, 6, 7, 14-18).

Severity of the Disease

Pirskanen et al.[12] found a significant increase of B8 in a subgroup of patients with ocular and milder forms of the disease (37.68% in 69 patients as compared with 17.5% in 326 controls, $p = 0.0005$). Similar results were also obtained by Safwenberg et al.[13] in 37 patients with the ocular and mild generalized form of the disease. In the Japanese study[4] B12 was present in 73.3% of the 15 patients with the ocular type as compared with 17% in 271 controls

TABLE 8.5. Myasthenia Gravis: Female

Country/Population	Patients n	Patients %+	Controls n	Controls %+	RR	χ^2	Ref.
HLA-A1							
U.S.A.	43	33	90	24	1.56	1.26	10
England	30	60	200	37	2.51	5.63	15
West Germany	33	52	600	23	3.61	13.31	11
Finland	112	42	326	17	3.52	27.61	12
	218	44	1216	24	2.92	44.21	
	Heterogeneity χ^2 (3 df)					3.60	
HLA-B8							
Caucasians (unspecified)	67	45	3184	16	4.30	35.01	6
U.S.A.	43	47	90	18	3.96	11.77	10
U.S.A.	16	43	855	18	3.49	6.68	17
	59	46	945	18	3.76	18.41	
	Heterogeneity χ^2 (1 df)					0.04	
England	30	57	200	28	3.36	9.68	15
West Germany	33	54	600	17	5.68	23.83	11
Finland	112	57	326	18	5.98	56.90	12
Sweden	37	68	100	31	4.59	14.36	39
	338	54	5355	17	4.67	155.48	
	Heterogeneity χ^2 (6 df)					2.76	
HLA-B12							
Japan	47	45	271	17	3.98	17.64	4
HLA-DW3							
Sweden	37	41	100	19	2.93	6.90	39
HLA-DR3							
U.S.A.	16	44	47	15	4.27	5.64	17
England	30	47	200	27	2.39	5.06	15
	46	46	247	25	2.83	10.07	
	Heterogeneity χ^2 (1 df)					0.64	

and 31.1% in 45 patients with the generalized disease type ($p < 0.05$).

In Safwenberg's data[13] 4 of the 23 patients (17.39%) with severe generalized disease had B8 as compared with 41.94% in 31 patients with the ocular and mild generalized type and 19% in 500 controls. The difference between severe and generalized types and controls was not significant. On the other hand, Pirskanen et al.[12] found the B8 frequency to be 37.2% in 43 patients with the severe form and 72.3% in 47 patients who improved with time. All these increases were significant (see also refs. 6, 18.).

Acetylcholine Receptor Antibody Titer

Edvard Smith et al.[16] measured acetylcholine receptor antibodies in 20 B8-positive and 20 B8-negative patients. The mean titers in these 2 groups were 2.82 and 3.27, respectively (no significant difference). These authors also studied antibody titers in subgroups of patients with thymic hyperplasia (n = 11), thymoma (n = 7), and normal thymus histology (n = 11). B8-positive and -negative patients were compared in each subgroup and between the subgroups. The only significant difference was between B8-negative patients with thymoma (n = 6, mean titer = 6.01) and B8-negative myasthenics with hyperplasia (n = 5, mean titer = 1.77) ($p < 0.02$).

Naeim et al.[17,19] also studied acetylcholine receptor antibodies in 28 patients (5 with and 23 without thymoma). The average antibody titer in patients without thymoma was $28 \pm 8.7 \times 10^{-9}$. The patients were then divided into groups with antibody titer > 28 and titer < 28. Each of these subgroups was further subdivided into B8-positive, B8-negative, DR3-positive, and DR3-negative subgroups. The analysis of the patients in these subgroups showed a highly significant association with high antibody titer (higher than average level) and B8 and DR3 positivity (for detailed data see refs. 17, 18). High antibody titers in B8-positive patients have also been reported by Dawkins[6] (see also refs. 40, 43).

Richman et al.[14] studied the association between cellular response to acetylcholine receptor and HLA-A and -B loci antigens in 28 patients with myasthenia gravis. There were 17 acetylcholine responders and 11 nonresponders. No HLA antigen was associated with positive cellular reponse to acetylcholine receptor.

In the study of Compston et al.[15] there was no association between A1, B8, or DR3 and titers of limb or ocular acetylcholine antibody.

Homozygosity for B8

In a small sample of 7 patients homozygous for B8, Van Den Berg-Loonen et al.[1] estimated the relative risk to be 4.67 times the relative risk for heterozygous individuals (no details of calculations are given).

Autoantibodies

Yoshida et al.[4] have determined the autoantibodies (the presence of one or more antibodies to skeletal muscle, nuclei, thyroid microsome thyroglobulin, and thymus) in 63 Japanese patients. B5 was present in 63.2% of the 19 patients positive for the antibodies as compared with 25.0% in 44 patients negative for the antibodies ($p < 0.05$). The frequency of B12 in the antibody-positive group was 26.3% and 45.5% in the antibody-negative group ($p < 0.05$). Compston et al.[15] did not find any association between A1, B8, and DR3 and the presence of striated muscle antibody or other autoantibodies.

Family Data

Family data are not available. However, Whiteley et al.[20] described 2 brothers with congenital myasthenia gravis. They had 2 different haplotypes and neither had the A1-B8-DW3 haplotype.

See also refs. 21–35 and 40–44.

References

1. Van Den Berg-Loonen EM, Nijenhuis LE, Engelfriet CP, Feltkamp JEW, Van Rossum AL, Oosterhuis HJG: Segregation of HLA haplotypes in 100 families with a myasthenia gravis patient. J Immunogenet 4:331-340, 1977
2. Kaakinen A, Pirskanen R, Tiilikainen A: LD antigens associated with HL-A8 and myasthenia gravis. Tissue Antigens 6:175-182, 1975
3. Moller E, Hammarstrom L, Smith E, Matell G: HL-A8 and LD-8A in patients with myasthenia gravis. Tissue Antigens 7:39-44, 1976
4. Yoshida T, Tsuchiya M, Ono A, Yoshimatsu H, Satoyoshi E, Tsuji K: HLA antigens and myasthenia gravis in Japan. J Neurol Sci 32:195-201, 1977
5. Ono A, Kurita K, Tsuchiya M, Yamanaka I, Tsuji K: HLA antigens of intrathymic and peripheral lymphocytes in autoimmune disease. Keio J Med 24:367-376, 1975
6. Dawkins R: Myasthenia gravis. In Terasaki PI (ed): Histocompatibility Testing 1980. UCLA Tissue Typing Laboratory, Los Angeles, 1981, pp 662-667
7. Mehra NK, Ahuja GK, Taneja V, Vaidya MC: HLA antigens and myasthenia gravis in north India. J Neurol Neurosurg Psychiatry 46:361-364, 1983
8. Nakao Y, Matsumoto H, Miyazaki T, Nishitani H, Ota K, Fujita T, et al: GM allotypes in myasthenia gravis. Lancet i:677-680, 1980
9. Hammarstrom L, Smith E, Moller E, Franksson C, Matell G, Von Reis G: Myasthenia gravis: Studies on HL-A antigens and lymphocyte subpopulations in patients with myasthenia gravis. Clin Exp Immunol 21:202-215, 1975
10. Fritze D, Herrmann C JR, Naeim F, Smith GS, Zeller E, Walford RL: The biologic significance of HL-A antigen markers in myasthenia gravis. Ann NY Acad Sci 274:440-450, 1976
11. Gross WL, Kruger J, Groschel-Stewart U, Friedrich H, Kunze K: Studies on HLA antigens and cellular and humoral autoimmune phenomena in patients with myasthenia gravis. Clin Exp Immunol 27:48-54, 1977
12. Pirskanen R: Genetic associations between myasthenia gravis and the HL-A system. J Neurol Neurosurg Psychiatry 39:23-33, 1976
13. Safwenberg S, Hammarstrom L, Lindblom JB, Matell G, Moller E, Osterman PO, et al.: LA-A, -B, -C, and -D antigens in male patients with myasthenia gravis. Tissue Antigens 12:136-142, 1978
14. Richman DP, Antel JP, Patrick JW, and Arnason BGW: Cellular immunity to acetylcholine receptor in myasthenia gravis: Relationship to histocompatibility type and antigenic site. Neurology 29:291-296, 1979
15. Compston DAS, Vincent A, Newsom-Davis J, Bathchelor JR: Clinical, pathological, HLA antigen and immunological evidence for disease heterogeneity in myasthenia gravis. Brain 103:579-601, 1980

16. Edvard Smith CIL, Hammarstrom L, Moller E, Lefvert AK, Matell G: No significant correlation of HLA-B8 and amount of antibodies directed to acetylcholine receptor protein in patients with myasthenia gravis. Tissue Antigens 12:387-395, 1978
17. Naeim F, Keesey JC, Herrmann C, Lindstrom J, Zeller E, Walford RL: Association of HLA-B8, DRW3, and anti-acetylcholine receptor antibiodies in myasthenia gravis. Tissue Antigens 12:381-386, 1979
18. Keesey J, Naiem F, Lindstrom J, Roe D, Herrmann C, Walford R: Acetylcholine receptor antibody titer and HLA-B8 antigen in myasthenia gravis. Arch Neurol 39:73-77, 1982
19. Keesey J, Naeim F, Lindstrom J, Zeller E, Herrmann C JR, Walford R: Correlation between acetylcholine receptor antibody titer and HLA-B8 and HLA-DRW3 antigens in myasthenia gravis. Trans Am Neurol Assoc 103:188-190, 1978
20. Whiteley AM, Schwartz MS, Sachs JA, Swash M: Congenital myasthenia gravis: Clinical and HLA studies in two brothers. J Neurol Neurosurg Psychiatry 39:1145-1150, 1976
21. Hoshino K, Inouye H, Unokuchi T, Ito M, Tamaoki N, Tsuji K: HLA and disease in Japanese. In Dausset J Svejgaard A (eds): HLA and Disease. De L'institut National De La Sante Et De La Recherche Medicale, Paris 1976, p 249
22. Okimoto K, Kosaka K: Myasthenia gravis and HLA. Nippon Rinsho 36:3164-3170, 1978
23. Oosterhuis HJ, Feltkamp TEW, Van Rossum AL, Van Den Berg-Loonen PM, Nijenhuis LE: HL-A antigens, autoantibody production, and associated diseases in thymoma patients, with and without myasthenia gravis. Ann NY Acad Sci 274:468-474, 1976
24. Pirskanen R: On the significance of HL-A and LD antigens in myasthenia gravis. Ann NY Acad Sci 274:451-460, 1976
25. Remuzzi G, Livio M, Donati MB, De Gaetano G: Myasthenia gravis, thrombocytopenia and HLA antigens. Ann Intern Med 87:250-251, 1977
26. Fritze D, Herrmann C, Walford RL: Myasthenia gravis: Familial occurrence and HL-A types. Compr Ther 3:19-25, 1977
27. Remuzzi G, Misiani R, Livio M, Dall'olio A, Donati MB, De Gaetano G: Possible role of HLA-B8 antigen as a genetic marker of autoimmune thrombocytopenia in a patient with myasthenia gravis. Thromb Haemost 38:593-594, 1977
28. Fritze D, Herrman C JR, Naeim F, Smith GS, Walford RL: HL-A antigens in myasthenia gravis. Lancet i:240-243, 1974
29. Pirskanen R, Tiilikainen A, Hokkanen E: Histocompatibility (HLA) antigens associated with myasthenia gravis. Ann Clin Res 4:304-306, 1972
30. Friedrich H, Samland O, Krueger J, Gross W, Hackell U, Kunze K, et al: HL-A antigene bei myasthenia gravis. Z Immunitaetsforsch BD 148:394-396, 1975
31. Keesey J, Novom S: HLA antigens in pencillamine-induced myasthenia gravis. Neurology 29:528-529, 1979
32. Naeim F, Stoddard A, Fritze D, Herrmann C, Zeller E, Walford RL: HL-A antigens on hyperplastic and neoplastic thymic tissue. Cancer Res 34:654-656, 1974
33. Feltkamp EW, Van Den Berg-Loonen PM, Engelfriet CP, Nijenhuis LE, Van Rossum AL, Van Loghem JJ, et al: HL-A typing en auto-antistoffen BIJ patienten met myasthenia gravis. Ned Tijdschr Geneeskd 118:895-896, 1974
34. Papatestas AE, Genkins G, Kornfeld P, Horowitz SH: HL-A antigens in myasthenia gravis. Lancet i:511-512, 1974
35. Fritze D, Herrmann C JR, Naeim F, Smith GS, Walford RL: HL-A antigens in myasthenia gravis. Lancet ii:43, 1974
36. Fritze D, Herrmann C JR, Smith GS, Walford RL: HL-A types in myasthenia gravis. Lancet ii:211, 1973
37. Behan PO, Simpson JA, and Dick H: Immune response genes in myasthenia gravis. Lancet ii:1033, 1973
38. Safwenberg J, Lindblom JB, Osterman PO: HL-A frequencies in patients with myasthenia gravis. Tissue Antigens 3:465-469, 1973
39. Moller E, Link H, Matell G, Olhagen B, Stendahl L: LD alleles in ankylosing, myasthenia gravis, multiple sclerosis and neuritis. In Kissmeyer-Nielsen F (ed): Histocompatiblity Testing 1975. Munksgaard, Copenhagen, 1975, pp 778-781
40. Christiansen FT, Houliston JB, Dawkins R: HLA, anti-DNA, and complement in myasthenia gravis. Muscle Nerve 1:467-470, 1978
41. Behan PO: Immune disease and HLA association with myasthenia gravis. J Neurol Neurosurg Psychiatry 43:611-621, 1980
42. Seybold ME, Lindstrom JM: Antiacetylcholine receptor antibody and its relationship to HLA type in asymptomatic siblings of a patient with myasthenia gravis. Neurology (NY) 31:778-780, 1981
43. Garlepp MJ, Dawkins RL, Christiansen FT: HLA antigens and acetylcholine receptor antibodies in penicillamine induced myasthenia gravis. Br Med J 286:338-340, 1983
44. Dawkins RL, Christiansen FT, Kay PH, Garlepp M, McCluskey J, Hollingsworth PN, et al: Disease associations with complotypes, supratypes and haplotypes. Immunol Rev 70:5-22, 1983

Spinocerebellar Ataxia

Family Data

Yakura et al.[1] first published HLA types of a small family (2 parents and 5 siblings) with the father and 3 female siblings affected by Marie's ataxia. This data suggested that a dominant ataxia might be linked to HLA. Later, Jackson et al.[2] studied a large kindred with spinocerebellar ataxia and, using the lod score method, estimated that this dominantly inherited ataxia locus was located on chromosome 6 at a distance of 12% recombination (lod score = 3.15). Following this, several other families with spinocerebellar ataxia and HLA data were reported[3–12].

Morton et al.[13] did segregation and linkage analysis of all of the 13 published pedigrees. (Five families with dominant and 3 with recessive ataxia, published later, are included in this review.) Segregation analysis of these pedigrees showed overwhelming evidence for a major locus. The linkage analysis produced estimates of distance between this locus and HLA as 22.3% and 32.7% recombination in males and females, respectively (lod score = 5.53). Thus, there is very strong evidence that the spinocerebellar ataxia locus is loosely linked to HLA.

It is important to note that the lod scores of 5 families with dominant ataxia studied by Koeppen et al.[8] and of 2 families by Van Rossum et al.[12] were negative for all values of recombinations (see also ref. 9). However, the total of this and 13 pedigrees analyzed by Morton et al.[13] would still produce a lod score of > 3.00, generally accepted as evidence for linkage.

The gene for this disease has been mapped on chromosome 6.

References

1. Yakura H, Wakisaka A, Fujimoto S, Itakura K: Hereditary ataxia and HL-A genotypes. N Engl J Med 291:154-155, 1974
2. Jackson JF, Currier RD, Terasaki PI, Morton NE: Spinocerebellar ataxia and HLA linkage. N Engl J Med 296:1138-1141, 1977
3. Noreen HJ, Nino HE, Dubey DP, Resch JA, Namboodiri K, Elston RC, Yunis EJ: Genetic linkage with HLA in spinocerebellar ataxia. Transplant Proc 11:1729-1731, 1979
4. Nino HE, Noreen HJ, Dubey DP, Resch JA, Namboodiri K, Elston RC, et al: A family with hereditary ataxia: HLA typing. Neurology 30:12-20, 1980
5. Jackson JF, Whittington JE, Currier RD, Terasaki PI, Morton NE, Keats BJB: Genetic linkage and spinocerebellar ataxia. Adv Neurol 21:315-318, 1978
6. Moller E, Hindfelt B, Olssol JE: HLA-determination in families with hereditary ataxia. Tissue Antigens 12:357-366, 1978
7. Wastiaux JP, Lamoureux G, Bouchard JP, Durivage A, Barbeau C, Barbeau A: HLA and complement typing in olivo-ponto-cerebellar atrophy. Can J Neurol Sci 5:75-81, 1978
8. Koeppen AH, Goedde HW, Hirth L, Benkmann H -G, Hiller C: Genetic linkage in hereditary ataxia. Lancet i:92-93, 1980
9. Albert ED, Zander H: Inherited ataxia. In Terasaki PI (ed): Histocompatibility Testing 1980. UCLA Tissue Typing Laboratory, Los Angeles, 1981, pp 732-733
10. Suciu-Foca N, Rohowsky C, Godfrey M, Khan R, O'Neill G, Starkman S, et al: HLA and spinocerebellar ataxia. In Terasaki PI (ed): Histocompatibility Testing 1980. UCLA Tissue Typing Laboratory, Los Angeles, 1981, p 943
11. Whittington JE, Keats BJB, Jackson JF, Currier RD, Terasaki PI: Linkage studies on glyoxalase I (GLO), pepsinogen (PG), spinocerebellar ataxia (SCA1), and HLA. Cytogenet Cell Genet 28:145-150, 1980
12. Van Rossum J, Veenema H, Went LN: Linkage investigations in two families with hereditary ataxia. J Neurol Neurosurg Psychiatry 44:516-522, 1981
13. Morton NE, Lalouel JM, Jackson JF, Currier RD, Yee S: Linkage studies in spinocerebellar ataxia(SCA). Am J Med Genet 6:251-257, 1980

Friedreich's Ataxia

Family Data

In 5 Canadian families studied by Chamberlain et al.[1] the segregation of the disease was found to be independent of the HLA system. All families were typed for the antigens of A, B, and C loci.

Reference

1. Chamberlain S, Walker JL, Sachs JA, Wolf E, Festenstein H: Non-association of Friedreich's ataxia and HLA based on five families. Can J Neurol Sci 6:451-452, 1979

Muscular Dystrophy

Population Association

Forty-six American Caucasian patients with non-sex-linked muscular dystrophy were typed for A and B loci antigens by Eckels et al.[1] They found no significant difference when compared with a control sample of 1405 individuals.

TABLE 8.6. Chronic Relapsing Idiopathic Inflammatory Polyneuropathy (Guillain-Barré Type)

	Patients		Controls				
Country/Population	n	%+	n	%+	RR	χ^2	Ref.
HLA-B8							
Australia	16	50	322	26	2.84	4.56	1
England	14	50	571	25	2.99	4.64	2
	30	50	893	25	2.91	9.19	
	Heterogeneity χ^2 (1 df)					0.01	
HLA-DW3							
Australia	13	46	59	14	5.04	6.62	1
England	14	37	99	17	2.91	3.43	2
	27	41	158	16	3.74	9.64	
	Heterogeneity χ^2 (1 df)					0.42	
HLA-DR3							
England	14	50	351	17	4.85	9.24	2

Reference

1. Eckels DD, Gershwin ME, Terasaki P, Fowler WM Jr, Taylor RG: HLA typing in the non-x-linked muscular dystrophies. Hum Genet 48:231-233, 1979

Myotonic Dystrophy

Family Data

Hsia et al.[1] have published HLA haplotypes of a 4-generation American Black family with a total of 29 members. Six individuals were affected with myotonic dystrophy.

In this family the disease was not found to be segregating with any particular HLA haplotype.

Reference

1. Hsia S, Ho CK, Aliffi VB, Doran DM, Hamilton D: Myotonic dystrophy: HLA antigens and mitogen stimulated lymphocyte responses of a black American family. Tissue Antigens 19:53-59, 1982

Neurolathyrism

Population Association

Forty-three Ashkenazi Jews suffering from chronic neurolathyrism were typed for A and B loci antigens.[1] When frequencies were compared with those in 130 controls (Ashkenazi Jews) there was no significant difference between the 2 groups.

Reference

1. Cohn DF, Streifler M, Zamir R, Kott E, Rinot Y: HLA antigens in neurolathyrism. Neurol India 26:55-57, 1978

Chronic Relapsing Idiopathic Inflammatory Polyneuropathy (Guillain-Barré Type)

Population Association

Stewart et al.[1] have reported a significant association with AW30/31 in 16 patients (38% vs. 4% in 322 controls, $p = 0.0001$). This, however, was not observed in the data from England and this apparent association may have been due to the small sample or serologic problems associated with the typing of AW30/31.[2]

In both studies, there was an increase in the frequencies of B8, DR3, and DW3 (Table 8.6) and in the combined analysis these associations were marginally significant if correction for multiple comparisons is considered.

Disease Heterogeneity

Stewart et al.[1] have also published data on a group of 6 patients with subacute polyneuritis (not included in 16 patients with chronic relapsive polyneuritis). There was no indication of any HLA associations.

References

1. Stewart GJ, Pollard JD, Mcleod JG, Wolnizer CM: HLA antigens in the Landry-Guillain-Barré syn-

TABLE 8.7. Guillain-Barré Syndrome

	Patients		Controls				
Country/Population	n	%+	n	%+	RR	χ^2	Ref.
HLA-DR3							
Mexico	38	32	100	11	3.74	8.38	4

drome and chronic relapsing polyneuritis. Ann Neurol 4:285-289, 1978
2. Adams D, Festenstein H, Gibson JD, Hughes RAC, Jaraquemada J, Papasteriadis C, et al: HLA antigens in chronic relapsing idiopathic inflammatory polyneuropathy. J Neurol Neurosurg Psychiatry 42:184-186, 1979

Guillain-Barré Syndrome

Population Association

In 59 patients from London typed for A and B loci antigens, no significant deviation was observed by Adams et al.[1] Similar results were also reported for 22 Australian[2] and 18 American Caucasian patients also studied for D locus antigens.[3] A recent report on 38 Mexican mestizo patients by Gorodezky et al.[4] showed a significant association with DR3 antigen (Table 8.7).

References

1. Adams D, Gibson JD, Thomas PK, Batchelor JR, Hughes RAC, Kennedy L, Festenstein H, Sachs J: HLA antigens in Guillain-Barré syndrome. Lancet ii:504-505, 1977
2. Stewart GJ, Pollard JD, Mcleod JG, Wolnizer CM: HLA antigens in the Landry-Guillain-Barré syndrome and chronic relapsing polyneuritis. Ann Neurol 4:285-289, 1978
3. Latovitzki N, Suciu-Foca N, Penn AS, Olarte MR, Chutorian AM: HLA typing and Guillain-Barré syndrome. Neurology 29:743-745, 1979
4. Gorodezky C, Varela B, Castro-Escobar LE, Chavez-Negrete A, Escobar-Gutierrez A, Martinex-Mata J: HLA-DR antigens in Mexican patients with Guillain-Barré syndrome. J Neuroimmunol 4:1-7, 1983

Bell's Palsy (Idiopathic Facial Palsy)

Population Association

Smith et al.[1] typed 50 Swedish patients (22 females and 28 males) for A, B, and C loci antigens. An increased frequency of A2 (70% vs. 50%, $\chi^2 = 6.00$) was observed. This, however, would not have been significant if the corresponding probability was multiplied by 29, the total number of A, B, and C antigens compared in the study.

Disease Heterogeneity

Subgrouping of patients on the basis of sex and age at onset ($\leq$ 47 years and $>$ 47 years) also did not produce any significant association.

Reference

1. Edvard Smith CI, Hammarstrom L, Siden A: No significant association between HLA and Bell's palsy. Tissue Antigens 12:404-406, 1978

Amyotrophic Lateral Sclerosis

Population Association

American and European Caucasians

Antel et al.[1] found a significant increase in the frequency of A3 in a sample of 44 American Caucasian patients (Table 8.8). Their study was done in 2 steps. The first 25 amyotrophic lateral sclerosis (ALS) cases were considered as 1 study and 15 subsequent cases were analyzed separately as a second independent study. Antigen A3 was increased in both samples.

The HLA types of 40 American Caucasian patients studied by Bartfeld et al.,[2] 25 patients from Denmark,[3] and 10 patients from Finland[4] did not show an increase in A3. In the combined analysis of American and Danish data no evidence of association of ALS with A3 was present (Table 8.8). No frequency data on controls were available for the Finnish study. The authors, however, did give frequency data for B40 which was somewhat increased (Table 8.8). Thus, these data revealed no indication of a strong association of ALS with HLA in this population. Danish patients were also tested for HLA-D locus antigens.

TABLE 8.8. Amyotrophic Lateral Sclerosis

	Patients		Controls				
Country/Population	n	%+	n	%+	RR	χ^2	Ref.
HLA-A3							
Jews (unspecified)	28	46	140	19	3.60	9.16	5
U.S.A.	40	20	262	19	1.11	0.06	2
U.S.A.	44	43	200	26	2.15	5.12	1
	84	32	462	22	1.64	3.61	
	Heterogeneity χ^2 (1 df)					1.57	
Denmark	25	20	1967	30	0.63	1.01	3
	109	29	2429	28	1.30	1.36	
	Heterogeneity χ^2 (2 df)					4.83	
HLA-B40							
U.S.A.	40	5	262	9	0.64	0.48	2
Denmark	25	20	1967	18	1.22	0.18	3
Finland	10	50	551	15	5.64	8.61	4
	75	16	2780	17	1.62	2.32	
	Heterogeneity χ^2 (2 df)					6.95	

Israeli Jews

Kott et al.[5] have studied 28 ALS patients and 1480 matched controls from Israel. The frequency of A3 was 46% in patients and 19% in controls, giving a relative risk value of 3.60 (Table 8.8). Nine of the 13 patients with A3 also had a positive index of "migration inhibition factor," suggesting an association between A3 and poliovirus in the pathogenesis of ALS.

Guamanians

Twenty-eight ALS patients from Guam were studied by Hoffman et al.[6] and they reported no significant increase in the frequency of any antigen.

Disease Heterogeneity

In Guamanians no difference in HLA antigen frequency with respect to age at onset, duration, or severity of disease was evident.

See also refs. 7 and 8.

References

1. Antel JP, Arnason BGW, Fuller TC, Lehrich JR: Histocompatibility typing in amyotrophic lateral sclerosis. Arch Neurol 33:423-425, 1976
2. Bartfeld H, Pollack MS, Cunningham-Rundles S, Donnenfeld H: HLA frequencies in amyotrophic lateral sclerosis. Arch Neurol 39:270-271, 1982
3. Pedersen L, Platz P, Jersild C, Thomsen M: HLA (SC and LD) in patients with amyotrophic lateral sclerosis (ALS). J Neurol Sci 31:313-318, 1977
4. Jokelainen M, Tiilikainen A, Lapinleimu K: Polio antibodies and HLA antigens in amyotrophic lateral sclerosis. Tissue Antigens 10:259-266, 1977
5. Kott E, Livni E, Zamir R, Kuritzky A: Cell-mediated immunity to polio and HLA antigens in amyotrophic lateral sclerosis. Neurology 29:1040-1044, 1979
6. Hoffman PM, Robbins DS, Gibbs CJ JR, Gajdusek DC, Carruto RM, Terasaki PI: Histocompatibility antigens in amyotrophic lateral sclerosis and Parkinsonism-dementia on Guam. Lancet ii:717, 1977
7. Behan PO, Dick HM, Durward WF: Histocompatibility antigens associated with motor neuron disease. J Neurol Sci 32:213-217, 1977
8. Hoffman PM, Robbins DS: Cell-mediated immunity to polio and HLA antigens in amyotrophic lateral sclerosis. Neurology 30:679-680, 1980

Migraine

Population Association

In 18 American Caucasian female patients with "classic" migraine, Kudrow[1] found a slightly increased frequency of B17 (17% vs. 4%, $\chi^2 = 4.79$).

This increase, however, was not evident in another study on a similar population (n = 21) by O'Neill et al.[2] Thus, classic migraine does not seem to be associated with the antigens of the A and B loci.

O'Neill et al.[2] also studied 29 patients with "common" migraine and again no HLA association was observed.

Disease Heterogeneity

In the study by O'Neill,[2] subdivision of migraine patients into "classic" and "common" groups (as well as in total, i.e., classic + common) did not reveal any significant association. The authors also grouped their patients into the categories of "positive family history" and "negative family history" and again no HLA association was found.

References

1. Kudrow L: HL-A antigens in cluster headache and classical migraine. Headache 18:167-168, 1978
2. O'Neill BP, Kapur JS, Good AE: HLA antigens in migraine. Headache 19:71-73, 1979

Infantile Spasms (West's Syndrome)

Population Association

The only report available is that by Howitz and Platz[1] on 21 Danish children. The HLA antigen frequencies, when compared with 196 blood donors, showed no significant deviations.

Disease Heterogeneity

When patients were divided into cryptogenic groups (normal pregnancy and birth, normal psychomotor development until the appearance of spasms, no abnormal laboratory findings) and symptomatic (abnormalities before the onset of spasms, infections or trauma during the pregnancy, epilepsy, psychomotor retardation, etc.), no differences in HLA frequencies were detected.

Reference

1. Howitz P, Platz P: Infantile spasms and HLA antigens. Arch Dis Child 53:680-682, 1978

Cluster Headache

Population Association

Kudrow et al.[1] studied 25 patients with episodic cluster headache. No association was found. Similar results were observed in 37 German patients typed for A, B, and C loci antigens by Cuypers and Altenkirch.[2] In the German study[2] there were 5 patients (4 males and 1 female) with the chronic type of cluster headache. Interestingly, all 5 were positive for A1.

References

1. Kudrow L: HL-A antigens in cluster headache and classical migraine. Headache 18:167-168, 1978
2. Cuypers J, Altenkirch H: HLA antigens in cluster headache. Headache 19:228-229, 1979

Epilepsy

Population Association

Twenty-three Swiss patients[1, 2] with low IgA serum concentrations were compared with 1765 controls (Table 8.9). The frequency of A2 was significantly increased in the patient group.

References

1. Fontana A, Joller H, Skvaril F, Grob P: Immunological abnormalities and HLA antigen frequencies in IGA deficient patients with epilepsy. J Neurol Neurosurg Psychiatry 41:593-597, 1978
2. Fontana A, Grob PJ: Immunoglobulin deficiency, HLA antigens, and seizures. Ann Intern Med 88:429, 1978

TABLE 8.9. Epilepsy

	Patients		Controls				
Country/Population	n	%+	n	%+	RR	χ^2	Ref.
HLA-A2							
Switzerland	25	96	1765	47	18.42	15.65	1

TABLE 8.10. Lennox-Gastaut Syndrome

	Patients		Controls				
Country/Population	n	%+	n	%+	RR	χ^2	Ref.
HLA-B7							
Italy	22	45	443	10	7.35	20.67	1

Lennox-Gastaut Syndrome

Population Association

In 22 Italian patients[1] B7 was found to be significantly increased (Table 8.10).

Family Data

In this Italian study[1] some families were also HLA-typed. The authors have claimed that the segregation of B7 diverged from the normal segregation in patients but was normal in healthy siblings. No pedigree data were given.

Reference

1. Smeraldi E, Smeraldi RS, Cazzullo CL, Cazzullo AG, Fabio G, Canger R: Immunogenetics of the Lennox-Gastaut syndrome: Frequency of HL-A antigens and haplotypes in patients and first-degree relatives. Epilepsia 16:699-703, 1975

Paraplegia and/or Quadriplegia

Population Association

In 54 randomly selected Canadian Caucasian patients with paraplegia or quadriplegia of more than 3 years duration no association with any of the HLA-A and B loci antigens was found.[1]

Disease Heterogeneity

When the patients in the study were divided into groups with abnormal sacroiliac joints (n = 24) and normal sacroiliac joints (n = 30), no association of HLA with the changes in sacroiliac joint was observed.

Reference

1. Hunter T, Hildahl CR, Smith NJ, Dubo HIC, Schroeder ML: Histocompatibiltiy antigens in paraplegic or quadriplegic patients with sacroiliac joint changes. J Rheumatol 6:92-95, 1979

Parkinson's Disease

Population Association

Emile et al.[1] have reported increased frequencies of B17 and B18 in 50 patients from France (no data are given). However in 64 patients from Scotland,[2] 52 from Finland,[3,4] and 64 American Caucasians from New York[5] no evidence of significant association was found. The patients in the Finnish study[3] were also typed for D locus antigens and those in the American study[5] were also investigated for the antigens of the DR locus. The disease in all these studies was classified as "idiopathic Parkinson's disease."

An increased frequency of BW16 has been reported in a study from Guam (Table 8.11). This increase, however, would not be significant if probability is corrected for the 34 antigens compared in this study.

Takagi et al.[6] have reported A and B loci antigens in 36 Japanese patients with idiopathic Parkinson's disease and 11 patients with Parkinson's syndrome

TABLE 8.11. Parkinson's Disease

	Patients		Controls				
Country/Population	n	%+	n	%+	RR	χ^2	Ref.
HLA-B14							
Jews (unspecified)	18	44	148	8	8.81	16.47	7
HLA-BW16							
Guam	51	28	65	9	3.73	6.81	9

with cerebrovascular disease. No significant deviations were found.

Elizan et al.[7] have studied 17 American Jewish patients with idiopathic Parkinson's disease and 18 with postencephalitic Parkinson's disease. A significant association with B14 was observed (Table 8.11) only in the idiopathic group. However, another report by Lees et al.[8] on 21 English patients with postencephalitic type of disease did not find any significant association with A, B, C, and DR loci antigens. The frequency of B14 in the patients was 5% and 9% in 153 controls.

Disease Heterogeneity

The report by Marttila et al.[4] on Finnish patients also included data on serum and cerebrospinal fluid antibodies against herpes simplex and measles viruses. No association of viral antibody levels with any particular HLA antigen was found.

In the Japanese study[6] subgrouping of patients according to age at onset, sex, clinical manifestations, and response to L-dopa therapy also did not show any HLA associations.

Family Data

Reed et al.[5] have given family information on 6 patients. Five of these had 1 affected sibling and 1 had 2 affected siblings. The distribution of HLA haplotypes in these 6 affected sibpairs was not significantly different from the random segregation of haplotypes and the disease.

References

1. Emile J, Truelle JL, Pouplard A, Hurez D: Association maladie de parkinson-antigenes HLA-B17 et B18. Nouv Presse Med 6:4144, 1977
2. Leheny WA, Davidson DLW, DeVane P, House AO, Lenman AR: HLA antigens in Parkinson's disease. Tissue Antigens 21:260-261, 1983
3. Marttila RJ, Rinne UK, Tiilikainen A: Histocompatibility types in Parkinson's disease. J Neurol Sci 51:217-221, 1981
4. Marttila RJ, Rinne UK, Tiilakainen A: Virus antibodies in Parkinson's disease. J Neurol Sci 54:227-238, 1982
5. Reed E, Lewison A, Mayeaux R, Suciu-Foca N: HLA antigens in Parkinson's disease. Tissue Antigens 21:161-163, 1983
6. Takagi S, Shinohara Y, Tsuji K: Histocompatibility antigens in Parkinson's disease. Acta Neurol Scand 66:590-593, 1982
7. Elizan TS, Terasaki PI, Yahr MD: HLA-B14 antigen and postencephalitic Parkinson's disease: Their association in an American-Jewish ethnic group. Arch Neurol 37:542-544, 1980
8. Lees AJ, Stern GM, Compston DAS: Histocompatibility antigens and post-encephalitic Parkinsonism. J Neurol Neurosurg Psychiatry 45:1060-1061, 1982
9. Hoffman PM, Robbins DS, Gibbs CJ JR, Gajdusek DC, Carruto RM, Terasaki PI: Histocompatibiblity antigens in amyotrophic lateral sclerosis and Parkinsonism-dementia on Guam. Lancet ii:717, 1977

Motor Neuron Disease

Population Association

Forty-four British patients and 342 controls were studied by Behan et al.[1, 2] and no significant difference in the frequency of A and B loci antigens was observed.

References

1. Behan PO, Durward WF, Dick H: Histocompatibility antigens associated with motor-neuron disease. Lancet ii:803, 1976
2. Behan PO, Dick HM, Durward WF: Histocompatibility antigens associated with motor neuron disease. J Neurol Sci 32:213-217, 1977

Spinal Muscular Atrophy

Population Association

The only data available on this disorder are on 55 patients from England.[1] A highly significant increase in B7 was observed (Table 8.12).

TABLE 8.12. Spinal Muscular Atrophy

	Patients		Controls				
Country/Population	n	%+	n	%+	RR	χ^2	Ref.
HLA-B7							
England	55	66	110	24	5.99	25.47	1

Disease Heterogeneity

In the aforementioned British study there were 26 type II and 23 type III patients. The frequency of B7 was similar in both groups of patients.

Reference

1. Upstill-Goddard G, Gardner-Medwin D, Roberts DF, Wentzel J: Spinal muscular atrophy associated with HLA-B7. Br Med J 1:720-721, 1979

Peroneal Muscular Atrophy (Charcot-Marie-Tooth Desease)

Population Association

In 24 American Caucasian patients typed for A, B, and C antigens, Williams[1] has noted a nonsignificant increase of A2 and B12 antigens.

Family Data

The segregation of haplotypes in 24 families studied by Williams[1] did not show any evidence of linkage of this disorder with the HLA complex. The probands of these 24 families were used in the analysis of population association.

Reference

1. Williams LL: HLA in Charcot-Marie-Tooth disease. Ann Neurol 8:452, 1980

Ataxia-Telangiectasia

Family Data

Analyses of 9 multiple-case families by lod score and sib pair methods did not provide any evidence of linkage between HLA and this autosomal recessive disorder.[1]

Reference

1. Hodge SE, Berkel AI, Gatti RA, Boder E, Spence MA: Ataxia-telangiectasia and xeroderma pigmentosum: No evidence of linkage to HLA. Tissue Antigens 15:313-317, 1980

Huntington's Disease

Population Association

HLA-A, -B, and -C typing of 17 German patients compared with 1,000 controls[1] showed an increase in the frequency of BW16 (24% vs. 6%, uncorrected $p \sim 0.01$).

Family Data

In the German study[1] 6 families were also investigated. There was no evidence of joint segregation of HLA and Huntington's disease.

Reference

1. Foerster K, Freudenberg J: HLA antigen frequencies in patients with Huntington's chorea and their relatives. J Neurol 223:119-125, 1980

Subacute Sclerosing Panencephalitis

Population Association

The results of 2 independent studies (Table 8.13) are not consistent. Kurent et al.[1] found a highly significant association with A29. This, however, was not confirmed in the German[2] and Turkish[3] studies. In

TABLE 8.13. Subacute Sclerosing Panencephalitis

Country/Population	Patients n	Patients %+	Controls n	Controls %+	RR	χ^2	Ref.
HLA-A29							
Turkey	24	13	300	5	3.12	3.65	3
U.S.A.	36	25	1085	7	4.56	15.39	1
West Germany	24	4	1000	4	1.47	0.26	2
	60	17	2085	6	3.61	13.88	
	Heterogeneity χ^2 (1 df)					1.76	

the pooled data the association with A29 was still significant and there was no indication of heterogeneity (Table 8.13).

See also ref. 4.

References

1. Kurent JE, Sever JL, Terasaki PI: HL-A W29 and subacute sclerosing panencephalitis. Lancet i:927-928, 1975
2. Kreth HW, Ter Meulen VT, Eckert G: HL-A and subacute sclerosing panencephalitis. Lancet ii:415-416, 1975
3. Aysun S, Ersoy F, Sanal O, Yalaz K, Ozdirim E, Berkel AI, et al: HLA antigens in subacute sclerosing panencephalitis. Arch Neurol 40:38-39, 1983
4. Furlan AJ, Rothner AD: S.S.P.E. and multiple sclerosis. Lancet i:1113, 1974

Paralytic Dementia

Paralytic dementia usually develops 10–20 years following primary infection with *Treponema pallidum*. It is the most severe neurological manifestation of untreated or inadequately treated latent syphilis.

Population Association

Whitsett et al.[1] typed 75 American Caucasian and 58 American Black institutionalized patients with paralytic dementia. In the Caucasian sample, the frequency of AW24 was decreased and that of B18 was increased (Table 8.14). In the Black group, A2 and BW40 were increased. The researchers concluded that the apparent decrease in AW24 in the Caucasian sample may have been the result of technical problems with respect to the reliability of sera, as there was no significant difference in the frequency of A9. Thus, these results are only marginally significant and need confirmation in additional studies.

TABLE 8.14. Paralytic Dementia

Country/ Population	Patients n	Patients %+	Controls n	Controls %+	RR	χ^2	Ref.
HLA-A2							
U.S.A.— Black	58	48	268	29	2.25	7.80	1
HLA-AW24							
U.S.A.	75	3	855	15	0.21	7.28	1
HLA-B18							
U.S.A.	75	19	855	10	2.16	6.24	1
HLA-B40							
U.S.A.— Black	58	10	268	1	9.99	12.01	1

Reference

1. Whitsett C, Turner WJ, Lee TD, Dupont B: HLA antigen frequencies in paralytic dementia. J Neurol Sci 30:417-420, 1976

Neurofibromatosis (Von Recklinghausen's Disease)

Population Association

Lepage et al.[1] have typed 16 unrelated French patients for A, B, C, and DR loci antigens. When compared with 106 normal controls, no significant deviations in the antigen frequencies were observed.

Family Data

In the above study[1] 7 multiple case families were also studied. Analysis of lod scores of these families showed no evidence of close linkage between the HLA complex and a disease susceptibility gene for neurofibromatosis.

Reference

1. Lepage V, Tongio MM, Mayer S, Groshans E, Ceccaldi C, Puissant A, et al: Neurofibromatosis (Von Recklinghausen's disease). In Terasaki PI (ed): Histocompatibility Testing 1980. UCLA Tissue Typing Laboratory, Los Angeles, 1981, pp 719-721

Idiopathic Torsion Dystonia

Population Association

Korein et al.[1] did not observe any association with A, B, C, and DR loci antigens in 67 American Caucasian patients from New York.

Family Data

In the above study[1] lod score analysis was performed in 9 families with either 1 or 2 affected individuals. The maximum lod score was 0.387 at a recombination frequency of 20%. Thus additional family data

TABLE 8.15. Syringomyelia

	Patients		Controls				
Country/Population	n	%+	n	%+	RR	χ^2	Ref.
HLA-A9							
England	53	36	500	14	3.47	16.35	1

would be necessary to either accept or reject the hypothesis of linkage with HLA.

Reference

1. Korein J, Willoughby E, Pollack MS, Levidow L, Dupont B: Human leukocyte antigens in torticollis and other idiopathic dystonic syndromes. Ann Neurol 10:573-575, 1981

Syringomyelia

Population Association

A significant association with A9 was observed by Newman et al.[1] in 53 British patients (Table 8.15). Forty of these patients had an associated Chiari anomaly. In these patients the frequency of A9 was 33%.

Reference

1. Newman PK, Wentzel J, Foster JB: HLA and syringomyelia. J Neuroimmunol 3:23-26, 1982

Sensorineural Hearing Loss

Population Association

In 103 German patients with moderate or severe bilateral sensorineural hearing loss, Gross and Arndt-Hanser[1] have observed a significant increase of BW16 and B18 antigens (Table 8.16).

Reference

1. Gross M, Arndt Hanser A: HLA-antigens and sensorineural deafness. Laryngol Rhinol Otol (Stuttg) 61:316-318, 1982

Anencephaly

Population Association

In an interesting report Feingold et al.[1] have studied the geographic correlation between the incidence of anencephaly and the HLA antigens. Data on the incidence of anencephaly at birth from 15 European countries, Israel, Japan, and Mexico and HLA antigen frequencies in these populations were analyzed for the correlation coefficient between the 2 variables.

Significant positive correlations with A1 (0.69) and B8 (0.78), and negative correlations with B5 (−0.69) and BW35 (−0.75) were found in the total sample of 15 European populations. These results were also similar for the combined data on 18 populations (15 European populations plus Israel, Japan, and Mexico). The level of significance of these varied from 0.05 to 0.001.

Family Data

Farb et al.[2] published a case report on an American Black with a twin pregnancy. Both infants were affected with anencephaly. She and her husband both

TABLE 8.16. Sensorineural Hearing Loss

	Patients		Controls				
Country/Population	n	%+	n	%+	RR	χ^2	Ref.
HLA-BW16							
West Germany	103	14	9999	6	2.62	11.95	1
HLA-B18							
West Germany	103	16	9999	7	2.59	12.91	1

TABLE 8.17 Narcolepsy

Country/Population	Patients n	Patients %+	Controls n	Controls %+	RR	χ^2	Ref.
HLA-B27							
England	42	67	200	22	7.01	29.14	5
France	38	53	300	15	6.31	26.95	4
	80	60	500	18	6.65	56.05	
	Heterogeneity χ^2 (1 df)					0.04	
HLA-BW35							
Japan	92	34	244	16	2.70	12.79	3
HLA-DR2							
Japan	92	100	244	34	358.08	33.61	3
England	37	100	200	22	263.76	29.46	5
France	8	100	110	22	59.40	14.35	6
	45	100	310	22	129.77	42.81	
	Heterogeneity χ^2 (1 df)					1.00	

were negative for B27, an antigen suggested to be involved in spinal development.

References

1. Feingold J, Feingold N, Bois E: Spina bifida and anencephaly: Geographic correlation with the HLA system. Tissue Antigens 15:318-324, 1980
2. Farb HF, Thomason J, Carandang FS, Sampson MB, Spellacy WN: Anencephaly, twins and HLA-B27. J Reprod Med 25:166-170, 1980

Narcolepsy

Population Association

The first report by Honda et al.[1] from Japan on 56 patients showed a significantly increased frequency of BW35 in 56 patients. A second report by the same group of authors[2] showed that all of the 40 patients tested for DR antigens were positive for DR2 antigen. These results were further confirmed in a third report[3] on 92 patients (Table 8.17). The frequency data in Table 8.17 were taken only from the third study with the largest sample size.

In 38 Caucasian patients from France, Seignalet and Billiard[4] found a significant association with HLA-B7. This association was confirmed in a second study from England by Langdon et al.[5] Like the Japanese study,[3] all patients in the British[5] and French[6] were also positive for DR2 (Table 8.17).

Thus, narcolepsy is one of very few diseases in which an HLA antigen was found to be present in almost all of the patients. This very important result may provide further clues to the genetic basis of this disease.

References

1. Honda Y, Asaka A, Tanaka Y, Juji T: Discrimination of narcoleptic patients by using genetic markers and HLA. Sleep Research 12:254, 1983
2. Juji T, Satake M, Honda Y, Doi Y: HLA antigens in Japanese patients with narcolepsy. Tissue Antigens 24:316–319, 1984
3. Juji T, Matsuki K, Nohara T, Satake M, Honda Y: HLA antigens in Japanese patients with narcolepsy. Lancet i:227, 1985
4. Seignalet J, Billiard M: Possible association between HLA-B7 and narcolepsy. Tissue Antigens 23:188–189, 1984
5. Langdon N, Welsh K, van Dam M, Vaughan RW, Parkes D: Genetic markers in narcolepsy. Lancet ii:1178–1180, 1984
6. Billiard M, Seignalet J: Extraordinary association between HLA-DR2 and narcolepsy. Lancet i:226–227, 1985

CHAPTER 9

Endocrinology

Juvenile Diabetes Mellitus (Insulin-Dependent)

Population Association

The first study in 1972 by Finkelstein et al.[1] on 28 Caucasian, 10 Mexican, and 6 American Black patients did not show any significant association with A and B loci antigens. A year later, Singal et al.[2] studied 50 Canadian patients and found a significantly increased frequency of B15 (36% in the patients vs. 10% in 100 controls). Subsequent reports from several countries have provided data on various racial groups showing an association of juvenile diabetes with several HLA antigens.

Caucasians

HLA-A, -B, -C, -D, and -DR frequency data available from a large number of studies on Caucasian populations revealed significant associations with B7, B8, B15, B18, CW3, DR2, DR3, DR4, DW2, DW3, and DW4 antigens (Table 9.1). There are significant linkage disequilibria between B8-DR3, B8-DW3, B15-DR4, and B15-DW4. The analyses of the combined data also showed higher relative risks for DR3, DR4, DW3, and DW4 antigens. Thus, the increased frequencies of B8 and B15 were most probably secondary to that of DR3 and DR4, respectively. In fact analysis of DW3 and DW4 antigens in the presence and absence of B8 and B15 by Sachs et al.[3] and of DR3 and DR4 antigens in the presence and absence of B8 and B15 by Farid et al.[4] and Solow et al.[5] showed that the primary association of the disease is with D and DR loci antigens.

The frequencies of B7, DR2, and DW2 antigens were significantly decreased in the patients (Table 9.1) and the relative risks for DR2 and DW2 were lower than that for B7. There were linkage disequilibria between B7-DR2 and B7-DW2. Thus this, as in the case of DR3 and DR4, may suggest the primary association with D/DR locus antigens. Sachs et al.[3] presented data indicating that the decreased frequency of DW2 was secondary to the increased frequency of DW3. This contradicted the hypothesis that the association with DW2 indicates "protection" or "resistance" to the disease.[6–9]

In Sachs' data[3] the frequency of DW3-DW4 heterozygotes was significantly increased in the patients (50% in 58 diabetics vs. 5% in 43 controls, relative risk = 16.6). A similar increase was also reported for DR3-DR4 heterozygotes by Farid et al.[4] (25% in 40 patients vs. 3.8% in the controls, relative risk = 7.62). The data of Ilonen et al.[10] on D locus antigens in Finnish patients also demonstrated an increased frequency for DW3-DW4 heterozygotes (see also refs. 5, 11–13). Similar results for DR3-DR4 heterozygotes have been reported by Svejgaard et al.,[14] Wolf et al.,[15] Platz et al.,[12] and Barbosa et al.[13]

American Blacks

In these patients the pattern of HLA associations is very similar to that in Caucasian patients (Table 9.1).

African Blacks

Hammond et al.[16] reported significant associations with B8, B14, and BW42 in Zulus from Durban, South Africa (Table 9.1). In another study from South Africa Briggs et al.[17] found that BW35 was increased

TABLE 9.1. Juvenile Diabetes Mellitus (Insulin-Dependent)

Country/Population	Patients n	Patients %+	Controls n	Controls %+	RR	χ^2	Ref.
HLA-A9							
Taiwan—Chinese	40	53	60	43	1.48	0.96	169
China	31	55	128	23	4.02	11.71	170
	71	54	188	29	2.43	9.63	
	Heterogeneity χ^2 (1 df)					3.04	
HLA-BFS 1							
India	57	21	342	4	6.35	20.10	171
HLA-BFF 1							
Canada	70	16	206	3	5.92	13.01	172
Canada	72	11	150	2	5.49	7.55	28
	142	13	356	3	5.75	20.56	
	Heterogeneity χ^2 (1 df)					0.01	
Australia	64	8	200	1	7.51	7.85	106
France	53	19	116	4	5.30	9.29	31
France	51	78	87	24	10.71	33.67	29
	104	48	203	13	8.32	41.90	
	Heterogeneity χ^2 (1 df)					1.06	
West Germany	510	6	536	2	3.04	10.20	173
Spain	62	39	330	9	6.41	34.08	32
	882	15	1625	5	5.71	109.68	
	Heterogeneity χ^2 (6 df)					5.97	
HLA-B5							
China	31	16	128	17	0.99	0.00	170
Japan	131	18	101	37	0.38	10.36	27
Japan	27	11	106	55	0.12	14.10	21
Japan	40	35	120	40	0.82	0.29	72
Japan	63	8	76	32	0.20	10.80	174
	261	17	403	42	0.37	25.30	
	Heterogeneity χ^2 (3 df)					10.25	
	292	17	531	36	0.42	22.04	
	Heterogeneity χ^2 (4 df)					13.51	
HLA-B7							
U.S.A.—Black	40	23	67	16	1.57	0.87	175
U.S.A.—Black	79	14	283	15	0.95	0.02	176
U.S.A.—Black	43	14	192	18	0.78	0.29	177
	162	16	542	16	1.02	0.01	
	Heterogeneity χ^2 (2 df)					1.18	
Zulu	57	23	756	16	1.60	2.17	16
South Africa—Xhosa	25	28	153	17	1.95	2.00	17
	244	19	1451	16	1.29	1.98	
	Heterogeneity χ^2 (4 df)					3.38	

TABLE 9.1. *(continued)*

Country/Population	Patients n	Patients %+	Controls n	Controls %+	RR	χ^2	Ref.
HLA-B7							
India	54	2	118	23	0.10	9.91	19
South Africa—Indian	44	11	632	13	0.90	0.06	178
	98	6	750	15	0.48	3.47	
	Heterogeneity χ^2 (1 df)					6.50	
Mexico	112	9	332	8	1.17	0.17	76
Canada	73	7	214	44	0.10	25.95	4
Canada	94	18	200	29	0.55	3.93	5
	167	13	414	37	0.32	20.39	
	Heterogeneity χ^2 (1 df)					9.49	
U.S.A.	249	14	481	22	0.58	6.57	13
U.S.A.	74	20	100	20	1.01	0.00	179
U.S.A.	110	14	217	13	1.10	0.09	180
U.S.A.	29	7	77	22	0.32	2.97	87
U.S.A.	90	10	282	31	0.26	14.22	60
	552	14	1157	22	0.61	12.17	
	Heterogeneity χ^2 (4 df)					11.67	
Australia	169	17	1460	22	0.74	2.11	181
U.S.S.R.	90	27	600	25	1.12	0.21	182
England	121	12	635	28	0.36	12.78	78
England	186	12	100	26	0.39	8.89	183
England	288	15	375	30	0.41	19.72	36
England	96	10	417	28	0.30	12.46	50
	691	13	1527	28	0.38	53.11	
	Heterogeneity χ^2 (3 df)					0.74	
France	53	6	116	11	0.57	0.91	31
France	51	6	50	18	0.32	3.31	54
France	100	14	270	16	0.87	0.18	184
	204	10	436	15	0.68	2.28	
	Heterogeneity χ^2 (2 df)					2.12	
West Germany	112	13	1000	26	0.44	8.60	73
West Germany	124	13	4302	27	0.41	11.28	66
	236	13	5302	27	0.42	19.86	
	Heterogeneity χ^2 (1 df)					0.02	
Italy	90	9	488	13	0.69	0.96	41
Switzerland	123	13	176	22	0.54	3.80	185
Ireland	113	22	200	34	0.55	4.87	63
Finland	75	13	96	40	0.23	14.11	71
Finland	121	7	900	24	0.25	15.87	40
Finland	63	16	218	33	0.40	6.47	10
	259	11	1214	27	0.29	35.14	
	Heterogeneity χ^2 (2 df)					1.30	

TABLE 9.1. *(continued)*

	Patients		Controls				
Country/Population	n	%+	n	%+	RR	χ^2	Ref.
HLA-B7							
Norway	126	19	1628	30	0.56	6.55	62
Sweden	102	14	500	28	0.43	8.23	35
Sweden	99	11	272	28	0.33	10.89	38
	201	13	772	28	0.38	18.77	
	Heterogeneity χ^2 (1 df)					0.36	
	3021	14	15374	26	0.49	145.76	
	Heterogeneity χ^2 (26 df)					60.15	
HLA-B8							
U.S.A.—Black	38	16	192	8	2.27	2.81	186
U.S.A.—Black	79	18	283	8	2.54	6.85	176
U.S.A.—Black	43	19	192	8	2.74	4.99	177
U.S.A.—Black	80	20	42	5	3.97	4.52	18
U.S.A.—Black	40	8	67	9	0.93	0.01	175
	280	17	776	8	2.38	16.35	
	Heterogeneity χ^2 (4 df)					2.84	
Zulu	57	30	756	14	2.67	10.61	16
	337	19	1532	11	2.47	26.86	
	Heterogeneity χ^2 (5 df)					2.93	
India	54	20	118	12	1.84	2.03	19
South Africa—Indian	44	14	632	6	2.69	5.07	178
	98	17	750	7	2.21	6.73	
	Heterogeneity χ^2 (1 df)					0.38	
Mexico	112	14	332	6	2.56	7.28	76
Mexico	74	24	42	10	2.62	3.22	18
Mexico	67	13	332	6	2.40	4.48	44
	253	17	706	6	2.52	14.95	
	Heterogeneity χ^2 (2 df)					0.02	
Caucasians (unspecified)	293	32	384	16	2.46	23.41	53
Canada	73	34	214	54	0.44	8.51	4
Canada	94	29	200	22	1.45	1.77	5
	167	31	414	39	0.80	1.28	
	Heterogeneity χ^2 (1 df)					8.99	
U.S.A.	74	24	100	28	0.82	0.34	179
U.S.A.	66	47	119	16	4.57	19.42	102
U.S.A.	249	36	481	15	3.18	40.03	13
U.S.A.	42	38	100	16	3.18	8.02	18
U.S.A.	110	46	217	21	3.18	21.22	180
U.S.A.	63	47	125	18	3.98	16.73	69
U.S.A.	90	60	282	20	5.93	47.29	60
U.S.A.	29	38	77	22	2.16	2.87	87
	723	41	1501	18	3.21	132.39	
	Heterogeneity χ^2 (7 df)					23.52	

TABLE 9.1. *(continued)*

Country/Population	Patients n	Patients %+	Controls n	Controls %+	RR	χ^2	Ref.
HLA-B8							
Australia	169	48	1460	24	2.92	42.30	181
Hungary	67	37	450	19	2.51	11.14	95
Hungary	286	39	352	16	3.34	41.04	187
	353	39	802	18	3.05	51.46	
	Heterogeneity χ^2 (1 df)					0.72	
U.S.S.R.	90	38	600	16	3.22	23.48	182
England	96	50	417	26	2.84	20.45	50
England	119	56	300	28	3.25	27.90	46
England	121	46	635	27	2.30	17.09	78
England	150	49	300	31	2.13	13.73	37
England	186	50	100	23	3.30	18.79	183
England	288	51	375	29	2.54	32.63	36
	960	50	2127	28	2.61	127.39	
	Heterogeneity χ^2 (5 df)					3.22	
France	53	13	116	8	1.74	1.20	31
France	100	23	270	16	1.58	2.55	184
France	51	16	50	6	2.71	2.47	39
	204	19	436	13	1.73	5.61	
	Heterogeneity χ^2 (2 df)					0.61	
West Germany	112	30	1000	21	1.62	4.94	73
West Germany	124	46	4302	19	3.63	49.78	66
	236	38	5302	19	2.60	46.69	
	Heterogeneity χ^2 (1 df)					8.03	
Italy	90	23	488	13	2.02	6.32	41
Italy	16	31	174	15	2.64	3.20	188
	106	24	662	14	2.14	9.32	
	Heterogeneity χ^2 (1 df)					0.19	
Austria	50	32	3000	18	2.18	6.75	189
Austria	64	44	450	18	3.58	21.27	42
	114	39	3450	18	2.85	26.54	
	Heterogeneity χ^2 (1 df)					1.48	
Switzerland	123	37	176	17	2.84	14.87	185
Ireland	113	46	200	35	1.58	3.68	63
Denmark	85	45	1967	24	2.60	18.48	190
Finland	75	30	96	12	3.07	8.22	71
Finland	63	37	216	11	4.71	21.56	10
Finland	121	38	900	20	2.46	19.54	40
	259	35	1212	18	2.95	46.54	
	Heterogeneity χ^2 (2 df)					2.78	

TABLE 9.1. *(continued)*

Country/Population	Patients n	Patients %+	Controls n	Controls %+	RR	χ^2	Ref.
HLA-B8							
Norway	126	44	1628	25	2.36	21.08	62
Sweden	99	49	272	25	2.87	18.84	38
Sweden	102	38	500	19	2.62	17.24	35
	201	43	772	21	2.73	36.01	
	Heterogeneity χ^2 (1 df)					0.08	
	4322	40	23093	21	2.57	578.84	
	Heterogeneity χ^2 (38 df)					101.34	
HLA-B14							
U.S.A.—Black	43	0	192	6	0.17	2.78	177
Zulu	57	18	756	6	3.53	12.00	16
	100	10	948	6	2.56	7.44	
	Heterogeneity χ^2 (1 df)					7.33	
HLA-B15							
U.S.A.—Black	79	10	283	2	5.29	9.91	176
U.S.A.—Black	43	12	192	7	1.90	1.56	177
U.S.A.—Black	80	11	42	0	11.03	5.06	18
U.S.A.—Black	40	5	67	4	1.32	0.12	175
	242	10	584	4	3.05	12.18	
	Heterogeneity χ^2 (3 df)					4.47	
Zulu	57	2	756	6	0.45	1.25	16
	299	8	1340	5	2.21	7.44	
	Heterogeneity χ^2 (4 df)					10.46	
India	54	17	118	17	1.02	0.00	19
South Africa—Indian	44	11	632	11	1.08	0.03	178
	98	14	750	12	1.05	0.02	
	Heterogeneity χ^2 (1 df)					0.01	
Mexico	112	9	332	9	1.03	0.01	76
Mexico	74	23	42	10	2.48	2.85	18
	186	15	374	9	1.36	1.03	
	Heterogeneity χ^2 (1 df)					1.82	
Caucasians (unspecified)	293	20	384	10	2.24	13.17	53
Canada	73	27	214	19	1.59	2.21	4
Canada	94	30	200	14	2.62	10.37	5
	167	29	414	17	2.06	11.23	
	Heterogeneity χ^2 (1 df)					1.35	

TABLE 9.1. *(continued)*

	Patients		Controls				
Country/Population	n	%+	n	%+	RR	χ^2	Ref.
HLA-B15							
U.S.A.	249	26	481	10	3.15	30.40	13
U.S.A.	42	24	100	9	3.14	5.67	18
U.S.A.	46	15	217	17	0.90	0.06	180
U.S.A.	63	8	125	7	1.20	0.11	69
U.S.A.	74	15	100	8	1.99	2.15	179
U.S.A.	90	16	282	12	1.42	1.10	60
U.S.A.	66	8	119	8	1.04	0.00	102
U.S.A.	29	31	77	12	3.24	5.32	87
	659	19	1501	11	2.10	31.44	
	Heterogeneity χ^2 (7 df)					13.38	
Australia	169	19	1460	8	2.72	21.43	181
Hungary	286	19	352	8	2.67	16.18	187
U.S.S.R.	90	12	600	15	0.80	0.45	182
England	119	13	300	14	0.93	0.05	46
England	288	18	375	10	1.97	8.79	36
England	96	26	417	13	2.36	10.10	50
England	186	18	100	10	1.91	3.07	183
England	121	20	635	8	2.89	15.92	78
England	150	21	300	10	2.38	10.06	37
	960	19	2127	11	2.04	39.31	
	Heterogeneity χ^2 (5 df)					8.67	
France	51	4	50	10	0.42	1.36	39
France	53	11	116	5	2.33	2.22	31
France	100	11	270	10	1.14	0.12	184
	204	9	436	9	1.17	0.32	
	Heterogeneity χ^2 (2 df)					3.39	
West Germany	112	25	1000	15	1.91	7.70	73
West Germany	124	33	4302	14	3.04	32.85	66
	236	29	5302	14	2.51	38.17	
	Heterogeneity χ^2 (1 df)					2.38	
Italy	90	4	488	8	0.54	1.52	41
Austria	64	23	450	10	2.72	9.33	42
Austria	50	26	3000	12	2.64	9.32	189
	114	24	3450	12	2.68	18.64	
	Heterogeneity χ^2 (1 df)					0.01	
Ireland	113	18	200	5	4.06	12.77	63
Denmark	85	33	1967	18	2.26	12.08	190
Finland	75	42	96	22	2.54	7.76	71
Finland	121	37	900	20	2.36	17.59	40
Finland	63	49	218	20	3.81	19.97	10
	259	41	1214	20	2.70	43.51	
	Heterogeneity χ^2 (2 df)					1.81	

TABLE 9.1. *(continued)*

Country/Population	Patients n	Patients %+	Controls n	Controls %+	RR	χ^2	Ref.
HLA-B15							
Norway	126	35	1628	20	2.16	15.63	62
Sweden	99	43	272	21	2.83	17.37	38
Sweden	102	31	500	26	1.29	1.15	35
	201	37	772	24	1.86	13.24	
	Heterogeneity χ^2 (1 df)					5.29	
	4052	22	22295	14	2.16	258.15	
	Heterogeneity χ^2 (35 df)					67.22	
HLA-B18							
U.S.A.—Black	79	11	283	6	1.98	2.64	176
India	54	0	118	4	0.20	2.16	19
South Africa—Indian	44	2	632	3	1.00	0.00	178
	98	1	750	3	0.58	0.73	
	Heterogeneity χ^2 (1 df)					1.43	
Mexico	112	15	332	6	2.77	8.81	76
Canada	73	10	214	12	0.85	0.15	4
U.S.A.	74	22	100	7	3.59	7.77	179
U.S.A.	110	4	217	6	0.70	0.48	180
U.S.A.	29	34	77	4	10.97	14.33	87
U.S.A.	90	10	282	8	1.31	0.47	60
U.S.A.	249	12	481	9	1.38	1.71	13
	552	13	1157	8	1.70	9.39	
	Heterogeneity χ^2 (4 df)					15.37	
Hungary	286	11	352	12	0.91	0.15	187
U.S.S.R.	90	22	600	9	2.88	13.62	182
England	96	11	417	6	1.98	3.35	50
England	121	11	635	8	1.45	1.40	78
England	186	7	100	5	1.35	0.36	183
England	288	12	375	5	2.56	10.33	36
	691	10	1527	7	1.89	13.23	
	Heterogeneity χ^2 (3 df)					2.21	
France	100	25	270	12	2.44	9.32	184
France	51	73	50	24	8.14	22.39	39
France	53	20	116	8	2.84	5.04	31
	204	36	436	12	3.36	31.44	
	Heterogeneity χ^2 (2 df)					5.30	
West Germany	124	15	4302	9	1.82	5.69	66
Italy	90	20	488	13	1.70	3.32	41
Spain	62	39	330	16	3.36	16.72	32
Austria	50	10	3000	11	0.98	0.00	189
Switzerland	123	18	176	10	1.96	4.01	185
Ireland	113	11	200	8	1.43	0.86	63
Finland	63	11	218	9	1.30	0.35	10
Finland	121	14	900	10	1.49	2.08	40
	184	13	1118	10	1.44	2.35	
	Heterogeneity χ^2 (1 df)					0.07	

TABLE 9.1. *(continued)*

Country/Population	Patients n	Patients %+	Controls n	Controls %+	RR	χ^2	Ref.
HLA-B18							
Norway	126	14	1628	5	3.15	17.40	62
Sweden	102	9	500	7	1.36	0.68	35
	2870	15	16028	9	1.86	84.78	
	Heterogeneity χ^2 (24 df)					57.18	
HLA-BW21							
India	54	35	118	4	11.88	23.42	19
South Africa—Indian	44	5	632	2	3.01	2.96	178
	98	22	750	2	6.96	23.57	
	Heterogeneity χ^2 (1 df)					2.80	
HLA-BW22							
Japan	34	38	123	15	3.45	8.60	53
Japan	32	22	150	25	0.88	0.08	24
	66	30	273	20	1.81	3.73	
	Heterogeneity χ^2 (1 df)					4.96	
HLA-BW35							
U.S.A.—Black	79	30	283	39	0.68	2.08	176
U.S.A.—Black	43	28	192	29	0.97	0.01	177
	122	29	475	35	0.77	1.46	
	Heterogeneity χ^2 (1 df)					0.63	
South Africa—Xhosa	25	20	153	4	5.97	8.84	17
	147	28	628	27	0.97	0.02	
	Heterogeneity χ^2 (2 df)					10.91	
HLA-BW42							
U.S.A.—Black	43	2	192	6	0.48	0.83	177
Zulu	57	9	756	28	0.28	8.79	16
South Africa—Xhosa	25	0	153	16	0.10	4.83	17
	125	5	1101	22	0.27	13.05	
	Heterogeneity χ^2 (2 df)					1.40	
HLA-BW52							
Japan	40	3	79	28	0.11	9.04	22
HLA-BW54							
Taiwan—Chinese	40	20	60	3	6.67	6.99	167
China	31	19	128	7	3.15	4.51	170
Japan	40	33	120	8	5.51	13.89	72
Japan	63	49	76	13	6.17	19.67	174
Japan	32	44	76	13	5.08	11.69	25
Japan	89	44	128	10	6.85	29.49	23
Japan	27	63	106	21	6.18	16.47	21
Japan	131	36	101	9	5.45	20.17	27
	382	42	607	12	5.92	111.01	
	Heterogeneity χ^2 (5 df)					0.37	
	453	39	795	11	5.65	121.21	
	Heterogeneity χ^2 (7 df)					1.66	

TABLE 9.1. *(continued)*

	Patients		Controls				
Country/Population	n	%+	n	%+	RR	χ^2	Ref.
HLA-CW3							
Mexico	112	21	332	25	0.81	0.68	76
Caucasians (unspecified)	293	32	384	19	2.00	14.92	53
Canada	94	28	200	14	2.38	8.23	5
Canada	28	13	60	14	0.97	0.00	4
	122	25	260	14	2.00	6.54	
	Heterogeneity χ^2 (1 df)					1.69	
England	121	46	635	25	2.55	21.40	78
England	119	27	300	30	0.87	0.35	46
	240	37	935	27	1.63	9.92	
	Heterogeneity χ^2 (1 df)					11.82	
France	53	17	116	8	2.34	3.17	31
France	51	8	50	14	0.56	0.92	39
	104	13	166	10	1.35	0.64	
	Heterogeneity χ^2 (1 df)					3.45	
Austria	64	38	450	19	2.62	11.85	42
Austria	50	34	3000	21	1.96	5.24	189
	114	36	3450	21	2.29	16.59	
	Heterogeneity χ^2 (1 df)					0.50	
Finland	75	58	96	40	2.05	5.41	71
Finland	121	38	900	32	1.31	1.81	40
Finland	62	57	83	37	2.23	5.66	10
	258	48	1079	33	1.61	10.22	
	Heterogeneity χ^2 (2 df)					2.66	
Sweden	102	44	500	40	1.18	0.58	35
	1233	35	6774	24	1.71	52.72	
	Heterogeneity χ^2 (12 df)					26.82	
HLA-CW4							
Japan	89	19	128	6	3.54	8.29	23
Mexico	112	21	332	31	0.60	3.98	76
Canada	94	21	200	11	2.15	5.29	5
England	121	4	635	11	0.37	5.11	78
France	51	18	50	20	0.88	0.07	39
France	53	9	116	13	0.70	0.46	31
	104	13	166	15	0.79	0.43	
	Heterogeneity χ^2 (1 df)					0.10	
Finland	75	10	96	26	0.33	6.64	71
Finland	63	8	79	24	0.29	5.99	10
Finland	121	9	900	19	0.44	6.79	40
	259	9	1075	20	0.37	18.86	
	Heterogeneity χ^2 (2 df)					0.56	
Sweden	102	12	500	19	0.60	2.64	35
	680	11	2576	17	0.62	11.47	
	Heterogeneity χ^2 (7 df)					21.51	

TABLE 9.1. *(continued)*

Country/Population	Patients n	Patients %+	Controls n	Controls %+	RR	χ^2	Ref.
HLA-DYT							
Japan	131	55	101	24	3.81	21.61	27
Japan	46	46	65	17	4.03	10.50	26
	177	53	166	21	3.88	32.09	
	Heterogeneity χ^2 (1 df)					0.01	
HLA-DW2							
U.S.A.—Black	41	3	79	25	0.13	7.93	186
U.S.A.—Black	41	5	79	25	0.19	6.57	191
	82	4	158	25	0.16	14.33	
	Heterogeneity χ^2 (1 df)					0.17	
U.S.A.	83	0	203	15	0.03	10.99	13
U.S.A.	66	2	119	20	0.11	9.81	102
	149	1	322	17	0.08	19.89	
	Heterogeneity χ^2 (1 df)					0.91	
England	58	10	43	23	0.39	3.15	3
Finland	75	1	96	30	0.04	16.72	71
Finland	32	3	104	30	0.11	8.52	10
	107	2	200	30	0.07	24.39	
	Heterogeneity χ^2 (1 df)					0.85	
	314	3	565	22	0.13	40.85	
	Heterogeneity χ^2 (4 df)					8.34	
HLA-DW3							
U.S.A.—Black	41	89	79	14	43.71	46.70	186
U.S.A.—Black	41	88	79	14	39.96	46.37	191
	82	89	158	14	41.75	93.05	
	Heterogeneity χ^2 (1 df)					0.01	
Japan	19	16	67	0	29.03	8.59	26
U.S.A.	66	59	119	17	6.85	31.45	102
U.S.A.	83	47	203	18	4.00	24.10	13
	149	52	322	18	4.97	54.08	
	Heterogeneity χ^2 (1 df)					1.46	
England	58	81	43	33	8.22	21.82	3
Norway	16	63	16	13	9.21	7.87	10
Sweden	74	30	176	19	1.83	3.72	38
	297	53	557	19	4.16	76.65	
	Heterogeneity χ^2 (4 df)					12.31	
HLA-DW4							
U.S.A.—Black	41	39	79	8	6.94	15.16	191
U.S.A.—Black	41	42	79	8	7.83	17.26	186
	82	41	158	8	7.37	32.39	
	Heterogeneity χ^2 (1 df)					0.03	

TABLE 9.1. *(continued)*

Country/Population	Patients n	Patients %+	Controls n	Controls %+	RR	χ^2	Ref.
HLA-DW4							
Caucasians (unspecified)	293	38	384	13	4.07	53.33	53
U.S.A.	66	23	119	20	1.20	0.26	102
U.S.A.	83	49	203	13	6.33	38.17	13
	149	37	322	16	3.24	25.96	
	Heterogeneity χ^2 (1 df)					12.47	
England	58	55	43	35	2.23	3.91	3
Finland	26	62	24	8	14.94	13.64	10
Finland	75	49	96	12	6.80	25.59	71
	101	52	120	11	8.03	38.31	
	Heterogeneity χ^3 (1 df)					0.91	
Sweden	79	52	133	19	4.55	23.70	38
	680	43	1002	15	4.02	137.83	
	Heterogeneity χ^2 (6 df)					20.77	
HLA-DR2							
U.S.A.—Black	34	3	145	36	0.08	11.47	44
U.S.A.—Black	61	2	137	34	0.06	16.84	176
U.S.A.—Black	40	0	67	37	0.02	13.79	175
U.S.A.—Black	50	0	55	44	0.01	17.57	192
	185	1	404	37	0.04	56.98	
	Heterogeneity χ^2 (3 df)					2.70	
Mexico	85	0	209	15	0.03	11.16	76
Canada	62	18	54	38	0.37	5.67	5
Canada	40	1	79	22	0.08	8.04	4
	102	11	133	28	0.28	11.28	
	Heterogeneity χ^2 (1 df)					2.43	
U.S.A.	68	9	404	27	0.29	9.28	193
U.S.A.	57	0	119	22	0.03	11.46	102
U.S.A.	140	4	253	26	0.13	23.57	13
	265	4	776	26	0.17	39.47	
	Heterogeneity χ^2 (2 df)					4.83	
England	122	4	110	28	0.12	20.78	15
France	53	5	116	14	0.37	2.72	31
Austria	51	10	160	22	0.42	3.34	189
Switzerland	123	7	160	22	0.28	11.03	185
	716	6	1455	24	0.23	82.53	
	Heterogeneity χ^2 (8 df)					13.37	
HLA-DR3							
U.S.A.—Black	61	51	137	25	3.09	12.54	176
U.S.A.—Black	40	73	67	30	6.05	17.40	175
U.S.A.—Black	34	47	145	30	2.06	3.65	44
	135	57	349	28	3.20	30.06	
	Heterogeneity χ^2 (2 df)					3.53	

TABLE 9.1. *(continued)*

Country/Population	Patients n	Patients %+	Controls n	Controls %+	RR	χ^2	Ref.
HLA-DR3							
Taiwan—Chinese	40	31	60	7	5.50	9.09	169
China	31	55	105	13	7.88	21.17	170
Japan	34	3	144	1	3.35	1.55	194
Japan	34	65	123	35	3.37	9.46	53
	68	34	267	17	3.36	11.01	
	Heterogeneity χ^2 (1 df)					0.00	
	139	38	432	14	4.87	39.05	
	Heterogeneity χ^2 (3 df)					2.22	
Mexico	85	39	209	22	2.26	8.81	76
Caucasians (unspecified)	293	27	384	17	1.80	9.81	53
Canada	62	39	54	18	2.82	5.95	5
Canada	40	20	79	18	1.16	0.10	4
	102	32	133	18	1.89	4.09	
	Heterogeneity χ^2 (1 df)					1.96	
U.S.A.	68	46	404	23	2.85	15.35	193
U.S.A.	140	44	253	25	2.35	14.77	13
U.S.A.	57	58	119	17	6.58	28.02	102
	265	48	776	23	3.04	52.03	
	Heterogeneity χ^2 (2 df)					6.11	
Australia	64	58	544	30	3.20	19.11	106
England	122	71	110	32	5.12	33.47	15
France	51	91	50	24	28.39	37.00	39
France	53	31	116	10	3.96	10.96	31
	104	60	166	14	8.10	39.80	
	Heterogeneity χ^2 (1 df)					8.16	
Austria	50	36	107	11	4.44	12.95	195
Austria	51	55	160	20	4.81	21.62	189
	101	46	267	16	4.66	34.55	
	Heterogeneity χ^2 (1 df)					0.02	
Switzerland	123	59	160	14	8.65	56.11	185
	1174	46	2540	22	3.39	212.61	
	Heterogeneity χ^2 (12 df)					52.60	
HLA-DR4							
U.S.A.—Black	61	30	137	8	4.81	14.83	176
U.S.A.—Black	40	73	67	25	7.73	21.60	175
U.S.A.—Black	34	41	145	7	8.93	22.66	44
	135	46	349	11	6.74	57.93	
	Heterogeneity χ^2 (2 df)					1.16	

TABLE 9.1. *(continued)*

Country/Population	Patients n	Patients %+	Controls n	Controls %+	RR	χ^2	Ref.
HLA-DR4							
Taiwan—Chinese	40	59	60	49	1.48	0.96	169
China	31	29	105	17	2.01	2.36	170
Japan	34	47	123	12	6.34	18.53	53
Japan	34	56	144	33	2.55	6.12	194
	68	52	267	23	3.80	22.13	
	Heterogeneity χ^2 (1 df)					2.53	
	139	49	432	25	2.60	21.40	
	Heterogeneity χ^2 (3 df)					6.57	
Mexico	60	52	186	38	1.76	3.67	44
Mexico	85	65	209	39	2.88	15.90	76
	145	60	395	39	2.31	18.04	
	Heterogeneity χ^2 (1 df)					1.53	
Caucasians (unspecified)	293	39	384	15	3.60	47.82	53
Canada	62	44	54	18	3.46	8.60	5
Canada	40	23	79	17	1.47	0.69	4
	102	36	133	17	2.34	7.44	
	Heterogeneity χ^2 (1 df)					1.86	
U.S.A.	68	60	404	30	3.47	21.78	193
U.S.A.	140	72	253	30	5.93	59.44	13
U.S.A.	57	53	119	27	3.01	11.10	102
	265	65	776	30	4.28	88.59	
	Heterogeneity χ^2 (2 df)					3.74	
Australia	64	42	544	33	1.48	2.15	106
England	122	78	110	34	6.75	42.42	15
France	51	38	50	16	3.09	5.96	45
France	53	31	116	7	5.74	15.06	31
	104	34	166	10	4.25	20.11	
	Heterogeneity χ^2 (1 df)					0.92	
Austria	50	32	107	16	2.45	5.24	195
Austria	51	75	160	26	8.26	34.28	189
	101	54	267	22	4.73	34.32	
	Heterogeneity χ^2 (1 df)					5.20	
	1051	51	2380	25	3.68	222.53	
	Heterogeneity χ^2 (11 df)					32.02	

in 25 patients of the Xhosa tribe (Table 9.1). In this group, as in the Zulus, the BW42 frequency was also decreased (Table 9.1).

Mexicans

Patel et al.[18] studied 74 Mexican patients and found no significant association with A and B loci antigens. Similarly, in another study on 67 patients, Zeidler et al.[44,76] reported no associations with A, B, and C loci antigens; however, DR4 was increased in the patients (Table 9.1). Analysis of the combined data from all the available studies revealed that B8, B18, DR2, DR3, and DR4, appeared to be associated with the disease (Table 9.1).

Indians
An association with B8 in South African Indians has been reported by Hammond et al.[16] In 54 patients from India Srikanta et al.[19] found a highly significant increase of BW21 (Table 9.1).

Japanese
Several studies from Japan[20–27] reported associations with B5, BW22, BW52, BW54, CW4, DR3, DR4, DW3, and DYT antigens (Table 9.1).

D/DR frequency data are available on Caucasian, American Black, Mexican, and Japanese patient populations. In all these groups there are significant associations with DR3 and DR4 antigens. This is also true for DW3 and DW4 wherever data are available. The relative risks associated with D/DR antigens were higher in all the groups studied for these antigens.

Highly significant associations with the BfF1 allele of the Bf gene[28–32] and 1 C4 complement allele[29] have also been reported (Table 9.1).

Chinese
In Chinese patients the disease appeared to be associated with DR3 (Table 9.1).

Disease Heterogeneity

Age at Onset
In several studies[12,15,33–40] patients were subdivided into various groups on the basis of age at onset (e.g., 0–5, 6–10, 11–15 . . . years). Although the groupings in these reports were not identical, the frequencies of B and D/DR loci antigens did not differ significantly among the groups. Only in the data of Illeni et al.[41] and Schernthaner et al.[42] was there some indication of increased frequencies of B8 and B15 in certain subgroups (see also refs. 14 and 43).

Zeidler et al.[44] reported DR locus typings on 60 Mexican and 33 American Black patients. In both races the patients were subdivided into 2 groups: group 1 consisted of ketosis-prone patients whose disease began before 19 years of age—none was overweight; group 2 consisted of patients between 19 and 31 years of age—they were not ketosis-prone and were more than 20% above their ideal weight. In group 1 (30 Mexican patients) DR4 frequency was 70% as compared with 38% in 189 controls (corrected $p = 0.016$). In 30 group 2 Mexican patients the frequency of 33% was not significantly different from that of the controls. Similar results were also found in American Black patients. DR4 was present in 52% of 21 group 1 patients as compared with 7% in 145 controls (corrected $p = 0.0001$) and 23% in 13 group 2 patients (not significant). None of the group 2 patients was positive for DR2 as compared with 36% in the controls (corrected $p = 0.016$) and 8% in 13 group 2 patients (not significant).

Pittman et al.[45] studied 140 American Caucasian patients who had onset of the disease after 40 years of age. As in the case of early-onset type of disease DR4 was significantly increased in the sample of patients.

Pancreatic Islet-Cell Antibodies
Morris and coworkers[46,47] reported a significant increase of B8 in 99 patients positive for pancreatic islet-cell antibodies. In this group the frequency of B8 was 61% as compared with 35% in 20 antibody-negative patients and 28% in 300 normal controls.[46] Similar differences were also reported by Nerup and associates.[48,49] However, in the studies of Richens et al.,[50,51] Lendrum et al.,[52] Batchelor and Morris,[53] Mustonen et al.,[54] and Sakurami et al.[27] no associations with these antibodies and any HLA antigens were observed. Batchelor's and Morris'[53] report also included data on DR3 and DR4 antigens. DR3 did not differ significantly between the antibody-positive and -negative groups. The frequency of DR4 in 37 antibody-positive patients was 62% as compared with 49% in 53 antibody-negative patients and 24% in 384 controls ($p < 0.05$) (See also ref. 55).

Retinopathy
Larkins et al.[56] reported an increased frequency of B8 in 16 patients with proliferative retinopathy. In Bertrams et al.'s data[57] an association between DR4 and proliferative retinopathy was also observed. However, studies by Barbosa et al.,[58,59] Moller et al.,[38] Becker et al.,[60] Cove et al.,[61] Jervell et al.,[62] Johnston et al.,[63] McCann et al.,[64] Danielsen et al.,[65] Standl et al.,[66] and Deckert et al.[67] showed no association of retinopathy with HLA antigens. Cove et al.[61] analyzed the pooled data from 5 of the above reports; no association was found.

Seasonal Variation
Rolles et al.[68] studied 56 children attending a diabetic clinic in whom HLA type and the month of diagnosis was available. Twenty-six (46%) were positive for B8 and of these 21 (81%) presented within the 5 months of October through February. Of the 30 non-B8 patients only 10 (33%) presented in the 5-month period in which the B8-positive group showed an

increased incidence. Illeni et al.[41] have also reported an increased frequency of B8 (26.19%) in 42 patients with onset between October and January as compared with 12.5% in 488 controls. The B8 frequency in 38 children with onset between February and September was 23.68%. Similar results have been observed in a small sample of patients studied by Farid et al.[4]

However, Garavoy et al.,[69] Richens et al.,[50,51] and Moller et al.[38] found no such association with B8.

Family History

Ludvigsson et al.,[35] Moller et al.,[38] Platz et al.,[12] Barbosa et al.,[13] and Bengsch et al.[70] found no significant HLA difference between the patients with and without a positive family history of the disease (See also ref. 71).

Kawa et al.[20] first observed an association of BW54 in Japanese patients with a positive family history. However, another report by Kikuchi et al.[72] on 40 Japanese patients did not find any association between BW54 and a family history of diabetes. In the group of patients without a family history this antigen was not increased.

Duration of the Disease

No significant association with any HLA antigens was observed.[35,38,40,47,58]

Insulin Antibodies

Bertrams et al.[73,74] studied 112 patients who could be subgrouped into responders and nonresponders to insulin on the basis of humoral immune response to insulin. In 39 nonresponders and 73 responders the frequencies of B8 were 41.0 and 24.7%, respectively. There was no significant difference between these 2 groups. Similar nonsignificant differences were also observed for B7 and B15 antigens. In the data of Schernthaner et al.[75] 3 of the 9 nonresponders (33%) and 26 of the 58 responders (44.8%) were B8-positive. Again, there was no significant difference between the 2 groups. The results were similar for B15. A third report by Deckert et al.[67] also did not find any association of B8 and B15 with a high insulin-binding capacity (see also ref. 35).

It should be noted that in the data of Zeidler et al.[76] on 112 Mexican-American patients IgG insulin antibody formation was found to be significantly increased in DR3- and DR4- negative patients.

Cell-Mediated Hypersensitivity Reactions Against Coxsackie B4 Virus

Richens et al.[50,51] measured, using leukocyte migration tests, cell-mediated hypersensitivity reactions against particles of coxsackie B4 virus in 49 patients. The mean migration indices for patients with B8, B15, B8 + B15, and non-B8, B15 were not significantly different from each other.

In 103 Japanese patients studied by Sakurami et al.[77] the titers of antibodies to coxsackie B group viruses did not show any association with HLA antigens.

Gastric Parietal Cell Antibody

No significant association with HLA antigens in patients with gastric parietal cell antibody was observed.[50,51,78]

Thyroid Antibody

No significant assocation with HLA antigens in patients with thyroid antibody was observed.[50,51,78]

Mitochondria, Smooth Muscle, Reticulum, and Antinuclear Antibodies

No association with HLA antigens in 18 patients positive for these non-organ-specific antibodies was observed.[50,51]

Infections Before Onset

No association with HLA was observed.[35]

C-Peptide

Ludvigsson et al.[35] reported that patients with B18 had detectable C-peptide more often than the groups of patients with B7, B8, and B15 antigens.

Total Serum Insulin

In the data of Ludvigsson et al.[35] there were relatively more cases with low serum insulin in the B8-positive patients.

Microangiopathy

Barbosa et al.[180] reported A and B loci frequency data on 110 juvenile-onset insulin-dependent diabetics with terminal glomerulosclerosis and retinopathy. These patients were kidney transplant recipients. Only the frequency of B8 was significantly increased (45.5% in the patients vs. 21.2% in 217 controls). B7, B15, and B18 were similar in both groups.

Antipancreatic Cell-Mediated Autoimmunity

Christy et al.[48] reported a B8 frequency of 89% in 18 patients with antipancreatic cell-mediated autoimmunity as measured by the leukocyte migration test. In 19 patients without this autoimmunity the frequency of B8 was 58% ($p = 0.04$).

Ketonuria at Onset
In Ludvigsson et al.'s[35] study of 102 patients the frequency of ketonuria at onset was similar in subgroups of patients with B7, B8, B15, and B18 antigens.

Serum Antibody to Bovine Serum Albumin
Singal et al.[79] measured antibody response to bovine serum albumin (a component of cow's milk) in 97 patients. In 38 patients positive for the antibody the frequencies of B8 and DR3 were 13.2% and 33.3%, respectively. The frequency of these 2 antigens in 59 patients without the antibody were 39% and 45.2%, respectively. Thus B8 and DR3 were increased in the patients without the antibody ($p < 0.05$). B15 was decreased in the antibody-negative group (16.9% vs. 44.7% in patients with the antibody, $p < 0.05$).

Lymphocytotoxic Antibodies
Serjeantson et al.[80] observed associations between cold-reacting serum lymphocytotoxic antibodies and B8 and B18 antigens.

Glucose Tolerance
Ludwig et al.[81] performed intravenous glucose tolerance tests in 19 families of diabetic patients. An abnormal glucose tolerance test was found in 13 of the 36 blood relatives (siblings, parents, and offspring) under age 35 years. The relative chances of glucose intolerance in blood relatives positive for B8, B15, and CW3 were 25, 1.6, and 1.8, respectively. In siblings, they were 3, 2.4, and 5.3, respectively. Four of the 13 relatives under age 35 with glucose intolerance had already developed diabetes (see also ref. 82).

Long-Term Diabetes
In the reports of Larkins et al.[83] and Deckert et al.[67] all the patients had the disease for 20 years or more. No HLA associations other than with B8, B15, and B18 were found.

Muscle Capillary Basement Membrane Thickness
Deckert et al.[67] reported HLA types and electron microscopic measurements of muscle capillary basement membrane thickness of 39 patients who had the disease for 20 years or more. They found no difference in basement membrane thickness between patients positive for B8 and/or B15.

Congenital Rubella
No data are available; however, see ref. 84.

Family Data

Diabetic patients and their families have been HLA-typed and analyzed in several studies.[8,10,11,31,37,50,52,70,81,82,85–105] In these studies the investigators have presented various methods of genetic analyses of the data, interpretation of the results, and hypotheses related to the mode of inheritance of the "diabetes gene" and its linkage with the HLA complex. However, the data from several studies agree on only 2 major findings:

Higher Relative Risk for DR3-DR4/DW3-DW4 Heterozygotes
The frequencies of DR3-DR4 and DW3-DW4 heterozygotes were higher in patients than in the controls and thus the relative risks associated with the heterozygotes were higher than those for the single antigens DR3, DR4, DW3, and DW4.[8,10,12–15,31,49,50,86,92,93,100,102,106] As an example, in Nerup's data[49,93] on 100–125 patients the relative risk values for DW3, DW4, and DW3-DW4 were 3.7, 4.9, and 9.4, respectively. DR locus typing data on 122 diabetic probands from 122 families reported by Wolf et al.[15] showed relative risks for DR3, DR4, and DR3-DR4 as 5.04, 6.80, and 14.26, respectively. It should be noted that these estimates varied from study to study but heterozygotes showed higher relative risks. Similar data were also reported for B8-B15 heterozygotes.[10,49,50,93]

Another interesting result reported by Christy et al.,[92] Suciu-Foca et al.,[102] and Barbosa et al.[13] was higher relative risk values for DR3, DR4, DW3, and DW4 homozygotes. (see also ref. 14.)

However, these results need confirmation in other studies. Deschamps et al.[13] did not find any increase of DR3 and DR4 homozygotes in 53 French families. Similar results were also observed in 122 diabetic probands studied by Wolf et al.[15]

Distorted Segregation of HLA Haplotypes and Diabetes in Affected Sib-Pairs
Similarity of the HLA haplotypes in affected sib-pairs has been investigated.[8,14,15,31,37,50,86,96,108] If the disease is segregating independently of HLA then the expected proportion of affected sib-pairs sharing 0, 1, and 2 haplotypes will be 25%, 50%, and 25%, respectively. (This would also be the proportion in normal sib-pairs.) However, if the susceptibility to diabetes is governed by one or more genes linked to

HLA then the proportion of sib-pairs sharing 2 haplotypes would be significantly increased and that of sharing 0 and 1 haplotype would be decreased. This segregation distortion from the expected proportions has been observed by several authors.[8,14,15,26,31,37,50,70,86,91–93,95,101,103,108] Ryder et al.[91] counted 118 affected sib-pairs from 6 different studies and presented the following results:

	Haplotypes Shared			
	0	1	2	
Observed	5 (4.2%)	44 (37.3%)	69 (58.5%)	
Expected (If disease is independent of HLA)	29.5 (25%)	59.0 (50%)	29.5 (25%)	$\chi^2 = 77.1$, 2 df $p < 10^{-15}$

As the χ^2 shows there was a highly significant departure from the expected proportions, indicating the joint segregation of diabetes and HLA. Thus, these data support the assumption that there is at least one major diabetic gene linked with HLA.

Beyond the increased frequency of DR3-DR4/DW3-DW4 heterozygotes in the patients and the distorted segregation of the disease and HLA haplotypes, the mode of inheritance of the diabetic gene and the nature of its linkage with HLA are not clear. The results and their interpretations are variable. All the hypotheses cannot be discussed in detail. However, it is informative to list some of the major ideas on this subject.

Recessive Inheritance

Rubinstein et al.[94,97,101–103,109] proposed, on the basis of their family data, a recessive gene closely linked with HLA-D and with 33–50% penetrance.[101,103] Stenszky et al.[95] studied 55 Hungarian families and also reported a recessive mode of inheritance with 4.8% penetrance. Similar results were also reported by Green et al.[110] and Dunsworth et al.[111] (see also ref. 112).

Dominant Inheritance

Spielman et al.[105] analyzed the pooled data from 3 studies and reported that "the data are more plausibly explained by a 1-dose (dominant) than by a 2-dose or 'recessive' hypothesis." The penetrance was 40%.

Intermediate Model of Inheritance

On the basis of an analysis of 92 Caucasian pedigrees from Europe Morton et al.[113] proposed an intermediate model in which morbid risk is increased by 1 HLA-linked diabetes determinant, and greatly increased by 2 determinants, which may by qualitively different in DR3 and DR4 haplotypes (see also refs. 14, 114).

Two Different Genes Associated with HLA

Christy et al.[92] suggested that 2 different genes associated with HLA are involved in the inheritance of diabetes. They argued that if susceptibility to diabetes is due to only 1 gene closely associated with either DW3 (DR3) or DW4 (DR4), the relative risk for heterozygotes DW3-DW4 (DR3-DR4) should be intermediate between the risk for the 2 homozygotes. The data showed, however, that the risk for heterozygotes was highest. Deschamps et al.[31] also proposed the hypothesis of 2 diabetogenic genes associated with 2 DR alleles (see also ref. 91).

Two Different Genes but Only One Linked with HLA

Thomson[115] proposed a model in which 2 disease susceptibility genes are involved. Only 1 of these genes is linked with HLA.

Three-Allele Model

Hodge et al.[116] postulated 1 susceptibility gene for diabetes. This gene is highly linked with HLA and has 2 mutant alleles. One is associated with B8 and the other is associated with B15.

Epistatic Model

Suarez et al.[117] and Clerget-Darpoux et al.[118] suggested a genetic model of diabetes in which the diabetes gene has an epistatic interaction with genes located in or near the HLA complex.

Other Models

Several other hypotheses on the mode of inheritance of diabetes have been proposed. For details see refs. 12, 15, 108, 114, and 119–124.

Linkage Analysis

Barbosa et al.[99] performed linkage analysis by calculating lod scores. Assuming an autosomal recessive mode of inheritance and 50% penetrance the maximum lod score for 21 multiplex families with normal parents was 3.98 at a recombination fraction of 18%.

Clerget-Darpoux et al.[104] also applied the lod score method on 28 families with at least 1 child with diabetes. The data from these 28 families were pooled with that of 21 other families from the literature. Assuming autosomal recessive inheritance the maximum lod scores (6.00–7.36) were obtained for recombination fractions from 4–16%, depending on the level of penetrance (10–90%). Although the evidence in favor of linkage was highly significant, the high estimates of recombination fraction were not consistent with the hypothesis of linkage disequilibrium between HLA alleles and a diabetic susceptibility gene.

Linkage Analysis of Families with Patients in Two Consecutive Generations

Barbosa et al.[100] reported lod score data on 28 families with insulin-dependent diabetics in 2 or more consecutive generations. These types of families were ascertained to maximize the likelihood of obtaining a homogeneous type of disease within a family and an autosomal mode of inheritance. Lod scores were calculated assuming an autosomal dominant mode of inheritance and several values of penetrance. The maximum lod score for 50% penetrance was 0.37 at the recombination fraction of 0.29.

It should be noted that these results were different from those reported by Barbosa et al.[99] in which 21 families with normal parents were analyzed. In this data the maximum lod score was 3.98 at a recombination fraction of 13%. The mode of inheritance was assumed to be recessive and the level of penetrance was 50%.

Intra-HLA Recombination in Juvenile Diabetes Mellitus

The frequency of recombination within the HLA region of the chromosome is < 1%. In a report on a group of 10 families with 37 children, 1 or more of whom had juvenile diabetes mellitus, Suciu-Foca and Rubinstein[125] observed a recombination frequency of 15%. The crossovers separated A and B in 3 cases and B and D in the other 3. On the basis of those results the authors suggested "the existence of a gene which increases the rate of recombination in at least a segment of human chromosome 6 and which, when homozygous, may be associated with the appearance of J.D.M. (juvenile diabetes mellitus)." This very interesting result, however, was not confirmed in several other reports.[8,10,70,90,93,94,126–128] In a later report on larger numbers of meiosis, Rubenstein and Suciu-Foca[103] also concluded that the recombination frequencies in diabetic families were not significantly different from those generally accepted for the general population.

See also refs. 101, 107, 129–168, and 196–215.

References

1. Finkelstein S, Zeller E, Walford RL: No relation between HL-A and juvenile diabetes. Tissue Antigens 2:74-77, 1972
2. Singal DP, Blajchman MA: Histocompatibility (HL-A) antigens, lymphocytotoxic antibodies and tissue antibodies in patients with diabetes mellitus. Diabetes 22:429-432, 1973
3. Sachs JA, Cudworth AG, Jaraquemada D, Gorsuch AN, Festenstein H: Type 1 diabetes and the HLA-D locus. Diabetologia 18:41-43, 1980
4. Farid NR, Sampson L, Noel P, Barnard JM, Davis AJ, Hillman DA: HLA-D-related (DRW) antigens in juvenile diabetes mellitus. Diabetes 28:552-557, 1979
5. Solow H, Hidalgo R, Singal DP: Juvenile-onset diabetes: HLA-A, -B, -C, and -DR alloantigens. Diabetes 28:1-4, 1979
6. Van De Putte I, Vermylen C, Decraene P, Vlietinck R, Van Den Berghe H: Segregation of HLA B7 in juvenile-onset diabetes mellitus. Lancet ii: 251, 1976
7. Ilonen J, Herva E, Tiilikainen A, Akerblom HK, Kaivukangas T, Kouvalaimen K: HLA-DW2 as a marker of resistance against juvenile diabetes mellitus. Tissue Antigens 11:144-146, 1978
8. Thomsen M, Platz P, Christy M, Nerup J, Ryder LP, Svejgaard A: HLA-D-associated resistance and susceptibility to insulin-dependent diabetes mellitus. Transplant Proc 11:1307-1308, 1979
9. Ludwig H, Schernthaner G, Mayr WR: Is HLA-B7 a marker associated with a protective gene in juvenile-onset diabetes mellitus? N Engl J Med 294:1066, 1976
10. Ilonen J, Herva E, Tiilikainen A, Akerblom HK, Mustonen A, Koivukangas T, et al: HLA genetics of insulin-dependent juvenile-onset diabetes mellitus in northern Finland. Tissue Antigens 15:381-388, 1980
11. Cudworth AG, Festenstein H: HLA genetic heterogeneity in diabetes mellitus. Br Med Bull 34:285-289, 1978
12. Platz P, Jakobsen BK, Morling N, Ryder LP, Svejgaard A, Thomsen M, et al: HLA-D and -DR antigens in genetic analysis of insulin dependent diabetes mellitus. Diabetologia 21:108-115, 1981
13. Barbosa J, Bach FH, Rich SS: Genetic heterogeneity of diabetes and HLA. Clin Genet 21:25-32, 1982
14. Svejgaard A, Platz P, Ryder LP: Insulin dependent diabetes mellitus. In Terasaki PI (ed): Histocompatibility Testing 1980. UCLA Tissue Typing Laboratory, Los Angeles, 1981, pp 638-656
15. Wolf E, Spencer KM, Cudworth AG: The genetic susceptibility to type 1 (insulin-dependent) diabetes: Analysis of the HLA-DR association. Diabetologia 24:224-230, 1983

16. Hammond MG, Asmal AC, Amar MAK: HLA and insulin-dependent diabetes in South African negroes. Diabetologia 19:101-102, 1980
17. Briggs BR, Jackson WPU, Dutoit ED, Botha MC: The histocompatibility (HLA) antigen distribution in diabetes in Southern African blacks (Xhosa). Diabetes 29:68-71, 1980
18. Patel R, Ansari A, Covarrubias CLP: Leukocyte antigens and disease: III. Association of HLA-B8 and HLA-BW15 with insulin-dependent diabetes in three different population groups. Metabolism 26:487-492, 1977
19. Srikanta S, Ahuja MMS, Malaviya AN, Mehra NK, Vaidya MC: Type I (insulin-requiring) diabetes mellitus in North India: HLA and autoimmunity. N Engl J Med 304:1175-1176, 1981
20. Kawa A, Nakazawa M, Sakaguchi S, Nakamura S, Komo Y, Hazeki H, et al: HLA system in Japanese patients with diabetes mellitus. Diabetes 26:591-595, 1977
21. Kawa A, Nakazawa M, Kono Y, Sakaguchi S, Nakamura S, Kanehisa T: HLA BW54 and B5 in Japanese diabetics with juvenile-onset and insulin-dependency (with special reference to the family history). Experientia 34:669-670, 1978
22. Kawa A, Nakamura S, Kono Y, Maeda Y, Kanehisa T: A negative association of HLA-BW52 with Graves' disease and insulin-dependent diabetes mellitus with juvenile onset among Japanese population. Experientia 35:547-548, 1979
23. Okimoto K, Juji T, Ishiba S, Maruyama H, Tohyama H, Kosaka K: HLA-BW54 (BW22-J, J-1) antigens in juvenile onset diabetes mellitus in Japan. Tissue Antigens 11:418-422, 1978
24. Nakao Y, Fukunishi T, Koide M, Akasawa K, Ikeda M, Yahata M, et al: HLA antigens in Japanese patients with diabetes mellitus. Diabetes 26:736-739, 1977
25. Wakisaka A, Aizawa M, Matsuura N, Nakagawa S, Nakayama E, Okuno A, et al: HLA and juvenile diabetes mellitus in the Japanese. Lancet ii:970, 1976
26. Sasazuki T, Kohno Y, Iwamoto I, Kosaba K, Okimoto K, Maruyama H, et al: HLA and Graves' disease or diabetes mellitus in Japan. N Engl J Med 298:630-631, 1978
27. Sakurami T, Nagaoka K, Nabeya N, Imura H, Kuno S: Islet-cell antibodies and HLA type in Japanese insulin-dependent diabetics. Endocrinol Jpn 27:149-152, 1980
28. Dornan J, Allan P, Noel EP, Larsen B, Farid NR: Properdin factor B(BF) allele BF(F1) specifies an HLA-B18 diabetogenic haplotype. Diabetes 29:423-427, 1980
29. De Mouzon A, Ohayon E, Ducos J: BF and C4 markers for insulin-dependent diabetes in Basques. Lancet ii:1364, 1979
30. Bertrams J, Baur MP, Gruneklee D, Gries FA: Association of BfF1, HLA-B18 and insulin-dependent diabetes mellitus. Lancet ii:98, 1979
31. Deschamps I, Lestradet H, Bonaiti C, Schmid M, Busson M, Benajam A, et al: HLA genotype studies in juvenile insulin-dependent diabetes. Diabetologia 19:189-193, 1980
32. Arnaiz-Villena A, Rodriguez De Cordoba S, Dujovne IL, Regueiro JR, Bootello A, Serrano-Rios M: HLA factors in non-insulin-dependent diabetes mellitus. N Engl J Med 303:1065, 1980
33. Farid NR, Barnard JM, Pepper B, Noel EP, Kelly F, Davis AJ, et al: The association of HLA with juvenile diabetes mellitus in Newfoundland. Tissue Antigens 12:215-222, 1978
34. Barta L, Simon S, Kosnai I: HLA B8 and BW15 antigens in diabetic children. Acta Paediatr Acad Sci Hung 19:41-44, 1978
35. Ludvigsson J, Safwenberg, Heding LG: HLA-types, C-peptide and insulin antibodies in juvenile diabetes. Diabetologia 13:13-17, 1977
36. Cudworth AG, Woodrow JC: Genetic susceptibility in diabetes mellitus: Analysis of the HLA association. Br Med J 2:846-848, 1976
37. Cudworth AG, Woodrow JC: Evidence for HL-A linked genes in "juvenile" diabetes mellitus. Br Med J 3:133-135, 1975
38. Moller E, Persson B, Sterky G: HLA phenotypes and diabetic retinopathy. Diabetologia 14:155-158, 1978
39. Cambon De-Mouzon A, Ohayon E, Hauptmann G, Sevin A, Abbal M, Sommer E, et al: HLA-A, -B, -C, -DR antigens Bf, C4 and glyoxalase I (GLO) polymorphisms in French Basques with insulin-dependent diabetes mellitus (IDDM). Tissue Antigens 19:366-379, 1982
40. Pitkanen E, Kuhlback B, Tiilikainen A, Lokki ML, Karkkainen J: HLA-antigen distribution in juvenile diabetics with end-stage nephropathy. Ann Clin Res 13:91-95, 1981
41. Illeni MT, Pellegris G, Del Guercio MJ, Tarantino A, Buseti F, Di Pietro C, et al: HLA antigens in diabetic children. Diabetes 26:870-873, 1977
42. Schernthaner G, Ludwig H, Mayr WR: Juvenile diabetes mellitus: HLA-antigen frequencies dependent on the age of onset of the disease. J Immunogenet 3:117-121, 1976
43. Bertrams J, Baur MP, Gruneklee D, Gries FA. Age-related association of insulin-dependent diabetes mellitus with BfF1 and HLA-B18, BfF1 haplotype. Diabetologia 21:47-49, 1981
44. Zeidler A, Loon J, Frasier SD, Kumar D, Renny R, Terasaki PI: HLA-DRW antigens in Mexican-American and Black-American diabetic patients. Diabetes 29:247-250, 1980
45. Pittman WB, Acton RT, Barger B, Bell DS, Go RCP, Murphy CC, et al: HLA-A, -B, and -DR as-

sociations in type 1 diabetes mellitus with onset after age forty. Diabetes 31:122-125, 1982

46. Morris PJ, Vaughan H, Irvine WJ, McCallum FJ, Gray RS, Campbell CJ, et al: HLA and pancreatic islet cell antibodies in diabetes. Lancet ii:652-653, 1976
47. Irvine WJ, McCallum CJ, Gray RS, Campbell CJ, Duncan LJP, et al: Pancreatic islet-cell antibodies in diabetes mellitus correlated with duration and type of diabetes, coexistent autoimmune disease, and HLA type. Diabetes 26:138-147, 1977
48. Christy M, Nerup J, Bottazzo GF, Donaich D, Platz P, Svejgaard A, et al: Association between HLA-B8 and autoimmunity in juvenile diabetes mellitus. Lancet ii:142-143, 1976
49. Nerup J, Platz P, Ryder LP, Thomsen M, Svejgaard A: HLA, islet cell antibodies, and types of diabetes mellitus. Diabetes 27(Suppl I):247-250, 1978
50. Richens ER, Quilley J, Hartog M: Immunological features of juvenile onset diabetic patients correlated to HLA type. Clin Exp Immunol 36:198-204, 1979
51. Richens ER, Quilley J, Hartog M: Studies on the frequency and associations of islet-cell antibodies in juvenile diabetes mellitus. Acta Diabetol Lat 15:229-235, 1978
52. Lendrum R, Walker G, Cudworth AG, Woodrow JC, Gamble DR: HLA-linked genes and islet-cell antibodies in diabetes. Br Med J 1:1565-1567, 1976
53. Batchelor JR, Morris PJ: Juvenile onset diabetes: Joint report. In Bodmer W et al. (eds): Histocompatibility Testing 1977. Munksgaard, Copenhagen, pp 211-213, 1978
54. Mustonen A, Ilonen J, Akerblom HK, Tiilikainen A: An islet cell antibody negative form of insulin-dependent diabetes mellitus (IDD) associated with HLA antigens A9 and Bw16. Clin Exp Immunol 48:213-217, 1982
55. Ginsberg-Fellner F, Dobersen MJ, Witt ME, Rayfield EJ, Rubinstein P, Notkins AL: HLA antigens, cytoplasmic islet cell antibodies, and carbohydrate tolerance in families of children with insulin-dependent diabetes mellitus. Diabetes 31:292-298,1982
56. Larkins RG, Martin FIR, Tait BD: HLA patterns and diabetic retinopathy. Br Med J 1:1111, 1978
57. Bertrams J, Dewald G, Spitznas M, Rittner CH: HLA-A, -B, -C, -DR, Bf, and C2 alleles in insulin-dependent diabetes mellitus with proliferative retinopathy. Immunobiology 158:113-118, 1980
58. Barbosa J, Ramsay RC, Knobloch WH, Cantrill HL, Noreen H, King R, et al.: Histocompatibility antigen frequencies in diabetic retinopathy. Am J Ophthalmol 90:148-153, 1985
59. Barbosa J: Is diabetic microangiopathy genetically heterogeneous? HLA and diabetic nephropathy. Horm Metab Res 11:77-80, 1981
60. Becker B, Shin DH, Burgess D, Kilo C, Miller WV: Histocompatibility antigens and diabetic retinopathy. Diabetes 26:997-999, 1977
61. Cove DH, Walker JM, Wells L, Mackintosh P, Wright AD: Are HLA types or BF alleles markers for diabetic retinopathy? Diabetologia 19:402-403, 1980
62. Jervell J, Solheim B: HLA-antigens in long standing insulin dependent diabetics with terminal nephropathy and retinopathy with and without loss of vision. Diabetologia 17:391, 1979
63. Johnston PB, Kidd M, Middleton D, Greenfield AA, Archer DB, Maguire CJF, Kennedy L: Analysis of HLA antigen association with proliferative diabetic retinopathy. Br J Ophthalmol 66:277-279, 1982
64. McCann VJ, McCluskey J, Kay PH, Zilko PJ, Christiansen FT, Dawkins RL: HLA and complement genetic markers in diabetic retinopathy. Diabetologia 24:221, 1983
65. Danielsen R, Helgason T, Arnason A, Jonasson F: HLA and retinopathy in type 1 (insulin-dependent) diabetic patients in Iceland. Diabetologia 22:297-298, 1982
66. Standl E, Dexel T, Lander T, Albert ED, Scholz S, Greite JH, et al: Association of HLA antigens with severity of diabetic retinopathy in southern Germany. Horm Metab Res 11:81-86, 1981
67. Deckert T, Egeberg J, Frimodt-Moller C, Sander E, Svejgaard A: Basement membrane thickness, insulin antibodies and HLA-antigens in long standing insulin dependent diabetics with and without severe retinopathy. Diabetologia 17:91-96, 1979
68. Rolles CJ, Rayner PHW, Mackintosh P: Aetiology of juvenile diabetes. Lancet ii:230, 1975
69. Garovoy MR, Carpenter CB, Myrberg SM, Gleason RE, Funk IB, Flood TM, et al: Increased incidence of HLA-B8 in jurenile-onset diabetes mellitus. Transplant Proc 9:177-179, 1977
70. Bengsch N, Kobberling J, Eckert G, Willms B: HLA-typing in juvenile diabetes with and without positive family history and in families with one and two diabetic siblings. Diabetologia 15:447-451, 1978
71. Ilonen J, Akerblom HK, Tiilikainen A, Mustonen A, Herva E, Koskimie S, et al: Increase of HLA haplotype A9-BW16 in familial insulin-dependent diabetes mellitus in Northern Finland. Acta Diabetol Lat 19:167, 1982
72. Kikuchi T, Toyota T, Ouchi E: HLA antigens in juvenile onset diabetes. Tohoku J Exp Med 132:289-293, 1980
73. Bertrams J, Jansen, Gruneklee D, Reis HE, Drosy H, and Beyer J, et al: HLA antigens and immuno-

responsiveness to insulin in insulin-dependent diabetes mellitus. Tissue Antigens 8:13-19, 1976
74. Bertrams J, Jansen FK, Gruneklee D, Reis HE, Drost H, Beyer J, et al: HLA antigen associated immuneresponsiveness to insulin in insulin-dependent diabetes mellitus. Z Immunitaetsforsch 152:309-313, 1976
75. Schernthaner G, Ludwig H, Mayr WR, Willvonseder R: Genetic factors on insulin antibodies in juvenile-onset diabetes. N Engl J Med 295:622, 1976
76. Zeidler A, Frasier SD, Kumar D, Loon J: Histocompatibility antigens and immunoglobulin G insulin antibodies in Mexican-American insulin-dependent diabetic patients. J Clin Endocrinol Metab 54:569-573, 1982
77. Sakurami T, Nabeya N, Nagaoka K, Matsumori A, Kuno S, Honda A: Antibodies to coxsackie B viruses and HLA in Japanese with juvenile-onset type 1 (insulin-dependent) diabetes mellitus. Diabetologia 22:375-377, 1982
78. Court S, Parkin M, Roberts DF, Wentzel J: HLA antigens and growth in diabetic children. Ann Hum Biol 9:329-336, 1982
79. Singal DP, Perets A, Dolovich J: HLA antigens and serum antibodies to bovine serum albumin. Transplant Proc 11:1864-1865, 1979
80. Serjeantson S, Theophilus J, Zimmet P, Court J, Crossley JR, Elliott RB: Lymphocytotoxic antibodies and histocompatibility antigens in juvenile-onset diabetes mellitus. Diabetes 30:26-29, 1981
81. Ludwig H, Mayr WR, Schernthaner G: Glucose-tolerance tests in HL-A-typed relatives of patients with juvenile onset diabetes mellitus. Lancet ii:1152-1153, 1975
82. Landgraf R, Landgraf-Leurs MMC, Lander T, Scholz S, Kuntz B, Albert ED: HLA haplotypes and glucose tolerance in families of patients with juvenile-onset diabetes mellitus. Lancet ii:1084-1085, 1976
83. Larkins RG, Martin FIR, Heding LG, Tait BD: Hormonal profile, blood sugar control and HLA patterns in long-term insulin dependent diabetes with and without vascular disease. Aust NZ J Med 8:465-471, 1978
84. Menser MA, Forrest JM, Honeyman MC, Burgess JA: Diabetes, HL-A antigens, and congenital rubella. Lancet ii:1508-1509, 1974
85. Cudworth AG, Woodrow JC: HL-A system and diabetes mellitus. Diabetes 24:345-349, 1975
86. Serjeantson S, Kirk RL, Dry PJ, Ryan DP, Court J, Zimmet P, et al: HLA studies in Australian multiple-case families of juvenile onset diabetes mellitus. Med J Aust 1:107-109, 1980
87. Krawisz JE, Palumbo PJ, Taswell HF, Elveback LR: HLA antigens in patients with juvenile diabetes and their first-degree relatives. Mayo Clin Proc 53:782-787, 1978
88. Cudworth AG, Gorsuch AN, Wolf E, Festenstein H: A new look at HLA genetics with particular reference to type-1 diabetes. Lancet ii:389-391, 1979
89. Nelson PG, Pyke DA, Cudworth AG, Woodrow JC, Batchelor JR: Histocompatibility antigens in diabetic identical twins. Lancet ii:193-194, 1975
90. Fitzgerald GA, Drury MI: HLA identity in juvenile onset diabetes. Ir J Med Sci 147:430-434, 1978
91. Ryder LP, Christy M, Nerup J, Platz P, Svejgaard A, Thomsen M: HLA studies in diabetics. Adv Exp Med Biol 119:41-50, 1979
92. Christy M, Green A, Christau B, Kronann H, Nerup J, Platz P, et al: Studies of the HLA system and insulin-dependent diabetes mellitus. Diabetes Care 2:209-214, 1979
93. Nerup J: HLA studies in diabetes mellitus: A review. Adv Metab Disord 9:263-277, 1978
94. Falk CT, Suciu-Foca N, Rubinstein P: Possible localization of the gene(s) for juvenile diabetes mellitus (JDM) to the HLA region of chromosome 6. Cytogenet Cell Genet 22:298-300, 1978
95. Stenszky V, Kozma L, Ambro I, Karmazsin L: Calculation of disease susceptibility gene frequency in insulin-dependent diabetes mellitus. Haematologia 12:141-148, 1978-1979
96. Barbosa J, King R, Noreen H, Yunis EJ: The histocompatibility system in juvenile, insulin-dependent diabetic multiplex kindreds. J Clin Invest 60:989-998, 1977
97. Rubinstein P, Suciu-Foca N, Nicholson JF, Fotino M, Molinaro A, Harisiadis L, et al: The HLA system in the families of patients with juvenile diabetes mellitus. J Exp Med 143:1277-1282, 1976
98. Barbosa J, Noreen H, King R, Yunis EJ: Genetics of juvenile diabetes. N Engl J Med 298:462, 1978
99. Barbosa J, Chern MM, Noreen H, Anderson VE, Yunis EJ: Analysis of linkage between the major histocompatibility system and juvenile, insulin-dependent diabetes in multiplex families. J Clin Invest 62:492-495, 1978
100. Barbosa J, Chern MM, Anderson VE, Noreen H, Johnson S, et al: Linkage analysis between the major histocompatibility system and insulin-dependent diabetes in families with patients in two consecutive generations. J Clin Invest 65:592-601, 1980
101. Rubinstein P, Suciu-Foca N, Nicholson JF: Genetics of juvenile diabetes mellitus: A recessive gene closely linked to HLA-D with 50 percent penetrance. N Engl J Med 297:1036-1040, 1977
102. Suciu-Foca N, Rubinstein P, Nicholson J, Susinno E, Weiner J, Godfrey M, et al: Juvenile diabetes

mellitus and the HLA system. Transplant Proc 11:1309-1313, 1979
103. Rubinstein P, Suciu-Foca N: HLA and the genetic aspects of the predisposition to juvenile diabetes mellitus. A follow-up. Adv Exp Med Biol 119:33-40, 1979
104. Clerget-Darpoux F, Bonaiti-Pellie C, Hors J, Deschamps I, Feingold N: Application of the lod score method to detection of linkage between HLA and juvenile insulin-depehndent diabetes. Clin Genet 18:51-57, 1980
105. Spielman RS, Baker L, Zmijewski CM: Inheritance of susceptiblity to juvenile onset diabetes. Prog Clin Biol Res 32:567-585, 1979
106. McCluskey J, McCann VJ, Kay PH, Zilko PJ, Christiansen FT, O'Neill GJ, et al: HLA and complement allotypes in type 1 (insulin-dependent) diabetes. Diabetologia 24:162-165, 1983
107. Johnston PB, Middleton D, Archer DB, Hadden DR: HLA antigens in proliferative diabetic retinopathy. Int Ophthalmol 3:87-89, 1981
108. Weitkamp LR: HLA and disease: Predictions for HLA haplotype sharing in families. Am J Hum Genet 33:776-784, 1981
109. Rubinstein P, Ginsberg-Fellner F, Falk C: Genetics of type I diabetes mellitus: A single, recessive, predisposition gene mapping between HLA-B and GLO. Am J Hum Genet 33:865-862, 1981
110. Green JR, Low HC, Woodrow JC: Inference on inheritance of disease using repetitions of HLA haplotypes in affected siblings. Ann Hum Genet 47:73-82, 1983
111. Dunsworth TS, Rich SS, Morton NE, Barbosa J: Heterogeneity of insulin-dependent diabetes-new evidence. Clin Genet 21:233-236, 1982
112. Barrai I, Cann HM: Segregation analysis of juvenile diabetes mellitus. J Med Genet 2:8-11, 1965
113. Morton NE, Green A, Dunsworth T, Svejgaard A, Barbosa J, Rich SS, et al: Heterozygous expression of insulin-dependent diabetes mellitus (IDDM) determinants in the HLA system. Am J Hum Genet 35:201-213, 1983
114. Green A, Morton NE, Iselius L, Svejgaard A, Platz P, Ryder LP, et al: Genetic studies of insulin-dependent diabetes mellitus: Segregation and linkage analysis. Tissue Antigens 19:213-221, 1982
115. Thomson G: A two locus model for juvenile diabetes. Ann Hum Genet 43:383-398, 1980
116. Hodge SE, Rotter JI, Lange KL: A three-allele model for heterogeneity of juvenile onset insulin-dependent diabetes. Ann Hum Genet 43:399-412, 1980
117. Suarez B, Hodge SE, Reich T: Is juvenile diabetes determined by a single gene closely linked to HLA? Diabetes 28:527-532, 1979
118. Clerget-Darpoux BF, Bonaiti-Peddie C, Deschamps I, Hors J, Feingold N: Juvenile insulin-dependent diabete: A possible susceptibility gene in interaction with HLA. Ann Hum Genet 45:199-206, 1981
119. Curie-Cohen M: HLA antigens and susceptibility to juvenile diabetes: Do additive relative risks imply genetic heterogeneity. Tissue Antigens 17:136-148, 1981
120. Rotter JI: The modes of inheritance of insulin-dependent diabetes mellitus or the genetics of IDDM, no longer a nightmare but still a headache. Am J Hum Genet 33:835-851, 1981
121. Svejgaard A, Ryder LP: HLA genotype distribution and genetic models of insulin-dependent diabetes mellitus. Ann Hum Genet 45:293-298, 1981
122. Contu L, Deschamps I, Lestradet H, Jors J, Schmid M, Busson M, et al: HLA haplotype study of 53 juvenile insulin-dependent diabetic (I.D.D.) families. Tissue Antigens 20:123-140, 1982
123. Bach FH, Segall M, Rich S, Barbosa J: HLA and susceptibility to type I diabetes. Tissue Antigens 20:28-32, 1982
124. Rotter JI, Anderson CE, Rubin R, Congleton JE, Terasaki PI, Rimoin DL: HLA genotypic study of insulin-dependent diabetes. Diabetes 32:169-174, 1983
125. Suciu-Foca N, Rubinstein P: Intra-HLA recombinations in juvenile diabetes mellitus. Lancet i:371-372, 1976
126. Mayr WR, Schernthaner G, Ludwig H: Intra-HLA recombination frequency in juvenile diabetes. Lancet i:865, 1976
127. Platz P, Thomsen M, Svejgaard A, Cudworth AG, Woodrow JC, Nerup J: More on the genetics of juvenile diabetes. N Engl J Med 298:1200-1201, 1978
128. Hsu SH, Hsu TH, Chase GA, Bias WB: Further data on HLA recombination in juvenile-onset diabetes. Transplant Proc 9:1855-1858, 1977
129. Neel JV: The genetics of juvenile-onset-type diabetes mellitus. N Engl J Med 297:1062-1063, 1977
130. Drash AL: The etiology of diabetes mellitus. N Engl J Med 300:1211-1213, 1979
131. Yoon JW, Austin M, Onodera T, Notkins AL: Virus-induced diabetes mellitus: Isolation of a virus from the pancreas of a child with diabetic ketoacidosis. N Engl J Med 30[illegible]:1173-1179, 1979
132. Barbosa J: HLA and diabetes mellitus. Lancet i:906-907, 1977
133. Solow H, Hidalgo R, Blajchman M, Singal DP: HLA-A, -B, -C and B-lymphocyte alloantigens in insulin-dependent diabetes. Tranplant Proc 9:1859-1861, 1977
134. Nerup J, Anderson OO, Christy M, Platz P, Ryder L, Thomsen M, et al: HLA autoimmunity,

viruses and the pathogenesis of juvenile diabetes mellitus. Acta Endocrinol (83 Suppl 205):167-175, 1976
135. Bottazzo GF, Doniach D: Pancreatic autoimmunity and HLA antigens. Lancet ii:800, 1976
136. Woodrow JC: HL-A and its association with clinical disease. Proc Roy Soc Med 68:18-20, 1975
137. Schernthaner G, Ludwig H, Eibl M, Erd W, Packer M, Mayr WK: HLA-system und diabetes mellitus. Schweiz Med Wochenschr 106:514-517, 1976
138. Cudworth AG, Woodrow JC: Genetic susceptibility in diabetic identical twins. Lancet ii:518-519, 1976
139. Nakazawa M, Hirata Y: Diabetes mellitus and HLA antigens. Nippon Rinsho 36:3193-3196, 1978
140. Cudworth AG: Type I diabetes mellitus. Diabetologia 14:281-291, 1978
141. Barta L, Simon S: Role of HLA-B8 and BW15 antigens in diabetic children. N Engl J Med 296:397, 1976
142. De Moerloose PH, Chardonnens X, Vassalli P, Jeannet M: Antigenes HLA-D des lymphocytes B et susceptibilite a certaines maladies. Schweiz Med Wochenschr 107:1461, 1977
143. Williams RM: Ia-like antigens in human autoimmune diseases: HLA and DRW antigens in chronic active hepatitis and diabetes mellitus. In Amos DB, Schwartz RS, Janichi BW (eds): Immune Mechanisms and Disease. Academic Press, New York, 1979, pp 163-177
144. Dippe SE, Bennett PH, Miller M, Maynard JE, Berquist KR: Lack of causal association between coxsackie B4 virus infection and diabetes. Lancet i:1314-1317, 1975
145. Woodrow JC, Cudworth AG: HL-A8 and W15 in diabetes mellitus. Lancet i:803, 1975
146. Cathelineau G, Cathelineau L, Hors J, Schmid M, Dausset J: Les groupes HLA dans le diabete a debut precoce. Nouv Presse Med 5:586, 1976
147. Tattersall RB, Pyke DA: Diabetes in identical twins. Lancet ii:1120-1125, 1972
148. Pyke DA, Tattersall RB: Diabetic retinopathy in identical twins. Diabetes 22:613-618, 1973
149. Maugh TH: Diabetes: Epidemiology suggests a viral connection. Science 188:347-351, 1975
150. Kromann H, Lernmark A, Vestergaard BF, Egeberg J, Nerup J: The influence of the major histocompatibility complex (H-2) on experimental diabetes in mice. Diabetologia 16:107-114, 1979
151. Dimopoulos C, Likourinas M, Melekos M: Diabetes insipidus and hydronephrosis. J Urol 121:689, 1979
152. MacDonald MJ, Curie-Cohen M: HLA in juvenile diabetes. N Engl J Med 302:405-406, 1980
153. Rotter JI, Rimon DL: Diabetes mellitus: The search for genetic markers. Diabetes Care 2:215-226, 1979
154. Serjeantson S: Distorted HLA segregation or biased ascertainment. Lancet i:40-41, 1980
155. Lajos B, Erzebet G, Zsuzsa MS: Juvenilis diabetes es addison-kor egyuettes eloefordulasa HLA-B8 antigen pozitivitassal. Orv Hetil 118:931-933, 1977
156. Pointel JP, Sauvanet JP, Dourin P, Debry G, Rafoux C, Streiff F: Diabete insulino-dependant: Frequence des antigenes HLA selon le sexe des malades. Nouv Presse Med 7:1747, 1978
157. Mirouze J, Seignalet J, Selam JL, Lapinski H, Jaffiol C: Antigenes HLA chez les diabetiques insulino-dependants. Nouv Presse Med 5:1628-1630, 1976
158. Schernthaner G, Mayr WR, Pacher M, Ludwig H, Erd W, Eibl M: HL-A8, W15 and T3 in juvenile onset diabetes mellitus. Horm Metab Res 7:521-522, 1975
159. O'Regan S: HLA-B8 autoimmune polyendocrinopathy and systemic lupus erythematosus. Can Med Assoc J 121:1168-1169, 1979
160. Cudworth AG Woodrow JC: HL-A antigens and diabetes mellitus. Lancet ii:1153, 1974
161. Dvorakova L, Majsky A: HLA antigens in offspring of both diabetic parents. Cas Lek Cesk 118:1294-1296, 1979
162. Neufeld MR, Maclaren NK, Riley WJ: HLA in American Blacks with juvenile diabetes. N Engl J Med 303:111-112, 1980
163. De Moor P, Louwagle A, Van Baelen H, Van De Putte I: Unexplained high transcortin levels in patients with various hematological disorders and in their relatives: A connection between these high transcortin levels and HLA antigen B12. J Clin Endrocrinol Metab 50:421-426, 1980
164. Serova LD: Changes in incidence of HL-A antigens in diabetes mellitus. Prob Endokrinol (Mosk) 26:12-15, 1980
165. Deschamps I, Hors J, Lestradet H: Inheritance of insulin-dependent diabetes mellitus in relation to the HLA system. Semin Hop Paris 58:153-157, 1982
166. Cahill GF Jr: Current concepts of diabetic complications with emphasis on hereditary factors: A brief review. Prog Clin Biol Res 32:113-125, 1979
167. Palumbo PJ: Classification of diabetes mellitus. Prog Clin Biol Res 32:127-134, 1979
168. Rotter JI: Genetic heterogeneity within diabetes mellitus: A review. Prog Clin Biol Res 32:135-155, 1979
169. Maeda H, Takeuchi F, Juji T, Akanuma Y, Kasuga M, Lee YS, Kosaka K, Tsai SH: HLA-DRW3 in juvenile onset diabetes mellitus in Chinese. Tissue Antigens 15:173-176, 1980

170. Zhao T, Chi Z, Wang H, Shen M, Zhou Z, Bu K, et al: HLA and diabetes mellitus in Chinese. Chin Med J 95:609-612, 1982
171. Kirk RL, Ranford PR, Theophilus J, Ahuja HMS, Mehra NK, Vaidya MC: The rare factor BfSl of the properdin system strongly associated with insulin-dependent diabetes in north India. Tissue Antigens 20:303-304, 1982
172. Walsh LJ, Cox DW, Ehrlich RM: The HLA-B18, BfF1 in haplotype in type I diabetes. Am J Med Genet 11:337-343, 1982
173. Bertrams J, Baur MP, Gruneklee D, Hintzen U: Association of BfF1 and haplotype HLA-B18,BfF1 with insulin-dependent diabetes mellitus. Immunobiology 158:129-133, 1980
174. Moriuchi J, Katagiri M, Wakisaka A, Matsuura N, Maruyama N, Ikeda H, et al: Association of B cell alloantigen with juvenile onset diabetes mellitus in the Japanese. Hum Immunol 4:357-362, 1980
175. Rodey GE, White N, Frazer TE, Duquesnoy RJ, Santiago JV: HLA-DR specificities among Black Americans with juvenile-onset diabetes. N Engl J Med 301:810-812, 1979
176. Reitnauer PJ, Roseman JM, Barger BO, Murphy CC, Kirk KA, Acton RT: HLA associations with insulin-dependent diabetes mellitus in a sample of the American Black population. Tissue Antigens 17:286-293, 1981
177. Duquesnoy RJ, MacDonald MJ, Mullins P, Hackbarth SA, Traisman HS, Levitsky LL: Increased frequency of HLA-DW3 in North-American Blacks with juvenile onset diabetes. Tissue Antigens 13:369-372, 1979
178. Hammond MG, Asmal AC: HLA and insulin dependent diabetes in South African Indians. Tissue Antigens 15:244-248, 1980
179. Slater LM, Kershnar A, Golden M, Mosier MA, Arquilla ER: Decreased incidence of HLA-A11 and increased incidence of HLA-B18 in North American population of insulin dependent diabetics. J Clin Lab Immunol 4:91-94, 1980
180. Barbosa J, Noreen H, Emme L, Goetz F, Simmons R, De Leiva A, et al: Histocompatibility (HLA) antigens and diabetic microangiopathy. Tissue Antigens 7:233-237, 1976
181. Zimmet P, Kiely P, Cross R, Court J, Bornstein J: HLA patterns in Australian patients with insulin dependent diabetes mellitus (IDDM). Aust NZ J Med 9:633-636, 1979
182. Vasyukova EA, Gulyaeva ES, Katsnelson LA, Knyazev YA, Mikhailova NA, Zefirova S: HLA-antigens, hormonal profile, insulin antibodies in patients with IDDM with retinopathy. Klin Med (Mosk) 59:42-46, 1981
183. Gray RS, Starkey IR, Rainbow S, Kurtz AB, Abdel-Khalik A, Urbaniak S, et al: HLA antigens and other risk factors in the development of retinopathy in type 1 diabetes. Br J Ophthalmol 66:280-285, 1982
184. Seignalet J, Mirouze J, Jaffiol C, Selam JL, Lapinski H: HL-A in Graves' disease and in diabetes mellitus insulin-dependent. Tissue Antigens 6:272-274, 1975
185. De Moerloose P, Jeannet M, Bally C, Raffoux C, Pointel JP, Sizomenbo P: HLA and DRW antigens in insulin-dependent diabetes. Br Med J 1:823-824, 1978
186. MacDonald MJ, Traisman HS, Levitsky LL, Duquesnoy RJ, Mullins P, Hackbarth SA: HLA types in American black juvenile diabetics strong associations with DW3 and DW4. Metabolism 30:533-536, 1981
187. Lajos B, Zsuzsa S, Eva GK: Osszefuggesek a HLA antigenek es a gyermekkori diabetes kozott. Orv Hetil 120:2061-2063, 1979
188. Savi M, Neri TM, Zavaroni I, Coscelli C: Marcatori genetici nel diabete giovaniole insulino dipendente. Minerva Med 69:3359-3365, 1978
189. Schober E, Schernthaner G, Mayr WR: HLA-DR antigens in insulin-dependent diabetes. Arch Dis Child 56:227-229, 1981
190. Nerup J, Platz P, Andersen OO, Christy M, Lyngsoe J, Poulsen JE, et al: HL-A antigens and diabetes mellitus. Lancet ii:864-866, 1974
191. Mullins P, Collins J, MacDonald MJ, Duquesnoy RJ: Unusual MLC responses of Black patients with juvenile-onset diabetes. Transplant Proc 11:1879-1881, 1979
192. Reitnauer PJ, Roseman JM, Barger BO, Murphy C, Acton RT: Juvenile onset diabetes in American Blacks. N Engl J Med 302:406, 1980
193. Garovoy MR, Barbosa J, Reddish M, Martin S, Noreen H, Yunis EJ, et al: HLA-DR antigens and unique serologic reactions in juvenile-onset diabetes mellitus. Transplant Proc 10:967-969, 1978
194. Sakurami T, Ueno Y, Nagaoka K, Kuno S, Iwaki Y, Park MS, et al: HLA-DR specifications in Japanese with juvenile-onset insulin-dependent diabetes mellitus. Diabetes 31:105-106, 1982
195. Schernthaner G, Ludwig H, Mayr WR: B-lymphocyte alloantigens and insulin-dependent diabetes mellitus. Lancet ii:1128, 1977
196. Standl E, Dexel T, Lander T, Albert ED, Scholz S: HLA- antigens and diabetic retinopathy: A different view warranted. Diabetologia 18:79-80, 1980
197. Bertrams J, Sodomann P, Grosse-Wilde H, Rittner Ch: Two HLA-B/D, DR recombinants in diabetic families: The susceptibility gene traveled with HLA-D, DR fragment. In Terasaki PI (ed): Histocompatibility Testing 1980. UCLA Tissue Typing Laboratory, 1980, pp 947
198. Berger W, Calabi F, Garotta G, Neri TM, Cep-

pellini R: HLA and insulin-dependent diabetes mellitus: High risk for DRW3/DRW4 heterozygous and segregation in a B/DR recombinant family. In Terasaki PI (ed): Histocompatibility Testing 1980. UCLA Tissue Typing Laboratory, 1980, pp 948

199. Barbosa J, Chavers B, Steffes M, Szalapski E, Cohen RA, Michael AF, et al: Muscle extracellular membrane immunofluorescence and HLA as possible markers of prediabetes. Lancet ii:330-333, 1980
200. Phillips WR, Pauli R: Simultaneous onset of insulin dependent diabetes mellitus in sibling. Lancet i:807, 1981
201. Asplund K: Diabetes, mumps and HLA antigens. Lancet ii:807, 1981
202. Miller AP, Rich S, Barbosa J: Insulin dependent diabetic families: Sex ratio and HLA haplotype segregation. Lancet i:388, 1981
203. Srikanta S, Mehra NK, Vaidya MC, Malaviya AN, Ahuja MS: HLA antigens in type 1 (insulin-dependent) diabetes mellitus in North India. Metabolism 30:992-993, 1981
204. Christy M, Nerup J, Platz P, Thomsen M, Ryder LP, Svejgard A: A review of HLA antigens in longstanding IDDM with and without severe retinopathy. Horm Metab Res 11:73-77, 1981
205. Joron GE, Shuster J, Webb JL: C-peptide and HLA antigens in long-standing juvenile diabetes. Diabetes Care 3:703-704, 1980
206. Bertrams J, Sodomann P, Gries FA, Sachsse B, Jahnke K. Die HLA-association des insulinpflichtigen diabetes mellitus, typ 1. Dtsch Med Wochenschr 106:927-932, 1981
207. Hollander PH, Asplin CM, Kniaz D, Hansen JA, Palmer JP: Beta-cell dysfunction in nondiabetic HLA identical siblings of insulin-dependent diabetics. Diabetes 31:149-153, 1982
208. Marks JF, Raskin P, Stastny P: Increase in capillary basement membrane width in parents of children with type 1 diabetes mellitus. Diabetes 30:475-480, 1981
209. Sakurami T, Ueno Y, Iwaki Y, Park MS, Terasaki PI, Saji H: HLA-DR specificities among Japanese with several autoimmune disease. Tissue Antigens 19:129-133, 1982
210. Valenta LJ, Bull RW, Hackel E, Bottazzo GF: Correlation of the HLA-A1, B8 haplotypes with circulating autoantibodies in a family with increased incidence of autoimmune disease. Acta Endocrinol 100:143-149, 1982
211. Cox JW, Bourke GM: Benefits of HLA typing a family with diabetes. Aust Paediatr J 17:224-225, 1981
212. Kay PH, McCluskey J, Christiansen FT, Feeney D, McCann VJ, Zilko PJ, et al: Complement allotyping reveals new genetic markers in rheumatoid arthritis and diabetes mellitus. Tissue Antigens 21:159-160, 1983
213. Suarez BK, Van Eerdewegh P: Type I (insulin dependent) diabetes mellitus: Is there strong evidence for a non-HLA linked gene? Diabetologia 20:524-529, 1981
214. Scholz S, Albert E: HLA and diseases: Involvement of more than one HLA-linked determinant of disease susceptibility. Immunol Rev 70:77-88, 1983
215. Dornan J, Allan P, Noel EP, Sampson L, Farid NR: Alleles of the second component of complement (C2) in insulin-dependent diabetes mellitus. Hum Hered 31:211-213, 1981

Maturity-Onset Diabetes Mellitus (Insulin-Independent)

Population Association

Caucasian

B8 was significantly increased in the patients (Table 9.2) in the pooled data from several independent studies.

Nelson et al.[1] reported HLA data on 22 pairs of maturity-onset diabetic twins. All were concordant and showed no deviations in A and B loci antigen frequencies.

Arnaiz-Villena et al.[2] studied 36 Spanish patients for HLA and Bf loci. The frequency of the B18-non-BfF1 haplotype in patients was 19.4% as compared with 7.27% in 330 healthy controls ($p < 0.02$). However, B18 and BfF1 in the patients were not significantly different from controls.

Mexican

Patel et al.[3] typed A and B loci antigens in 76 Mexican patients and 42 controls. No significant deviations were found.

Japanese

Several reports from Japan on Japanese patients showed no significant deviations of A and B loci antigens.[4-9]

American Blacks

Patel et al.[3] tested 74 American Black patients and 42 controls for A and B loci antigens and they found no significant associations.

African Blacks

Briggs et al.[10] studied 53 Xhosa patients from South Africa. As the data in Table 9.2 show, A2 and BW41

TABLE 9.2. Maturity-Onset Diabetes Mellitus (Insulin-Independent)

Country/Population	Patients n	Patients %+	Controls n	Controls %+	RR	χ^2	Ref.
HLA-A2							
South Africa—Xhosa	56	41	153	23	2.32	6.60	10
Pima—A.I.	191	81	69	65	2.29	7.26	12
HLA-B8							
U.S.A.	36	14	100	16	0.90	0.04	3
U.S.A.	160	31	282	20	1.80	6.77	13
U.S.A.	21	41	100	20	2.78	4.36	27
	217	29	482	19	1.75	8.63	
	Heterogeneity χ^2 (2 df)					2.55	
England	50	36	233	32	1.21	0.34	28
England	66	26	417	26	1.02	0.00	29
England	26	65	300	28	4.64	13.77	30
England	25	64	300	28	4.45	12.72	31
	167	41	1250	28	1.81	11.60	
	Heterogeneity χ^2 (3 df)					15.23	
Denmark	61	28	1967	24	1.25	0.63	32
	445	33	3699	25	1.68	19.55	
	Heterogeneity χ^2 (7 df)					19.09	
HLA-BW41							
South Africa—Xhosa	56	9	153	2	4.55	5.24	10
HLA-BW54							
China	50	18	128	7	2.89	4.85	33
HLA-BW61							
Fiji—Indian	58	31	47	9	4.17	7.01	11

were increased and A29 was decreased. These deviations were not highly significant, however.

Chinese
In the Chinese BW54 appeared to be increased in the patient group (Table 9.2).

Fiji Indians
Serjeantson et al.[11] reported A and B loci antigens in 58 Indians from Suva, Fiji. BW61 was increased in this sample (Table 9.2).

Pima Indians
Williams et al.[12] found an increased frequency of A2 (Table 9.2).

Disease Heterogeneity

In Becker et al.'s[13] study 76 patients were with and 84 without retinopathy. The frequency of B8 in the retinopathy group was 18% and in the nonretinopathy was 43%. Thus, there was a significant difference between the 2 groups ($p = 0.00087$). The frequency of B8 in 282 controls was 20%. The difference between the control and the group without retinopathy was also significant ($p = 0.00002$). Similar differences were also found for A1.

Family Data

See ref. 1.
See also refs. 14-26 and 34.

References

1. Nelson PG, Pyke DA, Cudworth AG, Woodrow JC, Batchelor JR: Histocompatibility antigens in diabetic identical twins. Lancet ii:193-194, 1975
2. Arnaiz-Villena A, Rodriguez De Cordoba S, Dujovne IL, Regueiro JR, Bootello A, Serrano-Rios

M: HLA factors in non-insulin-dependent diabetes mellitus. N Engl J Med 303:1065, 1980
3. Patel R, Ansari A, Covarrubias CLP: Leukocyte antigens and disease: III. Association of HLA-B8 and HLA-Bw15 with insulin-dependent diabetes in three different population groups. Metabolism 26:487-492, 1977
4. Sakurami T, Nagaoka K, Nabeya N, Imura H, Kuno S: Islet-cell antibodies and HLA type in Japanese insulin-dependent diabetics. Endocrinol Jpn 27:149-152, 1980
5. Kawa A, Nakazawa M, Sakaguchi S, Nakamura S, Komo Y, Hazeki H, et al: HLA system in Japanese patients with diabetes mellitus. Diabetes 26:591-595, 1977
6. Kawa A, Nakamura S, Kono Y, Maeda Y, Kanehisa T: A negative association of HLA-BW52 with Graves' disease and insulin-dependent diabetes mellitus with juvenile onset among Japanese population. Experientia 35:547-548, 1979
7. Nakao Y, Fukunishi T, Koide M, Akasawa K, Ikeda M, Yahata M, et al: HLA antigens in Japanese patients with diabetes mellitus. Diabetes 26:736-739, 1977
8. Nakazawa M, Hirata Y: Diabetes mellitus and HLA antigens. Nippon Rinsho 36:3193-3196, 1978
9. Moriuchi J, Katagiri M, Wakisaka A, Matsuura N, Maruyama N, Ikeda H, et al: Association of B cell alloantigen with juvenile onset diabetes mellitus in the Japanese. Hum Immunol 4:357-362, 1980
10. Briggs BR, Jackson WPU, Dutoit ED, Botha MC: The histocompatibility (HLA) antigen distribution in diabetes in Southern African blacks (Xhosa). Diabetes 29:68-71, 1980
11. Serjeantson SW, Ryan DP, Ram P, Zimmet P: HLA and noninsulin dependent diabetes in Fiji Indians. Med J Aust 1:462-463, 1981
12. Williams RC, Knowler WC, Butler WJ, Pettit DJ, Lisse JR, Bennett PH, et al: HLA-A2 and type 2 (insulin independent) diabetes mellitus in Pima Indians: An association of allele frequency with age. Diabetologia 21:460-463, 1981
13. Becker B, Shin DH, Burgess D, Kilo C, Miller WV: Histocompatibility antigens and diabetic retinopathy. Diabetes 26:997-999, 1977
14. Cudworth AG, Festenstein H: HLA genetic heterogeneity in diabetes mellitus. Br Med Bull 34:285-289, 1978
15. Cudworth AG, Woodrow JC: Genetic susceptibility in diabetes mellitus: Analysis of the HLA association. Br Med J 2:846-848, 1976
16. Tattersall RB, Pyke DA: Diabetes in identical twins. Lancet ii:1120-1125, 1972
17. Pyke DA, Tattersall RB: Diabetic retinopathy in identical twins. Diabetes 22:613-618, 1973
18. Maugh TH: Diabetes: Epidemiology suggests a viral connection. Science 188:347-351, 1975
19. Kromann H, Lernmark A, Vestergaard BF, Egeberg J, Nerup J: The influence of the major histocompatibility complex (H-2) on experimental diabetes in mice. Diabetologia 16:107-114, 1979
20. Richens ER, Quilley J, Hartog M: Studies on the frequency and associations of islet-cell antibodies in juvenile diabetes mellitus. Acta Diabetol Lat 15:229-235, 1978
21. Rotter JI, Rimon DL: Diabetes mellitus: The search for genetic markers. Diabetes Care 2:215-226, 1979
22. Serjeantson S: Distorted HLA segregation or biased ascertainment. Lancet i:40-41, 1980
23. Dvorakova L, Majsky A: HLA antigens in offspring of both diabetic parents. Cas Lek Cesk 118:1294-1296, 1979
24. Cahill GF Jr: Current concepts of diabetic complications with emphasis on hereditary factors: A brief review. Prog Clin Biol Res 32:113-125, 1979
25. Palumbo PJ: Classification of diabetes mellitus. Prog Clin Biol Res 32:127-134, 1979
26. Rotter JI: Genetic heterogeneity within diabetes mellitus: A review. Prog Clin Biol Res 32:135-155, 1979
27. Singal DP, Blajchman MA: Histocompatibility (HL-A) antigens, lymphocytotoxic antibodies and tissue antibodies in patients with diabetes mellitus. Diabetes 22:429-432, 1973
28. Cudworth AG, Woodrow JC: HL-A system and diabetes mellitus. Diabetes 24:345-349, 1975
29. Richens ER, Quilley J, Hartog M: Immunological features of juvenile onset diabetic patients correlated to HLA type. Clin Exp Immunol 36:198-204, 1979
30. Irvine WJ, McCallum CJ, Gray RS, Campbell CJ, Duncan LJP, et al: Pancreatic islet-cell antibodies in diabetes mellitus correlated with duration and type of diabetes, coexistent autoimmune disease, and HLA type. Diabetes 26:138-147, 1977
31. Morris PJ, Vaughan H, Irvine WJ, McCallum FJ, Gray RS, Campbell CJ, et al: HLA and pancreatic islet cell antibodies in diabetes. Lancet ii:652-653, 1976
32. Nerup J, Platz P, Andersen OO, Christy M, Lyngsoe J, Poulsen JE, et al: HL-A antigens and diabetes mellitus. Lancet ii:864-866, 1974
33. Zhao T, Chi Z, Wang H, Shen M, Zhou Z, Bu K, et al: HLA and diabetes mellitus in Chinese. Chin Med J 95:609-612, 1982
34. Majsky A, Dvorakova L: HLA und potentielle diabetoler (typ 2). Folia Haematol (Leipz) 107:61-64, 1980

Maturity-Onset Type Diabetes in Young

This form of diabetes appears to segregate like an autosomal dominant gene.[1]

Family Data

Nelson and Pyke[1] reported the inheritance of HLA haplotypes in 3 multiple- case families from England. The diabetics in each family did not share a common haplotype. Similar results were also found by Faber et al.[2] in a large pedigree from Denmark. There was no evidence of close linkage in this family. The segregation of the disease and HLA haplotypes was such that several recombinants between maturity-onset diabetes in young and HLA would have to be postulated to show close linkage.

A third report by Barbosa et al.[3] included data on a large pedigree from the United States showing some evidence of linkage. However, in a later report on the linkage analysis of 10 large pedigrees, Barbosa[4] also found no evidence of linkage.

The lod score calculations were not performed in the families studied by Nelson and Pyke[1] and Faber et al.[2] Since HLA haplotypes in these families did not segregate with the disease, the lod scores would probably provide evidence against linkage.

References

1. Nelson PG, Pyke DA: Genetic diabetes not linked to the HLA locus. Br Med J 1:196-197, 1976
2. Faber OK, Thomsen M, Binder C, Platz P, Svejgaard A: HLA antigens in a familiy with maturity-onset diabetes mellitus. Acta Endocrinol 88:329-338, 1978
3. Barbosa J, King R, Goetz FC, Noreen H, Yunis EJ. HLA in maturity-onset type of hyperglycemia in the young. Arch Intern Med 138:90-93, 1978
4. Barbosa J: No linkage between HLA and maturity onset hyperglycaemia in the young. Diabetologia 24:137, 1983

Gestational Diabetes

Population Association

Rubinstein et al.[1] compared the A, B, C, and DR loci antigens of 136 American patients (96 Puerto Rican and 40 American Blacks and Caucasians) and 417 controls. No significant difference between the two groups was found.

Reference

1. Rubinstein P, Walker M, Krassner J, Carrier C, Carpenter C, Dobersen MJ, et al: HLA antigens and islet cell antibodies in gestational diabetes. Hum Immunol 3:271-275, 1981

Wolfram Syndrome

Wolfram syndrome is an unusual inherited form of diabetes in juvenile patients (association of diabetes mellitus with diabetes insipidus, optic atrophy, and neural deafness).

Family Data

Stanley et al.[1] published data on HLA haplotypes of a family of 5 members in which all 3 siblings (ages 12, 13, and 15 years) were affected by this syndrome. Two affected siblings had identical haplotypes but the third did not share any haplotype. Both parents and 2 full siblings were not affected. A maternal half-brother, a maternal half-sister, and 5 paternal half-siblings were also said to be unaffected. However, HLA types were available only for the 3 affected siblings and the mother. Thus, these data were insufficient for any comment on the linkage between HLA and Wolfram syndrome.

See also ref. 2.

References

1. Stanley CA, Spielman RS, Zmijewski CM, Baker L: Wolfram syndrome not HLA linked. N Engl J Med 301:1398-1399, 1979
2. Van Eden W, Schreuder GMTH: Wolfram syndrome and HLA. N Engl J Med 302:1263-1264, 1980

Glucose Intolerance After the Use of Low-Estrogen Oral Contraceptive

Population Association

Spellacy et al.[1] studied glucose tolerance in 13 women who were taking low-estrogen oral contraceptives for 6 months. All of the women ingested a diet high in carbohydrates (> 250 g/day) for 3 days preceding the test and were fasting for at least 10 h before the test. A control glucose tolerance test was done on each woman in the fasting state at 0.5, 1, 2, and 3 h. The patients were then given a low-estrogen type oral contraceptive for 6 months. After 6 months of treatment all women returned for an identical glucose tolerance test. For the analysis the patients were grouped on the basis of HLA type into high- and low-risk groups for insulin-dependent diabetes mellitus. There were 6 women in the high-risk group (B8- and B15-positive) and 7 in the low-risk group (B7- and BW35-positive).

The 0.5-h control glucose value was significantly

lower in the low-risk group. There were no significant changes in any of the individual blood glucose values between the control and 6-month tests for either the low- or high-risk groups.

There was no significant difference in the plasma insulin values between the 2 groups.

Reference

1. Spellacy WN, Birk S, Buhi WC: Influence of HLA types on carbohydrate effects of a low-estrogen oral contraceptive. Fertil Steril 33:506-509, 1980

Glucose Intolerance After Renal Transplantation

Population Association

D'Apice et al.[1] reported A and B loci frequency and glucose intolerance data on 109 renal transplant patients from Australia. Patients were classified as glucose intolerant if they had exhibited glycosuria in the second 6-month period after the transplant or a random blood glucose > 8 mmol/liter or had received antidiabetic therapy.

There were 67 glucose-tolerant and 42 intolerant patients. A comparison of A and B loci antigens between these 2 groups did not show any significant deviations, especially for B8, B15, and B18 antigens which are associated with juvenile diabetes mellitus. However, if B8, B15, BW16, and B18 were considered as one "group" then this frequency was increased in the glucose intolerant patients (54.76% vs. 31.34% in the glucose-tolerant group, $p = 0.01$).

Reference

1. D'Apice AJF, Mathews JD, Tait BD, Kincaid-Smith P: Association of HLA antigens with glucose intolerance following renal transplantation. Tissue Antigens 11:423-426, 1978

Graves' Disease

Population Association

A combined analysis of all the frequency data on A and B loci antigens show that A1 and B8 are significantly associated with this disease in Caucasian populations of Europe and North America (Table 9.3).

Chan et al.[1] reported a significant increase of BW46 and a decrease of B15 in 86 Chinese patients from Singapore.

Three reports from Japan[2–4] revealed a significant positive association with BW35 and a negative association with BW52.

A strong association (as measured by the relative risk) with DW3 (Table 9.3) was first reported by Bech et al.[5] in 86 Danish patients. Later, Allanic et al.,[6] Farid et al.,[7] and Dahlberg et al.[8] reported similar data for DR3 (Table 9.3). A third study from Japan by Sasazuki et al.[9] also showed a stronger, but, like HLA-B, a different association with the D locus. In this study the frequency of DW12 (formerly DHO) was 48% in patients as compared with only 16% in the controls (Table 9.3).

Thus, a number of studies on 3 distinct populations provide very strong evidence of an HLA association with Graves' disease. On the basis of higher relative risks associated with DW3, DR3, and DW12 we can conclude that the primary association of the disease is probably with the D/DR locus.

Disease Heterogeneity

Antithyroglobulin and Antimicrosomal Antibodies
Thorsby et al.[10] reported a significant increase of B8 in patients with antithyroglobulin and/or antimicrosomal antibodies (no precise frequency data were given). Balazs et al.[11] subdivided their patients into groups with antibody titer 1–16 (n = 131) and with titer ≤ 64 (n = 40). The frequencies of A1 and B8 in the first subgroup were 37.4% and 35.1%, respectively. In the second subgroup A1 was present in 80% and B8 in 85% of the patients. Thus, there was a significant difference in the frequency of the 2 subgroups ($p < 0.001$). The studies on Caucasian populations by Grumet et al.,[12,13] Mather et al.,[14] Whittingham et al.,[15] Farid et al.,[16] Dahlberg et al.,[8] and Schernthaner et al.[17] and on Japanese patients by Nakao et al.[4] and Grumet et al.[3] did not find any association between antibody titer and HLA.

Bovine Serum Albumin Antibody
Singal et al.[18] studied patients with and without antibody to bovine serum albumin. B8 was present in 80% of the patients without the antibody as compared with only 23.5% of the patients with the antibody ($p < 0.001$). There was a total of 27 patients listed and the report does not give the number of patients in each subgroup.

Ophthalmopathy

In a study by Mayer et al.[19] the frequency of CW3 was 0% in 31 patients without endocrine ophthalmopathy as compared with 30.4% in 23 patients with endocrine opthalmopathy. The difference between the 2 groups was significant ($p < 0.0014$). B8 frequencies were similar in both groups. It should be noted that in a report on 77 patients from England, Irvine et al.[20] did not find any significant increase of CW3 in the patients. This antigen was typed with 2 well-defined antisera.

Another report from Hungary by Balazs et al.[11] found a significant difference in the frequencies of A1 and B8 in the patients with (n = 87) and without (n = 84) ophthalmopathy. In the group with ophthalmopathy these antigens were 71.3% and 80.5%, respectively. These 2 antigens were present in only 22.6% and 11.9% respectively, of the patients without opthalmopathy ($p < 0.001$).

In other reports by Bech et al.,[5] Jaffiol et al.,[21–23] Allanic et al.,[6,24] Grumet et al.,[3] Sergott et al.,[25] and Whittingham et al.,[15] HLA was not associated with opthalmopathy. Thus, in the existing data there is no strong evidence of HLA association with opthalmopathy.

Lymphocyte Transformation Index

An increased frequency of A1 and B8 in patients with lymphocyte transformation index ≤ 4 has been reported by Balazs et al.[11] This subgroup had 52 patients and A1 and B8 frequencies were 78.8% and 90.4%, respectively. In the group with an index between 1 and 3.9 there were 119 patients. A1 and B8 frequencies were 33.6% and 27.7%, respectively. The difference between the 2 groups was significant ($p < 0.001$).

Age

No association between HLA and various age subgroups of the patients was found in several studies.[4,8,15,16,24]

Age at Onset

In 4 reports,[11,21–23] there was no evidence of association between A1 and B8 and age at onset.

Irradiation

In the data of Grumet et al.[13] B8 was not present in any of the 5 patients in which disease occurred after neck irradiation. This zero frequency in the postirradiation patients was different from that of 47% in the general patient population ($p < 0.05$).

Yersinia *Antibody Titer*

Bech et al.[5] presented DW3 frequency data on 40 patients with *Yersinia* antibody titer ≥ 40 and 38 with titer < 10. The frequency of DW3 in both groups was 53%.

Sex

There was no evidence of association between sex of the patients and positivity for A1 or B8.[4,15,21–23]

Family History

There was no association between family history of the disease and HLA.[21–23]

Goiter

No association was evident between presence of the disease and HLA.[6,16,21–23]

Severity of the Disease

There was no evidence of association with HLA.[6,16,21–23]

Relapse

In the data of Bech et al.[5] the frequency of DW3 in 48 patients with relapse was 65% as compared with 33% in 18 patients without relapse ($p = 0.018$). However, no significant association was found in reports on 78 Swedish patients studied by Dahlberg et al.[8] and on 86 Irish patients studied by McKenna et al.[26]

Clinical Course of the Disease

Irvine et al.[20] studied patients who relapsed after withdrawal of antithyroid drug and those who at 5 years or more after withdrawal of therapy had a satisfactory or exaggerated serum thryroid-stimulating hormone response to intravenous thyroid-stimulating hormone. A1 and B8 frequency (%) data in these 2 groups and controls are given below:

	Graves' Disease		Control (Total)	
	Group I	Group II		
Antigen	n = 42	n = 35	n = 77	n = 100
A1	60	40	51	35
B8	69	40	56	28

The frequency of B8 in patients who relapsed after withdrawal of antithyroid drug was 69% as compared with 40% in patients who remained in remission and 28% in the controls. B8-positive patients were 1.8 times more likely to relapse after withdrawal of drug therapy than B8-negative patients. The authors also

TABLE 9.3. Graves' Disease

Country/Population	Patients n	Patients %+	Controls n	Controls %+	RR	χ^2	Ref.
HLA-A1							
Canada	47	45	128	29	2.00	4.00	16
U.S.A.	73	38	3896	31	1.37	1.75	46
U.S.A.	62	45	113	33	1.66	2.48	12
	135	41	4009	31	1.47	4.01	
	Heterogeneity χ^2 (1 df)					0.22	
Australia	67	33	700	34	0.97	0.02	36
Australia	64	34	700	34	1.01	0.00	15
	131	33	1400	34	0.99	0.00	
	Heterogeneity χ^2 (1 df)					0.01	
New Zealand	100	470	100	36	1.57	2.48	47
Hungary	171	47	450	28	2.28	19.81	11
England	60	47	60	30	2.04	3.62	48
England	77	51	300	35	1.93	6.61	20
England	105	43	117	29	1.84	4.70	14
	242	47	477	33	1.92	14.87	
	Heterogeneity χ^2 (2 df)					0.05	
France	86	41	356	29	1.70	4.70	6
France	100	26	270	20	1.41	1.63	21
	186	33	626	25	1.57	6.07	
	Heterogeneity χ^2 (1 df)					0.26	
Denmark	86	44	1967	31	1.75	6.50	5
Sweden	78	41	100	26	1.96	4.46	8
	1176	42	9257	31	1.65	49.95	
	Heterogeneity χ^2 (13 df)					12.80	
HLA-B8							
Canada	47	58	128	26	3.87	14.84	16
U.S.A.	62	47	113	21	3.29	12.43	12
U.S.A.	73	37	3896	21	2.23	10.93	46
	135	42	4009	21	2.54	22.47	
	Heterogeneity χ^2 (1 df)					0.89	
Australia	67	39	700	24	2.03	7.36	39
Australia	64	42	700	24	2.30	9.93	15
	131	40	1400	24	2.16	17.17	
	Heterogeneity χ^2 (1 df)					0.11	
New Zealand	100	40	100	25	1.98	5.06	47
Hungary	171	47	450	19	3.77	46.90	11
England	105	40	117	25	1.99	5.65	14
England	60	35	60	27	1.44	0.89	48
England	77	56	300	28	3.25	20.53	20
	242	44	477	27	2.32	23.61	
	Heterogeneity χ^2 (2 df)					3.46	

TABLE 9.3. *(continued)*

Country/Population	Patients n	Patients %+	Controls n	Controls %+	RR	χ^2	Ref.
HLA-B8							
France	100	35	270	16	2.82	15.36	21
France	86	44	356	23	2.63	15.09	6
	186	39	626	20	2.72	30.41	
	Heterogeneity χ^2 (1 df)					0.04	
Austria	54	19	450	18	1.10	0.08	19
Austria	48	31	450	18	2.07	4.97	17
	102	25	900	18	1.55	3.33	
	Heterogeneity χ^2 (1 df)					1.71	
Ireland	86	51	95	30	2.40	8.17	26
Denmark	86	47	1967	24	2.81	22.06	5
Norway	81	44	1628	25	2.36	14.17	10
Sweden	78	53	100	20	4.42	20.06	8
	1445	43	11880	22	2.56	213.54	
	Heterogeneity χ^2 (17 df)					20.92	
HLA-B15							
Singapore—Chinese	86	8	238	22	0.33	7.67	1
HLA-BW35							
Japan	85	36	150	13	3.71	16.21	4
Japan	33	39	106	11	5.05	12.57	2
Japan	44	57	83	20	5.15	16.78	3
	162	42	339	14	4.41	45.03	
	Heterogeneity χ^2 (2 df)					0.52	
HLA-BW46							
Singapore—Chinese	86	52	238	23	3.60	23.82	1
HLA-BW52							
Japan	58	2	79	28	0.07	12.61	49
HLA-DW3							
Denmark	86	51	157	21	3.87	22.09	5
HLA-DW12							
Japan	42	48	69	16	4.68	12.48	9
HLA-DR3							
Canada	83	64	80	24	5.49	24.89	7
France	86	51	100	20	4.09	18.79	6
Ireland	86	54	95	31	2.58	9.63	26
Sweden	78	55	100	24	3.81	17.27	8
	333	56	375	25	3.77	67.78	
	Heterogeneity χ^2 (3 df)					2.80	
HLA-DR5							
Japan	30	30	80	5	7.51	11.34	61

reported a significant correlation between B8 and the persistence of thyroid microsomal antibodies after therapy withdrawal.[20]

Gastric Antibodies
No association between B8 and the presence of gastric antibodies in the patients[15] was evident.

Recurrence of the Disease
No association with B8 was evident.[15]

Duration of the Disease
No association with B8 was evident.[15]

Hypothyroidism
No association with B8 was evident.[15]

Suppressor T Cell Activity
Balazs et al.[27] measured short-lived and concanavallin A (Con A) activated supressor T cell functions in 67 Hungarian patients. The activity of short-lived and Con-A-activated suppressor T cells in B8-positive patients was lower than those negative for B8.

Phenylthiocarbamide Tasting
Farid et al.[28] performed Phenylthiocarbamide (PTC) tasting studies in 18 B8 positive and 13 B8 negative patients. There was no evidence of association between PTC status and B8.

TSH-Receptor Antibodies
The data of Schernthaner et al.[17] on 48 Austrian patients showed no association between B8 and TSH-receptor antibodies (see also ref. 24).

In Graves' disease an association with Gm phenotype fnb/fb has also been reported by Farid et al.[29] Also, in a study of the gene frequency of a second component of complement (C2) in 60 patients and 800 controls by Noel et al.[30] no association of C2 with the disease was found (see also ref. 54).

Family Data

Pedigrees with 2 or more patients with Graves' disease have been published by Farid et al.,[31–33] Raffoux et al.,[34] Chan et al.,[35] Fernandez-Castener et al.,[36] Sasazuki et al.,[37] and Awashima et al.[38]

Farid et al.[33] tabulated the number of sib-pairs sharing 2, 1, and 0 haplotypes from 3 different studies. In a total of 14 sib-pairs 9 (64.3%) shared 2 haplotypes, 4 (28.6%) shared 1 haplotype, and 1 (7.1%) shared 0 haplotypes. This observed distribution, when compared with expected values of 25%, 50%, and 25%, respectively, was significant ($p < 0.005$). Similar results have been reported by Sasazuki et al.[37,61] Thus, there is significant evidence of linkage between HLA and Graves' disease. The statistical tests, however, could not differentiate between dominant and recessive modes of inheritance of the disease susceptibility gene.[33]

Uno et al.[61] also reported evidence of a second disease gene linked to the gene coding for the Gm allotype.

See also refs. 39–45 and 50–60.

References

1. Chan SH, Yeo PPB, Lui KF, Wee GB, Woo KT, Lim P, et al: HLA and thyrotoxicosis (Graves' disease) in Chinese. Tissue Antigens 12:109-114, 1978
2. Kawa A, Nakamura S, Nakazawa M, Sakaguchi S, Kawabata T, Maeda Y, et al: HLA-BW35 and B5 in Japanese patients with Graves' disease. Acta Endocrinol 86:754-757, 1977
3. Grumet FC, Payne RO, Konishi J, Mori T, Kriss JP: HL-A antigens in Japanese patients with Graves' disease. Tissue Antigens 6:347-352, 1975
4. Nakao Y, Kishihara M, Baba YH, Kuma K, Kubonishi T, Imura H: HLA antigens in autoimmune thyroid diseases. Arch Intern Med 138:567-570, 1978
5. Bech K, Lumholtz B, Nerup J, Thomson M, Platz P, Ryder LP, et al: HLA antigens in Graves' disease. Acta Endocrinol 86:510-516, 1977
6. Allanic H, Fauchet R, Lorcy Y, Heim J, Gueguen M, Leguerrier AM, et al: Maladie de Basedow: Predominance de l'antigene DRW3. Nouv Presse Med 9:1823-1826, 1980
7. Farid NR, Stone E, Johnson G: Graves' disease and HLA: Clinical and epidemiologic associations. Clin Endocrinol 13:535-544, 1980
8. Dahlberg PA, Holmlund G, Karlsson FA, Safwenberg J: HLA-A, -B, -C and -DR antigens in patients with Graves'disease and their correlation with signs and clinical course. Acta Endocrinol 97:42-47, 1981
9. Sasazuki T, Kohno Y, Iwamoto I, Kosaba K, Okimoto K, Maruyama H, et al: HLA and Graves' disease or diabetes mellitus in Japan. N Engl J Med 298:630-631, 1978
10. Thorsby E, Svejgaard E, Solem JH, Kornstad L: The frequency of major histocompatibility antigens (SD & LD) in thyrotoxicosis. Tissue Antigens 6:54-55, 1975
11. Balazs CS, Stenszky V, Kozma L, Leovey A: The

possible influence of HLA-A1, B8 antigens on the course of Graves' disease. Biomedicine 29:263-264, 1978
12. Grumet FC, Payne RO, Konishi J, Kriss JP: HL-A antigens as markers for disease susceptibility and autoimmunity in Graves' disease. J Clin Endocrinol Metab 39:1115-1119, 1974
13. Grumet FC, Payne RO, Konishi J, Kriss JP: HL-A antigen frequencies in Graves' disease. Transplant Proc 7:97-99, 1975
14. Mather BA, Roberts DF, Scalnon MF, Mukhtar ED, Davies TF, Smith BR, et al: HLA antigens and thyroid autoantibodies in patients with Graves' disease and their first degree relatives. Clin Endocrinol 12:155-163, 1980
15. Whittingham S, Morris PJ, Martin FIR: HL-A8: A genetic link with thyrotoxicosis. Tissue Antigens 6:23-27, 1975
16. Farid NR, Barnard JMP Marshall WH: The association of HLA with autoimmune thyroid disease in Newfoundland. The influence of HLA homozygosity in Graves' disease. Tissue Antigens 8:181-189, 1976
17. Schernthaner G, Ludwig H, Schleusener H, Finke R, Kotulla P, Mayr WR: TSH-receptor antibodies, HLA-B8 and thyroid autoantibodies in patients with Graves' disease in therapeutically induced euthyroidism. Experientia 35:1408-1409, 1979
18. Singal DP, Perets A, Dolovich J: HLA antigens and serum antibodies to bovine serum albumin. Transplant Proc 11:1864-1865, 1979
19. Mayr WR, Ludwig H, Schernthaner G, Hofer R: HLA CW3 in thyrotoxicosis patients with and without endocrine ophthalmopathy. Tissue Antigens 7:243-246, 1976
20. Irvine WJ, Gray RS, Morris PJ, Ting A: Correlation of HLA and thyroid antibodies with clinical course of thyrotoxicosis treated with antithyroid drugs. Lancet ii:898-900, 1977
21. Jaffiol C, Seignalet J, Baldet L, Robin M, Labinski H, Mirouze J: Systeme HLA et maladie de basedow. Ann Endocrinol (Paris) 37:219-226, 1976
22. Jaffiol C, Seignalet J, Baldet L, Robin M, Lapinski H, Mirouze J: Study of the HLA system in Basedow's disease. Ann Endocrinol 37:111-112, 1976
23. Jaffiol C, Seignalet J, Baldet L, Robin M, Lapinski H, Mirouze J: HLA B8 and Graves' disease. Ann Endocrinol 37:219-226, 1976
24. Allannic H, Fauchet R, Lorcy Y, Heim J, Gueguen M, Leguerrier AM, Genetet B: HLA and Graves' disease: An association with HLA-DRW3. J Clin Endocrinol Metab 51:863-867, 1980
25. Sergott RC, Felberg NT, Savino PJ, Blizzard JJ, Schatz NJ, Sanford CA: Association of HLA antigen BW35 with severe Graves' ophthalmopathy. Invest Ophthalmol Vis Sci 24:124-127, 1983
26. McKenna R, Kearns M, Sugrue D, Drury MI, McCarthy CF: HLA and hyperthyroidism in Ireland. Tissue Antigens 19:97-99, 1982
27. Balazs CS, Stenszky V, Kozma L, Szerze P, Leovey A: Connection between HLA-B8 antigen and suppressor T-cell activity in Graves' disease. Transplant Proc 11:1314, 1979
28. Farid NR, Barnard JM, Bryant DG: HLA and phenylthiocarbamide (PTC) tasting in autoimmune thyroid disease. Tissue Antigens 10:414-416, 1977
29. Farid NR, Newton RM, Noel EP, Barnard JM, Marshall WH: The operation of immunological networks in Graves' disease. Tissue Antigens 12:205-211, 1978
30. Noel EP, Sampson L, Pepper BM, Farid NR: Polymorphism of the second component of complement (C2) in Graves' disease. Hum Hered 30:245-247, 1980
31. Larsen B, Pepper B, Barnard JM, Farid NR: HLA/BF haplotypes in a Newfoundland family. Tissue Antigens 12:39-43, 1978
32. Farid NR, Barnard JM, Marshall WH, Woolfrey I, O'Driscoll RF: Thyroid autoimmune disease in a large Newfoundland family: The influence of HLA. J Clin Endocrinol Metab 45:1165-1172, 1977
33. Farid NR, Moens H, Larsen B, Payne R, Saltman K, Fifield F, et al: HLA haplotypes in familial Graves' disease. Tissue Antigens 15:492-500, 1980
34. Raffoux C, Thomas JL, Leclere J, Streiff F, Hartemann P: Lack of HLA association in a familiy with a high incidence of hyperthyroidism. Tissue Antigens 14:274-278, 1979
35. Chan SH, Yeo PPB, Cheah JS, Lim P: HLA haplotype sharing in affected siblings in multiple case Chinese families with thyrotoxicosis. Tissue Antigens 16:258-259, 1980
36. Castaner MF, Potau MA, Reus JC, Ercilla MG: HLA antigens in a family with both parents and several siblings affected by Graves' disease. Acta Endocrinol 102:535-538, 1983
37. Sasazuki T, Nishimura Y, Muto M, Ohta N: HLA-linked genes controlling immune response and disease susceptibility. Immunol Rev 70:51-75, 1983
38. Awashima F, Matsuo T, Akaza T, Kuzumaki N, Yoshida TO, Igarashi Y: Hashimoto's and Graves' diseases transmitted with the same HLA haplotype. In Terasaki PI (ed): Histocompatibility Testing 1980. UCLA Tissue Typing Laboratory, Los Angeles, 1980, pp 951
39. Morris PJ, Vaughan II, Tait BD, Mackay IR: Histocompatibility antigens (HLA): Association with immunopathic diseases and with response to microbial antigens. Aust NZ J Med 7:616-624, 1977
40. Remuzzi G, Livio M, Donati MB, De Gaetano G: Myasthenia gravis, thrombocytopenia and HLA antigens. Ann Intern Med 87:250-251, 1977
41. Seignalet J, Mirouze J, Jaffiol C, Selam JL, Lapinski H: HL-A in Graves' disease and in diabetes

mellitus insulin-dependent. Tissue Antigens 6:272-274, 1975
42. Grumet FC, Konishi J, Payne RO, Kriss JP: Association in Japanese of Graves' disease with the HL-A specificity W5. In Robbins J et al. (eds): Thyroid Research. Excerpta Medica, Amsterdam, 1976, pp 376-379
43. Farid NR, Barnard J, Kutas C, Noel EP, Marshall WH: HL-A antigens in Graves' disease and Hashimoto's thyroiditis. Int Arch Allergy Appl Immunol 49:837-842, 1975
44. Farid NR, Barnard JM, Sampson L, Noel EP, Marshall WH: The HLA BW4/W6 diallelic system in Graves' disease. Tissue Antigens 11:394-398, 1978
45. Allannic H, Fauchet R, Lorcy Y, Heim J, Gueguen M, Leguerrier A -M, et al: Systeme HLA et maladie de Basedow: Predominance de l'antigene DRW3. Ann Endocrinol (Paris) 41:70-72, 1980
46. Chopra IJ, Solomon DH, Chopra U, Yoshihara E, Terasaki PI, Smith F: Abnormalities in thyroid function in relatives of patients with Graves' disease and Hashimoto's thyroiditis. J Clin Endocrinol Metab 45:45-54, 1977
47. Ford D, Knight JG, Reeve JK, Stewart RDM: Histocompatibility antigens in Graves' disease. Aust NZ J Med 6:297-299, 1976
48. Nelson SD, Pollet JE: HL-A antigens and thyrotoxicosis. Tissue Antigens 5:38-40, 1975
49. Kawa A, Nakamura S, Kono Y, Maeda Y, Kanehisa T: A negative association of HLA-BW52 with Graves' disease and insulin-dependent diabetes mellitus with juvenile onset among Japanese population. Experientia 35:547-548, 1979
50. Kawahara K, Mitani H, Nokihara M, Mori H: Diseases of internal medicine and HL-A antigens: Basedow disease, Hashimoto's disease. Nippon Rinsho 36:3189-3192, 1978
51. Farid NR, Sampson L, Noel EP, Barnard JM, Mandeville R, Larsen B, et al: A study of human leukocyte D locus related antigens in Graves' disease. J Clin Invest 63:108-113, 1979
52. Dahlberg PA, Holmlund G, Karlsson FA, Safwenberg J: Prediction of relapse in Graves' disease. Lancet ii:1144, 1980
53. Farid NR, Bear JC: Two major genes linked to HLA and Gm, control susceptibility to Graves' disease. Nature 295:629, 1982
54. Tom W, Farid NR: Reduced C4 in HLA-B8 positive patients with Graves' disease. Hum Hered 31:227-231, 1981
55. Stenszky V, Balazs C, Kozma L, Leovey A, Farid NR: HLA control of thyroglobulin-induced blast-transformation in Graves' disease. Hum Hered 31:322-324, 1981
56. Briones-Urbina R, Bear JC, Farid NR: Association of hypergammaglobulinemia G with HLA-DR3 in Graves' disease. Tissue Antigens 19:20-24, 1982
57. Sakurami T, Ueno Y, Iwaki Y, Park MS, Terasaki PI, Saji H: HLA-DR specificities among Japanese with several autoimmune disease. Tissue Antigens 19:129-133, 1982
58. Davies TF, Platzer M, Farid NR: Prediction of therapeutic response to radioactive iodine in Graves' disease using TSH-receptor antibodies and HLA status. Clin Endocrinol 16:183-191, 1982
59. Schatz H: Die bedeutung der bestimmung von Schilddrusenantikorpern und der HLA-typisierung fur die prognose der hyperthyreose. Med Welt 32:649-652, 1981
60. Bech K, Nerup J, Thomsen M, Platz P, Svejgaard A: HLA and thyrotoxicosis. Lancet ii:1231, 1977
61. Uno H, Sasazuki T, Tamai H, Matsumoto H: Two major genes, linked to HLA and Gm, control susceptibility to Graves' disease. Nature 292:768-770, 1981

Congenital Hypothyroidism

Population Association

In 20 Japanese patients typed for A and B loci antigens Miyai et al.[1] found an increased frequency of AW24 (Table 9.4). A similar study of 20 American Caucasian patients by Cimino et al.[2] did not reveal any significant deviation in the frequencies of A and B loci antigens. (No frequency data are given.)

A report by Oxtoby et al.[3] has found a significant decrease of A11 in British patients (Table 9.4).

TABLE 9.4. Congenital Hypothyroidism

	Patients		Controls				
Country/Population	n	%+	n	%+	RR	χ^2	Ref.
HLA-A11							
England	97	1	635	11	0.12	8.26	3
HLA-AW24							
Japan	20	90	285	57	5.59	7.40	1

References

1. Miyai K, Mizuta H, Nose O, Fukunishi T, Hirai T, Matsuda S, et al: Increased frequency of HLA-AW24 in congenital hypothyroidism in Japan. N Engl J Med 303:226-227, 1980
2. Cimino P, Banks R, Maclaren N, Rosenbloom E, Riley W, Rosenbloom A, et al: HLA and congenital hypothyroidism. N Engl J Med 303:1177-1178, 1980
3. Oxtoby E, Roberts DF, Wentzel J, Frost G, Parkin JM: Congenital hypothyroidism and HLA. Tissue Antigens 19:1-5, 1982

Subacute Thyroiditis (De Quervain)

Population Association

From studies on several populations it is clear from Table 9.5 that BW35 and CW4 are significantly associated with this disease. Moreover, since there is strong linkage disequilibrium between BW35 and CW4, the association of CW4 is probably secondary to that of BW35.

The data on D locus antigens are available in only 2 studies[1,2] and in both of these studies the frequency of DW11 was higher in patients but it was not significant. Nyulassy et al.[10] compared DR locus antigens in 43 patients and 48 controls from Czechoslovakia. No significant deviations were found.

Disease Heterogeneity

Jenkins and Farid[3] reported HLA types of 14 patients with "subacute thyroiditis-like syndrome," a syndrome of transient hyperthyroidism, low radioiodine uptake, and lymphocytic infiltration of the thyroid. In this study 5 of these 14 patients were BW35.

See also ref. 10.

References

1. Buc M, Nyulassy S, Hnilica P, Busova B, Stefanovic: The frequency of HLA-DW11 determinants in subacute (De Quervain's) thyroiditis. Tissue Antigens 14:63-67, 1979
2. Bech K, Nerup J, Thomsen M, Platz P, Ryder LP, Svejgaard A, et al: Subacute thyroiditis De Quervain: A disease associated with a HLA-B antigen. Acta Endocrinol 86:504-509, 1977
3. Jenkins H, Farid NR: 'Subacute thyroiditis-like' syndromes-relation to HLA. Tissue Antigens 13:167-169, 1979
4. Nyulassy S, Hnilica P, Stefanovic J: The HL-A system and sub-acute thyroiditis. Tissue Antigens 6:105-106, 1975
5. Yeo PPB, Chan SH, Aw TC, Lui KF, Rauff A, Mathew T, et al: HLA and Chinese patients with subacute (De Quervain's) thyroiditis. Tissue Antigens 17:249-250, 1981

TABLE 9.5. Subacute Thyroiditis (De Quervain)

	Patients		Controls				
Country/Population	n	%+	n	%+	RR	χ^2	Ref.
HLA-BW35							
Singapore—Chinese	10	40	238	5	12.65	15.16	5
Czechoslovakia	16	63	231	14	9.99	19.64	6
Czechoslovakia	40	73	314	9	26.16	68.51	7
	56	70	545	11	18.40	85.98	
	Heterogeneity χ^2 (1 df)					2.18	
Austria	25	68	450	21	7.72	23.20	8
Switzerland	10	40	964	19	2.95	3.34	9
Denmark	24	71	1967	13	15.71	40.88	2
	115	67	3926	15	11.66	144.45	
	Heterogeneity χ^2 (4 df)					11.13	
HLA-CW4							
Austria	25	64	450	26	4.93	14.94	8
Denmark	24	54	426	17	5.66	17.57	2
	49	59	876	22	5.28	32.46	
	Heterogeneity χ^2 (1 df)					0.06	

6. Majsky A, Feix C: HLA Bw 35 antigen and subacute thyroiditis. Tissue Antigens 9:173, 1977
7. Nyulassy S, Hnilica P, Buc M, Guman M, Hirschova V, et al: Subacute (De Quervain's) thyroiditis: Association with HLA-BW35 antigen and abnormalities of complement system, immunoglobulins and other serum proteins. J Clin Endocrinol Metab 45:270-274, 1977
8. Aiginger P, Weissel M, Fritzsche H, Krioss A, Hofer R, Mayr WR: HLA antigens and De Quervain's thyroiditis. Tissue Antigens 11:59-60, 1978
9. Reiner M, Spengler H, Noseda G: HLA-antigene bei thyreoiditis De Quervain. Schweiz Med Wochenschr 106:1834-1836, 1976
10. Nyulassy S, Hnilica P, Hirschova V, and Buc M: Subacute De Quervain's thyroiditis. In Terasaki PI (ed): Histocompatibility Testing 1980. UCLA Tissue Typing Laboratory, Los Angeles, 1981, p 717

Painless Thyroiditis

Population Association

Hawe et al.[1] presented data on A, B, C, and DR loci antigens on 23 Canadian patients suffering from thyroid hyperthyroidism due to painless thyroiditis (unrelated to pregnancy). No significant associations were found.

Reference

1. Hawe BS, Walfish PG, Farid NR: HLA antigens in painless thyroiditis with transient hyperthyroidism. Tissue Antigens 19:311-312, 1982

Hashimoto's Thyroiditis

Population Association

Data on A and B loci antigen frequencies available in 4 studies (Table 9.6) on Caucasian populations showed that A1 and B8 may be associated with this disease. The association, however, was only marginally significant.

An increased frequency of BW16 in 56 Japanese patients has been reported by Nakao et al.[1] Another report from Japan by Kawahara et al.[2] on 24 patients showed an increase of A11 (45.8% in patients vs. 19.6% in 51 controls) and a decrease of B5 (12.5% in patients vs. 39.2% in controls). These deviations, however, were not highly significant. BW16 was not typed in this report.

DR Locus

An association with DR3 in 40 Canadian patients was first reported by Moens and Farid[3] (Table 9.6). This, however, was not confirmed in a second report from Austria by Weissel et al.[4] These investigators reported a highly significant association with DR5 (Table 9.6). The frequency data on DR5 were not available in the report of Moens and Farid[3] and thus a combined analysis is not possible. However, it should be added that the sample studied by Moens and Farid[3] included both atrophic and hypertrophic variants of the disease. All of Weissel's 39 patients[4] had a hypertrophic variant of the disease. Thus, the discrepancy may be due to the heterogeneity of the disease.

The second report by Farid et al.[5] subdivided the patients into groups of goiterous (n = 40) and atrophic (n = 50) thyroiditis. The data on DR5 in Table 9.6 are for the goiterous subgroup.

All patients studied by Thomsen et al.[6] for D locus antigens were females with the goiterous type of the disease. In this sample no significant association with A, B, and C loci was found.

Disease Heterogeneity

In the aforementioned study of Farid et al.[5] a highly significant association with DR3 was found in 50 patients with atrophic thyroiditis. This antigen was not increased in 40 patients with the goiterous subtype of disease. However, these results need to be confirmed in other independent studies.

An association between DW5 and thyroid-stimulating immunoglobulins has been observed in a study of 40 female patients with goiter by Bliddal et al.[19]

Family Data

Bode et al.[7] published data on 4 pedigrees with multiple cases of Hashimoto's thyroiditis. The segregation of HLA-A and -B haplotypes and the disease did not show any evidence of linkage with HLA. Similar results were also found in a large Finnish pedigree with 7 affected members studied by Gordin et al.[8] (See also ref. 9).

See also refs. 10–12 and 19.

References

1. Nakao Y, Kishihara M, Baba Y, Kuma K, Kuboni-shi T, Imura H: HLA antigens in autoimmune thyroid diseases. Arch Intern Med 138:567-570, 1978
2. Kawahara K, Mitani H, Nokihara M, Mori H: Dis-

TABLE 9.6. Hashimoto's Thyroiditis

	Patients		Controls				
Country/Population	n	%+	n	%+	RR	χ^2	Ref.
HLA-A1							
Canada	73	47	128	29	2.16	6.52	13
Canada	147	43	135	29	1.84	5.90	14
	220	44	263	29	1.96	12.26	
	Heterogeneity χ^2 (1 df)					0.17	
U.S.A.	31	42	3896	31	1.63	1.90	15
Australia	10	20	700	34	0.57	0.70	16
Australia	12	33	395	32	1.11	0.03	17
	22	27	1095	33	0.84	0.16	
	Heterogeneity χ^2 (1 df)					0.57	
	273	43	5254	31	1.69	11.11	
	Heterogeneity χ^2 (4 df)					3.95	
HLA-B8							
Canada	73	34	128	26	1.47	1.48	13
Canada	147	39	135	26	1.81	5.34	14
	220	37	263	26	1.66	6.55	
	Heterogeneity χ^2 (1 df)					0.27	
U.S.A.	31	42	3896	21	2.75	8.16	15
Australia	12	25	395	22	1.30	0.19	17
Australia	10	10	700	24	0.50	0.80	16
	22	18	1095	23	0.91	0.04	
	Heterogeneity χ^2 (1 df)					0.94	
	273	36	5254	22	1.72	11.18	
	Heterogeneity χ^2 (4 df)					4.79	
HLA-BW16							
Japan	56	14	150	3	5.00	8.05	1
HLA-DW3							
Denmark	41	10	389	29	0.30	6.16	6
HLA-DW5							
Denmark	41	22	389	12	2.13	3.71	6
HLA-DR2							
Japan	49	16	144	39	0.31	8.19	18
HLA-DR3							
Canada	40	55	54	26	3.38	7.95	3
Austria	39	15	160	20	0.75	0.40	4
	79	35	214	22	1.67	2.64	
	Heterogeneity χ^2 (1 df)					5.71	
HLA-DR5							
Canada	40	53	80	26	3.15	8.34	5
Austria	39	49	160	23	3.19	10.18	4
	79	51	240	24	3.17	18.52	
	Heterogeneity χ^2 (1 df)					0.00	

eases of internal medicine and HL-A antigens: Basedow disease, Hashimoto's disease. Nippon Rinsho 36:3189-3192, 1978
3. Moens H, Farid NR: Hashimoto's thyroiditis is associated with HLA-DRW3. N Engl J Med 299:133-134, 1978
4. Weissel M, Hofer R, Zasmeta H, Mayr WR: HLA-DR and Hashimoto's thyroiditis. Tissue Antigens 16:256-257, 1980
5. Farid NR, Sampson L, Moens H, Barnard JM: The association of goitrous autoimmune thyroiditis with HLA-DR5. Tissue Antigens 17:265-268, 1981
6. Thomsen M, Ryder LP, Bech K, Bliddal H, Feldt-Rasmussen U, Molholm J, et al: HLA-D in Hashimoto's thyroiditis. Tissue Antigens 21:173-175, 1983
7. Bode HH, Dorf ME, Forbes AP: Familial lymphocytic tyhroiditis: Analysis of linkage with histocompatibility and blood groups. J Clin Endocrinol Metab 37:692-697, 1973
8. Gordin A, Maenpaa J, Makinen T, Totterman TH, Tiilikainen A: Immunological and genetic markers in a family with Hashimoto's disease. Clin Endocrinol 11:425-435, 1979
9. Awashima F, Matsuo T, Akaza T, Kuzumaki N, Yoshida TO, Igarashi Y: Hashimoto's and Graves' diseases transmitted with the same HLA haplotype. In Terasaki PI (ed): Histocompatibility Testing 1980. UCLA Tissue Typing Laboratory, Los Angeles, 1981, pp 951
10. Hoshino K, Inouye H, Unokuchi T, Ito M, Tamaoki N, Tsuji K: HLA and disease in Japanese. In Dausset J, Svejgaard A (eds): HLA and Disease. De L'institut National De La Sante Et De La Recherche Medicale, Paris 1976, p 249
11. Farid NR, Barnard JM, Bryant DG: HLA and phenylthiocarbamide (PTC) tasting in autoimmune thyroid disease. Tissue Antigens 10:414-416, 1977
12. Farid NR, Barnard J, Kutas C, Noel EP, Marshall WH: HL-A antigens in Graves' disease and Hashimoto's thyroiditis. Int Arch Allergy Appl Immunol 49:837-842, 1975
13. Farid NR, Barnard JM, Marshall WH: The association of HLA with autoimmune thyroid disease in Newfoundland. The influence of HLA homozygosity in Graves' disease. Tissue Antigens 8:181-189, 1976
14. Moens H, Barnard JM, Bear J, Farid NR: The association of HLA-B8 with atrophic thyroiditis. Tissue Antigens 13:342-348, 1979
15. Chopra IJ, Solomon DH, Chopra U, Yoshihara E, Terasaki PI, Smith F: Abnormalities in thyroid function in relatives of patients with Graves' disease and Hashimoto's thyroiditis. J Clin Endocrinol Metab 45:45-54, 1977
16. Morris PJ, Vaughan H, Tait BD, Mackay IR: Histocompatibility antigens (HLA): Association with immunopathic diseases and with response to microbial antigens. Aust NZ J Med 7:616-624, 1977
17. Whittingham S, Youngchaiyud U, Mackay IR, Buckley JD, Morris PJ: Thyrogastric autoimmune disease: Studies on the cell-mediated immune system and histocompatibility antigens. Clin Exp Immunol 19:289-299, 1975
18. Sakurami T, Ueno Y, Iwaki Y, Park MS, Terasaki PI, Saji H: HLA-DR specificities among Japanese with several autoimmune disease. Tissue Antigens 19:129-133, 1982
19. Bliddal H, Bech K, Feldt-Rasmussen U, Thomsen M, Ryder L, Hansen JM, et al: Thyroid-stimulating immunoglobulins in Hashimoto's thyroiditis measured by radioreceptor assay and adenylate cyclase stimulation and their relationship to HLA-D alleles. J Clin Endocrinol Metab 55:995-998, 1982
20. Valenta LJ, Bull RW, Hackel E, Bottazzo GF: Correlation of the HLA-A1, B8 haplotypes with circulating autoantibodies in a family with increased incidence of autoimmune disease. Acta Endocrinol 100:143-149, 1982

Myxedema

Population Association

No HLA association has been observed in 22 patients from Czechoslovakia[1] who were typed for A and B loci antigens.

Disease Heterogeneity

In the Czechoslavakian study[1] when the patients were divided into 2 groups on the basis of a history of subacute thyroiditis, 14 had no history and none were positive for BW35. On the other hand, 6 out of 8 patients with a history of subacute thyroiditis were positive for BW35. This difference between the 2 groups was significant (corrected $p = 0.00836$).

Reference

1. Majsky A, Feix C: HLA antigens and myxedema. Tissue Antigens 10:119-120, 1977

Polyglandular Failure

Population Association

In a small sample of 25 patients from Newfoundland, Canada with polyglandular autoimmune disease (combinations of insulin-dependent diabetes, Graves' disease, atrophic thyroiditis, and goiterous thyroiditis) no association was evident.[1]

Family Data

Eisenbarth et al.[2] first published a pedigree with 6 individuals affected with polyglandular failure (thyroid disease, Addison's disease, hypogonad, and alopecia totalis). The proband and all the affected members of this pedigree had haplotype A1-B8. Only 1 person with this haplotype was unaffected. All the unaffected members did not have this haplotype, indicating possible transmission of the "disease gene" with A1-B8 haplotype in this pedigree. The second report[3] included a small family with 3 siblings. The 2 affected siblings did not share any haplotype and the haplotype of the healthy siblings was identical to one of the affected siblings.

Farid et al.[1] also studied 2 families with polyglandular autoimmune disease. In these 2 families there was some indication of the disease segregating with a haplotype. However, in both pedigrees there were several healthy members with the marker haplotype.

See also refs. 4 and 5.

References

1. Farid NR, Larsen B, Payne R, Noel EP, Sampson L: Polyglandular autoimmune disease and HLA. Tissue Antigens 16:23-29, 1980
2. Eisenbarth G, Wilson P, Ward F, Lebovitz HE: HLA type and occurrence of disease in familial polyglandular failure. N Engl J Med 298:92-94, 1978
3. Eisenbarth GS, Wilson PW, Ward F, Buchley C, Lebovitz H: The polyglandular failure syndrome: disease inheritance, HLA type, and immune function. Ann Intern Med 91:528-533, 1979
4. Farid NR: Polyglandular failure syndrome. Ann Intern Med 92:442-443, 1980
5. Brueton MJ, Chapel HM, Mackintosh LP: A study of genetic markers in a family with polyendocrine disease. Tissue Antigens 15:101-103, 1980

Congenital Adrenal Hyperplasia Due to 11-β-Hydroxylase Deficiency

Population Association

On the basis of data collected on 12 families (see below) Dupont et al.[1] reported no HLA association with this disease.

Family Data

Brautbar et al.[2] studied 9 Israeli Jewish families with 12 affected and 18 healthy siblings. In this family, on the basis of lod scores, the linkage of 11-β-hydroxylase deficiency gene with HLA could be excluded for recombination values of < 0.05%.

Two families from Denmark were also HLA typed by Glenthoj et al.[3] However, there was no strong evidence for or against the linkage in this material.

The report by Dupont et al.[1] presented lod score analysis of 12 additional families studied during the Eighth International Histocompatibility Workshop. In this data genetic linkage could be excluded for recombination values 0.00-0.20.

See also see ref. 4.

References

1. Dupont B, Pollack MS, Levine LS, O'Neill GJ, Hawkins BR, New MI: Congenital adrenal hyperplasia. In Terasaki PI (ed): Histocompatibility Testing 1980. UCLA Tissue Typing Laboratory, Los Angeles, 1981, pp. 693-706
2. Brautbar C, Roesler A, Landau H, Cohen I, Nelken D, Cohen T, et al: No linkage between HLA and congenital adrenal hyperplasia due to 11-β-hydroxylase deficiency. N Engl J Med 300:205-206, 1979
3. Glenthoj A, Dankjaer-Nielsen M, Starup J, Svejgaard A: HLA and congenital adrenal hyperplasia due to 11-hydroxylase deficiency. Tissue Antigens 14:181-182, 1979
4. Rochiccioli P, De Mouzon A, Gallegos D, Dutau G, Parra MT, Ohayon E: Liaison genetique entre HLA et hyperplasie virilisante des surrenales: Etude de 12 cas. J Hum Genet 28:201-205, 1980

Congenital Adrenal Hyperplasia Due to 17-α-Hydroxylase Deficiency

Family Data

Mantero et al.[1] first reported HLA typings in an Italian family with 3 affected members (1 male and 2 females) and 9 healthy siblings. The affected members differed from one another in 1 or 2 of their HLA haplotypes. The male patients and two healthy siblings had identical haplotypes. Similarly, an affected female and 2 normal siblings had identical haplotypes. The other healthy siblings had one haplotype that was also present in 2 of the affected members. Thus in this family the disease was not segregating with any specific haplotype.

In another Italian family studied by D'Armiento

et al.[2] 2 homozygous sisters were affected by the disease. However, they shared only 1 HLA haplotype. Since this disease is recessive, the affected siblings should have identical haplotypes. Thus the data from this family also seemed to exclude the linkage of this disease with HLA.

References

1. Mantero F, Scaroni C, Pasini CV, Fagiolo U: No linkage between HLA and congenital adrenal hyperplasia due to 17-alpha hydroxylase deficiency. N Engl J Med 303:530, 1980
2. D'Armiento M, Reda G, Bisignani G, Tabolli S, Cappellaci S, Lulli P, et al.: No linkage between HLA and congenital adrenal hyperplasia due to 17 alpha-hydroxylase deficiency. N Engl J Med 308:970-971, 1983

Congenital Adrenal Hyperplasia Due to 21-Hydroxylase Deficiency

Population Association

In the combined analysis of antigen frequency data from several reports on Caucasian patients, B8 and BW47 were significantly associated with this disease (Table 9.7).

Family Data

Dupont et al.[1] were the first to show evidence of very close linkage between 21-hydroxylase deficiency (an autosomal recessive disease) and HLA in 6 families. The total maximum lod score in these 6 families was 3.394 at the recombination value of 0%. Immediately after this report data from studies of families by several groups of investigators[2–18] confirmed the linkage between this disease and HLA. The gene for this disease has now been mapped on chromosome 6 in very close linkage with HLA.

The family data of Dupont et al.[1] included a patient who inherited a maternal HLA-A/B recombinant. The segregation of the disease and A and B loci antigens in this family indicated that the location of the disease gene was close to the HLA-B locus. This was also found in Weitkamp's,[3] Levine's,[4] and Yang's[19] data (see also ref. 9).

Disease Heterogeneity

Salt-Losing and Compensated Forms

The family data show that both forms of the disease were linked with HLA.[3, 20]

Late-Onset 21-Hydroxylase Deficiency

Laron et al.[21,22] reported data on 5 Ashkenazi families in which at least 1 patient had the late-onset type of disease. This form is characterized by elevated baseline levels of plasma 17-hydroxyprogesterone and urinary pregnanetriol and/or relatively high 17-hydroxyprogesterone following adrenocorticotropic hormone (ACTH) stimulation.[21] From the segregation of HLA haplotypes and the disease the authors[21] have concluded that the late-onset form is due to a new allele and the disease is seen in individuals either homozygous for this allele or heterozygous with other alleles for the congenital form of the disease.

Prenatal Diagnosis

Pollack et al.[23] HLA-typed amniotic cells in 2 at-risk families. In 1 family HLA typing showed that the fetus had the disease and this prediction was confirmed after birth. Both parents were known heterozygous carriers of the disease gene because they had an affected daughter.

In the second family, typing indicated that the fetus would be normal (carrier) and this prediction was also confirmed after birth. Similar results of prenatal diagnosis were reported by Couillin et al.,[24] Rosenmann et al.,[25] and Pollack et al.[26] (see also refs. 5 and 27). Thus HLA typing provides a useful tool in the prenatal diagnosis of this disease. Similar results have been reported by Rosenmann.[18]

In an interesting study Lorenzen et al.[28] showed that there was no difference in the steroidogenic adrenocortical function in heterozygotes for 21-hydroxylase deficiency in steroids of the 17-desoxy, 17-hydroxy, and C-19 pathways. However, the 17-hydroxyprogesterone responses in all males and prepubertal children confirmed the prediction of heterozygosity based on HLA genotyping.

See also refs. 29–33 and 38–44.

References

1. Dupont B, Oberfield SE, Smithwick EM, Lee TD, Levine LS: Close genetic linkage between HLA and congenital adrenal hyperplasia (21-hydroxylase deficiency). Lancet ii:1309-1312, 1977
2. Price DA, Klouda PT, Harris R: HLA and congenital adrenal hyperplasia linkage confirmed. Lancet i:930-932, 1978
3. Weitkamp LR, Bryson M, Bacon GE: HLA and congenital adrenal hyperplasia linkage confirmed. Lancet i:930-932, 1978
4. Levine LS, Zachmann M, New MI, Prader A, Pollack MS, O'Neill GJ, et al: Genetic mapping of the

TABLE 9.7. Congenital Adrenal Hyperplasia (21-Hydroxylase Deficiency)

	Patients		Controls				
Country/Population	n	%+	n	%+	RR	χ^2	Ref.
HLA-B8							
Caucasians (unspecified)	118	5	1504	15	0.32	8.10	14
U.S.A.	37	3	321	18	0.20	4.96	34
Czechoslovakia	25	0	130	17	0.09	5.12	35
England	22	0	230	28	0.06	7.72	6
France	52	4	106	17	0.24	4.86	36
Italy	40	3	522	12	0.32	2.68	37
Denmark	18	6	3301	25	0.27	3.15	15
	312	4	6114	21	0.24	33.06	
	Heterogeneity χ^2 (6 df)					3.53	
HLA-BW47							
Caucasians (unspecified)	118	9	1506	1	9.88	33.16	14
U.S.A.	37	11	321	1	11.73	12.97	34
Czechoslovakia	25	28	130	2	16.73	17.13	35
England	22	14	230	1	15.02	12.18	6
Italy	40	3	522	1	3.91	2.90	37
Denmark	18	11	3301	1	14.64	16.99	15
	260	11	6010	1	10.96	92.85	
	Heterogeneity χ^2 (5 df)					2.48	

21-hydroxylase-deficiency gene within the HLA linkage group. N Engl J Med 299:911-915, 1978

5. Sobel D, Gutai JP, Jones JC, Wagener DK, Smith W: Detection of heterozygote of 21-hydroxylase deficiency. Lancet i:47, 1980
6. Klouda PT, Harris R, Price DA: Linkage and association between HLA and 21-hydroxylase deficiency. J Med Genet 17:337-341, 1980
7. Betuel H, Fauchet R, Gebuhrer L, Freidel C, Bouhallier O: Informative families for the location of the congenital adrenal hyperplasia gene. In Terasaki PI (ed): Histocompatibility Testing 1980. UCLA Tissue Typing Laboratory, Los Angeles, 1981, pp 941
8. Bercovici JP, Khoury S, Le Fur JM, Saleun JP, Nahoul K, Scholler R: Hormonal profiles of heterozygotes in humans for 21-hydroxylase deficiency defined by HLA B typing. J Steroid Biochem 14:1049-1054, 1981
9. Bias WB, Urban MD, Migeon CJ, Hsu SH, Lee PA: Intra-HLA recombinations localizing the 21-hydroxylase deficiency gene within the HLA complex. Hum Immunol 2:139-145, 1981
10. Bercovici JP, Tater D, Khoury S, Le Fur JM, Saleun JP, Nahoul K, et al: Profil hormonal et typage HLA des sujets adultes de 7 familles d'hyperplasie congenitale des surrenales par deficit en 21-hydroxylase. Ann Endocrinol 43:203-211, 1982
11. Chrousos GP, Loriauz DL, Mann D, Cutler Jr GB: Late-onset 21-hydroxylase deficiency is an allelic variant of congenital adrenal hyperplasia characterized by attentuated clinical expression and different HLA haplotype associations. Horm Res 16:193-200, 1982
12. Cruz-Marin F, Raffoux C, Gilgenkrantz S, Janot C, Streiff F, Pierson M: Remarques sur la liaison entre l'hyperplasie congenitale des surrenales par deficit en 21 hydroxylase et des groupes d'histocompatibilite HLA. J Hum Genet 29:103-113, 1981
13. Boue A, Boue J, Couillin P: Hyperplasie congenitale des surrenales et antigenes HLA. J Hum Genet 28:195-200, 1980
14. Dupont B, Pollack MS, Levine LS, O'Neill GJ, Hawkins BR, New MI: Congenital adrenal hyperplasia. In Terasaki PI (ed): Histocompatibility Testing 1980. UCLA Tissue Typing Laboratory, Los Angeles, 1981, pp 693-706
15. Petersen KE, Svejgaard A, Nielsen MD, Dissing J: Heterozygotes and cryptic patients in families of patients with congenital adrenal hyperplasia (21-hydroxylase deficiency). Horm Res 16:151-159, 1982
16. Coullin P, Rappaport R, Kuttenn F, Canlorbe P, Hors J, Marcelli-Barge A, et al: HLA and 21-hydroxyrase deficiency in the French population. Tissue Antigens 19:100-107, 1982
17. Pollack MS, Levine LS, O'Neill GJ, Pang S, Lorenzen F, Kohn B, et al: HLA linkage and B14, DR1, BfS haplotype association with the genes for late onset and cryptic 21-hydroxylase deficiency. Am J Hum Genet 33:540-550, 1981
18. Rosenmann A, Schumert Z, Theodor R, Cohen T, Brautbar C: Amniotic 17 alpha hydroxyprogester-

one and HLA typing for the prenatal diagnosis of 21 alpha hydroxylase deficiency-congenital adrenal hyperplasia. Am J Med Genet 6:295-300, 1980
19. Yang SY, Levine LS, Zachmann M, New MI, Prader A, Oberfield SE, et al: Mapping of the 21-hydroxylase deficiency gene within the HLA linkage group. Transplant Proc 10:753-755, 1978
20. Murtaza LM, Hughes IA, Sibert JR, Balfour IC: HLA and congenital adrenal hyperplasia. Lancet ii:524, 1978
21. Laron Z, Pollack MS, Zamir R, Roitman A, Dickerman Z, Levine LS, et al: Late onset 21-hydroxylase deficiency and HLA in the Ashkenazi population: A new allele. Hum Immunol 1:55-66, 1980
22. Laron Z, Pollack MS, Zamir R, Roitman A, Dickerman Z, Kaufman H, et al: Late-onset 21-hydroxylase deficiency and HLA. Isr J Med Sci 16:411-412, 1982
23. Pollack MS, Levine LS, Pang S, Owens RP, Nitowsky HM, Maurer D, et al: Prenatal diagnosis of congenital adrenal hyperplasia (21-hydroxylase deficiency) by HLA typing. Lancet i:1107-1108, 1979
24. Couillin P, Nicolas H, Boue J, Boue A: HLA typing of amniotic-fluid cells applied to prenatal diagnosis of congential adrenal hyperplasia. Lancet i:1076, 1979
25. Rosenmann A, Schumert Z, Theodor R, Cohen T, Brautbar C: Amniotic 17-alpha hydroxyprogesterone and HLA typing for the prenatal diagnosis of 21 alpha hydroxylase deficiency - congenital adrenal hyperplasia. Am J Med Genet 6:295-300, 1980
26. Pollack MS, Maurer D, Levine LS, Mew MI, Pang S, Duchon MA, et al: HLA typing of amniotic cells: The prenatal diagnosis of congenital adrenal hyperplasia (21-OH-deficiency type). Transplant Proc 11:1726-1728, 1979
27. Zappacosta S, De Felice M, Minozzi M, Lombardi G, Valentino R, Vanacore G: HLA and congenital adrenal hyperplasia. Lancet ii:524, 1978
28. Lorenzen F, Pang S, New M, Pollack M, Oberfield S, Dupont B, et al: Studies of C-21 and C-19 steroids and HLA genotyping in siblings and parents of patients with congenital adrenal hyperplasia. J Clin Endocrinol Metab 50:572-577, 1980
29. Zachmann M, Prader A: Unusual heterozygotes of congenital adrenal hyperplasia due to 21-hydroxylase deficiency confirmed by HLA tissue typing. Acta Endocrinol 92:542-546, 1979
30. O'Neill GJ, Pollack MS, Yang SY, Levine LS, New MI, Dupont B: Gene frequencies and genetic linkage disequilibrium for the HLA-linked genes BF, C2, C4s, C4f, 21-hydroxylase deficiency, and glyoxalase I. Transplant Proc 11:1713-1715, 1979
31. Wurster KG, Clemens GE, Schunter F, Heilbronner H: Moglichkeit der pranatalen diagnostik eines adrenogenitalen syndroms durch HLA-typisierung kultivierter amnionzellen. Dtsch Med Wochenschr 104:526, 1979
32. Hughes IA, Laurence KM: Antenatal diagnosis of congenital adrenal hyperplasia. Lancet ii:7-8, 1979
33. Rubinstein P: Other markers in the HLA linkage group. Clin Immunobiol 4:183-194, 1980
34. Pollack MS, Levine L, Zachmann M, Prader A, New M, Oberfield S, et al: Possible genetic linkage disequilibrium between HLA and the 21-hydroxylase deficiency gene (congenital adrenal hyperplasia). Transplant Proc 11:1315-1316, 1979
35. Lisa L, Ivaskova E, Sajdlova H, Kupkova L: Congenital adrenogenital syndrome - its prognosis and immunogenetic relations. Cesk Pediatr 37:58-61, 1982
36. Couillin P, Kottler-Missonnier ML, Grisard MC, Hors J, Feingold J, Boue J, et al: HLA-A, B, C, DR alleles in congenital adrenal hyperplasia. Hum Genet 53:389-392, 1980
37. Pollack MS, New MI, O'Neill GJ, Levine LS, Callaway C, Pang S, et al: HLA genotypes and HLA-linked genetic markers in Italian patients with classical 21 hydroxylase deficiency. Hum Genet 58:331-337, 1981
38. Klouda PT, Harris R, Price DA: HLA and congenital adrenal hyperplasia. Lancet ii:1046, 1978
39. Stuckey MS, Boyne P, MacDonald WB, Christiansen FT, Houliston JB, Dawkins R: HLA typing and ACTH stimulation in the detection of carriers for 21-hydroxylase deficiency. Aust NZ Med 10:552-554, 1980
40. Mayer S, Tongio MM, Flori J, Bonardi JM, North ML, Klein J, et al: HLA and congenital adrenal hyperplasia. In Terasaki PI (ed): Histocompatibility Testing 1980. UCLA Tissue Typing Laboratory, Los Angeles, 1981, p 940
41. Mauseth RS, Hansen JA, Smith EK, Giblett ER, Kelley VC: Detection of heterozygotes for congenital adrenal hyperplasia: 21-Hydroxylase deficiency—a comparison of HLA typing and 17-OH progesterone to ACTH infusion. J Pediatr 97:749-753, 1980
42. Kauschansky A, Kaufman H, Zamir R, Elian E: Late onset adrenal hyperplasia (21-hydroxylase deficiency):17-OH progesterone response to ACTH stimulation and HLA typing. Hormone Res 14:73-78, 1981
43. Rochiccioli P, De Mouzon A, Gallegos D, Dutau G, Parra MT, Ohayon E: Liaison genetique entre HLA et hyperplasie virilisante des surrenales: Etude de 12 cas. J Hum Genet 28:201-205, 1980
44. Bercovici JP, Khoury S, Le Fur JM, Saleun JP, Nahoul K, Scholler R: Steroid pattern and HLA genotype in parents and siblings of patients with congenital adrenal hyperplasia due to 21-hydroxylase deficiency. Pathol Biol (Paris) 29:380-381, 1981

TABLE 9.8. Adrenocortical Hyperfunction

	Patients		Controls				
Country/Population	n	%+	n	%+	RR	χ^2	Ref.
HLA-A1							
Hungary	100	49	352	28	2.46	15.28	1
HLA-A3							
Hungary	100	9	352	26	0.29	11.91	1

Adrenocortical Hyperfunction

Population Association

Lada et al.[1] typed 100 Hungarian patients for A, B, and C loci antigens. When compared with 352 controls the data showed a significantly increased frequency of A1 and a decreased frequency of A3 (Table 9.8). A nonsignificant increase in B8 was also observed (27.4% in patients vs. 16.19% in controls).

Family Data

The same authors[1] also published the pedigrees of 2 families with several affected members in each family. The results did not show clear segregation of HLA haplotypes with the disease.

Reference

1. Lada G, Gyodi E, Glaz E: HLA antigens in patients with adrenocortical hyperfunction. Acta Med Acad Sci Hung 34:213-226, 1977

Idiopathic Addison's Disease

Population Association

Platz et al.[1] reported a significant increase in the frequency of B8 (Table 9.9). This, however, was not confirmed in 20 patients from Austria[2] and 25 patients from Belgium.[3] In the pooled data the increase of B8 was only marginally significant, and in addition there was significant heterogeneity in the material (Table 9.9).

See also see ref. 4.

References

1. Platz P, Ryder L, Staub Nielsen L, Svejgaard A, Thomsen M, Nerup J, et al: HL-A and idiopathic Addison's disease. Lancet ii:289, 1974
2. Ludwig H, Mayr WR, Pacher M, Schernthaner G, Koller K, Ebil M, et al: HL-A antigens in idiopathic Addison's disease. Z Immunitaetsforsch Bd 149:423-427, 1975
3. De Bruyere M, Vandeput Y, Crabbe J: Primary adrenocortical failure and the HLA system. Horm Res 16:345-352, 1982
4. Valenta LJ, Bull RW, Hackel E, Bottazzo GF: Correlation of the HLA-A1,B8 haplotypes with circulating autoantibodies in a family with increased incidence of autoimmune disease. Acta Endocrinol 100:143-149, 1982

Kallman's Syndrome (Hypogonadotropic Hypogonadism and Anosmia)

Family Data

Dornan et al.[1] published the HLA haplotypes of a family with 10 siblings (9 tested for HLA) in which 3 siblings suffered from hypogonadism. Two of these 3 siblings were anosmic. A fourth sibling was affected by hyposomia but was fertile.

In these data there was no indication of linkage of the syndrome with HLA.

See also ref. 2.

References

1. Dornan J, Barnard JM, Farid NR: Lack of close linkage of hypogonadotropic hypogonadism with HLA. Tissue Antigens 15:510-511, 1980
2. Klouda PT, Donnai D, Harris R: HLA study in a live-born infant with triploidy of paternal origin. Tissue Antigens 17:240-242, 1981

Multiple Endocrine Adenomatosis (Type I)

This disease is inherited as an autosomal dominant gene with incomplete penetrance.

TABLE 9.9. Idiopathic Addison's Disease

	Patients		Controls				
Country/Population	n	%+	n	%+	RR	χ^2	Ref.
HLA-B8							
Austria	20	20	450	18	1.24	0.16	2
Denmark	15	80	1967	24	11.30	17.83	1
	35	46	2417	23	3.37	9.89	
	Heterogeneity χ^2 (1 df)					8.11	

Family Data

The HLA types of a small 3-generation family from England were published by Jung et al.[1] Both parents were healthy but 3 of the 5 siblings were affected by the disease. The daughter of 1 of the affected siblings also had this disease. The affected siblings did not share a haplotype and thus there was no evidence of linkage with HLA in the data (see also ref. 2).

Farid et al.[3] reported HLA haplotypes of 4 families with more than 1 affected individual in each family. A lod score analysis produced a maximum lod score of 0.454 at the recombination frequency of 0.25. Thus in these data the possibility of linkage with HLA could not be excluded.

References

1. Jung RT, Joysey VC, Davie M, Chalmers TM: HLA in multiple endocrine adenomatosis (type I). Tissue Antigens 13:317-318, 1979
2. Groussin P, Renard JP, Chavanne D, Bertrand G, Avril J, Simier JL: Antigenes HLA d'une famille ayant une adenomatose polyendocrinienne de type 1. Nouv Presse Med 9:1033-1034, 1980
3. Farid NR, Buehler S, Russell NA, Maroun FB, Allerdice P, Smythe HS: Prolactinomas in familial multiple endocrine neoplasia syndrome type I: Relationship to HLA and carcinoid tumors. Am J Med 69:874-880, 1980

Cushing's Syndrome

Population Association

Luton et al.[1] did not find a significant association with any of the A and B loci antigens in 38 patients from France.

Reference

1. Luton JP, Baulieu F, Fumeron F, Hors J, Bricaire H: HLA tracers and Cushing's syndrome. Ann Endocrinol (Paris) 42:2-9, 1981

Aldosterone Biosynthetic Defect Due to Type 2 Corticosterone Methyl-Oxidase Deficiency

Family Data

This disorder is inherited as an autosomal recessive gene.

Brautbar et al.[1] performed lod score analysis of 9 Jewish families from Israel. There were a total of 18 affected and 12 healthy siblings in these families. In 8 of the 9 sibships parents were consanguineously related.

The maximum lod score was 1.128 at the recombination frequency of 5%. Thus there was some evidence of linkage between this disease and the HLA complex.

Reference

1. Brautbar C, Theodor R, Sack J, Levene C, Dupont B, Levine LS, et al: HLA in a selective aldosterone biosynthetic defect due to type 2 corticosterone methyl-oxidase deficiency. Tissue Antigens 17:212-216, 1981

Primary Ovarian Failure

Population Association

In 19 Canadian patients, Walfish et al.[1] observed an increase of DR3 antigen (Table 9.10). All patients had isolated secondary amenorrhoea before the age of 36, hypergonadotropic hypogonadism, and nor-

TABLE 9.10. Primary Ovarian Failure

	Patients		Controls				
Country/Population	n	%+	n	%+	RR	χ^2	Ref.
HLA-DR3							
Canada	19	58	80	23	4.46	8.54	1

mal chromosomal karyotypes. None had undergone surgical or medical gonadectomy.

Reference

1. Walfish PG, Gottesman IS, Shewchuk AB, Bain J, Hawe BS, Farid NR: Association of premature ovarian failure with HLA antigens. Tissue Antigens 21:168-169, 1983

Klinefelter's Syndrome

Population Association

Gautier et al.[1] did not find any significant deviations in the A or B loci antigens studied in 46 patients from France.

Reference

1. Gautier O, Petiteau PY, Lasfargues G, Hainault T, Fromantin M: Y a-t-il corrélation entre marqueurs HLA et syndrome de Klinefelter? Nouv Presse Med 11:130-131, 1982

Transcortin Level in Serum

Population Association

De Moor and Louwagie[1] measured basal transcortin levels in 60 male plasma donors from Belgium. HLA-A, -B, and -C loci antigens were typed in these individuals. The individuals with transcordin level > 0.70 mg/g protein were classified as "high transcortin group." In this group no individual antigen was significantly increased or decreased. However, authors have reported a significantly higher number of individuals with B12 and CW5 antigens in this subgroup with high transcortin levels.

Reference

1. De Moor P, Louwagie A: Association of aberrant transcortin levels with HLA antigens of the B and C loci. J Clin Endocrinol Metab 51:868-872, 1980

Testosterone Level in Serum

Population Association

Gerencer et al.[1] measured the concentration of testosterone in 59 Yugoslavian normal women and 63 women with recurrent spontaneous abortions of unknown etiology. The mean serum testosterone concentrations in these 2 groups were 38.9/100 ml and 41.1/100 ml, respectively. The difference between the 2 groups was not significant. Thus, the 2 groups were combined and then subdivided on the basis of testosterone concentration. There were 66 women with concentrations below the mean value and 56 with concentrations above the mean value. The frequency of B5 in the "below" group was found to be 16.67% as compared with 44.64% in the "above" group (χ^2 = 10.094). Only A and B loci antigens were typed in this study.

Reference

1. Gerencer M, Tajic M, Kerhin-Brkljacic V, Kastelan A: An association between serum testosterone level and HLA phenotype. Immunol Lett 4:155-158, 1982

CHAPTER 10

Gastroenterology

Idiopathic Hemochromatosis

Population Association

The first study by Simon et al.[1] on 20 French patients and 120 controls showed an association with A3 and B14. Since then many reports have confirmed these results. Later studies also reported an association with B7. Frequency data on these 3 antigens from all of the published studies and a combined analysis are given in Table 10.1. The highest relative risk was for A3, followed by B7 and B14.

Fauchet et al.[2] also reported an increase of DRW6 in 100 patients (Table 10.1). This was not confirmed in a report from Australia.[3] It should be noted that at present there is some difficulty in typing for DRW6; in addition, in a small sample of 23 patients, DW6 was not found to be increased.[2] Similar discrepant results were found for DR2 (Table 10.1). Thus, hemochromatosis is one of the very few diseases showing a stronger association with an A locus antigen.

Family Data

Simon et al.[4] reported first A and B loci haplotype data on 15 sibships with at least 2 patients with overt forms of hemochromatosis. There was a significant association ($p < 0.0001$) between the presence of hemochromatosis and the possession of the same 2 HLA haplotypes, indicating a recessive mode of transmission of the disease. The maximum lod score from 6 families available for study was 2.239 at a recombination frequency of 0.005. Thus, this study provided the first strong evidence supporting a recessive disease gene very closely linked with HLA (see also ref. 5, 6). These results were later confirmed by Lipinski et al.,[7] Cartwright et al.,[8] Doran et al.,[3,9] and Fauchet et al.[10] In the 14 families studied by Lipinski et al.,[7] the maximum lod score was 4.115 at 0.025 percent recombination frequency. The maximum lod score in 10 pedigrees reported by Cartwright et al.[8] was 9.8 at 0.0 % recombination. A second report on a large pedigree by the same group of authors[11] gave a lod score of 6.88 at 0.0 % recombination. The analysis of 10 families by Doran et al.[3] showed a maximum score of 4.578 at 0.0% recombination. Thus, these data provide very strong evidence in favor of a recessive gene linked with HLA (a maximum lod score of 3.00 is generally considered as evidence of linkage).

Edwards et al.[12] reported a pedigree with hereditary hemachromatosis in which a recombination between A and B loci was observed. In the pedigree the hemochromatosis locus segregated with the HLA-A locus and not with the HLA-B locus, indicating the position of the hemochromatosis locus close to the A locus.

Beaumont et al.[13] reported that the persons who shared both HLA haplotypes with the proband (homozygous for the hemochromatosis gene) differed significantly from those who shared only 1 haplotype (heterozygous) in terms of serum iron, unsaturated iron binding capacity, and serum ferritin. Pedigree data of Cartwright et al.[8] also showed that in heterozygotes over 20 years of age there was an intermediate increase in transferrin saturation and a limited increase in hepatic iron but no clinical manifestations. Thus, these data and those of Bassett et al.,[14] Lloyd et al.,[15] Simon et al.,[16] and of Valberg

TABLE 10.1. Idiopathic Hemochromatosis

	Patients		Controls				
Country/Population	n	%+	n	%+	RR	χ^2	Ref.
HLA-A3							
Canada	18	61	253	25	4.56	10.04	15
Australia	10	60	700	20	5.76	8.72	27
Australia	73	70	522	26	6.54	48.48	3
	83	69	1222	23	6.40	57.16	
	Heterogeneity χ^2 (1 df)					0.04	
BENELUX	12	83	40	25	11.96	11.34	28
England	35	69	95	31	4.79	14.26	29
France	154	73	439	30	6.25	77.92	2
France	66	78	444	26	9.82	54.88	30
France	48	75	591	26	8.29	39.71	7
	268	75	1474	27	7.41	170.89	
	Heterogeneity χ^2 (2 df)					1.62	
West Germany	22	73	5046	30	6.00	15.76	31
West Germany	35	74	100	21	10.17	27.71	32
	57	74	5146	30	7.86	42.77	
	Heterogeneity χ^2 (1 df)					0.70	
Ireland	20	60	143	24	4.61	10.36	33
	493	72	8373	28	6.77	313.57	
	Heterogeneity χ^2 (10 df)					5.62	
HLA-B7							
Canada	18	50	253	22	3.52	7.12	15
Australia	10	50	700	21	3.75	5.12	27
Australia	73	60	522	27	4.02	29.78	3
	83	59	1222	24	3.98	34.88	
	Heterogeneity χ^2 (1 df)					0.01	
BENELUX	12	75	40	15	14.41	13.65	28
England	35	34	95	20	2.06	2.87	29
France	154	39	439	27	1.73	7.81	2
France	48	38	591	19	2.63	9.81	7
France	66	53	444	20	4.48	30.85	30
	268	42	1474	22	2.45	40.26	
	Heterogeneity χ^2 (2 df)					8.22	
West Germany	35	60	100	22	5.17	16.05	32
West Germany	22	45	5046	27	2.23	3.81	31
	57	54	5146	27	3.40	17.77	
	Heterogeneity χ^2 (1 df)					2.10	
Ireland	20	60	143	27	3.94	8.45	33
	493	48	8373	25	2.98	115.33	
	Heterogeneity χ^2 (10 df)					20.00	

Table 10.1 *(continued)*

Country/Population	Patients n	Patients %+	Controls n	Controls %+	RR	χ^2	Ref.
HLA-B14							
Canada	18	17	253	8	2.59	2.52	15
Australia	10	20	700	7	3.87	3.93	27
Australia	73	10	522	8	1.34	0.53	3
	83	11	1222	7	1.76	2.67	
	Heterogeneity χ^2 (1 df)					1.79	
England	35	20	95	6	3.81	5.60	29
France	154	31	439	8	5.13	44.56	2
France	66	9	444	9	1.06	0.02	30
France	48	29	591	9	4.18	17.67	7
	268	25	1474	9	3.68	52.04	
	Heterogeneity χ^2 (2 df)					10.21	
West Germany	22	0	5046	5	0.42	0.71	31
West Germany	35	3	100	6	0.65	0.27	32
	57	2	5146	5	0.55	0.87	
	Heterogeneity χ^2 (1 df)					0.11	
Ireland	20	20	143	13	1.78	1.06	33
	481	19	8333	6	2.79	53.24	
	Heterogeneity χ^2 (9 df)					23.63	
HLA-DR2							
Australia	66	52	225	25	3.23	16.68	3
France	100	35	100	34	1.04	0.02	2
	166	42	325	28	1.86	9.17	
	Heterogeneity χ^2 (1 df)					7.54	
HLA-DRW6							
Australia	66	19	225	22	0.85	0.22	3
France	100	37	100	19	2.47	7.84	2
	166	30	325	21	1.50	2.95	
	Heterogeneity χ^2 (1 df)					5.12	

et al.[17] provide evidence for a recessive disease gene with partial biochemical expression in heterozygotes.

The gene for this disease has now been mapped on chromosome 6.

See also refs. 18–26, 34, and 35.

References

1. Simon M, Pawlotsky Y, Bourel M, Fauchet R, Genetet B: Hemochromatose idiopathique: Maladie associee a l'antigene tissulaire HL-A 3. Nouv Presse Med 4:1432, 1975
2. Fauchet R, Genetet N, Genetet B, Simon M, Bourel M: HLA determinants in idiopathic hemochromatosis. Tissue Antigens 14:10-14, 1979
3. Doran TJ, Bashir HV, Trejaut J, Bassett ML, Halliday JW, Powell LW. Idiopathic haemochromatosis in the Australian population: HLA linkage and recessivity. Hum Immunol 2:191-200, 1981
4. Simon M, Bourel M, Genetet B, Fauchet R: Idiopathic hemochromatosis: Demonstration of recessive transmission and early detection by family HLA typing. N Engl J Med 297:1017-1021, 1977
5. Simon M, Alexandre JL, Burel M, Marec BL, Scordia C: Heredity of idiopathic haemochromatosis: A study of 106 families. Clin Genet 11:327-341, 1977

6. Simon M, Hespel JP, Fauchet R, Brissot P, Hita de Nercy Y, Edan G, et al: Heredite recessive de l'hemochromatose idiopathique. Nouv Presse Med 8:421-424, 1979
7. Lipinski M, Hors J, Saleun JP, Saddi R, Passa P, Lafaurie S, et al: Idiopathic hemochromatosis: Linkage with HLA. Tissue Antigens 11:471-474, 1978
8. Cartwright GE, Edwards CQ, Kravitz K, Skolnick M, Amos DB, Johnson A, Bushjaer L: Hereditary haemochromatosis. N Engl J Med 301:175-179, 1979
9. Bassett ML, Doran TJ, Halliday JW, Bashir HV, Powell LW: Idiopathic hemochromatosis: Demonstration of homozygous-heterozygous mating by HLA typing of families. Hum Genet 60:352-356, 1982
10. Fauchet R, Simon M, Genetet B, Bourel M: Idiopathic hemochromatosis. In Terasaki PI (ed): Histocompatibility Testing 1980. UCLA Tissue Typing Laboratory, Los Angeles, 1981, pp 707-710
11. Kravitz K, Skolnick M, Cannings C, Carnelli D, Baty B, Amos B, et al: Genetic linkage between hereditary hemochromatosis and HLA. Am J Hum Genet 31:601-619, 1979
12. Edwards CQ, Cartwright GE, Skolnick MH, Amos DB: Genetic mapping of the hemochromatosis locus on chromosome six. Hum Immunol 1:19-22, 1980
13. Beaumont C, Simon M, Fauchet R, Hespel JP, Brisset P, Genetet B, Bourel M: Serum ferritin as a possible marker of the hemochromatosis allele. N Engl J Med 301:169-174, 1979
14. Bassett ML, Powell LW, Halliday JW, Doran T, Bashir H: Early detection of idiopathic haemochromatosis: Relative value of serum-ferritin and HLA typing. Lancet ii:4-7, 1979
15. Lloyd DA, Adams P, Sinclair NR, Stiller CR, Valberg LS: Histocompatibility antigens as markers of abnormal iron metabolism in idiopathic hemochromatosis. Can Med Assoc J 119: 1051-1056, 1978
16. Simon M, Fauchet R, Hespel JP, Beaumont C, Brissot P, et al: Idiopathic hemochromatosis: A study of biochemical expression in 247 heterozygous members of 63 families: Evidence for a single major HLA-linked gene. Gastroenterology 78:703-708, 1980
17. Valberg LS, Lloyd DA, Ghent CN, Flanagan PR, Sinclair NR, Stiller CR, et al: Clinical and biological expression of the genetic abnormality in idiopathic hemochromatosis. Gastroenterology 79:884-892, 1980
18. Eddleston ALWF, Williams R: HLA and liver disease. Br Med Bull 34:295-300, 1978
19. Simon M, Bourel M: Heredite de l'hemochromatoseidiopathique: Demonstration de la transmission recessive et mise en evidence du gene responsable porte par le chromosome 6. Gastroenterol Clin Biol 2:573-577, 1978
20. Simon M, Bourel M, Fauchet R, Genetet B: Association of HLA-A3 and HLA-B14 antigens with idiopathic haemochromatosis. Gut 17:332-334, 1976
21. Shewan WG, Mouat SA, Allan TM: HLA antigens in haemochromatosis. Br Med J 1:281-282, 1976
22. Simon M, Bourel M, Genetet B, Fauchet R, Edan G, Bisset P: Idiopathic hemochromatosis and iron overload in alcholic liver disease: Differentiation by HLA phenotype. Gastroenterology 73:655-658, 1977
23. Walters JM, Watt DW, Stevens FM, McCarthy CF: HLA antigens in haemochromatosis. Br Med J 4:520, 1975
24. Goossens JP, Schreuder I, Went LN: Inheritance of idiopathic haemochromatosis. Lancet i:1106-1107, 1977
25. Dyrszka H, Eberhardt G, Eckert G: The distribution of HLA-antigens in German patients with idiopathic hemochromatosis. Klin Wochenschr 57:529-531, 1979
26. Simon M, Bourel M, Fauchet R, Genetet B: HLA and "nonimmunological" disease: Idiopathic haemochromatosis. Lancet ii:973-974, 1976
27. Morris PJ, Vaughan H, Tait BD, Mackay IR: Histocompatibility antigens (HLA): Association with immunopathic diseases and with response to microbial antigens. Aust NZ J Med 7:616-624, 1977
28. Laukens P, Versieck J, De Potter E, Barbier F: Association of HLA antigens with idiopathic hemochromatosis. N Engl J Med 74:1351-1352, 1978
29. Bomford A, Eddleston ALWF, Kennedy LA, Batchelor JR, Williams R: Histocompatibility antigens as markers of abnormal iron metabolism in patients with idiopathic haemochromatosis and their relatives. Lancet i:327-329, 1977
30. Saddi R, Muller JY, Pouliquen A, Kaplan C, Sylvestre R: HLA-A3, B7 linkage disequilibrium in hemochromatotic patients with or without insulin dependent diabetes. Tissue Antigens 17:473-479, 1981
31. Dyrszka H, Eberhardt G, Eckert G: HLA-phenotype and hemochromatosis in Germany. Gastroenterology 75:555-556, 1978
32. Kuhnl P, Kaltwasser JP, Seidl S: HLA antigens in patients with idiopathic hemochromatosis (IH). Tissue Antigens 12:398-401,1978
33. McCarthy D, Fitzgerald GA, O'Connell LG: Histocompatibility antigens and haemochromatosis in Ireland. Irish J Med Sci 148:168-172, 1979
34. Edwards CQ, Skolnick MH, Kushner JP: Coincidental nontransfusional iron overload and thalassemia minor: Association with HLA-linked hemochromatosis. Blood 58:844-848, 1981

35. Edwards CQ, Skolnick MH, Dadone MM, Kushner JP: Iron overload in hereditary spherocytosis: Association with HLA-linked hemochromatosis. Am J Hematol 13:101-109, 1982

Celiac Disease

Population Association

The frequency data, available mostly for Caucasians, show that the antigens A1, B7, B8, DR3, DR7, DW3, and DW7 are significantly associated with this disease (Table 10.2). On the basis of lower relative risk for A1 and the well-established linkage disequilibrium between A1 and B8, the primary association of the disease appears to be with B8 (see also analyses in refs. 1, 2). In studies on Israeli Jews the increase of A1 was not significant (Table 10.2). Antigen B7 in Caucasian patients was significantly decreased with a combined relative risk of 0.41.

D and DR loci associations have also been studied in several reports. From these data, it is clear that DR3 and DW3 antigens are significatly increased in the patients (Table 10.2). The combined relative risk for DR3 was 11.67 and that for DW3 was 5.49. However, there was highly significant heterogeneity in the combined data for both of these antigens. In the case of DR3 the primary source of these heterogeneity data is that from Norway,[3] in which 95% of the patients were positive for DR3 (Table 10.2). The heterogeneity in DW3 estimates resulted from the data by Keuning et al.,[4] in which 96% of the patients were DW3 giving a relative risk of 45.17. The other 2 studies on both DR3 and DW3 were less heterogeneous. It is interesting to note that if these 2 studies[3,4] are excluded from the combined analysis then the relative risk for DR3 would be similar to that for B8. However, it would be much lower for DW3.

Keuning et al.[4] divided their patients and controls into DW3- and B8-positive and -negative groups. In the subgroupings based on DW3 (positive and negative), there were no associations with B8. On the other hand, in both positive and negative B8 subgroups there were significant associations with DW3. From these data, it appeared that the primary association of the disease was with DW3.

Several reports on DR7 and 1 on DW7[5] also showed a significant association of these antigens with celiac disease (Table 10.2). Thus, as in diabetes, the association was with 2 D and DR loci alleles, and this may provide insight into the genetic basis of the disease.

Disease Heterogeneity

In a study by Nelson et al.,[6] *in vitro* organ culture behavior of jejunal biopsies from B8-positive and B8-negative patients were compared. Biopsies were analyzed for alkaline phosphatase activity at the initiation and after 24–48 h of culture in the presence and absence of α-gliadin and a cyanogen bromide fraction of α-gliadin. When biopsies were cultured in the presence of α-gliadin the rise in alkaline phosphatase activity was inhibited in B8-positive patients. On the other hand, there was no inhibition in B8-negative patients. In the presence of a cyanogen bromide fragment of α-gliadin, inhibition of the rise in alkaline phosphatase activity was observed in both B8-positive and B8-negative groups of patients. The authors have suggested that celiac patients may have a binding site for gluten proteins on epithelial cells and/or on lymphocytes that depends on the gene product of the B8 allele.

Ferguson et al.[7] studied the presenting clinical features, hematologic and biochemical status, and morphologic parameters of immunologic reactivity in 19 B8-positive and 13 B8-negative celiac patients. The effect on these factors of gluten withdrawal of at least 1 year's duration was also examined. A significant increase in serum globulin levels and a decreased lymphocyte population in the lamina propria of the jejunum was observed in the B8-positive group when receiving gluten. This difference was not found on gluten withdrawal. These results suggest that there may be a difference in immunologic reactivity to gluten between B8-positive and B8- negative celiac patients.

Falchuk et al.[8] reported data on *in vitro* gluten-induced damage in the biopsies of B8-positive and -negative patients. Significantly more damage was observed in the B8-positive sample.

Simpson et al.[9] performed leukocyte migration inhibition tests (as an indicator of cell-mediated immunity to gluten fraction III) in 30 healthy controls and 58 patients. There was no significant difference between B8 and non-B8 patients and also no difference between patients and B8-positive controls.

Family Study

Data on families of celiac patients are available in several studies.[2,4,10–24] In most of these reports, however, the families have only 1 affected member.

TABLE 10.2. Celiac Disease

Country/Population	Patients n	Patients %+	Controls n	Controls %+	RR	χ^2	Ref.
HLA-A1							
Iraq	40	28	40	20	1.53	0.70	24
Jews—Ashkenazi	25	24	23	17	1.48	0.35	19
Jews—Ashkenazi	56	32	52	17	2.23	3.18	20
	81	30	75	17	1.96	3.27	
	Heterogeneity χ^2 (1 df)					0.26	
Jews—Non-Ashkenazi	56	27	38	37	0.63	1.08	20
Jews (unspecified)	18	39	27	22	2.19	1.55	41
Jews (unspecified)	33	33	395	29	1.23	0.31	42
	51	35	422	29	1.43	1.24	
	Heterogeneity χ^2 (1 df)					0.62	
	228	30	575	27	1.34	2.21	
	Heterogeneity χ^2 (5 df)					4.95	
African Caucasian	15	33	107	21	1.91	1.34	18
U.S.A.	24	67	200	35	3.64	8.70	14
West European (unspecified)	30	37	100	26	1.68	1.47	19
England	117	70	268	33	4.69	42.24	2
England	36	75	180	32	6.12	20.41	43
England	53	68	117	29	5.08	21.44	21
England	30	60	268	33	3.00	8.23	44 (
	236	69	833	32	4.60	90.47	
	Heterogeneity χ^2 (3 df)					1.85	
France	38	53	591	23	3.75	15.93	18
France	33	39	400	21	2.43	5.85	45
	71	46	991	22	3.09	21.01	
	Heterogeneity χ^2 (1 df)					0.78	
West Germany	53	64	462	27	4.74	27.11	16
Austria	54	57	240	30	3.06	13.58	17
Norway	57	54	1628	29	2.86	15.56	3
	540	60	4561	28	3.57	170.22	
	Heterogeneity χ^2 (11 df)					11.65	
HLA-B7							
Iraq	40	3	40	0	3.50	1.05	24
Jews—Ashkenazi	56	4	52	12	0.35	2.31	20
Jews—Ashkenazi	25	8	23	13	0.63	0.33	19
	81	5	75	12	0.44	2.34	
	Heterogeneity χ^2 (1 df)					0.30	
Jews—Non-Ashkenazi	56	5	38	8	0.62	0.42	20
Jews (unspecified)	18	0	27	11	0.19	2.04	41
Jews (unspecified)	33	0	395	8	0.17	2.97	42
	51	0	422	8	0.18	5.00	
	Heterogeneity χ^2 (1 df)					0.01	
	228	4	575	8	0.47	4.40	
	Heterogeneity χ^2 (5 df)					4.71	

TABLE 10.2. *(continued)*

Country/Population	Patients n	Patients %+	Controls n	Controls %+	RR	χ^2	Ref.
HLA-B7							
African Caucasian	15	7	107	14	0.64	0.31	18
U.S.A.	24	8	200	20	0.42	1.76	14
West European (unspecified)	30	10	100	16	0.65	0.51	19
England	117	24	268	44	0.41	13.39	2
England	36	11	180	22	0.48	2.03	43
England	53	13	117	27	0.42	3.86	21
	206	19	565	33	0.42	19.19	
	Heterogeneity χ^2 (2 df)					0.09	
France	38	13	591	19	0.69	0.67	18
France	33	0	400	22	0.05	8.30	45
	71	7	991	20	0.45	3.69	
	Heterogeneity χ^2 (1 df)					5.27	
Austria	54	6	240	29	0.18	10.83	17
	400	13	2203	24	0.41	32.78	
	Heterogeneity χ^2 (8 df)					8.88	
HLA-B8							
Iraq	40	40	40	5	10.37	11.95	24
Jews—Ashkenazi	56	34	52	10	4.33	8.31	20
Jews—Ashkenazi	25	32	23	0	22.83	8.10	19
	81	33	75	7	5.80	14.52	
	Heterogeneity χ^2 (1 df)					1.88	
Jews—Non-Ashkenazi	56	25	38	3	7.77	7.20	20
Jews (unspecified)	18	56	27	11	8.88	9.65	41
Jews (unspecified)	33	27	395	8	4.34	12.36	42
	51	37	422	8	5.23	21.25	
	Heterogeneity χ^2 (1 df)					0.77	
	228	33	575	7	6.15	54.01	
	Heterogeneity χ^2 (5 df)					3.56	
African Caucasian	15	33	107	12	3.67	4.94	18
U.S.A.	24	88	200	22	22.50	29.24	14
West European (unspecified)	30	60	100	12	10.48	25.35	19
BENELUX	28	79	100	31	7.82	18.07	4
England	30	77	268	30	7.42	21.62	44
England	36	89	180	26	20.62	35.19	43
England	21	76	253	27	8.00	17.69	46
England	53	70	117	25	6.80	28.33	21
England	117	80	268	30	9.15	70.91	2
	257	79	1086	28	8.94	170.23	
	Heterogeneity χ^2 (4 df)					3.51	
France	33	73	400	17	12.68	40.78	45
France	38	58	591	17	6.66	31.46	18
	71	65	991	17	8.72	70.72	
	Heterogeneity χ^2 (1 df)					1.52	

TABLE 10.2. *(continued)*

Country/Population	Patients n	Patients %+	Controls n	Controls %+	RR	χ^2	Ref.
HLA-B8							
West Germany	53	66	462	19	8.13	46.58	16
Italy	65	38	306	15	3.47	17.53	5
Austria	54	56	240	16	6.58	34.58	17
Finland	42	67	900	20	7.96	39.66	47
Norway	57	72	1624	25	7.56	47.60	3
	696	68	6116	22	7.69	490.47	
	Heterogeneity χ^2 (15 df)					19.05	
HLA-DW3							
BENELUX	28	96	100	27	45.17	26.08	4
Italy	44	57	58	24	4.07	11.09	5
Norway	25	52	213	22	3.80	10.17	3
	97	67	371	24	5.49	38.09	
	Heterogeneity χ^2 (2 df)					9.25	
HLA-DW7							
Italy	33	66	49	29	4.56	10.49	5
HLA-DR3							
Jews—Ashkenazi	18	33	23	13	3.01	2.34	19
Jews—Ashkenazi	17	35	52	17	2.61	2.62	20
	35	34	75	16	2.77	4.94	
	Heterogeneity χ^2 (1 df)					0.02	
Jews—Non-Ashkenazi	30	43	38	11	5.58	8.48	20
Jews (unspecified)	20	55	96	13	7.84	15.74	23
	85	42	209	14	4.64	26.76	
	Heterogeneity χ^2 (3 df)					2.42	
West European (unspecified)	29	79	100	18	15.84	30.83	19
France	22	64	100	21	6.40	14.58	45
Italy	45	60	63	22	5.14	15.26	5
Finland	41	85	88	24	16.57	34.61	47
Norway	57	95	120	25	48.41	46.87	3
	194	79	471	22	11.67	129.59	
	Heterogeneity χ^2 (4 df)					12.57	
HLA-DR7							
Jews—Ashkenazi	17	29	52	25	1.26	0.16	20
Jews—Ashkenazi	18	22	23	26	0.83	0.08	19
	35	25	75	25	1.06	0.02	
	Heterogeneity χ^2 (1 df)					0.22	
Jews—Non-Ashkenazi	30	67	38	24	6.05	11.94	20
Jews (unspecified)	20	60	96	23	4.85	10.18	23
	85	48	209	24	2.83	13.91	
	Heterogeneity χ^2 (3 df)					8.44	

TABLE 10.2. *(continued)*

Country/Population	Patients n	Patients %+	Controls n	Controls %+	RR	χ^2	Ref.
HLA-DR7							
West European (unspecified)	29	45	100	6	11.98	21.74	19
France	22	55	100	20	4.76	10.67	45
Italy	45	67	65	28	5.05	15.59	5
Finland	41	66	88	11	14.78	34.73	47
	137	60	353	15	7.73	77.94	
	Heterogeneity χ^2 (3 df)					4.80	

Therefore, no formal linkage analysis of multiple-case families is available in any of these reports, and thus no conclusions about the nature of the "disease susceptibility gene" and its relationship to HLA locus can be made.

Albert et al.,[16] Ludwig et al.,[17] and Mackintosh and Asquith[10] have examined the segregation of HLA in families in which 1 parent was heterozygous for an antigen and the other was negative for that antigen. In such back-cross matings the segregation of B8-positive and B8-negative offspring should be in a 1:1 ratio. In all 3 studies the ratio in celiac offspring was significantly different from 1:1, with more celiac offspring positive for B8. In healthy siblings of these patients the segregation ratio was not significantly different from 1:1.

In another report Scholz et al.[15] examined the joint segregation of HLA haplotypes in 19 families. The authors concluded that the inheritance patterns in these families were compatible with the assumption of joint segregation between HLA and the disease gene. In most cases, however, the penetrance was incomplete. If one of the patients in a family had the disease then all the offspring with this marker haplotype did not have the disease (no pedigree diagrams are available in this paper).

Mougenot et al.[18] published results on 6 small families in which 2 siblings were affected by the disease. In all 6 families the affected siblings shared at least 1 haplotype.

Keuning et al.[4] examined 4 families with only D-locus information. In 3 of these families there were at least 2 affected members. However, as would be expected, all the DW3-positive individuals were not suffering from the disease. Similar data have been presented by Falchuck et al.[13] in an organ culture study of 35 families (most of them with only 1 affected member). (See refs. 2, 11, 12, and 14.)

Thirty-four multiple-case families were studied during the 1980 Histocompatibility Workshop.[19] An analysis of the sib-pair data showed a significant excess of HLA haplotype-identical siblings. The segregation of the haplotypes in these families favored a recessive mode of inheritance. An analysis of the published affected sib-pair data by Greenberg et al.[25] also produced similar results.

Tiwari et al.[26] have done segregation and linkage analysis on 70 multiple-case families. This analysis favored a "celiac disease gene" that was additive on a continuous liability scale. The estimated frequency of this gene was 0.022. There was a significant excess of DR3/DR7 heterozygotes among patients. The linkage analysis of these pedigrees showed a highly significant evidence of linkage with the HLA complex. The maximum lod score was 10.90 at a recombination frequency of 8% in males.

See also refs. 27–40 and 48–56.

References

1. Falchuk ZM, Strober W: HL-A antigens and adult coeliac disease. Lancet ii:1310, 1972
2. Stokes PL, Asquith P, Holmes GKT, Mackintosh P, Cooke WT: Inheritance and influence of histocompatibility (HL-A) antigens in adult coeliac disease. Gut 14:627-630, 1973
3. Ek J, Albrechtsen D, Solheim BG, Thorsby E: Strong association between the HLA-DW3-related B cell alloantigen -DRW3 and coeliac disease. Scand J Gastroenterol 13:229-233, 1978
4. Keuning JJ, Pena AS, Van Leeuwen A, Van Hooff JP, Van Rood JJ: HLA-DW3 associated with coeliac disease. Lancet i:506-507, 1976
5. Demarchi M, Borelli I, Olivetti E, Richiardi P, Wright P, Ansaldi N, et al: Two HLA-D alleles are associated with coeliac disease. Tissue Antigens 14:309-316, 1979
6. Nelson DL, Falchuk ZM, Kasarda D, Strober W:

Gluten-sensitive enteropathy: Correlation of organ culture behavior with HL-A status. Clin Res 24:254a, 1976
7. Ferguson R, Asquith P, Cooke WT: Histocompatibility antigens in coeliac disease. Gut 15:834, 1974
8. Falchuk ZM, Nelson DL, Katz AJ, Bernardin JE, Kasarda DD, Hague NE, et al: Gluten-sensitive enteropathy: Influence of histocompatibility type on gluten sensitivity *in vitro*. J Clin Invest 66:227-233, 1980
9. Simpson FG, Bullen AW, Robertson DAF, Losowsky MS: HLA-B8 and cell-mediated immunity to gluten. Gut 22:633-636, 1981
10. Mackintosh P, Asquith P: HLA and coeliac disease. Br Med Bull 34:291-294, 1978
11. Dennis NR, Stokes CR: Risk of coeliac disease in children of patients and effect of HLA genotype. J Med Genet 15:20-22, 1978
12. Pena AS, Mann DL, Hague NE, Heck JA, Van Leeuwen A, Van Rood JJ, et al: Genetic basis of gluten-sensitive enteropathy. Gastroenterology 75:230-235, 1978
13. Falchuk ZM, Katz AJ, Shwachman H, Rogentine GN, Strober W: Gluten-sensitive enteropathy: Genetic analysis and organ culture study in 35 families. Scand J Gastroenterol 13:839-843, 1978
14. Falchuk ZM, Rogentine GN, Strober W: Predominance of histocompatibility antigen HL-A8 in patients with gluten-sensitive enteropathy. J Clin Invest 51:1602-1605, 1972
15. Scholz S, Schattenkirchner M, Harms K, Steinbauer-Rosenthal I, Albert ED: Family studies in HL-A associated diseases. Z Immun Forsch 148:387-388, 1975
16. Albert ED, Harms K, Wank R, Steinbauer-Rosenthal S, Scholz S: Segregation analysis of HL-A antigens and haplotypes in 50 families of patients with coeliac disease. Transplant Proc 5:1785-1789, 1973
17. Ludwig H, Granditsch G, Polymenidis Z: HL-A8 and haplotype HL-A1-8 in coeliac disease. J Immunogenet 1:91-97, 1974
18. Mougenot JF, Hors J, Schmid M, Cathelineau M, Navarro J, Polonovski C: Les antigenes HLA dans la maladie coeliaque et l'intolerance digestive aux proteines du lait de vache chez l'enfant. Gastroenterol Clin Biol 1:507-514, 1977
19. Betuel H, Gebuhrer L, Descos L, Bertrand J, Freycon F, Lepetit JC: Celiac disease and its association with HLA markers. In Terasaki PI (ed): Histocompatibility Testing 1980. UCLA Tissue Typing Laboratory, Los Angeles, 1981, pp 668-672
20. Brautbar C, Freier S, Ashkenazi A, Dekelbaum R, Tur-Kaspa I, Amar A, et al: Histocompatibility determinants in Israeli Jewish patients with coeliac disease: Population and family study. Tissue Antigens 17:313-323, 1981
21. Robinson BN, Roberts DF, Mather BA, Nelson R, Rowlatt AS: Coeliac disease and HLA: A family study. J Immunogenet 7:381-391, 1980
22. Lauras B, Freycon MT, Vial MT, Lepetit JC, Betuel H. Maladie coeliaque: Relations evec le groupe HL-A et formes familiales. Pediatrie 35:521-525, 1980
23. Orgad S, Avigad S, Jonas A, Mizrachi J, Gazit E: Immunogenetics of childhood celiac disease: The association with HLA DR3 and DR7 in unrelated patients and multiple affected families. Isr J Med Sci 17:1041-1044, 1981
24. Dawood FH, Jabbar AAR, Al-Mudaris AF, Al-Hasani MH: Association of HLA antigens with coeliac disease among Iraqi children. Tissue Antigens 18:35-39, 1981
25. Greenberg DA, Hodge SE, Rotter JI: Evidence for recessive and against dominant inheritance at the HLA-"linked" locus in coeliac disease. Am J Hum Genet 34:263-277, 1982
26. Tiwari JL, Betuel H, Gebuhrer L, Morton NE: Genetic epidemiology of coeliac disease. Genet Epidemiol 1:37-42, 1984
27. Ludwig H, Granditsch G: HL-A antigens and coeliac disease. Lancet ii:459, 1974
28. Mulder DJ: HL-A antigens and coeliac disease. Lancet ii:727, 1974
29. Strober W, Nelson DL, Rogentine GN, Falchuk ZM: HL-A antigens and coeliac disease. Lancet ii:459, 1974
30. Scott BB, Young S, Rajah SM, Marks J, Losowsky MS: The incidence of coeliac disease and HL-A8 in dermatitis herpetiformis. Gut 16:845, 1975
31. Rotthauwe HW, Rittner CH, Waiyawuth V, Becker M: HL-A Histokompatibilitatsantigene bei Kindern mit Coeliakie. Dtsch Med Wochenschr 101:849, 1976
32. Stokes PL, Asquith P, Holmes GKT, Mackintosh P, Cooke WT: Histocompatibility antigens associated with adult coeliac disease. Lancet ii:162-164, 1972
33. Gebhard RL, Falchuk ZM, Katz SI, Sessoms C, Rogentine GN, Strober W: Immunologic concomitants of small intestinal disease and relationship to histocompatibility antigen HL-A8. J Clin Invest 54:98-103, 1974
34. Scott BB, Swinburne LM, Rajah SM, Losowsky MS: The HLA system and the immunological response to dietary antigens. Gut 15:823, 1974
35. Ludwig H, Polymenidis Z, Granditsch G, Wick G: Association of HL-A1 and HL-A8 with childhood celiac disease. Z Immun Forsch 146:158-167, 1973
36. Granditsch G, Ludwig H, Polymenidis Z, Wick G: Coeliac disease and HL-A8. Lancet ii:908-909, 1973
37. Hobart MJ, Petrie A: HL-A8 and the immune response to gluten. Lancet ii:1573-1574, 1974

38. Scott H, Solheim BG, Brandtzaeg P, Thorsby E: HLA-DR-like antigens in the epithelium of the human small intestine. Scand J Immunol 12:77-82, 1980
39. Scott BB, Losowsky MS, Rajah SM: HL-A8 and HL-A12 in coeliac disease. Lancet ii:171, 1974
40. Scott BB, Swinburne ML, Rajah SM, Losowsky MS: HL-A8 and the immune response to gluten. Lancet ii:374-377, 1974
41. Ashkenazi A, Berrebi A, Levi R, Sakal E, Idar D: Frequency of HLA-B8 in Israeli children with celiac disease. Isr J Med Sci 15:826-828, 1979
42. Gazit E, Avigad S, Zfat Z, Efter T, Mizrachi Y, Rotem Y: The association of HL-A-B8 and childhood celiac disease in an Israeli population. Isr J Med Sci 13:400-404, 1977
43. Seah PP, Fry L, Kearney JW, Campbell E, Mowlray JF, Stewart JS, et al: A comparison of histocompatibility antigens in dermatitis herpetiformis and adult coeliac disease. Br J Dermatol 94:131-138, 1976
44. McNeish AS, Nelson R, Mackintosh P: HL-A 1 and 8 in childhood coeliac disease. Lancet i:668, 1973
45. Betuel H, Gebuhrer L, Descos L, Percebois H, Minaire Y, Bertrand J: Adult celiac disease associated with HLA-DRw3 and -DRw7. Tissue Antigens 15:231-238, 1980
46. Evans DAP: Coeliac disease and HL-A8. Lancet ii:1096, 1973
47. Verkasalo M, Tiilikainen A, Kuitunen P, Savilahti E, Backman A: HLA antigens and atopy in children with coeliac disease. Gut 24:306-310, 1983
48. Solheim BG, Ek J, Thune PO, Bablien K, Bratlie A, Rankin B, et al: HLA antigens in dermatitis herpetiformis and coeliac disease. Tissue Antigens 7:57-59, 1976
49. Mann DL, Nelson DL, Katz SI, Nelson DL, Abelson LD, Strober W: Specific B-cell antigens associated with gluten-sensitive enteropathy and dermatitis herpetiformis. Lancet i:110-111, 1976
50. Betuel H, Gebuhrer L, Percebois H, Descos L, Minaire Y, Bertrand J: Association de la maladie coeliaque de l'adulte avec HLA-DRW3 et -DRW7. Gastroenterol Clin Biol 3:605-606, 1979
51. Scott H, Brandtzaeg P, Solheim BG, Thorsby E: Relation between HLA-DR like antigens and secretory component (SC) in jejunal epithelium of patients with coeliac disease or dermatitis hepetiformis. Clin Exp Immunol 44:233-238, 1981
52. Malavasi F, De Marchi M, Borelli I, Richiardi P, Ansaldi N, Boschis D, et al: Properdin factor B and glyoxalase 1 polymorphism in celiac disease. N Engl J Med 303:530-531, 1980
53. Boyer J, Chouvet B, Gebuhrer L, Betuel H, Descos L, Thivolet J: Maladie coeliaque et lupus erythemateux dissemine: Association familiale et relation avec le systeme HLA-DR. Nouv Press Med 11:525-526, 1982
54. Scholz S, Albert E: HLA and diseases: Involvement of more than one HLA-linked determinant of disease susceptibility. Immunol Rev 70:77-88, 1983
55. Arnaud-Battandier F, Schmitz J, Muller JY, Jos J, Rey J: HLA and gluten cytotoxicity *in vitro*. Gastroenterology 84:201, 1983
56. O'Driscoll BRC, Stevens FM, O'Gorman TA, Finnegan P, McWeeney JJ, Little MPG, et al: HLA type of patients with coeliac disease and malignancy in the west of Ireland. Gut 23:662-665, 1982

Wilson's Disease (Hepatolenticular Degeneration)

This is an autosomal recessive disorder characterized by a metabolic disturbance associated with an abnormal copper balance.

Family Data

Tabacchi et al.[1] typed both parents and 9 siblings of an Italian family. Four of the 9 siblings were affected by this disease and they did not have any of the 4 parental haplotypes in common. Thus, in this family there was no indication of linkage between HLA and Wilson's disease.

Reference

1. Tabacchi PL, Bordini G, Barboni, Corazza GR, Gasbarrini G: Inheritance of HLA antigens in a family with Wilson's disease. In Bodmer W et al. (eds): Histocompatibility Testing 1977. Munksgaard, Copenhagen, 1977, pp 484-485

Alcoholic Liver Disease

Population Association

The available data on this disease do not show any consistency in the results. Bailey et al.[1] first reported an association with B8 in 63 English patients. In a Norwegian study Bell and Nordhagen[2,3] found an association with B40 and a third study from Chile[4] reported a significant increase of B13 in the patients. In several other reports given in the Table 10.3 there was no significant association with any HLA antigens. The data from each of these studies and a combined analysis of the frequencies of B8 and B40 are given in Table 10.3.

TABLE 10.3. Alcoholic Liver Disease

	Patients		Controls				
Country/Population	n	%+	n	%+	RR	χ^2	Ref.
HLA-B8							
Chile	58	17	186	11	1.69	1.66	4
Australia	32	34	700	24	1.66	1.89	10
England	18	28	900	27	1.11	0.05	11
England	63	40	95	25	1.99	3.98	1
England	92	29	191	23	1.37	1.24	5
	173	33	1186	26	1.50	4.13	
	Heterogeneity χ^2 (2 df)					1.14	
France	22	18	204	27	0.65	0.68	12
Denmark	45	29	3301	25	1.25	0.49	13
Norway	79	24	234	21	1.20	0.36	3
	351	30	5625	25	1.34	4.81	
	Heterogeneity χ^2 (6 df)					3.88	
HLA-B40							
Chile	58	2	186	4	0.65	0.30	4
Australia	32	16	700	16	1.07	0.02	10
England	18	17	900	11	1.86	1.20	11
France	22	9	204	8	1.35	0.20	12
Denmark	45	13	3301	18	0.73	0.58	13
Norway	79	33	234	18	2.24	7.80	3
	196	21	5339	16	1.47	4.16	
	Heterogeneity χ^2 (4 df)					5.64	
HLA-DR2							
Australia	57	47	119	26	2.50	7.61	14

Tait and Mackay[14] observed an increased frequency of DR2 in 57 Australian patients (Table 10.3).

Disease Heterogeneity

The HLA frequency data in Table 10.3 are for the patient total (i.e., with and without cirrhosis). In the study by Bailey et al.[1] 53 patients had alcoholic liver disease and cirrhosis and 10 were without cirrhosis. The frequencies of B8 in these 2 groups were 45% and 10%, respectively. Thus, the increase was noticeable in the cirrhosis group only. Similarily, in Bell's and Nordhagen's[3] data, 43 patients were with and 36 without cirrhosis. The B40 frequencies in the 2 groups were 49% and 14%, respectively. The data of Melendez et al.[4] were also subgrouped into 40 patients with and 18 without cirrhosis. B13 was present in 27.5% of the cirrhosis and in only 11.1% of the noncirrhosis group. Thus, the frequency of B13 was higher in the patients with cirrhosis. The difference between the 2 groups was not significant, however.

Morgan et al.[5] measured the rubella and measles antibody titers in B8-positive and B8-negative patients. There was no significant difference between the 2 groups.

See also refs. 6–9 and 15–21.

References

1. Bailey RJ, Krasner N, Eddelston ALWF, Williams IR, Tee DEM, Donaich D, et al: Histocompatibility antigens, autoantibodies, and immunoglobulins in alcoholic liver disease. Br Med J 2:727-729, 1976
2. Bell H, Nordhagen R: Association between HLA-BW40 and alcoholic liver disease with cirrhosis. Br Med J 1:822, 1978
3. Bell H, Nordhagen R: HLA antigens in alcoholics, with special reference to alcoholic cirrhosis. Scand J Gastroenterol 15:453-456, 1980
4. Melendez M, Vargas-Tank L, Fuentes C, Armas-

Merimo R, Castillo D, Wolff C, et al: Distribution of HLA histocompatibility antigens, ABO blood groups and RH antigens in alcoholic liver disease. Gut 20:288-290, 1979

5. Morgan MY, Ross MGR, Ng CM, Adams DM, Thomas HC, Sherlock S: HLA-B8, immunoglobulins, and antibody responses in alcohol-related liver disease. J Clin Pathol 33:488-492, 1980
6. Eddleston ALWF, Williams R: HLA and liver disease. Br Med Bull 34:295-300, 1978
7. Dyrszka H, Eberhardt G, Eckert G: HLA-phenotype and hemochromatosis in Germany. Gastroenterology 75:555-556, 1978
8. Petera V, Bufkova D, Kulich V: The HLA system and liver disease. Cas Lek Cesk 117:367-368, 1978
9. Seignalet J, Blanc F, Lapinski H: Groupes HLA des cirrhotiques alccoliques. Nouv Presse Med 9:712, 1980
10. Morris PJ, Vaughan H, Tait BD, Mackay IR: Histocompatibility antigens (HLA): Association with immunopathic diseases and with response to microbial antigens. Aust NZ J Med 7:616-624, 1977
11. Scott BB, Rajah SM, Losowsky MS: Histocompatibility antigens in chronic liver disease. Gastroenterology 72:122-125, 1977
12. Simon M, Bourel M, Genetet B, Fauchet R, Edan G, Bisset P: Idiopathic hemochromatosis and iron overload in alcholic liver disease: Differentiation by HLA phenotype. Gastroenterology 73:655-658, 1977
13. Gluud C, Aldershvile J, Dietrichson O, Hardt F, Iversen K, Juhl E, et al: Human leucocyte antigens in patients with alcoholic liver cirrhosis. Scand J Gastroenterol 15:337-341, 1980
14. Tait BD, Mackay IR: HLA and alcoholic cirrhosis. Tissue Antigens 19:6-10, 1982
15. Gluud C, Tage-Jensen U, Bahnsen M, Dietrichson O, Svejgaard A: Autoantibodies, histocompatibility antigens and testostorone in males with alcoholic liver cirrhosis. Clin Exp Immunol 44:31-37, 1981
16. Bell H, Nordhagen R, Orjasaeter H: Association between HLA-B40 and acute alcoholic hepatitis with cirrhosis and the lack of relation between carcinoembryonic antigen and HLA in alcoholic liver disease. Scand J Gastroenterol 18:267-271, 1983
17. Saunders JB, Wodak AD, Haines A, Powell-Jackson PR, Portmann B, Davis M, et al: Accelerated development of alcoholic cirrhosis in patients with HLA-B8. Lancet i:1381-1386, 1982
18. Barbatis C, Woods J, Morton JA, Fleming KA, McMichael A, McGee J O D: Immunohistochemical analysis of HLA (A,B,C) antigens in liver disease using a monoclonal antibody. Gut 22:985-991, 1981
19. Faizallah R, Krasner NK, Walker RJ, Morris AI: Are HLA antigens important in the developmnt of alcohol-induced liver disease? Br Med J 285:531, 1982
20. Kiernan TJ, Stevens FM, Bourke M, McCarthy CF: HLA types in liver disease in the west of Ireland. Irish J Med Sci 149:63-65, 1980
21. Thomas HC, Shipton U, Montano L: The HLA system: Its relevance to the pathogenesis of liver disease. Prog Liver Dis 7:517-527, 1982

Chronic Idiopathic Pancreatitis

Population Association

In 2 Japanese studies (1 sample of 21 patients from the western part and the other of 26 from the eastern part of Japan) an association with B5 (Table 10.4) antigen was found by Homma et al.[1,2]

TABLE 10.4. Chronic Idiopathic Pancreatitis

	Patients		Controls				
Country/Population	n	%+	n	%+	RR	χ^2	Ref.
HLA-B5							
Japan	26	81	120	34	7.65	16.55	1
Japan	21	38	140	28	1.60	1.02	1
	47	62	260	31	3.31	12.33	
	Heterogeneity χ^2 (1 df)					5.23	
HLA-B13							
Italy	39	10	824	5	2.32	2.76	4
Italy	64	22	425	8	3.28	12.06	3
	103	17	1249	6	2.94	14.50	
	Heterogeneity χ^2 (1 df)					0.32	

A third report from Italy by Gullo et al.[3] observed a significant increase of B13 (Table 10.4) in 64 patients. This result, however, was not confirmed in another Italian study by Venturi Pasini et al.[4] In the combined sample the association with B13 is significant, however.

Disease Heterogeneity

In the data of Gullo et al.[3] on 64 Italian patients, no relationship between B13 and sex, age at the clinical onset of disease, etiology, presence of pain, and diabetes was observed.

References

1. Homma T, Kubo K, Sato T: HLA antigens and chronic pancreatitis in Japan. Digestion 21:267-272, 1981
2. Homma T, Aizawa T, Nagata A, Oguchi H: HLA antigens in chronic idiopathic pancreatitis compared with chronic alcoholic panceratitis. Dig Dis Sci 26:449-452, 1981
3. Gullo L, Tabacchi PL, Corazza GR, Calanca F, Campione O, Labo G: HLA-B13 and chronic calcific pancreatitis. Digest Dis Sci 27:214-216, 1982
4. Venturi Pasini C, Fagiolo U, Settin A, Petrin P, Pedrazzoli S: Pancreatite chronique et antigenes HLA. Nouv Presse Med 10:2375, 1981

Chronic Alcoholic Pancreatitis

Population Association

Ninety alcoholic patients with chronic pancreatitis from the Brittany area were typed for A and B loci antigens by Fauchet et al.[1,2] B40 was significantly increased in the patients (Table 10.5).

Homma et al.[3] reported A, B, and C loci antigen frequencies in 38 Japanese patients with alcoholic pancreatitis and 120 controls. No significant difference was found.

Disease Heterogeneity

Subgroups of patients based on daily alcohol consumption, age at onset, and presence of diabetes did not show any significant increase or decrease in the B40 frequency.

B40 was found in 8 of the 43 (18%) patients with pancreatic calcification and in 11 of the 47 (23%) patients without calcification. Thus, the increase of B40 was slightly more pronounced in the group with pancreatic calcifications.

See also ref. 4.

References

1. Fauchet R, Genetet B, Gosselin M, Gastard J: HLA antigens in chronic alcholic pancreatitis. Tissue Antigens 13:163-166, 1979
2. Gosselin M, Fauchet R, Genetet B, Gastard J: Les antigenes HLA dans la pancreatite chronique alcoolique. Gastroenterol Clin Biol 2:883-886, 1978
3. Homma T, Aizawa T, Nagata A, Oguchi H: HLA antigens in chronic idiopathic pancreatitis compared with chronic alcoholic panceratitis. Dig Dis Sci 26:449-452, 1981
4. Homma T, Kubo K, Sato T: HLA antigens and chronic pancreatitis in Japan. Digestion 21:267-272, 1981

Cryptogenic Cirrhosis of the Liver

Population Association

Scott et al.[1] reported an increased frequency of B8 in 15 patients from England (53% in patients vs. 27% in 900 controls). This difference, however, would not be significant if corrections are made for 21 A and B loci antigens compared in this study. Morris et al.[2] observed an increased frequency of A10 in 16 Australian patients (25% in patients vs. 10% in 700 controls). The frequency of B8 in this study was 25% in the patients and 24% in the controls.

The only other study is on 11 Sephardic and 16

TABLE 10.5. Chronic Alcoholic Pancreatitis

	Patients		Controls				
Country/Population	n	%+	n	%+	RR	χ^2	Ref.
HLA-B40							
France	90	21	523	8	3.08	14.15	2

Ashkenazi Jews from Israel[3] in which no association with A or B loci antigens was found.

References

1. Scott BB, Rajah SM, Losowsky MS: Histocompatibility antigens in chronic liver disease. Gastroenterology 72:122-125, 1977
2. Morris PJ, Vaughan H, Tait BD, Mackay IR: Histocompatibility antigens (HLA): Association with immunopathic diseases and with response to microbial antigens. Aust NZ J Med 7:616-624, 1977
3. Enat R, Gideoni O, Barzilai D: Histocompatibility antigens in cryptogenic cirrhosis. Gastroenterology 76:432-434, 1979

Cirrhosis with Unknown Etiology

Population Association

Ohkubo et al.[1] typed 29 Japanese patients with hepatic cirrhosis of unknown etiology for A and B loci antigens. In this sample there was a significant association with B5 and BW54 (Table 10.6).

Reference

1. Ohkubo A, Okimoto K, Iwasaki Y, Kosaka K, Juji T, Tohyama H: Association of human leukocyte antigen (HLA)-B5 and -BW22-J with hepatic cirrhosis of apparently unknown etiology. Tohoku J Exp Med 123:257-263, 1977

Chronic Active Drug-Induced Hepatitis

Population Association

Lindberg et al.[1,2] reported A and B loci antigen frequencies in 12 Swedish patients with drug-induced chronic active hepatitis. These patients presented with a histologic picture of chronic active hepatitis at their first attack of jaundice and had a history of drug treatment in association with onset of symptoms. The drugs used by these patients were oxyphenisatin, sulphamethizole, sulphamethoxypyridazine, phenylbutazone, hydralazine, and nitrofurantoin. When compared with 690 healthy controls, there was no significant deviation in the antigen frequencies.

Eade et al.[3,4] also studied 17 patients (U.S.A. and England) who had clinical and biochemical features of hepatitis after halothane exposure. In some patients a liver biopsy was performed and histology showed features of acute hepatocellular injury. All patients were negative for hepatitis B surface antigen. In this small sample, there was no evidence of association with any HLA-A and -B loci antigens.

References

1. Lindberg J, Lindholm A, Lundin P, Iwarson S: Trigger factors and HL-A antigens in chronic active hepatitis. Br Med J 4:77-79, 1975
2. Lindberg J, Lindholm A, Iwarson S: Outcome of chronic active hepatitis: Influence of histocompatibility antigens and triggering factors. J Infect Dis 137:189-193, 1978
3. Eade OE, Krawitt EL, Grice D, Wright R, and Trowell J: HLA antigens and halothane hepatitis. Lancet ii:1384-1385, 1978
4. Eade OE, Grice D, Krawitt EL, Trowell J, Albertini R, Festenstein H, et al: HLA A and B locus antigens in patients with unexplained hepatitis following halothane anaesthesis. Tissue Antigens 17:428-432, 1981

Chronic Active Hepatitis Without Hepatitis B Surface Antigen

Population Association

Mackay and Morris[1] first reported significant associations with A1 and B8 in 37 Australian patients. The results in subsequent reports from several other

TABLE 10.6. Cirrhosis with Unknown Etiology

	Patients		Controls				
Country/Population	n	%+	n	%+	RR	χ^2	Ref.
HLA-B5							
Japan	29	72	128	32	5.24	14.39	1
HLA-BW54							
Japan	29	38	128	10	5.42	13.17	1

studies from Europe and the United States (Table 10.7) were not consistent. As the frequency data in the table show, only the studies of Galbraith et al.[2] and Freudenberg et al.[3] showed significant increases of A1 and B8 in the patients. In others, these 2 antigens were not significantly increased. Moreover, Majsky et al.'s data[4] from Czechoslovakia and that of Mazzilli et al.[5] indicated a decrease of these antigens in the patient groups.

In a combined analysis the association with A1 and B8 was highly significant (Table 10.7). It should be noted, however, that the analysis included data from reports by Mackay and Morris,[1] Morris et al.[6] and Mackay and Tait.[7] It is not known whether patients in these 3 studies were the same, overlapping, or different.

Ito et al.[8] reported no associations with A and B loci antigens in 45 Japanese patients.

Opelz et al.[9] studied D locus antigen frequencies in 34 patients and DW3 was determined to be significantly associated with the disease. (Table 10.7). Similarly, in Mackay's and Tait's data[7] on 43 Australian patients typed for the DR locus, DR3 was significantly increased.

The relative risk values in Table 10.7 for DR3 and DW3 are greater than that for B8. The relative risk for B8 is higher than that for A1. Thus the primary association of the disease is probably with DR3 and DW3 antigens. An analysis of the association with DW3 in B8-positive and -negative patients by Opelz et al.[9] also showed that the association was primarily with the D locus. The increased frequencies of A1 and B8 were most probably due to the linkage disequilibrium between these alleles.

Disease Heterogeneity

In Galbraith et al.'s study[10] there were 8 patients with and 49 without hepatitis B surface antigens. None of the patients with hepatitis antigen was positive for B8. In addition, the mean titers of antibodies to rubella, measles, smooth muscle, and nuclear antigens were significantly lower than the corresponding values in the patients without the hepatitis antigen.

Opelz et al.[9] found that the patients with and without DW3 were similar in age, sex, and incidence of viral or immunoserologic markers. Sixteen of 26 patients with DW3 had cirrhosis and/or were treatment failures compared with only 3 of the 12 patients without DW3 ($p < 0.0005$). A longer duration of treatment (23 months) was required in DW3-positive patients as compared with DW3-negative patients (13 months) ($p < 0.05$).

In 24 of the 43 patients studied by Mackay and Tait[7] disease started before age 30, and 23 of these patients were DR3-positive. On the other hand, of the 19 patients in whom disease started after age 30 only 9 were positive for DR3. The difference between the 2 groups was significant ($p < 0.0005$).

Whittingham et al.[11,12] reported an association of this disease with phenotype ax at the GM locus.

Family Data

Mackay and Tait[7] noted 1 family in which the 2 affected siblings (brother and sister) did not share any haplotype. In a second family there were 5 siblings with identical haplotypes but only 1 had acquired the disease. Thus, in these 2 families the disease did not seem to be segregating with the marker HLA haplotypes.

See also refs. 13–20, 26, and 27.

References

1. Mackay IR, Morris PJ: Association of autoimmune active chronic hepatitis with HL-A1,8. Lancet ii:793-795, 1972
2. Galbraith RM, Eddleston ALWF, Smith MGM, Williams R, McSween RNM, Watkinson G, et al: Histocompatibility antigens in active chronic hepatitis and primary biliary cirrhosis. Br Med J 3:604-605, 1974
3. Freudenberg J, Baumann H, Arnold W, Berger J, Meyer zum Buschenfelde KH: HLA in different forms of chronic active hepatitis. Digestion 15:260-270, 1977
4. Majsky A, Horejsi J, Cerhova M, Korinbova P, Mimra J, Novak J: Independent HBS antigen occurrence on HLA system. Tissue Antigens 13:170-171, 1979
5. Mazzilli MC, Trabace S, Di Raimondo F, Visco G, Gandini E: HLA and chronic active hepatitis. Digestion 15:278-285, 1977
6. Morris PJ, Vaughan H, Tait BD, Mackay IR: Histocompatibility antigens (HLA): Association with immunopathic diseases and with response to microbial antigens. Aust NZ J Med 7:616-624, 1977
7. Mackay IR, Tait BD: HLA associations with autoimmune-type chronic active hepatitis: Identification of B8-DRW3 haplotype by family studies. Gastroenterology 79:95-98, 1980
8. Ito K, Nakagawa J, Ikehara K, Sugiyama T: HL-A

TABLE 10.7. Chronic Active Hepatitis Without Hepatitis B Surface Antigen

	Patients		Controls				
Country/Population	n	%+	n	%+	RR	χ^2	Ref.
HLA-A1							
Australia	48	65	700	34	3.55	17.18	6
Australia	37	60	350	31	3.29	11.88	1
Australia	56	73	586	32	5.62	31.81	7
	141	67	1636	33	4.10	59.18	
	Heterogeneity χ^2 (2 df)					1.68	
Czechoslovakia	17	12	301	28	0.42	1.84	4
Hungary	28	29	352	28	1.08	0.04	21
England	45	53	89	22	3.92	12.58	2
England	35	40	900	34	1.31	0.62	22
	80	47	989	33	2.12	8.66	
	Heterogeneity χ^2 (1 df)					4.53	
West Germany	77	31	1000	29	1.11	0.18	23
West Germany	74	53	5046	28	2.89	21.00	3
	151	42	6046	28	1.87	13.36	
	Heterogeneity χ^2 (1 df)					7.81	
Italy	7	14	266	22	0.80	0.07	5
Ireland	20	55	105	49	1.26	0.24	24
	444	49	9695	29	2.20	58.36	
	Heterogeneity χ^2 (10 df)					39.06	
HLA-B8							
U.S.A.	34	32	91	24	1.50	0.90	9
Australia	48	69	700	24	6.91	37.33	6
Australia	56	73	586	27	7.15	40.93	7
Australia	37	68	350	18	9.41	37.19	1
	141	70	1636	24	7.60	114.97	
	Heterogeneity χ^2 (2 df)					0.47	
Czechoslovakia	17	6	301	17	0.45	1.12	4
Hungary	28	21	352	16	1.47	0.71	21
England	45	62	89	17	7.68	25.15	2
England	35	29	900	27	1.13	0.12	22
	80	48	989	26	2.67	13.05	
	Heterogeneity χ^2 (1 df)					12.22	
France	35	23	152	16	1.61	1.17	25
West Germany	74	57	5046	19	5.63	54.35	3
West Germany	77	30	1000	21	1.63	3.63	23
	151	43	6046	19	3.20	45.24	
	Heterogeneity χ^2 (1 df)					12.74	
Italy	7	0	266	8	0.75	0.07	5
Ireland	20	50	105	43	1.32	0.35	24
	513	46	9938	20	3.26	135.77	
	Heterogeneity χ^2 (12 df)					67.24	
HLA-CW7							
France	35	67	152	21	7.39	25.13	25

TABLE 10.7. *(continued)*

	Patients		Controls				
Country/Population	n	%+	n	%+	RR	χ^2	Ref.
HLA-DW3							
U.S.A.	34	71	91	24	7.42	21.14	9
HLA-DR3							
Australia	43	74	119	32	5.84	20.71	7
France	35	32	152	13	3.15	7.42	25
	78	55	271	21	4.40	26.97	
	Heterogeneity χ^2 (1 df)					1.16	

antigens, chronic active hepatitis, and idiopathic biliary cirrhosis. Nippon Rinsho 36:3181-3188, 1978
9. Opelz G, Vogten AJM, Summerskill WHJ, Schalm SW, Terasaki PI: HLA determinants in chronic active liver disease: Possible relation of HLA-DW3 to prognosis. Tissue Antigens 9:36-40, 1977
10. Galbraith RM, Eddleston ALWF, Williams R, Webster ADB, Pattison J, Doniach D, et al: Enhanced antibody responses in active chronic hepatitis: Relation to HLA-B8 and HLA-B12 and portosystemic shunting. Lancet i:930-934, 1976
11. Whittingham S, Mathews JD, Schanfield MS, Tait BD, Mackay IR: Effect of gene interaction on susceptibility to disease. Tissue Antigens 17:252-254, 1981
12. Whittingham S, Mathews JD, Schanfield MS, Tait BD, Mackay IR: Interaction of HLA and Gm in autoimmune chronic active hepatitis. Clin Exp Immunol 43:80-86, 1981
13. Eddleston ALWF, Williams R: HLA and liver disease. Br Med Bull 34:295-300, 1978
14. Vogten AJM, Shorter RG, Opelz G: HLA and cell-mediated immunity in HBsAg negative chronic active hepatitis. Gut 20:523-525, 1979
15. Freudenberg J, Meyer Zum Buschenfelde KH, Arnold W: Histokompatibilitats-(HLA) Antigene bei Patienten mit HBs AG-positiver und -negativer chronisch aktiver Hepatitis und gesunden Tragern von HBsAG und anti-HBs. Klin Wochenschr 54:579-583, 1976
16. Dumble LJ, Mackay IR: HLA and chronic active hepatitis (CAH). Digestion 15:254-259, 1977
17. Freudenberg J, Erdmann K, Berger J, Meyer Zum Buschenfelde KH, Forster E, Berger J: HL-A bei lebererkrankungen. Klin Wochenschr 51:1075-1076, 1973
18. Eddleston ALWF, Williams R: Inadequate antibody response to HBsAg or supressor T-cell defect in development of active chronic hepatitis. Lancet ii:1543-1545, 1974
19. Horejsi J, Cerhova M, Majsky A, Mimra J: HLA system and its association to chronic hepatitis and persistence of HBsAg in the organism. Tijdschr Gastroenterol 6:457-464, 1978
20. Bertrams J, Kuwert E, Reis HE, Selmair H, Wiese W: Australia Antigen, histokompatibilitats (HL-A) Antigene und Autolymphozytotoxine (cococy) bei verschiedenen Formen der Hepatitis und Zirrhose. Zbl Bakt Hyg 227:372-377, 1974
21. Par A, Bajtai G, Gyodi E, Ambrus M, Hernadi E, Tenyi I: HLA antigens in chronic active hepatitis. Acta Med Acad Sci Hung 37:17-24, 1980
22. Scott BB, Rajah SM, Losowsky MS: Histocompatibility antigens in chronic liver disease. Gastroenterology 72:122-125, 1977
23. Bertrams J, Reis HE, Kuwert E, Selmair H: Hepatitis associated antigen (HAA), HL-A antigens and auto-lymphocytotoxins (COCOCY) in chronic aggressive and chronic persistent hepatitis. Z Immun Forsch 146:300-307, 1974
24. Kiernan TJ, Stevens FM, Bourke M, McCarthy CF: HLA types in liver disease in the west of Ireland. Irish J Med Sci 149:63-65, 1980
25. Lepage V, Degos F, Carella G, De Lima M, Giraud MC, Degos L: HLA-Cw7 and HBsAg negative chronic active hepatitis. Tissue Antigens 18:105-107, 1981
26. Tait BD, MacKay IR, Kastelan A, Dausset J, Mayer S, Okochi K: Chronic liver disease including chronic active hepatitis. In Terasaki PI (ed): Histocompatibility Testing 1980. UCLA Tissue Typing Laboratory, Los Angeles, 1981, pp 657-661
27. Delpre G, Gazit E: HLA typing: An indicator of severity of disease. Gastroenterology 80:1083-1091, 1981

Chronic Active Hepatitis with Hepatitis B Surface Antigen

Population Association

HLA-A and -B loci frequency data available from Europe and the United States (1-5, and other references in Table 10.8) clearly show that this form

TABLE 10.8. Chronic Active Hepatitis with Hepatitis B Surface Antigen

Country/Population	Patients n	Patients %+	Controls n	Controls %+	RR	χ^2	Ref.
HLA-BW35							
Czechoslovakia	48	13	301	14	0.97	0.00	14
Hungary	47	26	352	23	1.20	0.28	15
England	9	22	89	14	1.96	0.83	16
West Germany	68	22	5046	17	1.41	1.42	17
Italy	35	46	266	33	1.73	2.40	18
Austria	16	56	450	21	4.70	10.06	2
Sweden	13	8	690	13	0.82	0.07	19
	236	26	7194	18	1.52	7.22	
	Heterogeneity χ^2 (6 df)					7.86	

of hepatitis is not associated with A1 and B8 antigens.

In Penner et al.'s[2] data a significant increased frequency of BW35 was also found (Table 10.8). However, as the data in the table show, other studies have not reported any association with this antigen. In the combined sample the association with BW35 was marginally significant, primarily because of the data of Penner et al.[2]

When Ito et al.[6] studied 20 Japanese patients and 114 controls, they found no significant deviations in A and B loci antigen frequencies.

Opelz et al.[1] did D locus typing on 4 patients. Two were positive for DW3 (Table 10.8). This antigen, however, was significantly associated in patients negative for hepatitis B surface antigen.

See also refs. 7–13 and 20–23.

References

1. Opelz G, Vogten AJM, Summerskill WHJ, Schalm SW, Terasaki PI: HLA determinants in chronic active liver disease: Possible relation of HLA-DW3 to prognosis. Tissue Antigens 9:36-40, 1977
2. Penner E, Grabner G, Dittrich H, Mayr WR: HLA antigen in HBS antigens positive chronic active hepatitis. Tissue Antigens 10:63-64, 1977
3. Tolentino P, Astaldi A: T cells, B cells, and HL-A8 in chronic active hepatitis. Lancet i:690, 1975
4. Giani G, Chiaramonte M, Pasini CV, Fagiolo U, Naccarato R: Hepatitis B surface antigenemia and HLA antigens. N Engl J Med 300:1056-1057, 1979
5. Lepage V, Degos F, Carella G, De Lima M, Giraud MC, Degos L: HLA-Cw7 and HBsAg negative chronic active hepatitis. Tissue Antigens 18:105-107, 1981
6. Ito K, Nakagawa J, Ikehara K, Sugiyama T: HL-A antigens, chronic active hepatitis, and idiopathic biliary cirrhosis. Nippon Rinsho 36:3181-3188, 1978
7. Eddleston ALWF, Williams R: HLA and liver disease. Br Med Bull 34:295-300, 1978
8. Freudenberg J, Meyer Zum Buschenfelde KH, Arnold W: Histokompatibilitats-(HLA) Antigene bei Patienten mit HBsAG-positiver und -negativer chronisch aktiver Hepatitis und gesunden Tragern von HBsAG und anti-HBs. Klin Wschr 54:579-583, 1976
9. Freudenberg J, Erdmann K, Berger J, Meyer Zum Buschenfelde KH, Forster E, Berger J: HL-A bei Lebererkrankungen. Klin Wochenschr 51:1075-1076, 1973
10. Galbraith RM, Eddleston ALWF, Williams R, Webster ADB, Pattison J, Doniach D, et al: Enhanced antibody responses in active chronic hepatitis: Relation to HLA-B8 and HLA-B12 and portosystemic shunting. Lancet i:930-934, 1976
11. Eddleston ALWF, Williams R: Inadequate antibody response to HBsAg or supressor T-cell defect in development of active chronic hepatitis. Lancet ii:1543-1545, 1974
12. Horejsi J, Cerhova M, Majsky A, Mimra J: HLA system and its association to chronic hepatitis and persistence of HBsAg in the organism. Tijdschr Gastroenterol 6:457-464, 1978
13. Lindberg J, Lindholm A, Iwarson S: Outcome of chronic active hepatitis: Influence of histocompatibility antigens and triggering factors. J Infect Dis 137:189-193, 1978
14. Majsky A, Horejsi J, Cerhova M, Korinbova P, Mimra J, Novak J: Independent HBS antigen occurrence on HLA system. Tissue Antigens 13:170-171, 1979
15. Par A, Bajtai G, Gyodi E, Ambrus M, Hernadi E, Tenyi I: HLA antigens in chronic active hepatitis. Acta Med Acad Sci Hung 37:17-24, 1980

16. Galbraith RM, Eddleston ALWF, Smith MGM, Williams R, McSween RNM, Watkinson G, et al.: Histocompatibility antigens in active chronic hepatitis and primary biliary cirrhosis. Br Med J 3:604-605, 1974
17. Freudenberg J, Baumann H, Arnold W, Berger J, Meyer zum Buschenfelde KH: HLA in different forms of chronic active hepatitis. Digestion 15:260-270, 1977
18. Mazzilli MC, Trabace S, Di Raimondo F, Visco G, Gandini E: HLA and chronic active hepatitis. Digestion 15:278-285, 1977
19. Lindberg J, Lindholm A, Lundin P, Iwarson S: Trigger factors and HL-A antigens in chronic active hepatitis. Br Med J 4:77-79, 1975
20. Tait BD, MacKay IR, Kastelan A, Dausset J, Mayer S, Okochi K: Chronic liver disease including chronic active hepatitis. In Terasaki PI (ed): Histocompatibility Testing 1980. UCLA Tissue Typing Laboratory, Los Angeles, 1981, pp 657-661
21. Whittingham S, Mathews JD, Schanfield MS, Tait BD, Mackay IR: Effect of gene interaction on susceptibility to disease. Tissue Antigens 17:252-254, 1981
22. Montano L, Miescher GC, Goodall AH, Wiedmann KH, Janossy G, Thomas HC: Hepatitis B virus and HLA antigen display in the liver during chronic hepatitis B virus infection. Hepatology 2:557-561, 1982
23. Thomas HC, Shipton U, Montano L: The HLA system: Its relevance to the pathogenesis of liver disease. Prog Liver Dis 7:517-527, 1982

Chronic Active Cryptogenic Hepatitis

Population Association

Lindberg et al.[1] first reported an increased frequency of B8 in 16 Swedish patients with histologically verified chronic active hepatitis at their first attack of jaundice. There was no serologic evidence of viral hepatitis and also no history of drug exposure. B8 was present in 62.5% of the patients as compared with 23.2% in 690 healthy controls ($p < 0.05$). In a later report by the same group of authors[2], 4 additional patients were included in the study. B8 was significantly increased (Table 10.9). In this sample 90% of the patients were females.

A third study by Freudenberg et al.[3] on 32 German patients also reported a nonsignificant increase of B8 in the patients (Table 10.9). In the combined sample the association with B8 was significant but there was also evidence of heterogeneity in the data (Table 10.9).

References

1. Lindberg J, Lindholm A, Lundin P, Iwarson S: Trigger factors and HL-A antigens in chronic active hepatitis. Br Med J 4:77-79, 1975
2. Lindberg J, Lindholm A, Iwarson S: Outcome of chronic active hepatitis: Influence of histocompatibility antigens and triggering factors. J Infect Dis 137:189-193, 1978
3. Freudenberg J, Baumann H, Arnold W, Berger J, Meyer zum Buschenfelde KH: HLA in different forms of chronic active hepatitis. Digestion 15:260-270, 1977

Chronic Active Hepatitis (Unspecified)

Population Association

The patients included in this category could not be classified in any of the 4 previously discussed types of hepatitis. As the combined analysis of the data from several studies from Europe and the United States in Table 10.10 show, A1 and B8 were significantly increased in the patients. In addition, DR3 and DW3 were also significantly associated in this group of patients. Williams et al.[1] found a significantly increased frequency of DR4 in 17 patients

TABLE 10.9. Chronic Active Cryptogenic Hepatitis

	Patients		Controls				
Country/Population	n	%+	n	%+	RR	χ^2	Ref.
HLA-B8							
West Germany	32	28	5046	19	1.71	2.02	3
Sweden	20	75	690	23	9.41	21.19	2
	52	46	5736	19	3.25	15.57	
	Heterogeneity χ^2 (1 df)					7.63	

TABLE 10.10. Chronic Active Hepatitis (Unspecified)

	Patients		Controls				
Country/Population	n	%+	n	%+	RR	χ^2	Ref.
HLA-A1							
U.S.A.	38	45	91	28	2.09	3.54	6
U.S.A.	21	48	216	24	2.91	5.75	2
U.S.A.	17	35	81	25	1.65	0.86	1
	76	44	388	25	2.21	9.44	
	Heterogeneity χ^2 (2 df)					0.70	
West European (unspecified)	50	56	332	26	3.59	17.49	7
West Germany	51	24	1000	29	0.79	0.51	8
West Germany	19	27	83	18	1.74	1.00	9
	70	25	1083	28	0.97	0.01	
	Heterogeneity χ^2 (1 df)					1.49	
Italy	42	19	266	22	0.87	0.13	10
	238	36	2069	26	1.72	13.23	
	Heterogeneity χ^2 (6 df)					16.04	
HLA-B8							
U.S.A.	21	62	216	18	7.19	18.24	2
U.S.A.	17	18	81	24	0.77	0.19	1
U.S.A.	38	34	91	24	1.64	1.44	6
	76	38	388	21	2.37	9.91	
	Heterogeneity χ^2 (2 df)					9.95	
West European (unspecified)	50	52	332	15	6.08	32.49	7
England	17	29	23	35	0.78	0.15	11
West Germany	51	22	1000	21	1.09	0.07	8
West Germany	19	16	83	17	1.02	0.00	9
	70	20	1083	21	1.08	0.06	
	Heterogeneity χ^2 (1 df)					0.01	
Italy	42	10	266	8	1.38	0.39	10
	255	31	2092	18	2.13	23.42	
	Heterogeneity χ^2 (7 df)					29.55	
HLA-DW3							
U.S.A.	38	68	91	24	6.49	20.41	6
HLA-DR3							
U.S.A.	17	24	81	22	1.19	0.09	1
West European (unspecified)	46	43	332	17	3.68	16.03	7
	63	38	413	18	2.81	13.23	
	Heterogeneity χ^2 (1 df)					2.89	
HLA-DR4							
U.S.A.	17	71	81	22	8.05	13.85	1

(Table 10.10). In this study, there was no association with DR3 (Table 10.10).

Page et al.[2] found 6 of 21 patients (28.6%) homozygous for B8 as compared with 2.8% in 216 controls ($p < 0.0001$). Similarly, 19.0% of the 21 patients were homozygous for A1 as compared with 0.9% of the controls ($p < 0.0001$). It should be noted that homozygosity for these antigens in the patients was determined by family study but in the controls individuals typed for only A1 or B8 antigens were counted as homozygous. Thus, homozygosity in the controls represented an overestimate.

Disease Heterogeneity

Page et al.[2] did not find any difference in severity of liver disease or associated vasculitis symptoms in the 6 patients homozygous for B8 when compared with other patients.

See also refs. 3-5.

References

1. Williams RM, Martin S, Falchuk KR, Trey C, Dubey DP, Cannady WG, et al: Increased frequency of HLA-DRW4 in chronic active hepatitis. Vox Sang 35:366-369, 1978
2. Page AR, Sharp HL, Greenberg LJ, Yunis EJ: Genetic analysis of patients with chronic active hepatitis. J Clin Invest 56:530-535, 1975
3. Hoshino K, Inouye H, Unokuchi T, Ito M, Tamaoki N, Tsuji K: HLA and disease in Japanese. In Dausset, Svejgaard A (eds): HLA and Disease. De L'institut National De La Sante Et De La Recherche Medicale, Paris 1976, p 249
4. Bertrams J, Kuwert E, Reis HE, Selmair H, Wiese W: Australia Antigen, histokompatibilitats (HL-A) Antigene und Autolymphozytotoxine (cococy) bei verschiedenen Formen der Hepatitis und Zirrhose. Zbl Bakt Hyg 227:372-377, 1974
5. Williams RM: Ia-like antigens in human autoimmune diseases: HLA and DRW antigens in chronic active hepatitis and diabetes mellitus. In Amos DB, Schwartz RS, Janichi BW (eds): Immune Mechanisms and Disease. Academic Press, New York, 1979, pp 163-177
6. Opelz G, Vogten AJM, Summerskill WHJ, Schalm SW, Terasaki PI: HLA determinants in chronic active liver disease: Possible relation of HLA-DW3 to prognosis. Tissue Antigens 9:36-40, 1977
7. Batchelor JR, Morris PJ: Active chronic hepatitis: Joint Report. In Bodmer W et al. (eds): Histocompatibility Testing 1977. Munksgaard, Copenhagen, 1978, pp 214-217
8. Bertrams J, Reis HE, Kuwert E, Selmair H: Hepatitis associated antigen (HAA), HL-A antigens and auto-lymphocytotoxins (COCOCY) in chronic aggressive and chronic persistent hepatitis. Z Immun-Forsch 146:300-307, 1974
9. Freudenberg J, Erdmann K, Berger J, Meyer Zum Buschenfelde KH, Forster E, Berger J: HL-A bei Lebererkrankungen. Klin Wochenschr 51:1075-1076, 1973
10. Mazzilli MC, Trabace S, Di Raimondo F, Visco G, Gandini E: HLA and chronic active hepatitis. Digestion 15:278-285, 1977
11. Scott BB, Swinburne ML, Rajah SM, Losowsky MS: HL-A8 and the immune response to gluten. Lancet ii:374-377, 1974

Acute Hepatitis

Population Association

In a study of 124 German patients and 83 controls no association with A and B loci antigens was observed by Freudenberg et al.[1]

Reference

1. Freudenberg J, Erdmann K, Berger J, Meyer Zum Buschenfelde KH, Forster E, Berger J: HL-A bei Lebererkrankungen. Klin Wochenschr 51:1075-1076, 1973

Crohn's Disease

Population Association

Van Den Berg-Loonen et al.[1] reported a significant association with B18 in 51 patients from the Netherlands. However, in several studies (before and after this report) this association was not confirmed. In the analysis of pooled data in the Table 10.11 there was a marginally significant association with B15.

DR locus antigens were studied by Pena et al.,[2] Smolen et al.,[3] and Caruso et al.[4] In the combined sample there was no evidence of association with any of these antigens.

In a small sample of Japanese patients (Table 10.11) an increased frequency of B27 was reported by Hiwatashi et al.[5]

Delpre et al.[6] reported no significant association wth A and B loci antigens in 18 patients from Israel.

TABLE 10.11. Crohn's Disease

Country/Population	Patients n	Patients %+	Controls n	Controls %+	RR	χ^2	Ref.
HLA-B15							
Canada	77	17	600	11	1.70	2.70	23
BENELUX	57	26	478	16	1.87	3.88	24
BENELUX	149	20	4000	16	1.33	1.89	2
	206	22	4478	16	1.47	4.95	
	Heterogeneity χ^2 (1 df)					0.82	
England	64	8	100	14	0.56	1.27	9
England	18	22	50	12	2.10	1.27	25
England	43	7	375	10	0.77	0.22	24
England	100	18	283	10	1.99	4.59	26
	225	13	808	11	1.32	1.48	
	Heterogeneity χ^2 (3 df)					5.87	
West Germany	74	8	350	5	1.73	1.40	27
West Germany	56	11	268	12	0.96	0.01	28
	130	9	618	8	1.27	0.55	
	Heterogeneity χ^2 (1 df)					0.86	
Austria	27	11	450	10	1.26	0.17	3
Norway	19	21	527	20	1.15	0.07	29
Sweden	62	24	335	21	1.21	0.35	30
	746	16	7816	15	1.38	9.30	
	Heterogeneity χ^2 (11 df)					8.52	
HLA-B27							
Japan	10	10	120	0	38.05	8.23	5

Family Data

Segregation of HLA haplotypes has been studied in 9 families by Pena et al.,[2] 1 family by Achord et al.,[7] 5 families by Schwartz et al.,[8] and in 5 families by Eade et al.[9] In these 20 multiple-case families the segregation was not significantly different from the expected Mendelian segregation[7] and thus there was no evidence for linkage between Crohn's disease and HLA.

See also refs. 10–22 and 31–34.

References

1. Van Den Berg-Loonen EM, Dekker-Saeys BJ, Meuwissen SGM, Nijenhuis LE, Engelfriet CP: Histocompatibility antigens and other genetic markers in ankylosing spondylitis and inflammatory bowel diseases. J Immunogenet 4:167-175, 1977
2. Pena AS, Biemond I, Kuiper G, Weterman IT, Van Leeuwen A, Schreuder I, et al: HLA antigen distribution and HLA haplotype segregation in Crohn's disease. Tissue Antigens 16:56-61, 1982
3. Smolen JS, Gangl A, Polterauer P, Menzel EJ, Mayr WR. HLA antigens in inflammatory bowel disease. Gastroenterology 82:34-38, 1982
4. Caruso C, Oliva L, Palmeri P, Cottone M: B cell alloantigens in Sicilian patients with Crohn's disease. Tissue Antigens 21:170-172, 1983
5. Hiwatashi N, Kikuchi T, Masamune O, Ouchi E, Watanabe H, Goyo Y: HLA antigens in inflammatory bowel disease. Tohoku J Exp Med 131:381-385, 1980
6. Delpre G, Kadish U, Gazit E, Joshua H, Zamir R: HLA antigens in ulcerative colitis and Crohn's disease in Israel. Gastroenterology 79:1452-1457, 1980
7. Achord JL, Gunn CH, Jackson JF: Regional enteritis and HLA concordance in multiple siblings. Digest Dis Sci 27:330-332, 1982
8. Schwartz SE, Siegelbaum SP, Fazio TL, Hubbell C, Henry JB: Regional enteritis: Evidence for genetic transmission by HLA typing. Ann Intern Med 93:424-427, 1980

9. Eade OE, Moulton C, MacPherson BR, Andre-Ukena SST, Albertini RJ, Beeken WL: Discordant HLA haplotype segregation in familial Crohn's disease. Gastroenterology 79:271-275, 1980
10. Huaux J, Fiasse R, De Bruyere M, De Deuxchaisnes CN: HLA B27 in regional enteritis with and without ankylosing spondylitis or sacroiliitis. J Rheumatol 4(Suppl 3):60-63, 1977
11. Monconduit M, Cavelier B, Deshayes P, Haebetsweiler P, Colim R, Geffrey Y, et al: Rheumatic symptoms in Crohn's disease and the HLA system. Biomedicine 27:41-42, 1977
12. Tsuchiya M, Ono A, Asakura H, Mizuno Y, Aiso S: Major histocompatibility complex in ulcerative colitis and Crohn's disease. Nippon Rinsho 36:3151-3158, 1978
13. Ono A, Kurita K, Tsuchiya M, Yamanaka I, Tsuji K: HLA antigens of intrathymic and peripheral lymphocytes in autoimmune disease. Keio J Med 24:367-376, 1975
14. Russell AS, Schlaut J, Percy JS, Dossetor JB: HL-A (transplantation) antigens in ankylosing spondylitis and Crohn's disease. J Rheumatol 1:203-209, 1974
15. Bluestone R, Morris RI, Metzger AL, Terasaki PI: (HLA) W27 and the spondylitis of chronic inflammatory bowel disease and psoriasis. Ann Rheum Dis 34:31-32, 1975
16. Morris RI, Metzger AL, Bluestone R, Terasaki PI: HL-A-W27-A useful discriminator in the arthropathies of inflammatory bowel disease. N Engl J Med 290:1117-1119, 1974
17. Russell AS, Schlaut JW: HL A antigens in inflammatory bowel disease. Lancet i:451, 1974
18. De Deuxchaisnes CN, Huaux JP, Fiasse R, De Bruyere M: Ankylosing spondylitis, sacroiliitis, regional enteritis, and HL-A27. Lancet i:1238-1239, 1974
19. Morris RI, Metzger AL, Bluestone MB, Terasaki PI: HL-A W27, spondylitis, and enteritis. N Engl J Med 291:681, 1974
20. Herd JK: HL-A W27, spondylitis, and enteritis. N Engl J Med 291:680-681, 1974
21. Lewkonia RM, Woodrow JC, Mcconnell RB, Price-Evans DA: HL-A antigens in inflammatory bowel disease. Lancet i:574-575, 1974
22. Van Den Berg-Loonen PM, Dekker-Saeys AJ, Meuwissen SGM, Nijenhuis LE: Histocompatibility antigens and other markers in ankylosing spondylitis and inflammatory bowel disease. J Rheumatol 4(Suppl 3):57-59, 1977
23. Russell AS, Percy JS, Schlaut J, Sartor VE, Goodhart JM, Sherbaniuk RW, et al: Transplantation antigens in Crohn's disease: Linkage of associated ankylosing spondylitis with HL-AW27. Am J Dig Dis 20:359-361, 1975
24. Woodrow JC, Lewkonia RM, McConnell RB, Van Den Berg-Loonen EM, Meuwissen SGM, Dekker-Saeys BJ, et al: HLA antigens in inflammatory bowel disease. Tissue Antigens 11:147-152, 1978
25. Gleeson MH, Walker JS, Wentzel J, Chapman JA, Harris R: Human leucocyte antigens in Crohn's disease and ulcerative colitis. Gut 13:438-440, 1972
26. Mallas EG, Mackintosh P, Asquith P, Cooke WT: Histocompatibility antigens in inflammatory bowel disease. Gut 17:906-910, 1976
27. Jacoby RK, Jayson MIV: HL-A27 in Crohn's disease. Ann Rheum Dis 33:422-424, 1974
28. Asquith P, Mackintosh P, Stokes PL, Holmes GKT, Cooke WT: Histocompatibility antigens in patients with inflammatory-bowel disease. Lancet i:113-115, 1974
29. Thorsby E, Lie SO: Relationship between the HL-A system and susceptibility to disease. Tranplant Proc 3:1305-1307, 1971
30. Bergman L, Lindblom JB, Safwenberg J, Krause U: HL-A frequencies in Crohn's disease and ulcerative colitis. Tissue Antigens 7:145-150, 1976
31. Tiwari JL, Betuel H, Gebuhrer L, Morton NE: Genetic epidemiology of coeliac disease. Genet Epidemiol 1:37-42, 1984
32. Rossen RD: HLA and disease: A postulated role for HLA in gastrointestinal diseases. Gastroenterology 78:1629-1635, 1980
33. Arnaud-Battandier F, Schmitz J, Muller JY, Jos J, Rey J: HLA and gluten cytotoxicity *in vitro*. Gastroenterology 84:201, 1983
34. Holdstock G, Macpherson B, Beeken WL: HLA B8 and granuloma formation in Crohn's disease. Gut 23:600-602, 1982

Crohn's Disease with Ankylosing Spondylitis

Population Association

The data from 4 independent studies showed that antigen B27 was significantly increased in patients with Crohn's disease and ankylosing spondylitis (Table 10.12). However, it should be noted that the association of B27 was not as strong as in the case of patients with only ankylosing spondylitis. The relative risk was only 9.79. (See Ankylosing Spondylitis.)

See also refs. 1 and 2.

References

1. Russell AS, Schlaut J, Percy JS, Dossetor JB: HL-A (transplantation) antigens in ankylosing spondylitis and Crohn's disease. J Rheumatol 1:203-209, 1974
2. De Deuxchaisnes CN, Huaux JP, Fiasse R, De Bruyere M: Ankylosing spondylitis, sacroiliitis, re-

TABLE 10.12. Crohn's Disease with Ankylosing Spondylitis

	Patients		Controls				
Country/Population	n	%+	n	%+	RR	χ^2	Ref.
HLA-B27							
Canada	11	91	600	9	70.73	29.57	3
BENELUX	19	26	250	8	4.20	7.19	4
BENELUX	30	50	778	10	8.95	34.52	5
	49	41	1028	10	6.99	40.37	
	Heterogeneity χ^2 (1 df)					1.34	
France	6	67	336	13	12.08	11.07	6
	66	51	1964	10	9.79	73.35	
	Heterogeneity χ^2 (3 df)					9.01	

gional enteritis, and HL-A27. Lancet i:1238-1239, 1974
3. Russell AS, Percy JS, Schlaut J, Sartor VE, Goodhart JM, Sherbaniuk RW, et al: Transplantation antigens in Crohn's disease: Linkage of associated ankylosing spondylitis with HL-AW27. Am J Dig Dis 20:359-361, 1975
4. Huaux J, Fiasse R, De Bruyere M, De Deuxchaisnes CN: HLA B27 in regional enteritis with and without ankylosing spondylitis or sacroiliitis. J Rheumatol 4(Suppl 3):60-63, 1977
5. Van Den Berg-Loonen EM, Dekker-Saeys BJ, Meuwissen SGM, Nijenhuis LE, Engelfriet CP: Histocompatibility antigens and other genetic markers in ankylosing spondylitis and inflammatory bowel diseases. J Immunogenet 4:167-175, 1977
6. Monconduit M, Cavelier B, Deshayes P, Haebetsweiler P, Colim R, Geffrey Y, et al: Rheumatic symptoms in Crohn's disease and the HLA system. Biomedicine 27:41-42, 1977

Crohn's Disease with Peripheral Arthritis

Population Association

In a small sample of 13 French patients studied by Monconduit et al.,[1] B17 was significantly increased (Table 10.13). All patients had Crohn's disease and acute or peripheral arthritis.

Reference

1. Monconduit M, Cavelier B, Deshayes P, Haebetsweiler P, Colim R, Geffrey Y, et al: Rheumatic symptoms in Crohn's discasc and thc HLA system. Biomedicine 27:41-42, 1977

Ulcerative Colitis

Population Association

A combined analysis of A and B loci frequency data from several studies on Caucasian populations showed a significant association with B27 (Table 10.14).

Schrumpf et al.[1] reported DR antigen frequencies in 34 Norwegian patients. DR3 was present in 35% of the patients as compared with 19% of the controls (sample size unknown).

Nahir et al.[2] and Delpre et al.[3] reported A and B loci antigen data on Ashkenazi Jews from Israel. In the pooled sample BW35 was significantly increased (Table 10.14).

TABLE 10.13. Crohn's Disease with Peripheral Arthritis

	Patients		Controls				
Country/Population	n	%+	n	%+	RR	χ^2	Ref.
HLA-B17							
France	13	54	336	7	15.12	23.65	1

The 3 studies from Japan[4–6] showed significant associations with AW19 and B5.

Disease Heterogeneity

Mallas et al.[7] noted a significantly increased incidence of total colonic involvement in patients positive for B27. In the report of Smolen et al.[8], no correlation between HLA antigens and clinical parameters, such as activity, number of exacerbations, or extent of the disease was observed.

Tsuchiya et al.[4] and Hiwatashi et al.[5] subdivided their patients on the basis of the extent of lesion: proctitis and total colitis. In the study by Tsuchiya et al.[4] there were 8 patients with proctitis and 36 with total colitis (extending over the rectum). The frequencies of B5 in these 2 groups were 37.5% and 80.6%, respectively. There was no significant difference between those with proctitis and controls (Table 10.14). Similarly, the report by Hiwatashi et al.[5] included 14 patients with proctitis and 46 with left-sided and total colitis. The frequencies of B5 in these 2 groups were 50.9% and 65.2%, respectively. There was no significant difference between the proctitis group and controls (Table 10.14). In both studies the subdivision of patients on the basis of age at onset and sex did not show any clear association in any particular subgroup.

In the data of Delpre et al.[3] subdivision of patients on the basis of age at onset and severity of the disease did not produce any significant difference in the frequency of BW38.

Family Data

Tsuchiya et al.[4] reported a small family in which both parents and 3 siblings were typed for A and B loci antigens. The 2 affected siblings did not share

TABLE 10.14. Ulcerative Colitis

	Patients		Controls				
Country/Population	n	%+	n	%+	RR	χ^2	Ref.
HLA-AW19							
Japan	44	0	271	21	0.04	9.62	4
HLA-B5							
Japan	44	73	271	41	3.79	14.42	4
Japan	60	62	120	40	2.42	7.63	5
	104	67	391	41	2.96	21.15	
	Heterogeneity χ^2 (1 df)					0.89	
HLA-B27							
BENELUX	58	19	778	10	2.17	5.09	17
England	36	22	180	9	2.90	5.37	18
England	51	12	375	8	1.65	1.28	18
England	100	14	283	7	2.18	4.65	7
	187	15	838	8	2.17	10.53	
	Heterogeneity χ^2 (2 df)					0.77	
Austria	30	13	450	8	1.88	1.47	8
Sweden	51	16	335	13	1.32	0.50	19
	326	16	2401	9	1.96	16.33	
	Heterogeneity χ^2 (5 df)					2.03	
HLA-BW35							
Jews (unspecified)	60	53	631	31	2.50	11.66	3
Jews (unspecified)	30	37	100	23	1.97	2.46	2
	90	48	731	30	2.34	13.90	
	Heterogeneity χ^2 (1 df)					0.22	

a haplotype. The haplotypes of 1 affected and 1 healthy sibling were identical.

See also refs. 9–16 and 20–22.

References

1. Schrumpf E, Fausa O, Forre O, Dobloug JH, Ritland S, Thorsby E: HLA antigens and immunoregulatory T cells in ulcerative colitis associated with hepatobiliary disease. Scand J Gastroenterol 17:187-191, 1982
2. Nahir M, Gideoni O, Eidelman S, Barzilai A: HLA antigens in ulcerative colitis. Lancet ii:573, 1976
3. Delpre G, Kadish U, Gazit E, Joshua H, Zamir R: HLA antigens in ulcerative colitis and Crohn's disease in Israel. Gastroenterology 79:1452-1457, 1980
4. Tsuchiya M, Yoshida T, Asakura H, Hibi T, Omoa T, Mizumo Y, et al: HLA antigens and ulcerative colitis in Japan. Digestion 15:286-294, 1977
5. Hiwatashi N, Kikuchi T, Masamune O, Ouchi E, Watanabe H, Goyo Y: HLA antigens in inflammatory bowel disease. Tohoku J Exp Med 131:381-385, 1980
6. Ono A, Kurita K, Tsuchiya M, Yamanaka I, Tsuji K: HLA antigens of intrathymic and peripheral lymphocytes in autoimmune disease. Keio J Med 24:367-376, 1975
7. Mallas EG, Mackintosh P, Asquith P, Cooke WT: Histocompatibility antigens in inflammatory bowel disease. Gut 17:906-910, 1976
8. Smolen JS, Gangl A, Polterauer P, Menzel EJ, Mayr WR: HLA antigens in inflammatory bowel disease. Gastroenterology 82:34-38, 1982
9. Tsuchiya M, Ono A, Asakura H, Mizuno Y, Aiso S: Major histocompatibility complex in ulcerative colitis and Crohn's disease. Nippon Rinsho 36:3151-3158, 1978
10. Gleeson MH, Walker JS, Wentzel J, Chapman JA, Harris R: Human leucocyte antigens in Crohn's disease and ulcerative colitis. Gut 13:438-440, 1972
11. Bluestone R, Morris RI, Metzger AL, Terasaki PI: (HLA) W27 and the spondylitis of chronic inflammatory bowel disease and psoriasis. Ann Rheum Dis 34:31-32, 1975
12. Morris RI, Metzger AL, Bluestone R, Terasaki PI: HL-A-W27-A useful discriminator in the arthropathies of inflammatory bowel disease. N Engl J Med 290:1117-1119, 1974
13. Macrae I, Wright V: A family study of ulcerative colitis. Ann Rheum Dis 32:16-20, 1973
14. Brewerton DA, Caffrey M, Nicholls AN, Walters D, James DCO: HL-A27 and arthropathies associated with ulcerative colitis and psoriasis. Lancet i:956-957, 1974
15. Asquith P, Mackintosh P, Stokes PL, Holmes GKT, Cooke WT: Histocompatibility antigens in patients with inflammatory-bowel disease. Lancet i:113-115, 1974
16. Van Den Berg-Loonen PM, Dekker-Saeys AJ, Meuwissen SGM, Nijenhuis LE: Histocompatibility antigens and other markers in ankylosing spondylitis and inflammatory bowel disease. J Rheumatol 4 (Suppl 3):57-59, 1977
17. Van Den Berg-Loonen EM, Dekker-Saeys BJ, Meuwissen SGM, Nijenhuis LE, Engelfriet CP: Histocompatibility antigens and other genetic markers in ankylosing spondylitis and inflammatory bowel diseases. J Immunogenet 4:167-175, 1977
18. Woodrow JC, Lewkonia RM, McConnell RB, Van Den Berg-Loonen EM, Meuwissen SGM, Dekker-Saeys BJ, et al: HLA antigens in inflammatory bowel disease. Tissue Antigens 11:147-152, 1978
19. Bergman L, Lindblom JB, Safwenberg J, Krause U: HL-A frequencies in Crohn's disease and ulcerative colitis. Tissue Antigens 7:145-150, 1976
20. Lewkonia RM, Woodrow JC, Mcconnell RB, Pr ice-Evans DA: HL-A antigens in inflammatory bowel disease. Lancet i:574-575, 1974
21. Rossen RD: HLA and disease: A postulated role for HLA in gastrointestinal diseases. Gastroenterology 78:1629-1635, 1980
22. Selby WS, Poulter LW, Hobbs S, Jewell DP, Janossy G: Heterogeneity of HLA-DR-positive histiocytes in human intestinal lamina propria: A combined histochemical and immunohistological analysis. J Clin Pathol 36:379-384, 1983

Primary Biliary Cirrhosis

Population Association

HLA-A and B-antigen frequencies are available in reports from England[1,2] and Australia.[3] There was no evidence of significant association with any of the antigens.

Disease Heterogeneity

Galbraith et al.[1] also studied their patients for smooth muscle and antinuclear antibodies. There was no correlation between HLA type and the presence of these 2 antibodies. Similar negative results were also observed for age and sex variables. Also, in the data of Hamlyn et al.[2] A and B loci antigens did not show any association with disease severity, sex, age at onset, autoantibody titer, DNA binding, or immunoglobulin concentration.

See also ref. 4.

References

1. Galbraith RM, Eddleston ALWF, Smith MGM, Williams R, McSween RNM, Watkinson G, et al: Histocompatibility antigens in active chronic hepatitis and primary biliary cirrhosis. Br Med J 3:604-605, 1974
2. Hamlyn AN, Adams D, Sherlock S: Primary or secondary sicca complex? Investigation in primary biliary cirrhosis by histocompatibility testing. Br Med J 281:425-426, 1980
3. Morris PJ, Vaughan H, Tait BD, Mackay IR: Histocompatibility antigens (HLA): Association with immunopathic diseases and with response to microbial antigens. Aust NZ J Med 7:616-624, 1977
4. McFarlane IG, McFarlane BM, Haines AJ, Eddleston ALWF, Williams R: Relationship between primary biliary cirrhosis and chronic GVH disease: Investigation of HLA antigenic determinants in biliary tract antigens. Clin Sci 64:113-116, 1983

Immunoproliferative Small Intestinal Disease (Mediterranean Abdominal Lymphoma)

Population Association

Nikbin et al.[1] studied 21 Iranian patients and 120 controls and reported a significant association with AW19 and B12 (Table 10.15). There was also a significant increase of an AW19-B12 combination in the patients.

Disease Heterogeneity

The 21 patients's sera were also tested for the presence of α-chain protein (IgA). Thus, 10 patients with α heavy chain paraproteinemia and 11 without did not show significant differences in HLA antigen frequencies.

Reference

1. Nikbin B, Banisadre M, Ala F, Mojtabai A: HLA, AW19, B12 in immunoproliferative small intestinal disease. Gut 20:226-228, 1979

Pyloric Stenosis

Population Association

Darke et al.[1] found no evidence of an association in 105 children with infantile pyloric stenosis typed for A and B loci antigens.

Reference

1. Drake C, Orellana W, Dodge JA: HLA types and ABO blood groups in infants with pyloric stenosis and their mothers. Tissue Antigens 7:189-190, 1976

Atrophic Gastritis

Population Association

Whittingham et al.[1] observed increased frequencies of A3 and B7 in 27 Australian patients. There was no evidence of any association with these antigens in 2 other studies from England.[2,3]

References

1. Whittingham S, Youngchaiyud U, Mackay IR, Buckley JD, Morris PJ: Thyrogastric autoimmune disease: Studies on the cell-mediated immune system and histocompatibility antigens. Clin Exp Immunol 19:289-299, 1975
2. Mawhinney H, Lawton JWM, White AG, Irvine WJ: HL-A3 and HL-A7 in pernicious anaemia and autoimmune atrophic gastritis. Clin Exp Immunol 22:47-53, 1975

TABLE 10.15. Immunoproliferative Small Intestinal Disease (Mediterranean Abdominal Lymphoma)

	Patients		Controls				
Country/Population	n	%+	n	%+	RR	χ^2	Ref.
HLA-AW19							
Iran	21	33	120	3	14.54	17.13	1
HLA-B12							
Iran	21	33	120	11	3.99	7.05	1

3. Ungar B, Mathews JD, Tait BD, Cowling DC: HLA patterns in pernicious anaemia. Br Med J 1:798-800, 1977

Duodenal Ulcer

Population Association

Rotter et al.[1] first reported an association with B5 in American Caucasian patients. However, subsequent studies from England,[2,3] Canada,[4] and Australia[5] did not confirm this result. In the pooled data from all these studies the association with B5 is marginally significant (Table 10.16). Similar negative results were also reported by Hammond and Moshal[6] in a report on 94 Indian patients from South Africa.

In 1 British study[2] a highly significant increase in the frequency of B12 was reported. This antigen was also typed in a second report from England[3] in which no significant associations were found (Table 10.16).

References

1. Rotter JI, Rimoin DL, Gursky JM, Terasaki P, Sturdevant RAA: HLA-B5 associated with duodenal ulcer. Gastroenterology 73:438-440, 1977
2. Ellis A, Woodrow JC: HLA and duodenal ulcer. Gut 20:760-762, 1979
3. Gough MJ, Rajah SM, Giles GR: HLA antigens in relationship to duodenal ulceration, gastric acid secretion and the clinical result following vagotomy. Br J Surg 69:105-107, 1982
4. O'Brien BD, Thomson ABR, Dossetor JB: HLA and peptic ulcer. Dig Dis Sci 24:314-315, 1979
5. Kang JY, Doran T, Crampton R, McClenehan W,

TABLE 10.16. Duodenal Ulcer

Country/Population	Patients n	Patients %+	Controls n	Controls %+	RR	χ^2	Ref.
HLA-B5							
South Africa—Indian	94	26	632	34	0.69	2.27	6
Canada	46	12	733	24	0.46	3.18	4
U.S.A.	54	24	3895	10	2.91	11.63	1
Australia	52	20	496	10	2.31	5.26	5
England	100	12	229	7	1.82	2.38	3
England	101	12	500	10	1.26	0.49	2
	201	12	729	9	1.47	2.35	
	Heterogeneity χ^2 (1 df)					0.53	
	353	15	5853	12	1.63	9.39	
	Heterogeneity χ^2 (4 df)					13.56	
HLA-B12							
Australia	52	27	496	26	1.07	0.05	5
England	101	47	500	29	2.17	12.33	2
England	100	35	229	28	1.39	1.66	3
	201	41	729	29	1.79	12.23	
	Heterogeneity χ^2 (1 df)					1.77	
	253	38	1225	28	1.61	10.27	
	Heterogeneity χ^2 (2 df)					3.78	
HLA-BW35							
England	100	22	229	10	2.53	8.39	3
England	101	11	500	11	1.03	0.01	2
	201	16	729	11	1.65	4.67	
	Heterogeneity χ^2 (1 df)					3.72	

Piper DW: HLA antigens and peptic ulcer disease. Digestion 26:99-104, 1983
6. Hammond MG, Moshal MG: HLA and duodenal ulcer in South African indians. Tissue Antigens 15:508-509, 1980

Gastric Ulcer

Population Association

In 43 Canadian patients[1] there was no significant association with A and B loci antigens. This study also reported similar results for 22 patients with gastric body ulcer, 18 with gastric antral ulcer, and 39 with gastric ulcer not associated with aspirin ingestion.

Another study from Australia by Kang et al.[2] also did not find any significant associations with A, B, and DR loci antigens.

References

1. O'Brien BD, Thomson ABR, Dossetor JB: HLA and peptic ulcer. Dig Dis Sci 24:314-315, 1979
2. Kang JY, Doran T, Crampton R, McClenehan W, Piper DW: HLA antigens and peptic ulcer disease. Digestion 26:99-104, 1983

Porphyria Cutanea Tarda

Population Association

The reported increased frequencies of A29 and B7 in Spanish patients,[1] of AW32 in Italian patients, and of A3 and B7 in German patients[2] are given in Table 10.17. These reports do not give frequencies of other antigens and thus a combined analysis of all the data cannot be done. However, the data on the frequency of B7 from Spain and Germany show a highly significant association with this disease (Table 10.17).

Family Data

In a family of 6 affected individuals 5 patients had the haplotype A3-B14.[3] It is interesting that A3 and B14 were also associated with hemochromatosis, another disease of abnormal iron metabolism. If these results for porphyria cutanea tarda are confirmed then there may be a common genetic mechanism for susceptibility to porphyria cutanea tarda and hemochromatosis.

The authors also mention that HLA typings of 2 other unrelated porphyria cutanea tarda patients revealed that both had antigen A3.

See also ref. 5.

References

1. Liorente L, De Salamanca RE, Campillo F, Pena ML: HLA and porphyria cutanea tarda. Arch Dermatol Res 269:209-210, 1980
2. Kuntz BME, Sonneborn HH, Lissner R: HLA-types in porphyria cutanea tarda. Lancet i:155, 1981
3. Benedetto AV, Braun WE, Taylor JS: HLA antigens in a family with porphyria cutanea tarda and low uroporphyrinogen decarboxylase. Clin Res 26:567a, 1978
4. Santoianni P, De Felice M, Ayala F, Budillon G, Zappacosta S: A novel association between HLA and

TABLE 10.17. Porphyria Cutanea Tarda

Country/Population	Patients n	Patients %+	Controls n	Controls %+	RR	χ^2	Ref.
HLA-A3							
West Germany	50	46	600	29	2.09	6.35	2
HLA-A29							
Spain	105	25	1000	12	2.47	13.90	1
HLA-AW32							
Italy	28	27	148	8	4.26	8.45	4
HLA-B7							
West Germany	50	44	600	25	2.36	8.52	2
Spain	105	26	1000	12	2.60	15.86	1
	155	32	1600	17	2.50	24.32	
	Heterogeneity χ^2 (1 df)					0.06	

TABLE 10.18. Intestinal Adenomatous Polyposis

	Patients		Controls				
Country/Population	n	%+	n	%+	RR	χ^2	Ref.
HLA-BW22							
Italy	51	14	730	1	15.97	28.75	1

disease: Porphyria cutanea tarda and HLA-AW32. Dermatologica 160:371-375, 1980
5. Cervinka J, Kalab M, Kordac V: HLA system in symptomatic hepatic porphyria. Cas Lek Cesk 120:1404-1411, 1981

Gilbert's Syndrome

Population Association

Penner et al.[1] found no significant association in 18 unrelated Austrian patients typed for A, B, and C loci antigens.

Family Data

In this study,[1] 3 families were also investigated. The disease did not segregate with the marker haplotypes in these families.

Reference

1. Penner E, Mayr WR, Pacher M, Djawan S, Seyfried H, Pantucek F: Gilbert's syndrome HL-A. Z Immunitaetsforsch 150:90-92, 1975

Acute Intermittent Porphyria

Population Association

HLA-A and -B loci data on 20 German patients studied by Teuber et al.[1] showed no evidence of association.

Family Data

A large pedigree of 46 members in which several individuals were affected by the disease was typed for GLO, Bf, and HLA-A, -B, and -C loci antigens.[2] The linkage analysis by the lod score method did not reveal any evidence of linkage with the HLA system.

References

1. Teuber J, Druschky F, Franzke W, Baenkler HW: HLA frequencies in intermittent acute porphyria. Int Arch Allergy Appl Immunol 54:473-474, 1977
2. Tongio MM, Mayer S, Hauptmann G, North ML, Koehl C, Abecassis J, et al.: Lack of linkage between acute intermittent porphyria and the A and B loci of the HLA system. Tissue Antigens 13:273-277, 1979

Intestinal Adenomatous Polyposis

Population Association

An association with BW22 in 51 Italian patients has been found by Spinelli et al.[1] (Table 10.18).

Reference

1. Spinelli P, Pellegris G, Illeni MT, Zella M, Musci R, Pizzetti P, et al.: Intestinal adenomatous polyposis: Association with BW22 and with some IA determinants. In Bodmer W, et al. (eds): Histcompatibility Testing 1977. Munksgaard, 1977, pp 486-487

Plummer-Vinson Stricture

The Plummer-Vinson stricture is a simple, painless, permanent stricture of the cervical esophagus, which causes dysphasia.

Population Association

Middleton et al.[1] studied 50 women from Northern Ireland. When compared with 200 normal controls, no difference in the frequency of A and B loci antigens was found.

Reference

1. Middleton D, Logan JS, Magennis BP, Nelson SD: HLA-antigen frequencies in patients with a Plum-

TABLE 10.19. Primary Sclerosing Cholangitis

	Patients		Controls				
Country/Population	n	%+	n	%+	RR	χ^2	Ref.
HLA-B8							
England	25	60	561	25	4.42	13.55	1

mer-Vinson stricture. Tissue Antigens 12:200-204, 1978

Intrahepatic Cholestasis of Pregnancy

Population Association

Reyes et al.[1] typed A and B antigens in 50 Chilean Caucasian and 50 Chilean Araucanian Indian women with intrahepatic cholestasis of pregnancy. For comparison 50 controls (females) in each of the 2 groups were also typed.

No significant association in any of the groups was found.

Reference

1. Reyes H, Wegmann ME, Segovia N, Cuchacovich M, Jadresic E, Contador M, et al: HLA in Chileans with intrahepatic cholestasis of pregnancy. Hepatology 2:463-466, 1982

Primary Sclerosing Cholangitis

Population Association

In a study of 25 patients from England, Chapman et al.[1] reported an association with HLA-B8 (Table 10.19). These patients were not typed for DR antigens.

Disease Heterogeneity

The concentrations of serum immunoglobulins IgM and IgG and the presence of low titers of antinuclear factors and smooth muscle antibody, and piecemeal necrosis on liver biopsy were not significantly different in B8-positive and -negative patients.

Reference

1. Chapman RW, Varghese Z, Gaul R, Patel G, Kokinon N, Sherlock S: Association of primary sclerosing cholangitis with HLA-B8. Gut 24:38-41, 1983

CHAPTER 11

Ophthalmology

Optic Neuritis

Population Association

All the available data on B7 and DW2 are given in Table 11.1.

In 2 independent studies from Sweden, the results were not consistent (Table 11.1). The data of Sandberg-Wollheim et al.[1,2] showed an association with B7 and more strongly with DW2 (primarily with DW2). This was not evident in the study by Stendahl-Brodin et al.[3] In the combined data only the increase in DW2 was significant. However, there was some indication of heterogeneity in the data.

In 88 patients from England,[4,5] the frequency of DR2 (BT101) was 58% as compared with 35% in the normal population (sample size unknown). The authors state that this difference was significant with a $\chi^2 = 11.40$ ($p < 0.001$, RR = 3.95).

No difference in the frequency of A and B loci antigens in 38 Japanese patients has been observed by Mimura et al.[6]

Disease Heterogeneity

Association between HLA (A3, B7, and DW2) and optic neuritis patients with and without oligoclonal IgG in cerebrospinal fluid (CSF) has been studied by Swedish investigators and the results were negative in both studies.

Optic neuritis patients with pleocytosis of the CSF also had higher (but nonsignificant) frequencies of A3, B7, and DW2.[1]

Arnason et al.[7] studied antimeasles antibody titiers in 30 American Caucasian patients and 100 controls; no significant difference was found.

Also see refs. 9 and 10.

References

1. Sandberg-Wollheim M, Platz P, Ryder LP, Nielsen LS, Thomsen M: HL-A histocompatibility antigens in optic neuritis. Acta Neurol Scand 52:161-166, 1975
2. Platz P, Ryder LP, Staub Nielsen L, Svejgaard A, Thomsen M, Wolheim MS: HL-A and idiopathic optic neuritis. Lancet i:520-521, 1975
3. Stendahl-Brodin L, Link H, Moller E, Norrby E: Optic neuritis and distribution of genetic markers of the HLA system. Acta Neurol Scand 57:418-431, 1978
4. Compston DAS, Batchelor JR, Earl CJ, McDonald WI: Factors influencing the risk of multiple sclerosis developing in patients with optic neuritis. Brain 101:495-511, 1978
5. Editorial: Multiple sclerosis and optic neuritis. Lancet i:85-86, 1979
6. Mimura O, Okamoto N, Shimo-Oku M, Imachi J, Taniwaki K: HL-A antigens in optic neuritis. Nippon Ganka Gakkai Zasshi 83:244-248, 1979
7. Arnason BGW, Fuller TC, Lehrich JR, Wray SH: Histocompatibility types and measles antibodies in multiple sclerosis and optic neuritis. J Neurol Sci 22:419-428, 1974
8. Dieckhues B, Junemann G, Kuchle HJ, Puttman T: HLA-Antigene bei Augenerkrankungen. Klin Monatsbl Augenheilkd 175:681-685, 1979
9. Moller E, Link H, Matell G, Olhagen B, Stendahl L: LD alleles in ankylosing, myasthenia gravis, multiple sclerosis and neuritis. In Kissmeyer-Niel-

TABLE 11.1. Optic Neuritis

Country/Population	Patients n	Patients %+	Controls n	Controls %+	RR	χ^2	Ref.
HLA-B7							
U.S.A.	30	27	100	21	1.42	0.58	7
West Germany	5	60	5046	27	3.78	3.03	8
Sweden	30	33	100	29	1.22	0.22	3
Sweden	54	39	1967	27	1.74	3.98	1
	84	37	2067	27	1.57	3.73	
	Heterogeneity χ^2 (1 df)					0.47	
	119	35	7213	27	1.64	6.01	
	Heterogeneity χ^2 (3 df)					1.80	
HLA-DW2							
Sweden	54	50	132	18	4.48	18.60	1
Sweden	30	33	45	27	1.33	0.33	3
	84	44	177	20	3.00	14.91	
	Heterogeneity χ^2 (1 df)					4.03	

sen F (ed): Histocompatiblity Testing 1975. Munksgaard, Copenhagen, 1975, pp 778-781

10. Stendahl-Brodin L: Studies on humoral immunity and HLA antigens in multiple sclerosis, optic neuritis and hereditary optic atrophy. Acta Ophthalmol 149 (Suppl):1-111, 1982

Acute Anterior Uveitis

Population Association

Brewerton et al.[1] first reported an association with B27. Since then in several independent studies similar associations with B27 have been observed (Table 11.2). In the combined data, this association was highly significant with a relative risk of 8.43.

Disease Heterogeneity

Acute Anterior Uveitis Associated with Yersinia *Infection*

Saari et al.[2] reported 100% B27 frequency in 17 Finnish patients who developed the disease after *Yersinia* infection.

Granulomatous Uveitis

The reports of Woodrow et al.[3,4] included data on 10 patients with granulomatous uveitis (characterized by the presence of muttonfat keratic precipitates). All 10 patients were negative for B27.

Clinical Manifestations

Zervas et al.[5] reported higher frequencies of exudates, hyaloid precipitations, recurrent attacks, and disease duration of more than 3 weeks in 12 B27-positive as compared with 21 B27-negative patients.

Crossreaction with Klebsiella pneumoniae

Holland et al.[6] tested the lymphocytes of B27-positive and -negative patients for cross-reactivity with isolates of *Klebsiella pneumoniae*. Unlike in ankylosing spondylitis (associated with B27) no evidence of cross-reactivity was found.

Family Data

Saari et al.[7–9] performed HLA typings in 12 Finnish families with at least 2 patients in each family. In all families affected siblings shared 1 or both haplotypes. The most frequent haplotype associated with the disease was A2-B27. No formal linkage analysis was done, however.

See also refs. 10–14 and 22–31.

References

1. Brewerton DA, Caffrey M, Nicholls A, Walters D, James DCO: Acute anterior uveitis and HL-A27. Lancet ii:994-996, 1973
2. Saari KM, Laitinen O, Leirisalo M, Saari R: Ocular inflammation associated with *Yersinia* infection. Am J Ophthalmol 89:84-95, 1980

TABLE 11.2. Acute Anterior Uveitis

Country/Population	Patients n	Patients %+	Controls n	Controls %+	RR	χ^2	Ref.
HLA-B8							
U.S.A.—Black	39	26	89	7	4.48	8.23	15
HLA-B27							
Australia	39	39	600	10	5.78	25.58	10
England	90	56	233	8	14.25	70.83	4
England	44	55	44	4	23.01	20.78	1
	134	56	277	7	15.49	91.21	
	Heterogeneity χ^2 (1 df)					0.40	
West Germany	100	36	1000	10	5.07	49.33	16
West Germany	26	23	5046	10	2.84	5.64	17
West Germany	101	37	1402	9	5.95	63.38	18
	227	35	7448	10	5.09	116.10	
	Heterogeneity χ^2 (2 df)					2.25	
Greek	33	36	233	5	10.46	26.69	5
Denmark	17	71	562	8	26.35	39.81	19
Finland	37	84	114	13	32.01	48.27	20
Norway	33	67	788	10	17.77	58.58	21
	520	47	10022	10	8.24	373.34	
	Heterogeneity χ^2 (9 df)					35.57	

3. Woodrow JC, Mapstone R, Anderson J, Usher N: HL-A27 and anterior uveitis. Tissue Antigens 6:116-120, 1975
4. Mapstone R, Woodrow JC: HL-A27 and acute anterior uveitis. Br J Ophthalmol 59:270-275, 1975
5. Zervas J, Tsokos G, Papadakis G, Kabouklis E, Papadopoulos D: HLA-B27 frequency in Greek patients with acute anterior uveitis. Br J Ophthalmol 61:699-701, 1977
6. Holland EJ, Loren AB, O'Donnell MJ, Spence DJ, Tessler HH, Yokoyama MM: HLA-B27, *Klebsiella pneumoniae*, and the relation to acute anterior uveitis. Invest Ophthalmol Vis Sci 22:213-219, 1982
7. Saari M, Miettinen R, Tiilikainen A, Herva E, Lahti R: Acute anterior uveitis and HLA-B27 in families. Can J Ophthalmol 12:4-11, 1977
8. Saari M, Miettinen R, Herva E, Tiilikainen A: Inheritance of acute anterior uveitis and HL-A antigen 27. Albrecht Von Graefes Arch Klin Ophthalmol 198:1-5, 1976
9. Saari KM, Solja J, Hakli J, Seppanen S, Tiilikainen A, Koskimies S, et al: Genetic background of acute anterior uveitis. Am J Ophthalmol 91:711-720, 1981
10. Andrews BS, Mcintosh J, Petts V, Penny R: Circulating immune complexes in acute uveitis: A possible association with the histocompatibility complex locus antigen B27. Int Arch Allergy Appl Immunol 58:313-321, 1979
11. Brewerton DA: HL-A27 and acute anterior uveitis. Ann Rheum Dis 34(Suppl):33-35, 1975
12. Scharf J, Nahir M, Scharf J, Briek R, Gidoni O, Brazilai A, et al: Anterior uveitis in ankylosing spondylitis: A histocompatibility study. Ann Ophthalmol 11:1061-1062, 1979
13. Mapstone R, Woodrow JC: Acute anterior uveitis and HL-A27. Lancet i:681-682, 1974
14. Edwards WM, Ferguson J, Owen DS JR: Arthritis, uveitis, and HL-A27. Arthritis Rheum 18:185-186, 1975
15. Nussenblatt RB, Mittal KK: Association of anterior uveitis in American blacks with HLA-B8 and not B27. In Terasaki PI (ed): Histocompatibility Testing 1980. UCLA Tissue Typing Laboratory, Los Angeles, 1981, p 942
16. Bertrams J, Rommelfanger M, Spitznas M, Kuwert E: HL A27 and acute anterior uveitis. Z Immun Forsch 148:389-391, 1975
17. Dieckhues B, Junemann G, Kuchle HJ, Puttman T: HLA-Antigene bei Augenerkrankungen. Klin Monatsbl Augenheilkd 175:681-685, 1979
18. Wenk HF, Ruprech KW, Schunter F: HLA-Antigene bei Uveitis anterior. Albrecht Von Graefes Arch Klin Exp Ophthalmol 215:137-143, 1980

19. Ehlers N, Kissmeyer-Neilsen F, Kjerbye KE, Lamm LU: HL-A27 in acute and chronic uveitis. Lancet i:99, 1974
20. Saari KM, Hakli J, Solja J, Kaakinen A, Seppanen S, Kallio S, et al: HLA-B27 frequency and MLC reactions in acute anterior uveitis. Albrecht Von Graefes Arch Klin Ophthalmol 216:23-29, 1981
21. Moller P, Berg K, Vinje O: HLA phenotypes and joint affection in psoriasis, acute anterior uveitis and chronic prostatitis. Clin Genet 19:266-270, 1981
22. Saraux H, Lebuisson DA, Offret H: Antigene tissulaire HLA-B 7 chez les malades ayant une uveite anterieure aigue. Nouv Presse Med 5:1257, 1976
23. Brewerton DA: The histocompatibility antigen (HL-A27) and acute anterior uveitis. Trans Ophthalmol Soc UK 94:735-741, 1974
24. Lods F: Interet pratique du groupage tissulaire dans les uveites. Bull Soc Opththalmol Fr 76:789-790, 1976
25. Kean WF, Anastassiades TP, Ford PM: Aortic incompetence in HLA B27-positive juvenile arthritis. Ann Rheum Dis 39:294-295, 1982
26. Rosenbaum JT: Why HLA-B27: An analysis based on two animal models. Ann Intern Med 94:261-263, 1981
27. Moller P, Vinje O, Olsen EG: HLA B27, sacro-ilitis peripheral arthropathy in acute anterior uveitis. Scand J Rheumatol 9:234-236, 1980
28. Colin J, Baikoff G: Interet de la recherche de l'antigene HLA-B27 dans le bilan O etiologique des uveites. Bull Soc Opthtalmol Fr 79:919-920, 1979
29. Moller P, Vinje O, Berg K: HLA antigens, psoriasis and acute anterior uveitis in Bechterew's syndrome (ankylosing spondylitis). Clin Genet 21:215-221, 1982
30. Ozyazgan Y, Pazarli H, Yazici H, Yurdakul S, Tuzun Y, Altac M, et al: Usefulness of HLA determination and pathergy test in diagnosis of uveitis in Turkey. Br J Ophthalmol 65:798-799, 1981
31. Saari KM: Ocular inflammations in rheumatic diseases: Relationship to HLA antigens. Scand J Rheumatol 42:10, 1982

Chronic Uveitis

Population Association

No significant A and B loci (specifically B27) associations were observed in 13 Danish[1] and 20 American Caucasian[2] patients.

References

1. Ehlers N, Kissmeyer-Neilsen F, Kjerbye KE, Lamm LU: HL-A27 in acute and chronic uveitis. Lancet i:99, 1974
2. Ohno S, Kimura SJ, O'Connor GR, Char DH: HLA antigens and uveitis. Br J Ophthalmol:62-64, 1977

Uveitis (Unspecified)

Population Association

Ohno et al.[1] reported a significant association with B27. This, however, was not observed in the French data[2] (Table 11.3). There was an increase in B12 in 24 Japanese patients (Table 11.3).

Family Data

Family data are not available (however, see refs. 3 and 4).

See also refs. 5–7.

TABLE 11.3. Uveitis (Unspecified)

	Patients		Controls				
Country/Population	n	%+	n	%+	RR	χ^2	Ref.
HLA-B12							
Japan	24	29	114	11	3.33	5.46	8
HLA-B27							
U.S.A.	33	55	72	7	14.79	24.56	1
France	56	20	368	13	1.71	2.28	2
	89	33	440	12	3.28	15.85	
	Heterogeneity χ^2 (1 df)					10.99	

References

1. Ohno S, Kimura SJ, O'Connor GR, Char DH: HLA antigens and uveitis. Br J Ophthalmol 61:62-64, 1977
2. Urvoy M: Groupes tissulaires et ophtalmologie. Bull Soc Ophtalmol Fr 76:785-788, 1976
3. Scharf J, Miller B, Zonis S, Scharf J, Nahir M, Gidoni O, et al: HL-A27 antigen associated with uveitis and ankylosing spondylitis in a family. Am J Ophthalmol 82:139-140, 1976
4. Saari KM: Family studies on uveitis and ankylosing spondylitis. Am J Ophthalmol 83:424-425, 1977
5. Verdet R, Vingtain P, Mercier P, Sirol J, Chovet M: Groupe tissulaire et uveite interet de la recherche de l'antigene B27. Bull Soc Ophtalmol Fr 76:479-483, 1976
6. Scharf Y, Zonis S: Histocompatibility antigens (HLA) and uveitis. Surv Ophthalmol 24:220-228, 1980
7. Crews SJ, Mackintosh P, Barry DR, Willshaw HE: HLA antigens and certain types of uveitis. Trans Ophthalmol Soc UK 99:156-159, 1979
8. Okinami S, Hayashi M, Uyama M, Nakagawa J, Ikehara Y: HLA antigens in the patients with Behcet's disease, sarcoid-uveitis, and endogenous uveitis. Nippon Ganka Gakkai Zasshi 81:43-47, 1977
9. Ozyazgan Y, Pazarli H, Yazici H, Yurdakul S, Tuzun Y, Altac M, et al: Usefulness of HLA determination and pathergy test in diagnosis of uveitis in Turkey. Br J Ophthalmol 65:798-799, 1981

Primary Open-Angle Glaucoma

Population Association

In a series of papers Shin and coworkers[1–12] reported associations of the disease with A3, B7, B12, and BW35 antigens. However, in a further study with a larger patient population they could not confirm these results either in American Caucasian or American Black patients.[13]

A report by Aviner et al.[14] in 1976 showed a frequency of 46.9% in 49 patients (46 Caucasian and 3 Blacks) and 22.8% in 250 controls (corrected $p < 0.012$). However, studies by Grabner and Mayr on 70 Austrian patients,[15,16] Ritch et al.[17] on 35 American Caucasians, Brown et al.[18] on 24 American Caucasians, David et al.[19] on 32 South African Caucasians and 41 South African Blacks, Damgaard-Jensen and Kissmeyer-Nielsen[20] on 125 Danish, Slagsvold and Nordhagen[21] on 43 Norwegian, Cordier et al.[22] on 30 French, Gabriel et al.[23] on 50 Greek, Rosenthal et al.[24] on 55 American Caucasians, Shaw et al.[25] on 48 American Blacks, Scharf et al.[26] on 70 Israeli Jews, and Ticho et al.[27] on 37 Israeli Jews (43 Ashkenazi and 14 non-Ashkenazi) have not confirmed any significant association with A, B, and C loci antigens.

Thus, in the data published from independent studies there was no evidence of any significant association with HLA in American and European Caucasians, Israeli Jews, and American and South African Blacks.

Disease Heterogeneity

In the aforementioned studies of Shin and coworkers B7 and B12 were found to be associated with cup/disk ratio, family history, and intraocular pressure. However, in a second study involving a larger sample size[13] these workers were not able to confirm their earlier reported association of B7 and B12 with primary open-angle glaucoma. Thus, the validity of their other results on heterogeneity parameters remains in question. Furthermore, Mayr and Grabner[15] also reported no associations of B7 and B12 patients with or without glaucomatous optic disk cupping, or in the patients with or without visual field defects. The comparison of the frequency of B7 and/or B12 between patients with and without glaucomatous optic disk cupping, or between patients with or without visual field defects also showed no significant difference.

Positive family history was also not found to be associated with B7 or B12 in the studies of Mayr and Grabner and Rosenthal and Payne.[24]

See also refs. 28–30.

References

1. Shin DH, Becker B: The prognostic value of HLA-B12 and HLA-B7 antigens in patients with increased intraocular pressure. Am J Ophthalmol 82:871-874, 1976
2. Becker B, Palmberg PF, Shin DH: Glucocorticoid responsiveness associated with HLA-B12. Invest Ophthalmol Vis Sci 16:61-63, 1977
3. Shin DH, Kass MA, Becker B: Intraocular pressure response to topical epinephrine and HLA-B12. Arch Ophthalmol 96:1012-1013, 1978
4. Shin DH, Becker B, Waltman SR, Palmberg PF, Bell CE: The prevalence of HLA-B12 and HLA-B7 antigens in primary open-angle glaucoma. Arch Ophthalmol 95:224-225, 1977

5. Becker B, Shin DH: HLA antigens and primary open-angle glaucoma in black Americans. Invest Ophthalmol Vis Sci 16:175-176, 1977
6. Waltman SR, Palmberg P, Newton W, Becker B: Glaucoma and HL-A antigens. Lancet i:927, 1975
7. Shin DH, Becker B, Kolker AE: Family history in primary open-angle glaucoma. Arch Ophthalmol 95:598-600, 1977
8. Becker B, Shin DH: Prognostic value of HLA-A3, BW35, B7, and B12 in ocular hypertension. Int Arch Allergy Appl Immunol 54:187-190, 1977
9. Shin DH, Becker B, Bell CE: HLA in primary open-angle glaucoma. Int Arch Allergy Appl Immunol 55:546-550, 1977
10. Shin DH, Kass MA, Becker B: The association of HLA-B7 and HLA-B12 antigens with cup/disk ratio, family history of glaucoma, and intraocular pressure. Am J Ophthalmol 83:347-349, 1977
11. Shin DH, Becker B: HLA-A11 and HLA-BW35 and resistance to glaucoma in white patients with ocular hypertension. Arch Ophthalmol 95:423-424, 1977
12. Shin DH, Sugar HS: HLA in pigment dispersion and glaucoma. Tissue Antigens 19:301-305, 1982
13. Kass MA, Palmberg P, Becker B, Miller JP: Histocompatibility antigens and primary open-angle glaucoma. Arch Ophthalmol 96:2207-2208, 1978
14. Aviner Z, Henley WL, Fotino M, Leopold IH: Histocompatibility (HL-A) antigens and primary open-angle glaucoma. Tissue Antigens 7:193-200, 1976
15. Mayr WR, Grabner G: HLA antigens-risk factors for primary open-angle glaucoma? Albrecht Von Graefes Arch Klin Ophthalmol 207:291-297, 1978
16. Grabner G, Mayr WR: Histokompatibilitatsantigene (HLA-A Atigene) und offenwinkel-Gaukom. Albrecht Von Graefes Arch Klin Ophthalmol 202:75-79, 1977
17. Ritch R, Podos SM, Henley W, Moss A, Southren AL, Fatino M: Lack of association of histocompatibility antigens with primary open-angle glaucoma. Arch Opthalmol 96:2204-2206, 1978
18. Brown RH, Lichter PR, Haines RF: The HLA system and primary open-angle glaucoma. Tissue Antigens 12:151-152, 1978
19. David R, Maier G, Baumgarten I, Abrahams C: HLA antigens in glaucoma and ocular hypertension. Br J Ophthalmol 63:293-296, 1979
20. Damgaard-Jensen L, Kissmeyer-Nielsen F: HLA histocompatibility antigens in open-angle glaucoma. Acta Ophthalmol 56:384-388, 1978
21. Slagsvold JE, Nordhagen R: The HLA system in primary open angle glaucoma and in patients with pseudoexfoliation of the lens capsule. Acta Ophthalmol 58:188-192, 1979
22. Cordier J, Lardenet F, Raffouz C, Raspiller A: Glaucome chronique et systeme HLA. Bull Soc Ophtalmol Fr 81:841-846, 1981
23. Gabriel L, Renieri N, Stavropoulos C: Frequency of HLA antigens in Greek patients with open-angle glaucoma. Ophthalmologica 182:49-53, 1981
24. Rosenthal AR, Payne R: Association of HLA antigens and primary open-angle glaucoma. Am J Ophthalmol 88:479-482, 1979
25. Shaw JF, Levene RZ, Sowell JG: The incidence of HLA antigens in black primary open-angle glaucoma patients. Am J Ophthalmol 86:501-505, 1978
26. Scharf J, Gideoni O, Zonis S, Barzilai A: Histocompatibility antigens (HLA) and open angle glaucoma. Ann Ophthalmol 10:914-916, 1978
27. Ticho U, Cohen T, Brautbar C: Absence of association between HLA antigens and primary open angle glaucoma in Israel. Isr J Med Sci 15:124-127, 1979
28. Leopold IH: The HLA system and glaucoma. Am J Ophthalmol 87:578-582, 1979
29. Henley WL, Leopold IH, Aviner Z: Glaucoma and HL-A antigens. Lancet ii:1273, 1974
30. Olivius E, Polland W: Histocompatibility (HLA) antigens in capsular glaucoma and simplex glaucoma. Acta Ophthalmol 58:406-410, 1980

Acute Angle-Closure Glaucoma

Population Association

In 2 studies[1,2] involving a total of 43 American Caucasian patients there was no evidence of association with any of the A and B loci antigens.

References

1. Ritch R, Podos SM, Henley W, Moss A, Southren AL, Fotino M: Lack of association of histocompatibility antigens with primary open-angle glaucoma. Arch Ophthalmol 96:2204-2206, 1978
2. Gieser DK, Wilensky JT: HLA antigens and acute angle-closure glaucoma. Am J Ophthalmol 88:232-235, 1979

Capsular Glaucoma

In 39 Swedish patients with capsular glaucoma, Olivius and Polland[1] found an increased frequency of BW35 (28% in patients vs. 9% in 985 controls, corrected $p < 0.0075$). This antigen was present in 18% of the 40 patients with simplex glaucoma. However, these results were not confirmed in another study on 45 Norwegian patients by Slagsvold and Nordhagen[2] (Table 11.4).

TABLE 11.4. Capsular Glaucoma

	Patients		Controls				
Country/Population	n	%+	n	%+	RR	χ^2	Ref.
HLA-BW35							
Norway	45	6	45	6	1.00	0.00	2
Sweden	39	28	985	9	4.02	14.83	1
	84	16	1030	9	3.12	12.13	
	Heterogeneity χ^2 (1 df)					2.70	

References

1. Olivius E, Polland W: Histocompatibility (HLA) antigens in capsular glaucoma and simplex glaucoma. Acta Ophthalmol 58:406-410, 1980
2. Slagsvold JE, Nordhagen R: The HLA system in primary open angle glaucoma and in patients with pseuodexfoliation of the lens capsule. Acta Ophthalmol 58:188-192, 1979

Pigmentary Glaucoma

Population Association

In a study of 21 French patients no significant association was found by Plane et al.[1]

Reference

1. Plane C, Bidet JM, Greae JF, Jouan JP: Groupes tissulares HLA et dispersion pigmentaire. Bull Soc Ophtalmol Fr 79:581-587, 1979

Ocular Hypertension

Population Association

Adhikary et al.[1] reported A and B loci antigen frequencies in 6 patients from England who had received allogeneic renal transplants. No significant deviations were found.

Reference

1. Adhikary HP, Sells RA, Basu PK: Ocular complications of systemic steroid after renal transplantation and their association with HLA. Br J Ophthalmol 66:290-291, 1982

Pigment Dispersion Syndrome

Population Association

Becker et al.[1] studied 21 American Caucasian and 9 American Black patients and compared the A and B loci frequencies with that of a group of patients without pigment dispersion syndrome (130 Caucasians and 73 Blacks). In the Caucasian patients (with pigment dispersion syndrome) a significant increase in the frequencies of B13 and B17 was found. The investigators also pooled the Black and Caucasian patients and compared them with a similarly pooled group of patients without pigment dispersion syndrome. The results were similar to those obtained without pooling the patients of the 2 different races. A second report by Shin and Sugar[2] on 12 American Caucasian patients was unable to confirm the results observed by Shin and coworkers.[1]

In another report on 27 American Caucasian patients with pigment dispersion syndrome and 323 healthy unselected controls, Kaiser-Kupfer and Mittal[2] did not find any significant difference in the frequencies of 36 A, B, and C loci antigens. Similar results have also been reported in a French study by Plane et al.[4]

Thus, in the available data there is no indication of an association of pigment dispersion syndrome with HLA-A, -B, and probably -C loci antigens.

See also refs. 3 and 4.

References

1. Becker B, Shin DH, Cooper DG, Kass MA: The pigment dispersion syndrome. Am J Ophthalmol 83:161-166, 1977
2. Shin DH, Sugar HS: HLA in pigment dispersion and glaucoma. Tissue Antigens 19:301-305, 1982
3. Kaiser-Kupfer MI, Mittal KK: The HLA and ABO

antigens in pigment dispersion syndrome. Am J Ophthalmol 85:368-372, 1978
4. Plane C, Bidet JM, Greae JF, Jouan JP: Groupes tissulares HLA et dispersion pigmentaire. Bull Soc Ophtalmol Fr 79:581-587, 1979

Eales' Disease

Population Association

In a sample of 48 patients and 1000 controls from Germany no significant deviation of any of the A and B loci antigens was found by Bertrams et al.[1]

See also ref. 2.

References

1. Bertrams J, Spitznas M, Rommelfanger M: Missing evidence for HLA antigen association with Eales' disease, chorioretinitis, central serous retinopathy, and malignant choroidal melanoma. Invest Ophthalmol Vis Sci 17:918-920, 1978
2. Urvoy M: Groupes tissulaires et ophtalmologie. Bull Soc Ophtalmol Fr 76:785-788, 1976

Stromal Dystrophy

Population Association

In 13 Danish patients compared with 2856 controls Damgaard-Jensen et al.[1] found no evidence of significant deviations in A and B loci antigens.

Reference

1. Damgaard-Jensen L, Ehlers N, Kissmeyer-Nielsen F: HLA types in corneal disease. Acta Ophthalmol 57:982-985, 1979

Fuchs' Endothelial Dystrophy

Population Association

Damgaard-Jensen et al.[1] reported no significant association with A and B loci antigens in 24 Danish patients compared with 2857 controls.

Reference

1. Damgaard-Jensen L, Ehlers N, Kissmeyer-Nielsen F: HLA types in corneal disease. Acta Ophthalmol 57:982-985, 1979

Keratoconus

Population Association

In 2 studies involving 56 Finnish patients[1,2] and 42 Danish patients,[3] no significant association with A or B loci antigens has been observed. Similar results have also been reported in 34 Japanese patients by Ohno.[4]

Family Data

In a small family of 4 members (parents and 2 offspring), only the father was not affected by keratoconus. Both offspring had inherited the haplotype A3-B27 from the affected mother.[5]

References

1. Vannas S, Vannas A, Tiilikainen A: Corneal transplantation reaction in avascular keratoconus patients due to HLA-associated immune aberration against infection: A hypothesis. Invest Ophthalmol Vis Sci 16:644-646, 1977
2. Vannas S, Vannas A, Karjalainen K: HLA-Atigene und allograf Teaktion bei Keratokonus. Klin Monatsbl Augenheilkd 170:391-396, 1977
3. Damgaard-Jensen L, Ehlers N, Kissmeyer-Nielsen F: HLA types in corneal disease. Acta Ophthalmol 57:982-985, 1979
4. Ohno S: Immunogenetic studies on various ocular diseases. Nippon Ganka Gakkai Zasshi 83:1875-1908, 1980
5. Gasset AR, Richman AV, Frias JL: HLA antigens and keratoconus. Ann Ophthalmol 9:767-768, 1977

Cogan's Syndrome

Population Association

Char et al.[1] typed 4 American Caucasian multiparous female patients: 3 were positive for B17. This antigen was also reported to be present in another patient studied by Del Carpio et al.[2] Later Cheson and Garovoy[3] reported the HLA types of a patient, his brother, and their parents. None was positive for B17 or any of the cross-reacting antigens.

In an interesting report on 10 patients with well-documented Cogan's syndrome and 469 controls, Kaiser-Kupfer et al.[4,5] did not find any significant difference in the frequency of B17 (10% in patients vs. 9.17% in controls). The 4 patients previously typed by Char et al.[1] were retyped and were included in this study. All 4 were negative for B17. Furthermore, 2 of the 3 patients who had been reported by Char et al.[1] to have B17 were HLA-typed by 2 other laboratories. They also did not find B17 in these patients (see ref. 6).

References

1. Char DH, Cogan DG, Sullivan WR: Immunologic study of nonsyphilitic interstitial keratitis with vestibuloauditory symptoms. Am J Ophthalmol 80:491-494, 1975
2. Del Carpio J, Espinoza LR, Osterland CK: Cogan's syndrome and HLA Bw17. N Engl J Med 295:1262-1263, 1976
3. Cheson BD, Garovoy MR: Cogan's syndrome and Bw17 revisited. N Engl J Med 297:62-63, 1977
4. Kaiser-Kupfer MI, Del Valle LA, Mittal KK, Haynes BF: HLA and Cogan's syndrome. N Engl J Med 298:1094-1095, 1978
5. Kaiser-Kupfer MI, Mittal KK, Del Valkle LA, and Haynes BF: The HLA antigens in Cogan's syndrome. Am J Ophthalmol 86:314-316, 1978
6. Char DH: HLA antigens in Cogan's syndrome. Am J Ophthalmol 86:850, 1978

Scleritis

Population Association

Joysey et al.[1] observed a significant association with B15 in 54 patients (Table 11.5). However, in the same study when the patients were compared with 2 other control groups of kidney donors (with a sample size of 371 and 100) there was no significant deviation in the frequency of B15. The authors attributed this association of B15 to the low frequency of this antigen in the control population of 1036 blood donors. In the other 2 control groups the frequency was much higher (9.2% and 12%). They suggest that the control group of blood donors was not as representative of the whole population as the other 2 control groups.

Reference

1. Joysey VC, Roger JH, Ashworth F, Bullman W, Hazleman BL, Lachman SM, Watson PG: Parallel studies of HLA antigens in patients with rheumatic heart disease and scleritis. J Rheumatol 4(Suppl 3):84-88, 1977

Toxoplasmic Retinochoroiditis

Population Association

In 20 American Caucasian patients and 72 controls typed for A and B loci antigens, no significant deviations in the frequencies were observed.[1]

Disease Heterogeneity

In this study[1] antibody against *Toxoplasma gondii*, an intracellular protozoan parasite, was also measured in all of the patients. There was no association between antibody titer and any HLA antigens.

Reference

1. Ohno S, O'Connor GR, Kimura SJ: HLA antigens and toxoplasmic retinochoroiditis. Tohoku J Exp Med 123:91-94, 1977

Retinitis Centralis Serosa (Central Serous Retinopathy)

Population Association

Bertrams et al.[1] found no significant deviations in A and B loci antigens in 67 German patients.

Reference

1. Bertrams J, Spitznas M, Rommelfanger M: Missing evidence for HLA antigen association with Eales' disease, chorioretinitis, central serous retinopathy, and malignant choroidal melanoma. Invest Ophthalmol Vis Sci 17:918-920, 1978

TABLE 11.5. Scleritis

	Patients		Controls				
Country/Population	n	%+	n	%+	RR	χ^2	Ref.
HLA-B15							
England	54	17	1036	5	4.02	13.83	1

Chorioretinitis

Population Association

In a report on 48 German patients and 1000 controls, Bertrams et al.[1] noted an increase in B13 (14.6% vs. 4.3%) and a decreased frequency of B5 (2.1% vs. 14.2%). None of these, however, would be significant if the probabilities were corrected for the 26 A and B loci antigens compared in the study.

Reference

1. Bertrams J, Spitznas M, Rommelfanger M: Missing evidence for HLA antigen association with Eales' disease, chorioretinitis, central serous retinopathy, and malignant choroidal melanoma. Invest Ophthalmol Vis Sci 17:918-920, 1978

Senile Cataract

Population Association

Hida and Kuwahara[1] studied A and B antigen frequencies in 60 Japanese patients and 355 controls. The frequency of blanks at the A locus was 61.7% in patients and 39.2% in controls (corrected $p <$ 0.051).

Reference

1. Hida M, Kuwahara K: Cataract and HLA antigen. Nippon Ganka Gakkai Zasshi 82:751-754, 1978

Steroid Induced Cataract

Population Association

In 36 British patients who had received allogeneic renal transplants, Adhikary et al.[1] have not found any significant association with A and B loci antigens.

Reference

1. Adhikary HP, Sells RA, Basu PK: Ocular complications of systemic steroid after renal transplantation and their association with HLA. Br J Ophthalmol 66:290-291, 1982

Juvenile Chronic Iridocyclitis

Population Association

Forty-three American Caucasian patients with juvenile chronic iridocyclitis and 72 controls were typed for A and B loci antigens by Ohno et al.[1] and no significant difference was observed between the 2 groups.

Disease Heterogeneity

The authors[1] subdivided the total sample into those with chronic iridocyclitis associated with juvenile rheumatoid arthritis (n = 23) and those with chronic iridocyclitis in young girls (n = 20). Antinuclear antibodies were also measured in both subgroups. There was no evidence of HLA association in the subgroups or between the antinuclear antibodies and HLA.

Reference

1. Ohno S, Char DH, Kimura SJ, O'Connor GR: HLA antigens and antinuclear antibody titres in juvenile chronic iridocyclitis. Br J Ophthalmol 61:59-61, 1977

Adult Iridocyclitis

Population Association

In a study of 33 American Caucasian patients from San Francisco, Ohno[1] observed a significantly increased frequency of B27 (Table 11.6).

TABLE 11.6. Adult Iridocyclitis

	Patients		Controls				
Country/Population	n	%+	n	%+	RR	χ^2	Ref.
HLA-B8							
U.S.A.—Black	42	26	129	6	5.34	11.82	2
HLA-B27							
U.S.A.	33	55	72	7	14.79	24.56	1

Another report by Nussenblatt and Mittal[2] showed a highly significant association with B8 in 42 American Black patients (Table 11.6). These patients were also typed for DR antigens.

References

1. Ohno S: Immunogenetic studies on various ocular diseases. Nippon Ganka Gakkai Zasshi 83:1875-1908, 1980
2. Nussenblatt RB, Mittal KK: Iridocyclitis in black Americans: Association with HLA B8 suggests an autoimmune aetiology. Br J Ophthalmol 65:329-332, 1981

Degenerative Choroidopathy

The disciform degeneration in this disease is morphologically the same as the presumed ocular histoplasmosis syndrome disciform scars. However, the etiology may be different.

Population Association

In a study by Meredith et al.,[1] 18 American Caucasian patients were tested for A, B, C, and DR loci antigens. When compared with 3240 controls (only 60 for DR), no significant deviations in the frequencies were observed.

Reference

1. Meredith TA, Smith RE, Duquesnoy RJ: Association of HLA-DRW2 antigen with presumed ocular histoplasmosis. Am J Ophthalmol 89:70-76, 1980

Retinitis Pigmentosa

Population Association

In 18 American Caucasian patients typed for A, B, and C loci antigens no association was reported by Chen et al.[1] The disease in this study was the autosomal recessive type.

Heckenlively et al.[2] also reported no significant associations with A, B, and C loci antigens in 24 patients with autosomal dominant, 143 with autosomal recessive, and 6 with sex-linked types of retinitis pigmentosa. All patients in this study were Caucasian. Similarly, in the data of Rocha and Antunes[3] on 70 Brazilian patients A and B loci antigens did not show any significant deviations.

Family Data

HLA typing (A, B, and C) of 2 families with autosomal recessive retinitis pigmentosa and 1 family with autosomal dominant retinitis pigmentosa, studied by Mayr et al.[4] did not show any evidence of close linkage with HLA.

Rocha and Antunes[3] reported HLA haplotypes in 2 small families with retinitis pigmentosa. In 1 family with 4 affected siblings, 3 shared 1 haplotype. The second family had only 2 affected siblings with 1 common haplotype.

See also refs. 3 and 4.

References

1. Chen MC, Marak GE, Pilkerton AR: The incidence of HLA-SD antigens in recessive retinitis pigmentosa. Br J Ophthalmol 62:172-173, 197
2. Heckenlively JR, Bastek JV, Pearlman JT, Gladden J, Terasaki P: HLA typing in retinitis pigmentosa. Br J Ophthalmol 65:131-132, 1981
3. Rocha H, Antunes L: Primary retinitis pigmentosa—autoimmunity. Metab Ophthalmol 1:153-156, 1977
4. Mayr WR, Grabner G, Thaler A, Heilig P: HLA in autosomal dominant and recessive retinitis pigmentosa. Ophthalmic Res 12:270-276, 1980

Rhegmatogenous Retinal Detachment

Population Association

Bertrams et al.[1,2] typed 132 German patients with rhegmatogenous retinal detachment for A, B, and C loci antigens. When the frequencies in patients were compared with those in 1000 controls no significant deviations were found.

Disease Heterogeneity

The studies of Bertrams et al.[1,2] consisted of 76 patients with myope and 51 with emmetrope forms of the disease. There was no HLA association in either of these 2 forms. Subdivision of patients on the basis of positive or negative family history of the disease also did not show any evidence of association with HLA antigens.

References

1. Bertrams J, Spitznas M, Vieira De Souza N: HLA-antigens in patients with rhegmatogenous retinal detachmant. Klin Monatsbl Augenheilkd 173:786-790, 1978

2. Grabner G: Stellungnahme zur Argeit: "HLA-Antigene bei Patienten mit ablatio Retinae." Klin Monatsbl Augenheilkd 175:428, 1975

Sympathetic Ophthalmia

Population Association

Ohno[1] has not observed any significant association in 8 Japanese patients typed for A, B, C, and DR antigens.

In another study of 20 patients (2 Mexicans, 16 American Caucasian, and 2 American Blacks) Reynard et al.[2] noted an increased frequency of A11. However, in view of the racially heterogeneous nature of this small sample, this deviation may be an artifact.

References

1. Ohno S: Immunogenetic studies on various ocular diseases. Nippon Ganka Gakkai Zasshi 83:1875-1908, 1980
2. Reynard M, Shulman IA, Azen SP, Minckler DS: Histocompatibility antigens in sympathetic ophthalmia. Am J Ophthalmol 95:216-221, 1983

Birdshot Retinochoroidopathy

Population Association

An association with A29 has been reported in 20 American Caucasian patients (Table 11.7) studied by Nussenblatt et al.[1] All these patients were typed for A, B, C, and DR antigens.

Reference

1. Nussenblatt RB, Mittal KK, Ryan S, Green WR, Maumenee AE: Birdshot retinochoroidopathy associated with HLA-A29 antigen and immune responsivenes to retinal S-antigen. Am J Ophthalmol 94:147-158, 1982

Pseudoexfoliation of the Lens Capsule

Population Association

In 43 Norwegian patients studied by Slagsvold and Nordhagen[1] no significant deviation of A or B loci antigen frequency was found.

Reference

1. Slagsvold JE, Nordhagen R: The HLA system in primary open angle glaucoma and in patients with pseudodexfoliation of the lens capsule. Acta Ophthalmol 58:188-192, 1979

Thygeson's Superficial Punctate Keratitis

Population Association

Antigen frequency data are available from only one study on 20 American Caucasian patients from New York.[1] In this report a significant association with DR3 was found (Table 11.8). The frequencies of A,

TABLE 11.7. Birdshot Retinochoroidopathy

	Patients		Controls				
Country/Population	n	%+	n	%+	RR	χ^2	Ref.
HLA-A29							
U.S.A.	20	80	418	7	47.96	50.87	1

TABLE 11.8. Thygeson's Superficial Punctate Keratitis

	Patients		Controls				
Country/Population	n	%+	n	%+	RR	χ^2	Ref.
HLA-DR3							
U.S.A.	20	50	133	15	5.55	12.33	1

B, and C antigens in patients did not differ from those observed in controls.

Reference

1. Darrell RW, Suciu-Foca N: HLA DR3 in Thygeson's superficial punctate keratitis. Tissue Antigens 18:203-204, 1981

Hereditary Optic Atrophy

Family Data

Stendahl-Brodin[1] has published a 3-generation pedigree in which 4 individuals were affected by optic atrophy. All 4 patients had A2-B8 haplotype. A lod score analysis of this pedigree showed a maximum lod score of 1.2.

Reference

1. Stendahl-Brodin L: Studies on humoral immunity and HLA antigens in multiple sclerosis, optic neuritis and hereditary optic atrophy. Acta Ophthalmol Suppl 149:1-111, 1982

Adie's Syndrome

Population Association

Ohno[1] has published A and B loci antigen frequencies in 15 Japanese patients and 130 controls. No significant deviations were found.

Reference

1. Ohno S: Immunogenetic studies on various ocular diseases. Nippon Ganka Gakkai Zasshi 83:1875-1908, 1980

CHAPTER 12

Malignancy

Carcinoma of the Thyroid Gland

Population Association

There was no indication of any association of the A and B loci antigens in 40 Czechoslovakian patients and 301 controls.[1] However, a highly significant association with DR1 has been reported by Panza et al.[2](Table 12.1).

References

1. Majsky VA, Feix C, Nemec J: Thyroid carcinoma and HLA-system. Z Gesamte Inn Med 33:797-798, 1978.
2. Panza N, Del Vecchio L, Maio M, De Felice M, Lombardi G, Minozzi M, et al: Strong association between HLA-DR antigen and thyroid carcinoma. Tissue Antigens 20:155-158, 1982

Carcinoma of the Mouth

Population Association

The A and B loci frequency data are available on 61 American Caucasian patients studied by Terasaki et al.[1] and 42 by Tarpley et al.[2] No significant association was found.

References

1. Terasaki PI, Perdue ST, Mickey MR: HLA frequencies in cancer: A second study. In Mulvihill JJ, Miller RW, Fraumeni JF Jr (eds): Genetics of Human Cancer. Raven Press, New York, 1977, p 321
2. Tarpley JL, Chretien PB, Rogentine N, Twomey PL, Dellon AL: Histocompatibility antigens and solid malignant neoplasms. Arch Surg 110:269-271, 1975

Carcinoma of the Brain

Population Association

Terasaki et al.[1] reported A and B loci frequencies in 35 American Caucasian patients. There was no significant difference between patients and 3896 controls (see also ref. 2).

References

1. Terasaki PI, Perdue ST, Mickey MR: HLA frequencies in cancer: A second study. In Mulvihill JJ, Miller RW, Fraumeni JF Jr (eds): Genetics of Human Cancer. Raven Press, New York, 1977, p 321
2. Hirschberg H, Endresen L, Wikeby P: Histocompatibility antigens on astrocytoma cells. J Neurol Neurosurg Psychiatry 45:193-198, 1982

TABLE 12.1. Carcinoma of the Thyroid Gland

	Patients		Controls				
Country/Population	n	%+	n	%+	RR	χ^2	Ref.
HLA-DR1							
Italy	20	80	120	18	16.41	25.00	2

Carcinoma of the Bladder

Population Association

In 139 American Caucasian patients Takasugi et al.[1] reported a nonsignificant decrease in B5. Later in a second report by Terasaki et al.[2](which included the patients in the first study) this deviation was not confirmed.

Braf et al.[3] published A and B loci frequency data on 44 Israeli patients with transitional cell carcinoma of the bladder. There was no indication of any HLA association.

Arce et al.[4] found a significant association with A9 in 40 Cuban patients with transitional cell carcinoma of the bladder (Table 12.2). The previously mentioned studies by Terasaki et al.[2] and Braf et al.[3] do not support these results. The data for A9 from all 3 studies are given in Table 12.2.

Obata et al.[5] have observed no significant association with A and B loci antigens in 86 Japanese patients.

Disease Heterogeneity

The Israeli patients[3] were subdivided into 5 categories according to the disease stage. Again there was no HLA difference among the 5 subgroups.

References

1. Takasugi M, Terasaki PI, Henderson B, Mickey MR, Menck H, Thompson RW: HL-A antigens in solid tumors. Cancer Res 33:648-650, 1973
2. Terasaki PI, Perdue ST, Mickey MR: HLA frequencies in cancer: A second study. In Mulvihill JJ, Miller RW, Fraumeni JF Jr (eds): Genetics of Human Cancer. Raven Press, New York, 1977, p 321
3. Braf ZF, Gazit E, Many M: HLA-A and HLA-B antigens in transitional cell carcinoma of the bladder. J Urol 122:465-466, 1979
4. Arce S, Lopez R, Almaguer M, Ballester JM, Filgueiras E, Vstariz C, et al.: HL-A antigens and transitional-cell carcinoma of the bladder. Mater Med Pol 10:98-100, 1978
5. Obata K, Ohno Y, Murase T, Aoki K, Tsuji K: Bladder cancer and HLA antigens. Nagoya J Med Sci 43:65-70, 1981

Carcinoma of the Prostate

Population Association

In 214 American Caucasian patients tested for A and B loci antigens Takasugi et al.[1]did not find any significant association. Later in a second and updated report on 299 patients (including the 214 in the first report) Terasaki et al.[2] noted interesting deviations in the frequencies of A1, A28, B8, and BW22 (Table 12.3). However, in 100 patients with prostatic adenocarcinoma Barry et al.[3] have not found any significant associations with A and B loci antigens.

Feingold et al.[4] measured correlation coefficients between the death rate for prostate carcinoma and A and B loci antigens. The data from a period of 10 years on 22 Caucasian populations showed a negative correlation with A10 and a positive correlation with B12 ($p < 0.01$).

See also ref. 5.

References

1. Takasugi M, Terasaki PI, Henderson B, Mickey MR, Menck H, Thompson RW: HL A antigens in solid tumors. Cancer Res 33:648-650, 1973
2. Terasaki PI, Perdue ST, Mickey MR: HLA frequencies in cancer: A second study. In Mulvihill JJ, Miller RW, and Fraumeni JF Jr (eds): Genetics of Human Cancer. Raven Press, New York, 1977, p 321
3. Barry JM, Goldstein A, Hubbard M: Human leukocyte A and B antigens in patients with prostatic adenocarcinoma. J Urol 124:847-848, 1980
4. Feingold N, Degos L, Feingold J: HLA in populations: An approach for genetical susceptibility to cancer. J Immunogenet 6:29-35, 1979
5. Claas FHJ, Van Steenbrugge GJ: Expression of HLA-like structures on a permanent human tumor line PC-93. Tissue Antigens 21:227-232, 1983

TABLE 12.2. Carcinoma of the Bladder

Country/Population	Patients n	Patients %+	Controls n	Controls %+	RR	χ^2	Ref.
HLA-A9							
Jews (unspecified)	44	32	400	26	1.36	0.85	3
Cuba	40	40	109	14	4.03	11.36	4
U.S.A.	264	22	3896	20	1.13	0.68	2

TABLE 12.3. Carcinoma of the Prostate

	Patients		Controls				
Country/Population	n	%+	n	%+	RR	χ^2	Ref.
HLA-A1							
U.S.A.	299	22	3896	31	0.63	10.37	2
U.S.A.	100	27	169	36	0.66	2.27	3
	399	23	4065	31	0.64	12.61	
	Heterogeneity χ^2 (1 df)					0.03	
HLA-A28							
U.S.A.	100	6	169	8	0.77	0.31	3
U.S.A.	299	13	3896	8	1.73	9.37	2
	399	11	4065	8	1.57	7.11	
	Heterogeneity χ^2 (1 df)					2.57	
HLA-B8							
U.S.A.	299	13	3896	21	0.57	10.50	2
U.S.A.	100	25	169	25	1.01	0.00	3
	399	16	4065	21	0.66	7.62	
	Heterogeneity χ^2 (1 df)					2.88	
HLA-BW22							
U.S.A.	100	1	169	8	0.17	5.45	3
U.S.A.	299	8	3896	4	2.12	11.21	2
	399	6	4065	4	1.73	6.53	
	Heterogeneity χ^2 (1 df)					10.13	

Carcinoma of the Ovary

Population Association

In the first report by Takasugi et al.[1] 69 American Caucasian patients were typed for A and B loci antigens and no significant deviations were found. The second report by Terasaki et al.[2] on 138 patients (including the 69 in the first study[1]) noted a decrease in B12 (Table 12.4).

Another report by Bertrams et al.[3] on 20 German patients showed increased frequencies of A9 and B18.

A combined analysis of the data for these 3 antigens are presented in Table 12.4. None of the 3 antigens show any significant association.

See also ref. 4.

References

1. Takasugi M, Terasaki PI, Henderson B, Mickey MR, Menck H, Thompson RW: HL-A antigens in solid tumors. Cancer Res 33:648-650, 1973
2. Terasaki PI, Perdue ST, Mickey MR: HLA frequencies in cancer: A second study. In Mulvihill JJ, Miller RW, and Fraumeni JF Jr (eds): Genetics of Human Cancer. Raven Press, New York, 1977, p 321
3. Bertrams J, Thraenhart O, Feldmann U, Kuwert E: HL-A antigens in carcinoma of the breast, ovarium, cervix and endometrium: Possible association of haplotype HL-A10-W18 with carcinoma of the breast. Z Krebsforsch 83:219-222, 1975
4. Tsuji K, Ito M, Miyamoto H, Yamashita H: HL-A antigenic loss in a cancer patient—A case report. Gan 63:495-497, 1972

Carcinoma of the Uterus

Population Association

The A and B loci frequency data of Twomey et al.[1] on 12 patients with adenocarcinoma of the uterus and that of Terasaki et al.[2] on 29 patients with carcinoma of the uterus (not specified) showed no significant deviations in the antigen frequencies. In both of these studies the patients were American Caucasians.

References

1. Twomey PL, Rogentine GN, Chretien PB: Lymphocyte function and HL-A antigen frequency in gynecologic squamous cancer. Int Surg 59:468-472, 1974
2. Terasaki PI, Perdue ST, Mickey MR: HLA frequencies in cancer: A second study. In Mulvihill JJ, Miller RW, Fraumeni JF Jr (eds): Genetics of Human Cancer. Raven Press, New York, 1977, p 321

Carcinoma of the Endometrium

Population Association

Takasugi et al.[1] first reported data on 68 American Caucasian patients. No association with A and B loci antigens were found. Later, in an updated version of the report, Terasaki et al.[2] again reported no association in 102 patients.

Similar nonsignificant results have also been obtained by Bertrams et al.[3] on 19 German patients and by Sniecinski et al.[4] on 17 American Caucasian patients.

References

1. Takasugi M, Terasaki PI, Henderson B, Mickey MR, Menck H, Thompson RW: HL-A antigens in solid tumors. Cancer Res 33:648-650, 1973
2. Terasaki PI, Perdue ST, Mickey MR: HLA frequencies in cancer: A second study. In Mulvihill JJ, Miller RW, Fraumeni JF Jr (eds): Genetics of Human Cancer. Raven Press, New York, 1977, p 321
3. Bertrams J, Thraenhart O, Feldmann U, Kuwert E: HL-A antigens in carcinoma of the breast, ovarium, cervix and endometrium: Possible association of haplotype HL-A10-W18 with carcinoma of the breast. Z Krebsforsch 83:219-222, 1975
4. Sniecinski I, Haley J, Morgan-Byrne J, Van Nagell J Jr: Histocompatibility-antigen distribution in patients with cervical endometrial carcinomas. Gynecol Oncol 11:68-74, 1981

Carcinoma of the Cervix

Population Association

A and B loci typings are available on 391 Caucasian patients from the United States[1-5] and 64 patients from Germany[6,7]. There was no evidence of strong HLA-A and -B loci associations in these studies.

The largest study is Terasaki's,[1] in which 253 patients were HLA-typed. HLA-A11 was significantly decreased in the patients. However, in the previous report[2] deviations in the frequencies of A1, A9, and B12 were noted. These were not confirmed in the larger study[1].

TABLE 12.4. Carcinoma of the Ovary

	Patients		Controls				
Country/Population	n	%+	n	%+	RR	χ^2	Ref.
HLA-A9							
U.S.A.	138	26	3896	20	1.42	3.17	2
West Germany	20	45	1000	18	3.76	9.21	3
	158	28	4896	20	1.67	8.22	
	Heterogeneity χ^2 (1 df)					4.15	
HLA-B12							
U.S.A.	138	16	3896	26	0.55	6.64	2
West Germany	20	25	1000	22	1.26	0.22	3
	158	17	4896	25	0.64	4.52	
	Heterogeneity χ^2 (1 df)					2.35	
HLA-B18							
U.S.A.	138	7	3896	8	0.91	0.09	2
West Germany	20	35	1000	10	4.98	12.42	3
	158	11	4896	8	1.61	3.22	
	Heterogeneity χ^2 (1 df)					9.30	

The data of Tarpley et al.[3] on 67 patients showed an increase in the frequency of B5 but other reports did not confirm this. Similarly, B8 was increased in 33 patients studied by Twomey et al.[4] In the combined analysis of all the data on Caucasian patients, B8 was not significantly increased.

There are 2 reports from South Africa on Indian[8] and Black[9] populations. The Indian patients (n = 249) were from Durban and consisted of 4 ethnic groups (Tamil, Telegu, Hindu, and Muslim). No significant deviations were found in the total groups and also when each of the 4 ethnic groups was considered separately.

Hammond et al.[9] also typed A, B and C loci antigens in 143 South African Black patients. Again in this population there was no indication of any HLA association.

Disease Heterogeneity

Koenig et al.[10] examined the sera of 89 German patients for antibodies against herpes simplex type 1 and type 2 viruses. The antibody titer for type 1 virus did not differ significantly between groups of individuals with and without a specific HLA antigen. The titer for type 2 virus was significantly higher in patients positive for B12.

The authors note that in their study of 120 patients, B12 was associated with cervical carcinoma. This result was similar to that reported earlier by Takasugi et al.[2] However, as mentioned in the previous section, this association was not confirmed in the larger data reported by Terasaki et al.[1] Thus, the validity of this result and its significance remain in question.

See also refs. 11–13.

References

1. Terasaki PI, Perdue ST, Mickey MR: HLA frequencies in cancer: A second study. In Mulvihill JJ, Miller RW, Fraumeni JF Jr (eds): Raven Press, New York, 1977, p 321
2. Takasugi M, Terasaki PI, Henderson B, Mickey MR, Menck H, Thompson RW: HL-A antigens in solid tumors. Cancer Res 33:648-650, 1973
3. Tarpley JL, Chretien PB, Rogentine N, Twomey PL, Dellon AL: Histocompatibility antigens and solid malignant neoplasms. Arch Surg 110:269-271, 1975
4. Twomey PL, Rogentine GN, Chretien PB: Lymphocyte function and HL-A antigen frequency in gynecologic squamous cancer. Int Surg 59:468-472, 1974
5. Sniecinski I, Haley J, Morgan-Byrne J, Van Nagell J Jr: Histocompatibility-antigen distribution in patients with cervical endometrial carcinomas. Gynecol Oncol 11:68-74, 1981
6. Bertrams J, Thraenhart O, Feldman U, Kuwert E: HL-A antigens in cancer of the breast and the collum uteri. Z Immun Forsch 148:391-394, 1975
7. Bertrams J, Thraenhart O, Feldmann U, Kuwert E: HL-A antigens in carcinoma of the breast, ovarium, cervix and endometrium: Possible association of haplotype HL-A10-W18 with carcinoma of the breast. Z Krebsforsch 83:219-222, 1975
8. Hammond MG, Appadoo B, Brain P: HLA and cancer in South African Indians. Tissue Antigens 14:296-302, 1979
9. Hammond MG, Appadoo B, Brain P: HLA and cancer in South African negroes. Tissue Antigens 9:1-7, 1977
10. Koenig UD, Muller N, Schneweis KE: Herpes-simplex-type-2 antibodies and HLA-B12 in cervical cancer. Lancet ii:857, 1976
11. Koenig UD, Muller N: Zur Wertigeit der Untersuchungen von HL-A Antigenen und lymphozytotoxischen Antiporperm bei Cervixcarcinom-Apatientinnen. Arch Gynaekol 224:473-474, 1977
12. Koenig UD, Muller N: Untersuchungen zur Bedeutung der Histokompatibilitatsantigene bei Zervixkarzinompatientinnen. Geburtshilfe Frauenheilkd 36:416-420, 1976
13. Truia CI, Truia M, Iosub A, Mudric V, Costachel O: Variation of the HL-A antigens during neoplasm evolution. Physiologie 17:239-245, 1980

Carcinoma of the Breast

Population Association

The first report by Patel et al.[1] showed a marginally significant increase in the frequency of B7 in 52 American Caucasian patients (Table 12.5). However, in 7 subsequent reports from several countries,[2–8] this association with B7 was not confirmed. The largest study is that by Terasaki et al.,[2,9] in which 705 patients were typed for A and B loci antigens. No significant association was observed. The authors, however, have noted a decrease of A3 in the patients (23% in 705 patients vs. 27% in 3896 controls).

In 1979 Bouillenne and Deneufbourg[6] reported an increased frequency of BW35 in 141 patients from Belgium (Table 12.5). It is interesting that none of the 7 reports was able to confirm this association. Yet, in the combined analysis of all the data the association with BW35 was significant (Table 12.5) and there was no evidence of heterogeneity in the data.

Two reports are also available from South Africa on Black[10] and Indian[11] populations. In 61 Black patients Hammond et al.[10] found no association with A, B, and C loci antigens. The same authors[11] also studied 249 patients from 6 Indian ethnic groups living in Durban. BW52 was determined to be significantly increased in a small sample of the Telegu ethnic group (Table 12.5).

In an interesting but different type of study, Feingold et al.[12] calculated correlation coefficients between the death rate from breast carcinoma and HLA antigens. There were positive correlations with A1, B8, and B12 in 22 different Caucasian populations. Interestingly, there was a negative correlation with BW35.

Disease Heterogeneity

Bouillenne and Deneufbourg[6] have grouped the patients according to hormonal status and parity. BW35 was increased in menopausal (n = 87), nulliparous (n = 34), and menopausal and nulliparous (n = 23) groups. A28 was also significantly increased in the nulliparous and menopausal groups.

De Jong-Bakker et al.[5] also subdivided their 200 patients with respect to age, parity, familial occurrence of breast cancer, bilateral cancer, axillary node involvement, type of spread, symptom-free interval after surgery, and histologic tumor type. None of these subgroups showed any significant deviations in antigen frequencies.

Family Data

See ref. 13.

See also refs. 14–18.

References

1. Patel R, Habal MB, Wilson RE, Birtch AG, Moore FD: Histocompatibility (HL-A) antigens and cancer of the breast: Association with HL-A7. Am J Surg 124:31-34, 1972
2. Terasaki PI, Perdue ST, Mickey MR: HLA frequencies in cancer: A second study. In Mulvihill JJ, Miller RW, Fraumeni JF Jr (eds): Genetics of Human Cancer. Raven Press, New York, 1977, p 321
3. Martz E, Benacerraf B: Lack of association between carcinoma of the breast and HL-A specificities. Tissue Antigens 3:30-38, 1973
4. Tarpley JL, Chretien PB, Rogentine N, Twomey PL, Dellon AL: Histocompatibility antigens and

TABLE 12.5. Carcinoma of the Breast

Country/Population	Patients n	Patients %+	Controls n	Controls %+	RR	χ^2	Ref.
HLA-BW35							
U.S.A.	52	27	123	26	1.07	0.03	1
U.S.A.	705	22	3896	19	1.20	3.50	2
U.S.A.	24	12	389	14	0.95	0.01	3
U.S.A.	40	13	80	13	1.04	0.00	4
	821	22	4488	19	1.18	3.23	
	Heterogeneity χ^2 (3 df)					0.32	
BENELUX	141	31	198	17	2.18	9.02	6
BENELUX	200	35	200	26	1.53	3.80	5
	341	33	398	22	1.77	11.72	
	Heterogeneity χ^2 (1 df)					1.10	
England	97	13	107	5	2.70	3.90	7
West Germany	60	15	1000	17	0.90	0.09	8
	1319	24	5993	18	1.30	11.29	
	Heterogeneity χ^2 (7 df)					9.07	
HLA-BW52							
South Africa—Indian	14	43	122	6	11.32	15.39	11

solid malignant neoplasms. Arch Surg 110:269-271, 1975
5. De Jong-Bakker M, Cleton FJ, D'Amaro J, Keuning JJ, Van Rood JJ: HL-A antigens and breast cancer. Eur J Cancer 10:555-558, 1974
6. Bouillenne C, Deneufbourg JM: Positive correlation between breast cancer incidence and HLA antigens. Oncology 36:156-159, 1979
7. Cordon AL, James DCO: HL-A and carcinoma of the breast. Lancet ii:565, 1973
8. Bertrams J, Thraenhart O, Feldman U, Kuwert E: HL-A antigens in cancer of the breast and the collum uteri. Z Immun Forsch 148:391-394, 1975
9. Takasugi M, Terasaki PI, Henderson B, Mickey MR, Menck H, Thompson RW: HL-A antigens in solid tumors. Cancer Res 33:648-650, 1973
10. Hammond MG, Appadoo B, Brain P: HLA and cancer in South African negroes. Tissue Antigens 9:1-7, 1977
11. Hammond MG, Appadoo B, Brain P: HLA and cancer in South African Indians. Tissue Antigens 14:296-302, 1979
12. Feingold N, Degos L, Feingold J: HLA in populations: An approach for genetical susceptibility to cancer. J Immunogenet 6:29-35, 1979
13. Hors J, Dausset J: Maladies malignes identiques au sein d'une meme famille. Nouv Presse Med 3:1237, 1974
14. Bertrams J, Thraenhart O, Feldmann U, Kuwert E: HL-A antigens in carcinoma of the breast, ovarium, cervix and endometrium: Possible association of haplotype HL-A10-W18 with carcinoma of the breast. Z Krebsforsch 83:219-222, 1975
15. Noulinier J, Hoerni B, Durand M, Chauvergne J: Antigenes HL-A et cancer du sein. Nouv Presse Med 2:1072, 1973
16. Fleming KA, McMichael A, Morton JA, Woods, J, McGee JOD: Distribution of HLA class 1 antigens in normal human tissue and in mammary cancer. J Clin Pathol 34:779-784, 1981
17. Truia CI, Truia M, Iosub A, Mudric V, Costachel O: Variation of the HL-A antigens during neoplasm evolution. Physiologie 17:239-245, 1980
18. Natali PG, Giacomini P, Bigotti A, Imai K, Nicotra MR, Ng AK, et al: Heterogeneity in the expression of HLA and tumor-associated antigens by surgically removed and cultured breast carcinoma cells. Cancer Res 43:660-668, 1983

Carcinoma of the Lung and Larynx

Population Association

There is only 1 study by Hammond et al.[1] in which 41 African Black patients with carcinoma of the lung and larynx were typed for A, B, and C loci antigens. When antigen frequencies were compared with those in 500 controls no significant deviations were found.

Reference

1. Hammond MG, Appadoo B, Brain P: HLA and cancer in South African negroes. Tissue Antigens 9:1-7, 1977

Carcinoma of the Lung

Population Association

The first report on lung carcinoma by Takasugi et al.[1] noted a decrease of B5 in American Caucasian patients. This antigen was present in 16% of the 250 patients as compared with 22% in 906 controls. In a second updated report by Terasaki et al.[2] in which 405 lung cancer patients were studied, the frequency of B5 was 10% in the patients compared with 10% in 3896 controls. In this study the authors noted an interesting increase of AW29 in the patients. In another report on 38 American Caucasian patients with small cell carcinoma Markman et al.[3] observed an increased frequency of BW44.

In a study by Tarpley et al.,[4] 44 lung cancer patients were typed for A and B loci antigens and interesting deviations (nonsignificant) in the frequencies of B13, BW15, and B17 were noted. In addition, there was no difference in 24 breast adenocarcinoma, 20 oat cell lung carcinoma, and 10 undifferentiated lung carcinoma patients.

The report by Tarpley et al.[4] also included data on 47 patients with lung carcinoma (25 squamous cell carcinoma and 13 adenocarcinoma). In this group there was a nonsignificant increase of B5 in the patients (34% in 47 patients vs. 15% in 100 controls).

Thus, from these 4 reports there is no consistent and strong evidence for any HLA association with lung cancer. (See also below.)

Disease Heterogeneity

Bronchogenic Carcinoma

Tongio et al.[5] have found an increased frequency of B12 in a study of French patients with primary bronchial carcinoma.

Dellon et al.[6,7] compared the A and B loci antigen frequencies at the time of diagnosis in 100 American Caucasian patients with bronchogenic carcinoma. Of these, 38 had squamous cell carcinoma, 32 had adenocarcinoma, 20 had oat cell carcinoma, and 10 patients had undifferentiated bronchogenic carcinoma. There was no significant difference between the total group and controls. The antigen frequencies in each of the subgroups of patients were also not different from the controls.

Sengar et al.[8,9] have also reported data on 37 Caucasian bronchogenic cell carcinoma patients from Canada. Twenty patients (13 squamous carcinoma, 5 adenocarcinoma, and 2 anaplastic carcinoma) were studied retrospectively. Another group of 17 patients (8 squamous cell carcinoma, 6 adenocarcinoma, and 3 anaplastic carcinoma) were HLA-typed prospectively.

The authors noted a decrease of A2 in the total patients (27% in 37 patients vs. 48.8% in 176 controls, $\chi^2 = 5.03$) and an increase of B8 in the retrospective group (45% in 20 patients vs. 18.7% in 176 controls, $\chi^2 = 5.07$). These 2 deviations, however, were not significant.

Thus, again on the basis of these 2 reports, bronchogenic carcinoma in North American Caucasians is not associated with HLA-A and -B loci antigens.

Disease-Free Survival

The report by Dellon et al.[6] compared the antigen frequencies in 14 Caucasian patients surgically treated for bronchogenic carcinoma (9 squamous cell carcinoma and 5 adenocarcinoma). The average time after treatment was 6.2 years and this retrospective group was considered cured. The second group of 100 patients was studied prospectively (the composition of the group is discussed in the previous section).

The frequencies of AW19 and B5 in the retrospective group were 36% and 43%, respectively. The AW19 frequency in this group was higher than that of the 10% in the prospective group and 11% in 184 controls (p for both comparisons < 0.025). Similarly, B5 was present in 17% of the patients in the prospective group and in 12% of the controls. Thus, B5 was slightly higher in the retrospective group compared with the controls ($p < 0.01$).

Of the 100 patients in the prospective group 60 were categorized as "prolonged survival" (without evidence of tumor at 1 year after surgery and/or radiation therapy). AW19 and B5 were significantly increased in the prolonged survival group as compared with the group in which tumor was present less than 1 year after treatment.

In a second report by the same group of authors,[7] 76 prospectively studied bronchogenic carcinoma (38 with squamous cell carcinoma and 32 with adenocarcinoma) patients were followed for 2 years. Again in this group disease-free status at 2 years was significantly associated with the presence of either AW19 or B5 (for detailed analysis of the data see ref. 7).

In another report on 20 American Caucasian patients with bronchogenic carcinoma (11 squamous cell carcinoma, 4 adenocarcinoma, and 5 undifferentiated carcinoma), Weiss et al.[10] also found a positive association between AW19 and/or B5 and a disease-free survival for at least 1 year from the time of diagnosis. Fifty percent of the patients were positive for AW19 and/or B5 as compared with 28.3% in 173 controls ($p < 0.08$).

The report by Sengar et al.[8,9] also had data on 20 patients studied retrospectively. These patients had a median survival time of 24 months after surgery. The B8 antigen was present in 45% of the patients compared with 18.7% in 176 controls ($\chi^2 = 5.07$). This study did not confirm the increased frequency of AW19 and B5 reported by Dellon et al.[6,7] and later by Weiss et al.[10] The difference in results may be a result of the heterogeneity of the bronchogenic carcinoma patients.

In an interesting study by Feingold et al.[11] correlation coefficients were obtained for the death rate from lung carcinoma and HLA antigens. There was no significant correlation in the data for 22 Caucasian populations.

In summary, available data do not reflect strong evidence for association between HLA-A and -B loci antigens and lung carcinoma.

See also ref. 12.

References

1. Takasugi M, Terasaki PI, Henderson B, Mickey MR, Menck H, Thompson RW: HL-A antigens in solid tumors. Cancer Res 33:648-650, 1973
2. Terasaki PI, Perdue ST, Mickey MR: HLA frequencies in cancer: A second study. In Mulvihill JJ, Miller RW, Fraumeni JF Jr (eds): Genetics of Human Cancer. Raven Press, New York, 1977, p 321
3. Markman M, Braine HG, Bias WB, Abeloff MD: Association between HLA-Bw44 and small-cell carcinoma of the lung. N Engl J Med 307:1087, 1982
4. Tarpley JL, Chretien PB, Rogentine N, Twomey PL, Dellon AL: Histocompatibility antigens and solid malignant neoplasms. Arch Surg 110:269-271, 1975
5. Tongio MM, Kerschen C, Pauli G, Roeslin N, Grange D, Mayer S: HLA antigens and primary bronchial carcinoma. Cancer 49:2485-2488, 1982
6. Dellon AL, Rogentine GN, Chretien PB: Prolonged

survival in bronchogenic carcinoma associated with HLA antigens W-19 and HL-A5: A preliminary report. J Natl Cancer Inst 54:1283-1286, 1975
7. Rogentine GN Jr, Dellon AL, Chretien PB: Prolonged disease-free survival in bronchogenic carcinoma associated with HLA-AW19 and HLA-B5. Cancer 39:2345-2347, 1977
8. Sengar DPS, McLeish WA, Stewart THM, Harris JE: HLA antigens in bronchogenic carcinoma. Oncology 34:143-145, 1977
9. Sengar DPS, McLeish WA, Stewart THM, Harris JE: HLA-Antigene beim Bronchuskarzinom. Onkologie 1:63-65, 1978
10. Weiss GB, Nawrocki LB, Daniels JC: HLA type and survival in lung cancer. Cancer 46:38-40, 1980
11. Feingold N, Degos L, Feingold J: HLA in populations: An approach for genetical susceptibility to cancer. J Immunogenet 6:29-35, 1979
12. Truia CI, Truia M, Iosub A, Mudric V, Costachel O: Variation of the HL-A antigens during neoplasm evolution. Physiologie 17:239-245, 1980

Carcinoma of the Larynx

Population Association

Terasaki et al.[1] reported a probable association with BW21 in American Caucasian patients (Table 12.6). However, in 64 American Caucasian[2] and in 110 French patients[3] no significant associations with any A and B loci antigens were found. BW21 was not typed in these studies.

References

1. Terasaki PI, Perdue ST, Mickey MR: HLA frequencies in cancer: A second study. In Mulvihill JJ, Miller RW, Fraumeni JF Jr (eds): Genetics of Human Cancer. Raven Press, New York, 1977, p 321
2. Tarpley JL, Chretien PB, Rogentine N, Twomey PL, Dellon AL: Histocompatibility antigens and solid malignant neoplasms. Arch Surg 110:269-271, 1975
3. Deneufbourg JM, Bouillenne C: Relationship of HLA antigens to larynx carcinoma: Incidence and five-year survival. Bull Cancer (Paris) 67:531-534, 1980

Carcinoma of the Pancreas

Population Association

Terasaki et al.[1] found no association with A and B loci antigens in 40 American Caucasian patients.

Reference

1. Terasaki PI, Perdue ST, Mickey MR: HLA frequencies in cancer: A second study. In Mulvihill JJ, Miller RW, Fraumeni JF Jr (eds): Genetics of Human Cancer. Raven Press, New York, 1977, p 321

Carcinoma of the Liver

Population Association

An association with A29 in American Caucasian patients was first reported by Terasaki et al.[1] Another report[2] found a significant increase of B12 in Greek patients. The frequency data from these two reports are given in Table 12.7.

In a small sample of Black patients from South Africa (Table 12.7) Hammond et al.[3] found an increased frequency of A1. However, in 102 South African Black patients with hepatocellular carcinoma, Kew et al.[4] found this antigen decreased in the patients (Table 12.7). In the combined sample the deviation of A1 was not significant and there was evidence of significant heterogeneity between these 2 patient groups.

AW36 was another antigen showing an interesting deviation in the data of Kew et al.[4] It was present in 5.9% of 102 patients and in only 0.5% of the 208 controls ($p < 0.05$ without correction). This antigen was not typed in Hammond et al.'s study.[3]

A third report from Singapore[5] on 114 Chinese patients (hepatocellular carcinoma) did not reveal any significant association with A and B loci antigens in the total sample.

TABLE 12.6. Carcinoma of the Larynx

	Patients		Controls				
Country/Population	n	%+	n	%+	RR	χ^2	Ref.
HLA-BW21							
U.S.A.	109	10	3896	5	2.19	6.19	1

TABLE 12.7. Carcinoma of the Liver

Country/Population	Patients n	Patients %+	Controls n	Controls %+	RR	χ^2	Ref.
HLA-A1							
Africa—Black (unspecified)	35	17	500	5	4.07	9.05	3
Africa—Black (unspecified)	102	1	208	8	0.17	5.63	4
	137	5	708	6	1.68	1.71	
	Heterogeneity χ^2 (1 df)					12.97	
HLA-A29							
U.S.A.	56	16	3896	6	3.11	10.24	1
Greece	52	4	290	4	1.18	0.06	2
	108	10	4186	6	2.50	8.61	
	Heterogeneity χ^2 (1 df)					1.70	
HLA-B12							
U.S.A.	56	36	3896	26	1.62	3.05	1
Greece	52	42	400	19	3.09	13.85	2
	108	39	4296	25	2.17	14.40	
	Heterogeneity χ^2 (1 df)					2.50	

Disease Heterogeneity

In the South African study by Kew et al.[4] 50 patients were positive and 50 were negative for HBsAg. The A29 frequency was 24% in the HBsAg-negative group and 6% in the HBsAg-positive group. This antigen was present in 12.5% of the 208 controls. The difference between HBsAg-negative and the controls and between HBsAg-positive and -negative groups was significant ($p < 0.05$).

The Chinese patients from Singapore[5] were subdivided into groups of α-fetoprotein-positive (n = 87), and α-fetoprotein- negative (n = 27), HBsAg-positive (n = 74), and HBsAg-negative (n = 40) persons. The frequencies of B15 in these 4 subgroups were 27.6%, 55.6%, 32.4%, and 37.5%, respectively. This antigen was present in 34.5% of the total patients (n = 114) and 22.3% of the 238 controls. Thus, the most pronounced difference was between the α-fetoprotein-negative (55.6% of 27 patients) and control (22.3% of 238) groups.

References

1. Terasaki PI, Perdue ST, Mickey MR: HLA frequencies in cancer: A second study. In Mulvihill JJ, Miller RW, Fraumeni JF Jr (eds): Genetics of Human Cancer. Raven Press, New York, 1977, p 321
2. Zervas J, Karvountzis G, Theodoropoulos G: HLA antigens and hepatocellular carcinoma. Gastroenterology 79:601, 1980
3. Hammond MG, Appadoo B, Brain P: HLA and cancer in South African negroes. Tissue Antigens 9:1-7, 1977
4. Kew MC, Gear AJ, Baumgarten I, Dusheiko GM, Maier G: Histocompatibility antigens in patients with hepatocellular carcinoma and their relationship to chronic hepatitis B virus infection in these patients. Gastroenterology 77:537-539, 1979
5. Chan SH, Simons MJ, Oon CJ: HLA antigen in Chinese patients with hepatocellular carcinomas. J Natl Cancer Inst 65: 21-23, 1980

Carcinoma of the Rectum

Population Association

In a sample of 88 American Caucasian patients, Terasaki et al.[1,2] found no association with A and B loci antigens. A second report by Alcalay et al.[3] found an increased frequency of B27 in 81 patients (19.75% in the patients vs. 8.5% in 319 controls). In Terasaki et al.'s data[1] B27 was actually decreased in the patients.

However, in a study of 22 Caucasians, A1, B8, and B12 were found to be correlated with the death rate for colorectal carcinoma[4].

Hiwatashi et al.[5] reported a probable association with BW35 in a small sample of Japanese patients (Table 12.8).

See also ref. 6.

TABLE 12.8. Carcinoma of the Rectum

	Patients		Controls				
Country/Population	n	%+	n	%+	RR	χ^2	Ref.
HLA-BW35							
Japan	25	28	120	10	3.52	6.00	5

References

1. Terasaki PI, Perdue ST, Mickey MR: HLA frequencies in cancer: A second study. In Mulvihill JJ, Miller RW, Fraumeni JF Jr (eds): Genetics of Human Cancer. Raven Press, New York, 1977, p 321
2. Takasugi M, Terasaki PI, Henderson B, Mickey MR, Menck H, Thompson RW: HL-A antigens in solid tumors. Cancer Res 33:648-650, 1973
3. Alcalay M, Bontoux D, Maire P, Matuchansky C, Alcalay D, Tanzer J: HLA-B27 and colorectal cancer. N Engl J Med 307:443-444, 1982
4. Feingold N, Degos L, Feingold J: HLA in populations: An approach for genetical susceptibility to cancer. J Immunogenet 6:29-35, 1979
5. Hiwatashi N, Kikuchi T, Masamune O, Ouchi E, Watanabe H, Goto Y: HLA antigens in colorectal cancers and adenomas. Tohoku J Exp Med 131:257-260, 1980
6. Daar AS, Fuggle SV, Ting A, Fabre JW: Anomolous expression of HLA-DR antigens on human colorectal cancer cells. J Immunol 129:447-449, 1982

Carcinoma of the Colon

Population Association

Terasaki et al.[1,2] found no evidence of an association with A and B loci antigens in 189 American Caucasian patients.

A report from Japan,[3] based on a small sample of 35 patients, however, did show some evidence of a probable association with BW35 (Table 12.9).

Correlation coefficients between death rates for various types of carcinoma and HLA antigens have been calculated by Feingold et al.[4] Data from 22 Caucasian populations showed a significant correlation ($p < 0.01$) between colorectal carcinoma and A1, B8, and B12 antigens.

Family Data

Sivak et al.[5] published a large pedigree with several affected individuals. The lod score analysis of this pedigree showed a maximum score of 1.06 at a recombination frequency of 20%.

See also refs. 6 and 7.

References

1. Terasaki PI, Perdue ST, Mickey MR: HLA frequencies in cancer: A second study. In Mulvihill JJ, Miller RW, Fraumeni JF Jr, (eds): Genetics of Human Cancer. Raven Press, New York, 1977, p 321
2. Takasugi M, Terasaki PI, Henderson B, Mickey MR, Menck H, Thompson RW: HL-A antigens in solid tumors. Cancer Res 33:648-650, 1973
3. Hiwatashi N, Kikuchi T, Masamune O, Ouchi E, Watanabe H, Goto Y: HLA antigens in colorectal cancers and adenomas. Tohoku J Exp Med 131:257-260, 1980
4. Feingold N, Degos L, Feingold J: HLA in populations: An approach for genetical susceptibility to cancer. J Immunogenet 6:29-35, 1979
5. Sivak MV, Sivak DS, Braun WA, Sullivan BH: A linkage study of HLA and inherited adenocarcinoma of the colon. Cancer 48:76-81, 1981
6. Daar AS, Fuggle SV, Ting A, Fabre JW: Anomolous expression of HLA-DR antigens on human colorectal cancer cells. J Immunol 129:447-449, 1982

TABLE 12.9. Carcinoma of the Colon

	Patients		Controls				
Country/Population	n	%+	n	%+	RR	χ^2	Ref.
HLA-BW35							
Japan	35	29	120	10	3.65	7.81	3

7. Alcalay M, Bontoux D, Maire P, Matuchansky C, Alcalay D, Tanzer J: HLA-B27 and colorectal cancer. N Engl J Med 307:443-444, 1982

Carcinoma of the Stomach

Population Association

Tsuji et al.[1] reported a decreased frequency of A9 in Japanese patients (Table 12.10). An analysis of A and B loci antigen frequencies in 99 Japanese patients from Hawaii (66 with intestinal and other histologic types of stomach cancer and 31 patients with the diffuse type) also showed a nonsignificant decrease in A9 (only the AW24 frequency is given; Table 12.10).

In American Caucasian patients, Terasaki et al.[2,3] reported deviations in the frequencies of A10 and A11 (Table 12.10).

References

1. Tsuji K, Miyamoto H, Motoaki I. HL-A and its clinical application. Keio J Med 21:159-169, 1972
2. Terasaki PI, Perdue ST, and Mickey MR: HLA frequencies in cancer: A second study. In Mulvihill JJ, Miller RW, Fraumeni JF Jr, (eds): Genetics of Human Cancer. Raven Press, New York, 1977, p 321
3. Takasugi M, Terasaki PI, Henderson B, Mickey MR, Menck H, Thompson RW: HL-A antigens in solid tumors. Cancer Res 33:648-650, 1973
4. Nomura A, Glober GA, Terasaki PI, Stemmermann GN: HLA antigens in stomach cancer. Int J Cancer 25:195-196, 1980

Carcinoma of the Esophagus

Population Association

The first report by Tarpley et al.[1] on 17 American Caucasian patients revealed an increased but not highly significant frequency of B12 in the patient group (Table 12.11). In a later report by Terasaki et al.,[2] a similar association with B12 was observed in 47 American Caucasian patients (Table 12.11). In their first study, Hammond et al.[3] found an association with BW45 (a split of B12) in South African Blacks (15.8% in 101 patients vs. 7.2% in 500 con-

TABLE 12.10. Carcinoma of the Stomach

	Patients		Controls				
Country/Population	n	%+	n	%+	RR	χ^2	Ref.
HLA-A9							
Japan	67	16	128	38	0.32	9.53	1
U.S.A. (Hawaii)—Japanese	99	48	222	60	0.62	4.00	4
	166	35	350	52	0.51	11.33	
	Heterogeneity χ^2 (1 df)					2.20	
HLA-A10							
U.S.A.	58	24	3896	13	2.16	6.51	2

TABLE 12.11. Carcinoma of the Esophagus

	Patients		Controls				
Country/Population	n	%+	n	%+	RR	χ^2	Ref.
HLA-B12							
U.S.A.	17	53	389	24	3.53	7.08	1
U.S.A.	47	40	3896	26	1.91	4.89	2
	64	43	4285	26	2.27	10.76	
	Heterogeneity χ^2 (1 df)					1.21	

trols). In the second study with additional patients, the frequency of BW45 was 10.6% in 254 patients compared with 6.4% in 756 controls. BW44, the second split of B12, was present in 16.9% of the patients and in 16.0% of the controls. The frequency of B12 (BW44 and BW45) in the total sample (2488) was not significantly different from the controls.[4]

The data of Tarpley et al.[1] showed a slight decrease of B12 in 22 American Black patients.

See also ref. 4.

References

1. Tarpley JL, Chretien PB, Rogentine N, Twomey PL, Dellon AL: Histocompatibility antigens and solid malignant neoplasms. Arch Surg 110:269-271, 1975
2. Terasaki PI, Perdue ST, and Mickey MR: HLA frequencies in cancer: A second study. In Mulvihill JJ, Miller RW, Fraumeni JF Jr, (eds): Genetics of Human Cancer. Raven Press, New York, 1977, p. 321
3. Hammond MG, Appadoo B, Brain P: HLA and cancer in South African negroes. Tissue Antigens 9:1-7, 1977
4. Hammond MG, Angorn B: HLA and cancer of the esophagus in South African Negroes. Tissue Antigens 16:254-255, 1980

Carcinoma of the Pharynx

Population Association

In 16 American patients (of unknown race), there was no association with A and B loci antigens.[1]

Reference

1. Tarpley JL, Chretien PB, Rogentine N, Twomey PL, Dellon AL: Histocompatibility antigens and solid malignant neoplasms. Arch Surg 110:269-271, 1975

Carcinoma of the Nasopharynx

Population Association

In their first report, Simons et al.[1] reported increased frequencies of A2 and a B locus antigen, Sin 2 (Singapore 2), now called BW46, in 31 Singapore Chinese patients. In subsequent reports by the same authors,[2–4] the study was expanded and more patients were HLA-typed. The increase of A2 and BW46 was observed in a later study[5] based on 153 patients (Table 12.12). It should be noted, however, that the increase of A2 was not significant and that of BW46 was significant only if corrections for multiple comparisons were not considered.

In 3 other studies from Tunisia[5] and from the United States on American Chinese[6] and on Alaskan Eskimos, Indians, and Aleuts,[7] no association with A2 was observed (Table 12.12).

Jing et al.[6] also reported an increase in A1 and a decrease in A2 in American Caucasian patients (Table 12.12).

The data of Simon et al.[3] showed that the frequency of the A2-BW46 haplotype in 130 Singapore Chinese patients was 34.6% as compared with 17.8% in 73 controls. This increase of the A2-BW46 haplotype was significant ($p = 0.007$, relative risk = 2.23). It should also be noted that A2 and BW46 are in linkage disequilibrium in healthy Chinese (see

TABLE 12.12. Carcinoma of the Nasopharynx

	Patients		Controls				
Country/Population	n	%+	n	%+	RR	χ^2	Ref.
HLA-A2							
Singapore—Chinese	153	63	91	52	1.57	2.86	3
U.S.A.—Chinese	37	76	48	42	4.19	9.42	6
U.S.A.—Eskimo	16	44	21	38	1.27	0.14	7
	206	64	160	47	1.89	8.63	
	Heterogeneity χ^2 (2 df)					3.79	
Tunisia	109	29	84	42	0.57	3.53	5
U.S.A.	39	31	49	47	0.52	2.28	6
HLA-BW46							
Singapore—Chinese	153	39	91	25	1.90	4.90	3

studies cited in ref. 3), and the demonstration of disease association with a haplotype requires detailed analyses.

Family Data

See ref. 8.

References

1. Simons MJ, Wee GB, Chan SH, Shanmugaratnam K, Day NE, De-The GB: Probable identification of an HL-A second-locus antigen associated with a high risk of nasopharyngeal carcinoma. Lancet i:142-143, 1975
2. Simons MJ, Day NE: Histocompatibility leukocyte antigen patterns and nasopharyngeal carcinoma. Natl Cancer Inst Monogr 47:143-146, 1977
3. Simons MJ, Wee GB, Singh D, Dharmalingham S, Yong NK, Chau JCW, et al: Immunogenetic aspects of nasopharyngeal carcinoma. V. Confirmation of a Chinese-related HLA profile (A2, Singapore 2). Natl Cancer Inst Monogr 47:147-151, 1977
4. Simons MJ, Wee GB, Goh EH, Chan SH, et al: Immunogenetic aspects of nasopharyngeal carcinoma. IV. Increased risk in Chinese of nasopharyngeal carcinoma associated with a Chinese-related HLA profile (A2 Sin 2). J Natl Cancer Inst 57:977-980, 1976
5. Betuel H, Camoun M, Colombani J, Day NE, Ellouz R, De-The G: The relationship between nasopharyngeal carcinoma and the HL-A system among Tunisians. Int J Cancer 16:249-254, 1975
6. Jing J, Louie E, Henderson BE, Terasaki PI: Histocompatibility leukocyte antigen patterns in nasopharyngeal carcinoma cases from California. Natl Cancer Inst Monogr 47:153-156, 1977
7. Lanier A, Bender T, Talbot M, Wilmeth S, Tschopp C, Henle W, et al: Nasopharyngeal carcinoma in Alaskan Eskimos, Indians, and Aleuts. Cancer 46:2100-2106, 1980
8. Joncas JH, Rioux E, Wastiaux JP, Leyritz M, Robillard L, Menezes J: Nasopharyngeal carcinoma and Burkitt's lymphoma in a Canadian family. I. HLA typing, EBV antibodies and serum immunoglobulins. Can Med Assoc J 115:858-860, 1976

Carcinoma of the Salivary Gland

Population Association

Tarpley et al.[1] reported A and B loci frequency data in a small sample of 18 American Caucasian patients with adenocarcinoma of the salivary gland. The noticeable observations were increased frequencies of B8 and B12 (Table 12.13).

Reference

1. Tarpley JL, Chretien PB, Rogentine N, Twomey PL, Dellon AL: Histocompatibility antigens and solid malignant neoplasms. Arch Surg 110:269-271, 1975

Carcinoma of the Pituitary Gland

Population Association

In a study of 22 Canadian patients with prolactin secretive adenomata, Farid et al.[1] observed an increase of B8 (Table 12.14).

Reference

1. Farid NR, Noel EP, Sampson L, Russell NA: Prolactin secreting pituitary adenomata are possibly associated with HLA-B8. Tissue Antigens 15:333-335, 1980

Testicular Cancer

Population Association

Carr and Bach[1] reported an increased frequency of AW24 (Table 12.15) in 9 patients with teratocar-

TABLE 12.13. Carcinoma of the Salivary Gland

	Patients		Controls				
Country/Population	n	%+	n	%+	RR	χ^2	Ref.
HLA-B8							
U.S.A.	18	67	389	17	9.47	21.17	1
HLA-B12							
U.S.A.	18	50	389	24	3.16	6.17	1

TABLE 12.14. Carcinoma of the Pituitary Gland

	Patients		Controls				
Country/Population	n	%+	n	%+	RR	χ^2	Ref.
HLA-B8							
Canada	22	55	214	25	3.61	8.56	1

cinoma (nonseminomatous). This, however, was not confirmed in another study of 145 patients by Pollack et al.[2] A report by Majsky et al.[3] from Czechoslovakia on 40 patients with testicular germinative tumors also did not show any significant increase in the A and B loci antigen frequencies. The frequencies in 22 patients with nonseminomatous tumors were also not different from controls.

DeWolf et al.[4] studied A, B, and D loci antigen frequencies in 26 patients with teratocarcinoma. A and B loci antigens did not differ from those of the control group but DW7 was significantly increased in the patients (Table 12.15). It is interesting to note that in Pollack et al.'s report[2] 105 patients were typed for DR locus antigens. The frequency of DR7 in the patients was not significantly different from the controls. In these data DR3 was found to be decreased (nonsignificant after correction).

Disease Heterogeneity

In DeWolf et al.'s data[4] A, B and D loci antigens were also studied in 24 patients with seminoma, 7 with choriocarcinoma, and 24 with embryonal cell carcinoma. No significant deviations were found.

Majsky et al.[3] subdivided their patients into seminoma (n = 40) and nonseminoma (n = 22) groups. No HLA association was found in either group. Nonseminoma patients were also subdivided on the basis of survival (less and greater than 5 years). Again no significant association was observed.

Similar nonsignificant results were also reported by Pollack et al.[2] in various subgroups of American Caucasian patients.

Family Data

Pollack et al.[2] reported HLA haplotypes in 3 small pedigrees with more than 1 affected sibling. In these families the affected sibpairs shared at least 1 HLA haplotype.

See also refs. 5-7.

References

1. Carr BI, Bach FH: Possible association between HLA-AW24 and metastatic testicular germ cell tumours. Lancet i:1346-1347, 1979
2. Pollack MS, Vugrin D, Hennessy W, Herr HW, Dupont B, Whitmore WF Jr: HLA antigens in patients with germ cell cancers of the testis. Cancer Res 42:2470-2473, 1982
3. Majsky A, Abrahamova J, Korinkova P, Bek V: HLA system and testicular germinative tumours. Oncology 36:228-231, 1979
4. DeWolf WC, Lange PH, Einarson ME, Yunis EJ: HLA and testicular cancer. Nature 277:216-217, 1979
5. Abrahamova J, Majsky A, Koutecky J, Bek V: HLA system a germinalni nadory gonadalni a extragonadalni. Cas Lek Cesk 119:51-54, 1980
6. Majsky A, Abrahamova J: Pritomnost HLA-A2 antigenu na lymfocytech: Ochrana pred vznikem nadoru? Cas Lek Cesk 119:47-50, 1980
7. Majsky A, Abrahamova J: Schutzen die HLA-A2-Gene vor der Entwicklung eines Tumors? Eine Hypothese. Folia Haematol (Leipz) 108:90-96, 1981

TABLE 12.15. Testicular Cancer

	Patients		Controls				
Country/Population	n	%+	n	%+	RR	χ^2	Ref.
HLA-DW7							
U.S.A.	26	46	150	9	8.39	20.57	4

Renal Cell Carcinoma

Population Association

Terasaki et al.[1] and DeWolf et al.[2] have found no association with A and B loci antigens in American Caucasian patients. However, in another report from Germany, Kuntz et al.[3] typed 44 hypernephroma patients and found a significant association with AW30 and AW31 (Table 12.16). The AW30 frequency for this study also included AW31 (i.e., in Table 12.16 AW30 = AW30 + AW31). The authors noted that the association was probably with AW30. In the early stages of this study it was not possible to type for AW30 and AW31 and thus in the analysis these 2 antigens were combined.

The report by Terasaki et al.[1] gives frequency data only for AW30, which was not significantly increased in the patients. Also, in the combined data, the association with AW30 was not significant (Table 12.16). DeWolf et al.[2] do not give data on A, B, and C loci antigens.

A highly significant increase of DR5 in patients (Table 12.16) has been observed by DeWolf et al.[2]

Family Data

In a French family[4] of 7 siblings, 4 had cancer of the left kidney (carcinomas with eosinophilic cells, diagnosed at an advanced stage with widespread lymph node involvement). All 4 affected siblings had the A2-B12 haplotype. However, the 3 affected siblings also had this particular haplotype.

Braun et al.[5] reported 3 families with 2 affected individuals in each (1 family had 4 affected individuals but 2 were deceased). In 2 of these families the affected individuals were 1 parent and 1 offspring. Thus, in these 3 families there was no strong evidence in favor of linkage between HLA and renal cell carcinoma. It should be noted that all the patients in this study had B17.

A third family with 2 affected and 4 healthy siblings was reported by Pilepich et al.[6] The 2 affected and 1 healthy siblings had the A2-BW21 haplotype in common. Three healthy siblings did not have this haplotype. Furthermore, the son of 1 of the affected siblings, had A2-BW21 but was disease-free. Thus, again there was no strong evidence to support the hypothesis of linkage in this family.

See also refs. 7 and 8.

References

1. Terasaki PI, Perdue ST, Mickey MR: HLA frequencies in cancer: A second study. In Mulvihill JJ, Miller RW, Fraumeni JF Jr, (eds): Genetics of Human Cancer. Raven Press, New York, 1977, p 321
2. DeWolf WC, Lange PH, Shepherd R, Martin-Alosco S, Yunis EJ: Association of HLA and renal cell carcinoma. Hum Immunol 1:41-44, 1981
3. Kuntz BME, Schmidt GD, Scholz S, Albert ED: HLA-antigens and hypernephroma. Tissue Antigens 12:407-408, 1978
4. Valleteau de Moulliac M, Ganansia R, Hors J, Letexier A, Morin M: Familial cancer of the kidney and the HLA sysyem (four cases of cancer of the left kidney in a sibship). Nouv Presse Med 3:1539-1542, 1974
5. Braun WE, Strimlan CV, Negron AG, Straffon MRA, Zachary AA, Bartee SL, et al: The association of W17 with familial renal cell carcinoma. Tissue Antigens 6:101-104, 1975
6. Pilepich MV, Berkman EM, Goodchild NT: HLA typing in familial renal carcinoma. Tissue Antigens 11:487-488, 1978
7. Schacter B, Braun WE, Bukowski R, Deodhar S:

TABLE 12.16. Renal Cell Carcinoma

	Patients		Controls				
Country/Population	n	%+	n	%+	RR	χ^2	Ref.
HLA-AW30							
U.S.A.	79	11	3896	10	1.17	0.20	1
West Germany	44	25	300	7	4.46	13.83	3
	123	16	4196	10	2.07	7.64	
	Heterogeneity χ^2 (1 df)					6.39	
HLA-DR5							
U.S.A.	26	54	124	20	4.60	12.10	2

HLA-B7 association with low spontaneous cell-mediated cytotoxicity (SP-CMC) to renal cell carcinoma cell lines. Transplant Proc 9:1849-1851, 1977
8. Hors J, Dausset J: Maladies malignes identiques au sein d'une meme famille. Nouv Presse Med 3:1237, 1974

Carcinoma (Unspecified)

Population Association

Jeannet and Magnin[1] reported a significant increase of A9 in 27 carcinoma (mainly lung and breast) patients. This antigen was present in 44% of the patients and in 21% of the 305 healthy controls ($p < 0.001$).

Family Data

Lynch et al.[2] HLA-typed 115 members of a large kindred in which approximately 1000 members were ascertained. An extraordinarily high frequency of cancer was observed in this family. Endometrium and colon carcinomas were predominant. In the cancer-prone line of the family, 11 of the 12 HLA-typed patients had the haplotype A2-B12 (relative odds = 6.06). Some of the patients were not typed but their haplotypes were assigned on the basis of information on relatives. When these patients were counted 20 of the 21 patients had the A2-B12 haplotype (relative odds = 6.30).

Gatti et al.[3] reported the lod score analysis of a pedigree in which more than 40% of the members of two generations have had breast, endometrial, and gastrointestinal cancer. The maximum lod score was 0.638 at a recombination frequency of 1% in females and 30% in males.

See also refs. 4–8.

References

1. Jeannet M, Magnin C: HL-A antigens in malignant diseases. Transplant Proc 3:1301-1303, 1971
2. Lynch HT, Thomas RJ, Terasaki PI, Ting A, Guirgis HA, Kaplan AR, et al: HL-A in cancer family "N." Cancer 36:1315-1320, 1975
3. Gatti RA, Sparkes RD, Field LL, Spence MA, Harris NS, Freidin M: Genetic linkage analysis in a high-risk cancer family: HLA and 24 other markers. Cancer Genet Cytogenet 8:9-18, 1983
4. Kersey JH, Yunis EJ, Todaro GJ, Aaronson SA: HL-A antigens of human tumor-derived cell lines and viral transformed fibroblasts in culture. Proc Soc Exp Biol Med 143:453-456, 1973
5. Kourilsky FM: Symposium international sur les relations entre les antigenes de tumeurs et les systemes d'histocompatibilite. Bull Cancer 58:315-324, 1977
6. Dellon AL, Chretien PB, Potvin C, Rogentine GN JR: Multiple primary malignant neoplasms: A search for an immunogenetic basis. Arch Surg 110:156-160, 1975
7. Pedersen-Bjergaard J, Philip P, Mortensen BT, Ersboll J, Jensen G, Panduro J, et al: Acute nonlymphocytic leukemia, preleukemia, and acute myeloproliferative syndrome secondary to treatment of other malignant disease. Blood 57:712-723, 1981
8. Ferrone S, Pellegrino MA, Callahan GN: Human and murine tumours: Changes in cell surface structures coded by the major histocompatibility complex region. J Immunogenet 7:71-79, 1980

Leukemia (Unspecified)

Population Association

Dickson[1] reported a highly significant increased frequency of A9 in a mixed sample of 54 patients with several types of leukemia (Table 12.17). In an earlier study of 24 patients by Pegrum et al.[2] and a later one by Terasaki et al.[3] of 140 patients this was not confirmed. In the combined sample (Table 12.17) the association was not highly significant and there was evidence of heterogeneity in the data.

In view of the mixed nature of each of the samples this marginally significant association with A9 was probably due to the artifact of serology and disease heterogeneity.

Terasaki et al.[3] also noted an increased frequency of AW32 in their 140 patients (12% in patients vs. 7% in 3896 controls, $p = 0.05$).

In a different type of study Feingold et al.[4] calculated correlation coefficients between death rate due to leukemia and HLA-A and -B loci antigens in 26 Caucasians. No significant correlation was found.

Family Data

No pedigree data are available. However, in a study of 30 couples with 1 child suffering with acute leukemia, Werner-Favre and Jeannet[5,6] reported an increased frequency of couples sharing 2 common HLA antigens (30% in 30 couples with an affected child vs. 8% in 58 healthy control couples, $p = 0.02$).

See also refs. 7–16.

TABLE 12.17. Leukemia (Unspecified)

Country/Population	Patients n	Patients %+	Controls n	Controls %+	RR	χ^2	Ref.
HLA-A9							
U.S.A.	140	24	3896	20	1.28	1.49	3
England	26	19	180	20	1.00	0.00	2
England	54	42	145	16	3.76	14.30	1
	80	35	325	18	2.42	9.55	
	Heterogeneity χ^2 (1 df)					4.74	
	220	28	4221	20	1.57	7.66	
	Heterogeneity χ^2 (2 df)					8.13	

References

1. Dickson A: A raised incidence of HL-A2 plus HL-A9 and other anomalies of the HL-A antigens of patients with leukemia. Acta Haematol 54:143-151, 1975
2. Pegrum GD, Balfour IC, Evans CA, Middleton VL: HL-A antigens on leukemia cells. Br J Haematol 19:493-498, 1970
3. Terasaki PI, Perdue ST, Mickey MR: HLA frequencies in cancer: A second study. In Mulvihill JJ, Miller RW, Fraumeni JF Jr, (eds): Genetics of Human Cancer. Raven Press, New York, 1977, p 321
4. Feingold N, Degos L, Feingold J: HLA in populations: An approach for genetical susceptibility to cancer. J Immunogenet 6:29-35, 1979
5. Werner-Favre CH, Jeannet M: HLA compatibility in couples with children suffering from acute leukemia or aplastic anemia. Tissue Antigens 13:307-309, 1979
6. Werner-Favre CH, Von Fliedner W, Jeannet M: Similitude des antigenes HLA chez les parents de patients atteints de leucemie aigue ou d'anemie aplastique. Schweiz Med Wochenschr 109:1399, 1979
7. Tsuji K: Neoplasms, leukemia, and HLA antigens. Nippon Rinsho 36:3137-3142, 1978
8. Editorial: Discussion on HLA by Drs. Laurber, Kourilsky, Walford, Thorsby, Sachs, and Morris. Transplant Proc 3:1311-1312, 1971
9. Billing RJ, Terasaki PI, Honig R, Peterson P: The absence of B-cell antigen B2 from leukaemia cells and lymphoblastoid cell lines. Lancet i:1365-1367, 1976
10. Ellman L, Green I, Martin WJ: Histocompatibility genes, immmune responsiveness, and leukaemia. Lancet i:1104-1106, 1970
11. Nedelkova M, Iliev D, Seratimov-Dimitrov W: Ueber die HL-A-Spezifitaet der Immunreaktion bei Parablastenleukosen. Folia Haematol 104:324-329, 1977
12. Kourilsky FM: Symposium international sur les relations entre les antigenes de tumeurs et les systemes d'histocompatibilite. Bull Cancer 58:315-324, 1977
13. Truia CI, Truia M, Iosub A, Mudric V, Costachel O: Variation of the HL-A antigens during neoplasm evolution. Physiologie 17:239-245, 1980
14. Oliver RTD, Lee SK: Histocompatibility antigens and T cell responses to leukemia antigens. Haematol Bluttranfus 23:377-379, 1979
15. Newman RA, Delia D, Greaves MF, Navarrete C, Fainboim L, Festenstein H: Differential expression of HLA-DR-linked determinants on human leukemias and lymphoid cells. Eur J Immunol 13:172-176, 1983
16. Morishima Y, Kawashima K, Yamada K, Minami S, Akaza T: Anomalous expression of histocompatibility antigens on human leukemia cells. Nippon Ketsueki Gakkai Zasshi 44:53-60, 1981

Granulocytic Leukemia

Population Association

In a small sample of 24 American Caucasian patients Terasaki et al.[1] noted an increased frequency of B27 (Table 12.18).

Reference

1. Terasaki PI, Perdue ST, Mickey MR: HLA frequencies in cancer: A second study. In Mulvihill JJ, Miller RW, Fraumeni JF Jr, (eds): Genetics of Human Cancer. Raven Press, New York, 1977, p 321

TABLE 12.18. Granulocytic Leukemia

	Patients		Controls				
Country/Population	n	%+	n	%+	RR	χ^2	Ref.
HLA-B27							
U.S.A.	24	21	3896	7	3.78	8.04	1

Chronic Myeloid Leukemia

Population Association

A and B loci frequency data available on 300 patients from 7 different studies on Caucasian patients from Europe and the United States do not show any consistent pattern of associations. Degos et al.[1] reported a higher frequency of A3 and a lower frequency of B12 in 47 French patients. Another study from France by Mayer et al.[2] reported an increase of A2 in 36 patients (75% vs. 54.77% in controls). The study by Jeannet and Magnin[3,4] noted an increase of A1 in 15 Swiss patients (60% in patients vs. 27% in 305 controls).

The results of 4 studies from the Unites States are also variable. Sixty patients studied by Pollack et al.[5] and a small sample of 7 patients studied by Miller[6] did not show any significant deviation. Another study by Hester et al.[7] on 43 patients showed an increase of A11, B5, and B17 and a decrease of B7 and BW35. A third report by Terasaki et al.[8] noted an increased frequency of B7 in 37 patients.

One study from the Soviet Union[9] did not find any significant association with A and B loci antigens.

In all of the above studies none of the deviations was significant if probabilities are corrected for multiple comparisons. Furthermore, the analysis of the pooled data does not show any significant association with A and B loci antigens.

See also refs. 10–14.

References

1. Degos L, Drolet Y, Dausett J: HL-A antigens in chronic myeloid leukemia (CML) and chronic lymphoid leukemia (CLL). Transplant Proc 3:1309-1310, 1971
2. Mayer S, Tongio MM, Bigel P: Etude des antigens HL-A dans la leucemie myeloide chronique. Nouv Rev Fr Hematol 15:284-288, 1975
3. Jeannet M, Magnin C: HL-A antigens in haematological malignant diseases. Eur J Clin Invest 2:39-42, 1976
4. Jeannet M, Magnin C: HL-A antigens in malignant diseases. Transplant Proc 3:1301-1303, 1971
5. Pollack MS, Dubois D: Possible effects of non-HLA antibodies in common typing sera on HLA antigen frequency data in leukemia. Cancer 39:2348-2354, 1977
6. Miller WV: HL-A antigens and hematologic malignancy. Arch Intern Med 133:397-399, 1974
7. Hester JP, Rossen R, Trujillo J, McCredie KB, Freireich EJ: Frequency of HLA antigens in chronic myelocytic leukemia. South Med J 70:691-693, 1977
8. Terasaki PI, Perdue ST, Mickey MR: HLA frequencies in cancer: A second study. In Mulvihill JJ, Miller RW, Fraumeni JF Jr, (eds): Genetics of Human Cancer. Raven Press, New York, 1977, p 321
9. Tananov AT, Kutyina RM, Turbina NS, Abakumov EM, Polyanskaya AM, Isaev VG, et al: HLA antigens in patients with blood pathology. Probl Gematol Pereliv Krovi 26:8-12, 1981
10. Morozova LF, Belyanchikova NI, Radzikhovskaya RM, Baryshnikov AYU, Volkova MA, Vinogradova MA et al: Discovery of B cell antigen on blast cells of patients with chronic myeloid leukemia. Biull Eksp Biol Med 87:574-576, 1979
11. Fingold N: Critical analysis of relationships between HL-A system and susceptibility to disease. Transplant Proc 3:1317-1320, 1971
12. Walford RL, Smith GS, Waters H: Histocompatibility systems and disease states with particular reference to cancer. Transplant Rev 7:78-111, 1971
13. Dickson A: A raised incidence of HL-A2 plus HL-A9 and other anomalies of the HL-A antigens of patients with leukemia. Acta Haematol 54:143-151, 1975
14. Billing RJ, Terasaki PI, Honig R, Peterson P: The absence of B-cell antigen B2 from leukaemia cells and lymphoblastoid cell lines. Lancet i:1365-1367, 1976

Acute Myeloid Leukemia

Population Association

A and B loci antigen frequencies have been studied in 4035 patients from the United States,[1–4] 32 from

Table 12.19. Acute Myeloid Leukemia

Country/Population	Patients n	Patients %+	Controls n	Controls %+	RR	χ^2	Ref.
HLA-DR3							
Switzerland	38	29	123	11	3.29	7.19	14

Germany,[5] 292 from England,[6,7] and 63 from Switzerland,[8–10] and 54 from the Soviet Union.[11] In the pooled data from all these studies there is no evidence of a significant association with A and B loci antigens.

In 1977 some DR groups were typed in 24 French patients by de Mouzon et al.[12] and none of them was associated with this disease. However, in 1980, when DR antigens were more accurately characterized, Von Fliedner et al.[13,14] reported a significant increase of DR3 (Table 12.19).

Warren et al.[15,16] studied leukocyte group 5, which segregates independently of the HLA complex, in 15 American Caucasian patients. The frequencies of the 2 alleles (5a and 5b) were not different from those in 72 controls.

Disease Heterogeneity

Survival

Harris et al.[6] subdivided their patients into groups with 1, 2, and 3 or more years of survival. The frequencies of B12 in these 3 groups were 27%, 29%, and 44%, respectively. In the total sample of 142 patients before the treatment this frequency was 20%. In 100 controls it was 35%. Thus B12 appeared to be associated with survival. Similar trends were also observed for A2, A3, and B15.

Greater survival rates for patients with A2 and B12 antigens were also reported by Oliver et al.[7] and Von Fliedner et al.[10] In the data of Oliver et al.[7] the frequency of B12 at 12-month survival was 32% (n = 100), at 12–24 months 42% (n = 21), and at 24 months 45% (n = 29). In a group of 15 patients with survival time of more than 3 years the frequency was 53%. These authors also calculated the survival rates for patients with A1/B8, A2/B12, and other phenotypes. Actuarial survival of patients at 12 months with A1/B8 and A2/B12 phenotypes was > 60%. The patients with other phenotypes had only 43% survival.

Contradictory results have been reported by Heise et al.[3] No HLA phenotype or haplotype was found to be associated with prolonged survival. However, patients with A1-B17, A29-B12, and A3-B7 haplotypes survived < 11 months.

Age

Heise et al.[3] grouped their patients on the basis of age at diagnosis. In 46 patients 41 years or older, B17 was present in 17.4%. This antigen was found in only 3% of the 33 patients to age 40 or less ($p < 0.05$).

Remission Status

Harris et al.[6] reported the remission rates in 45 patients with phenotypic combinations A1 with B8, A2 with B12, and A3 with B15 to be 47% compared with 28% for 97 patients with other phenotypes ($p < 0.05$). In the data of Heise et al.[3] B17 was found in 8 of the 39 (20.5%) nonremission patients as compared with 2 of the 40 (5.0%) remission patients ($p = 0.047$). The distribution of all other antigens was similar in remission and nonremission groups.

Thus, for these data there is no evidence of HLA association with remission status of the patients.

Family Data

See ref. 17.

See also refs. 18–26.

References

1. Terasaki PI, Perdue ST, Mickey MR: HLA frequencies in cancer: A second study. In Mulvihill JJ, Miller RW, Fraumeni JF Jr, (eds): Genetics of Human Cancer. Raven Press, New York, 1977, p 321
2. Pollack MS, Dubois D: Possible effects of non-HLA antibodies in common typing sera on HLA antigen frequency data in leukemia. Cancer 39:2348-2354, 1977
3. Heise E, Parrish E, Cooper R: HLA-B17 and the

HLA-A1, B17 haplotype in acute myelogenous leukemia. Tissue Antigens 14:98-104, 1979
4. Albert ED, Nisperos B, Thomas ED: HLA antigens and haplotypes in acute leukemia. Leukemia Res 1:261-269, 1977
5. Richter KV, Fischer G, Menzel GR, Langfeld M, Aigte H, Ruckwarth G, et al: HL-A antigene und Disposition für hamatologische Maligne Erkrankungen. Haematologia 7:203-209, 1973
6. Harris R, Zuhrie SR, Taylor GM, Freeman CB, Wentzel J, Geary C, et al: Influence of HLA, ABO, and RH(D) on survival after remission in acute myelogenous leukaemia. Lancet ii:653, 1977
7. Oliver RTD, Pillai A, Klouda PT, Lawler SD: HLA linked resistance factors and survival in acute myelogenous leukemia. Cancer 39:2337-2341, 1977
8. Jeannet M, Magnin C: HL-A antigens in haematological malignant diseases. Eur J Clin Invest 2:39-42, 1976
9. Jeannet M, Magnin C: HL-A antigens in malignant diseases. Transplant Proc 3:1301-1303, 1971
10. Von Fliedner VE, Khan ZS, Jeannet M: HLA-A and HLA-B antigens in acute leukemia: A2-B12 phenotypes correlate with longer survival in acute myelogenous leukemia. Acta Haematol 65:73-78, 1981
11. Tananov AT, Kutyina RM, Turbina NS, Abakumov EM, Polyanskaya AM, Isaev VG, et al: HLA antigens in patients with blood pathology. Prob Gematol Pereliv Krovi 26:8-12, 1981
12. De Mouzon A, Tongio MM, Jeannet M, Betuel H, De Boissezon JF, De Moerloose PH, et al: IA like serology in leukemia. Tissue Antigens 10:211, 1977
13. Von Fliedner V, Sultan-Khan Z, Jeannet M: HLA DRW antigens associated with acute leukemia. Blut 41:244-245, 1980
14. Von Fliedner VE, Sultan-Khan Z, Jeannet M: HLA-DRW antigens associated with acute leukemia. Tissue Antigens 16:399-404, 1980
15. Warren RP, Strob R, Nguyen DD, Thomas ED: Association between leucocyte group-5A antigen and acute lymphoblastic leukaemia. Lancet i:509-510, 1977
16. Warren RP, Storb R, Nelson NJ, Sale GE, Thomas ED: Increased frequency of the group 5a antigen in patients with hematologic malignancies. Tissue Antigens 18:85-91, 1981
17. Chan KW, Pollack MS, Braun D, O'Reilly RJ, Dupont B: Distribution of HLA genotypes in families of patients with acute leukemia. Implications for transplantation. Transplantation 33:613-615, 1982
18. Harris R, Lawler SD, Oliver RTD: The HLA system in acute leukaemia and Hodgkin's disease. Br Med Bull 34:301-304, 1978
19. Pendergrass TW, Stoller RG, Mann DL, Halterman RH, Fraumeni JF: Acute myelocytic leukaemia and leukaemia-associated antigens in sisters. Lancet ii:429-431, 1975
20. Zebrowski A, Billing R, Mikulski SM, Gale RP, Terasaki PI: Human B-lymphocyte antigens expressed by lymphocytic and myelocytic leukemia cells: Lymphocyte-dependent antibody studies with rabbit antisera. Leukemia Res 1:13-18, 1977
21. Fingold N: Critical analysis of relationships between HL-A system and susceptibility to disease. Transplant Proc 3:1317-1320, 1971
22. Zier KS, Huber C, Albert E, Braunsteiner H: Cell-mediated immune responses between HLA-identical siblings: Recognition of antigenic changes associated with acute myelogenous leukaemia. Clin Exp Immunol 40:136-146, 1980
23. Dickson A: A raised incidence of HL-A2 plus HL-A9 and other anomalies of the HL-A antigens of patients with leukemia. Acta Haematol 54:143-151, 1975
24. Billing RJ, Terasaki PI, Honig R, Peterson P: The absence of B-cell antigen B2 from leukaemia cells and lymphoblastoid cell lines. Lancet i:1365-1367, 1976
25. Mayer S, Tongio MM, Falkenrodt A, Pfeiffer B, Bergerat JP: Expression of HLA antigens on leukaemia cells. J Immunogenet 9:111-120, 1982
26. Morisima Y, Yamada K, Minami S, Kawashima K, Akaza T: HLA-A, B antigens in acute leukemia. Nippon Ketsueki Gakkae Zasshi 48:805-808, 1980

Acute Lymphatic Leukemia

Population Association

The first study by Kourilsky et al.[1] on 100 acute lymphatic leukemia patients in remission did not find any association with A and B loci antigens. In 1970 Walford et al.[2] published data on 10 families in which 1 child was afflicted with acute leukemia and in which at least 1 other sibling was available for HLA typing. Six of the 10 leukemic children had haplotype A2-B12. This observed frequency was calculated to be significantly greater than a frequency of 5 in the normal population ($p < 0.0025$). In subsequent reports data by Lawler et al.,[3] Batchelor et al.,[4] and others, the increase of haplotype A2-B12 in the patients was not confirmed. In subsequent reports from Europe and North America the results were variable. There was no consistent pattern of association with HLA. However, in the combined data (Table 12.20) the association with A2 and B12 antigens appears to be significant with some evidence of heterogeneity. As the data in Table 12.20 indicate, there are

TABLE 12.20. Acute Lymphatic Leukemia

Country/Population	Patients n	Patients %+	Controls n	Controls %+	RR	χ^2	Ref.
HLA-A2							
Japan	20	40	122	44	0.86	0.10	44
U.S.A.	85	65	401	44	2.34	12.02	6
U.S.A.	98	63	182	37	2.87	16.87	8
U.S.A.	198	60	1070	51	1.44	5.38	5
U.S.A.	24	46	98	60	0.57	1.57	45
U.S.A.	42	62	1942	43	2.14	5.88	43
U.S.A.	16	50	100	42	1.38	0.39	9
U.S.A.	215	56	1536	47	1.43	6.09	7
U.S.A.	30	50	383	57	0.75	0.58	46
	708	59	5712	47	1.57	29.74	
	Heterogeneity χ^2 (7 df)					19.05	
USSR	60	57	600	51	1.27	0.78	47
BENELUX	116	52	868	50	1.08	0.16	20
England	118	50	558	48	1.08	0.16	19
Switzerland	31	55	176	43	1.61	1.55	21
Switzerland	34	50	305	48	1.08	0.05	48
	65	52	481	46	1.30	1.02	
	Heterogeneity χ^2 (1 df)					0.58	
Norway	28	68	891	58	1.50	1.05	49
	1095	57	9110	48	1.41	27.40	
	Heterogeneity χ^2 (13 df)					25.13	
HLA-B12							
Japan	20	30	122	12	3.19	4.77	44
U.S.A.	98	40	182	17	3.23	17.27	8
U.S.A.	198	30	1070	26	1.22	1.43	5
U.S.A.	215	28	1536	24	1.24	1.71	7
U.S.A.	16	75	100	29	6.73	11.22	9
U.S.A.	85	22	401	27	0.77	0.83	6
U.S.A.	30	17	383	22	0.78	0.29	46
U.S.A.	24	42	98	29	1.78	1.61	45
U.S.A.	42	29	1942	23	1.40	1.01	43
	708	31	5712	24	1.36	11.53	
	Heterogeneity χ^2 (7 df)					23.85	
USSR	60	12	600	13	0.96	0.01	47
BENELUX	116	27	868	24	1.18	0.57	20
England	118	32	558	30	1.10	0.21	19
Switzerland	34	32	305	23	1.60	1.56	48
Switzerland	31	26	176	21	1.36	0.51	21
	65	29	481	22	1.49	1.98	
	Heterogeneity χ^2 (1 df)					0.08	
Norway	28	25	891	26	0.99	0.00	49
	1095	29	9110	24	1.29	12.03	
	Heterogeneity χ^2 (13 df)					26.20	

only 4 out of 10 studies[5-8] in which the association of A2 is significant ($\chi^2 > 3.84$). In the case of B12 only the studies by Walford et al.[9] and Sanderson et al.[8] found a significant association.

D/DR Locus

De Moerloose et al.[10] reported D locus typing in 49 patients from Switzerland. The frequency of DW7 in patients was 43% and only 21% in a control population of unknown size ($p < 0.05$).

DR locus frequencies were studied by Von Fliedner et al.[11,12] in 31 Swiss patients. No significant deviations were found. Similar results have also been reported by Michel et al.,[13] De Jongh et al.,[14] and Casper et al.[15]

The 2 dominant alleles (5a and 5b) of leukocyte group 5 were typed by Warren et al.[16,17] in 39 acute lymphatic leukemia patients and 72 controls. The 5a gene frequency was 38% in patients and only 9% in the controls ($p < 0.001$). (This leukocyte group segregated independently of the major histocompatibility complex.)

Disease Heterogeneity

Survival

The available data are variable and inconsistent. In 1 report on 58 acute lymphatic leukemia patients Lawler et al.[18,19] calculated the median lengths of survival from the date of diagnosis to the end of November 1973, at which time only 18 patients were alive. The patients positive for A9 had the longest median survival times (340 weeks) and the lowest median age at diagnosis (44 months).

In a somewhat similar report by Albert et al.[5] 118 patients were subdivided according to the time interval between diagnosis and HLA typing. There were 31 patients in the interval 0–6 months, 37 in 7–24 months, and 50 in > 25 months. The frequencies of A9 in these 3 subgroups were 22.6%, 8.1%, and 28.0%, respectively, which was not significant.

Rogentine et al.[6] also subdivided their patients into 2 subgroups: Survival > 1500 days and < 1500 days. Fifteen of the 18 patients (83%) in the first subgroup had A2 as compared with 62% (18/29) in the second subgroup and 44% in 401 normal controls. Thus A2 was found to be significantly increased in the group with longer survival as compared with the normal controls ($p < 0.005$). Another subgrouping was done based on the total normal peripheral blood lymphocyte count. Twenty-four of the 31 patients (77%) with a lymphocyte count of 1000–4000/mm³ (normal range) were positive for A2. Again, this frequency was significantly different ($p < 0.001$) from the normal controls. Interestingly, in contrast to Lawler's[18,19] and Albert's[5] data A9 was not found to be associated either in the total sample or in the longer survival subgroup.

De Bruyere et al.[20] performed survival analysis in 116 children with acute lymphatic leukemia. The patients with A2, B12 were found to have a long survival time (see also ref. 21). However, Davey et al.[22] have not found any A and B loci antigen deviation in 26 patients with survival < 3 years and 44 patients who survived > 3 years.

Associations of D/DR loci antigens have also been examined in several reports. However, the results are not consistent. Casper et al.[15] found an association of DR7 with disease-free remission during chemotherapy. In these data life table analysis showed that DR5 was significantly associated with a decrease in disease-free survival.

Michel et al.[13] noted that in a sample of 21 patients duration of first remission and duration of survival (for the first year) were longer for the patients negative for DR3.

De Bruyere et al.[23] reported a highly significant increase of DR2 in 32 patients with survival of > 8 years. However, De Jongh et al.[14] did not find any significant deviations in 41 patients in continuous complete remission for 2 years and 29 patients in remission for 5-7 years.

BCG Treatment and Survival

A significant increased frequency of B17 was reported by Tursz et al.[24,25] in 13 children who survived without relapse for > 6 years and were treated with bacille Calmette Guerin (BCG) immunotherapy. The patients were all Caucasians under age 20 at the time of diagnosis. The BCG immunotherapy lasted 4–10 years. All the patients were alive without any relapse 6–14 years after the initiation of BCG immunotherapy. The frequency of B17 was 46.1% in this group of patients as compared with 7.3% in 591 controls ($p < 0.001$). AW33 was present in 30.8% of the patients and in 1.2% of the controls ($p < 0.001$). This study also had 14 long-term survivors treated only with chemotherapy. The frequencies of AW33 and B17 in the chemotherapy group were not different from those in the controls.

Family Data

No multiple-case family data are available (however, see refs. 26, 27). MacSween et al.[28] HLA-typed the parents of 30 acute lymphatic leukemia patients and found that 26 parents shared a common haplotype. This was different from an expected incidence of 90.7 per 1,000 calculated from haplotype frequencies in a North American population ($\chi^2 = 7.61$, $p < 0.01$). The authors have suggested that this may be an indication of restricted genetic heterogeneity of acute lymphatic leukemia patients. This may also indicate the expression of a recessive gene for leukemia.

Albert et al.[5] also calculated the observed and expected number of families in which the parents shared 1 haplotype. Their results showed that there was no significant excess of families sharing an HLA-A, -B haplotype. This is in contradiction with the results of MacSween et al.[28]

See also refs. 29–43 and 50–54.

References

1. Kourilsky FM, Dausset J, Feingold N, Duput JM, Bernard J: Etude de la repartition des antigenes leucocytaires chez des malades atteints de leucemie aigue en remission. In J Dausset, J Hamburger, G Mathe (eds): Advances in Transplantation. Munksgaard, Copenhagen, 1967, pp 515-522
2. Walford RL, Finkelstein S, Neerhout R, Konrad P, Shanbrom E: Acute childhood leukaemia in relation to the HL-A human transplantation genes. Nature 225:461-462, 1970
3. Lawler SD, Klouda PT, Hardisty RM, Till MM: Histocompatibility and acute lymphoblastic leukaemia. Lancet i:699, 1971
4. Batchelor JR, Edwards JH, Stuart J: Histocompatibility and acute lymphoblastic leukaemia. Lancet i:699, 1971
5. Albert ED, Nisperos B, Thomas ED: HLA antigens and haplotypes in acute leukemia. Leukemia Res 1:261-269, 1977
6. Rogentine GN, Trapani RJ, Yankee RA, Henderson ES: HL-A antigens and acute lymphocytic leukemia: The nature of the HL-A2 association. Tissue Antigens 3:470-476, 1973
7. Terasaki PI, Perdue ST, Mickey MR: HLA frequencies in cancer: A second study. In Mulvihill JJ, Miller RW, Fraumeni JF Jr (eds): Genetics of Human Cancer. Raven Press, New York, 1977, p 321
8. Sanderson AR, Mahour GH, Jaffe N, Das L: Incidence of HL-A antigens in acute lymphocytic leukemia. Tranplantation 16: 672-673, 1973
9. Walford RL, Zeller E, Combs L, Konrad P: HL-A specificities in acute and chronic leukemia. Transplant Proc 3:1297-1300, 1971
10. De Moerloose PH, Chardonnens X, Vassalli P, Jeannet M: Antigenes HLA-D des lymphocytes B et susceptibilite a certaines maladies. Schweiz Med Wochenschr 107:1461, 1977
11. Von Fliedner V, Sultan-Khan Z, Jeannet M: HLA DRW antigens associated with acute leukemia. Blut 41:244-245, 1980
12. Von Fliedner VE, Sultan-Khan Z, Jeannet M: HLA-DRW antigens associated with acute leukemia. Tissue Anigens 16:399-404, 1980
13. Michel K, Hubbel C, Dock NL, Davey FR: Correlation of HLA-DRw3 with childhood acute lymphocytic leukemia. Arch Pathol Lab Med 105:560, 1981
14. De Jongh BM, Van Der Does-Van Den Berg A, Schreuder GM: Random HLA-DR distribution in children with acute lymphocytic leukaemia in long-term continuous remission. Br J Haematol 52:161-169, 1982
15. Casper JT, Marrari M, Piaskowski V, Lauer SJ, Dequesnoy RJ: Association between HLA-D region antigens and disease-free survival in childhood non-T, non-B acute lymphocytic leukemia. Blood 60:698-702, 1982
16. Warren RP, Strob R, Nguyen DD, Thomas ED: Association between leucocyte group-5A antigen and acute lymphoblastic leukaemia. Lancet i:509-510, 1977
17. Warren RP, Storb R, Nelson NJ, Sale GE, Thomas ED: Increased frequency of the group 5a antigen in patients with hematologic malignancies. Tissue Antigens 18:85-91, 1981
18. Lawler SD, Klouda PT, Smith PG, Till MM, Hardisty RM: Survival and the HL-A system in acute lymphoblastic leukemia. Br Med J 1:547-548, 1974
19. Klouda PT, Lawler SD, Till MM, Hardisty RM: Acute lymphoblastic leukemia and HL-A: A prospective study. Tissue Antigens 4:262-265, 1974
20. De Bruyere M, Cornu G, Heremans-Bracke T, Malchaire J, Sokal G: HLA haplotypes and long survival in childhood acute lymphoblastic leukaemia treated with transfer factor. Br J Haematol 44:243-251, 1980
21. Von Fliedner VE, Khan ZS, Jeannet M: HLA-A and HLA-B antigens in acute leukemia: A2-B12 phenotypes correlate with longer survival in acute myelogenous leukemia. Acta Haematol 65:73-78, 1981
22. Davey FR, Lachant NA, Dock NL, Hubbel C, Stockman JA, Henry JB: HLA antigens and childhood acute lymphocytic leukaemia. Br J Haematol 47:211-220, 1981
23. De Bruyere M, Cornu G, Ninane J, Latinne D, Lebacq AM, Sokal G: HLA-DR antigens in childhood acute lymphoblastic leukaemia long survival. Br J Haematol 51:659-665, 1982
24. Tursz T, Hors J, Lipinski M, Amiel JL: Phenotypes HLA des malades survivants a long terme apres im-

munotherapie par le BCG dans la leucemie aigue lymphoblastique de l'enfant. C R Acad Sci Paris 285:1585-1586, 1977
25. Tursz T, Hors J, Lipinski M, Aamiel JL: HLA phenotypes in long-term survivors treated with BCG immunotherapy for childhood all. Br Med J 1:1250-1251, 1978
26. Hors J, Dausset J: Maladies malignes identiques au sein d'une meme famille. Nouv Presse Med 3:1237, 1974
27. Chan KW, Pollack MS, Braun D, O'Reilly RJ, Dupont B: Distribution of HLA genotypes in families of patients with acute leukemia. Implications for transplantation. Transplantation 33:613-615, 1982
28. MacSween JM, Fernandez LA, Eastwood SL, Pyesmany AF: Restricted genetic heterogeneity in families of patients with acute lymphocytic leukemia. Tissue Antigens 16:70-72, 1980
29. Fu SM, Winchester RJ, Kunkel HG: The occurrence of the HL-B alloantigens on the cells of unclassified acute lymphoblastic leukemias. J Exp Med 142:1334-1338, 1975
30. Zebrowski A, Billing R, Mikulski SM, Gale RP, Terasaki PI: Human B-lymphocyte antigens expressed by lymphocytic and myelocytic leukemia cells: Lymphocyte-dependent antibody studies with rabbit antisera. Leukemia Res 1:13-18, 1977
31. Morozova LF, Belyanchikova NI, Radzikhovskaya RM, Baryshnikov AYU, Volkova MA, Vinogradova MA, et al: Discovery of B cell antigen on blast cells of patients with chronic myeloid leukemia. Biull Eksp Biol Med 87:574-576, 1979
32. Jeannet M, Magnin C: HL-A antigens in malignant diseases. Transplant Proc 3:1301-1303, 1971
33. Fingold N: Critical analysis of relationships between HL-A system and susceptibility to disease. Transplant Proc 3:1317-1320, 1971
34. Thorsby E, Engeset A, Lie SO: HL-A antigens and susceptibility to disease. Tissue Antigens 1:147-152, 1971
35. Pegrum GD, Balfour IC, Evans CA, Middleton VL: HL-A typing of "leukaemic" cells. Lancet i:852-853, 1971
36. Walford RL, Smith GS, Waters H: Histocompatibility systems and disease states with particular reference to cancer. Transplant Rev 7:78-111, 1971
37. Lawler SD, Klouda PT, Hardisty RM, Till MM: The HL-A system in lymphoblastic leukaemia. Br J Haematol 21:595-605, 1971
38. Urcan S, Cote GB, Edwards JH: HL-A and susceptibility to acute lymphoblastic leukaemia. Ann Genet 17:73-76, 1974
39. Rogentine GN Jr, Yankee RA, Gart JJ, Nam J, Trapani RJ: HL-A antigens and disease: Acute lymphocytic leukemia. J Clin Invest 51:2420-2428, 1972
40. Davey FR, Henry JB, Gottlieb AJ: HL-A antigens in lymphatic leukaemia. Lancet ii:802, 1973
41. Bradstock KF, Janossy G, Bollum FJ, Milstein C: Anomalous phenotype in thymic acute lymphoblastic leukaemia. Nature 284:455-457, 1980
42. Dickson A: A raised incidence of HL-A2 plus HL-A9 and other anomalies of the HL-A antigens of patients with leukemia. Acta Haematol 54:143-151, 1975
43. Pollack MS, Dubois D: Possible effects of non-HLA antibodies in common typing sera on HLA antigen frequency data in leukemia. Cancer 39:2348-2354, 1977
44. Morisima Y, Yamada K, Minami S, Kawashima K, Akaza T: HLA-A, B antigens in acute leukemia. Nippon Ketsueki Gakkae Zasshi 48:805-808, 1980
45. Davey FR, Henry JB, Gottlieb AJ: HL-A antigens and acute lymphocytic leukemia. Am J Clin Pathol 61:662-665, 1974
46. Dick FR, Fortuny I, Theologides A, Greally J, Wood N, Yunis E: HL-A and lymphoid tumors. Cancer Res 32:2608-2611, 1972
47. Tananov AT, Kutyina RM, Turbina NS, Abakumov EM, Polyanskaya AM, Isaev VG, et al: HLA antigens in patients with blood pathology. Prob Gematol Pereliv Krovi 26:8-12, 1981
48. Jeannet M, Magnin C: HL-A antigens in haematological malignant diseases. Eur J Clin Invest 2:39-42, 1976
49. Thorsby E, Lie SO: Relationship between the HL-A system and susceptibility to disease. Tranplant Proc 3:1305-1307, 1971
50. Billing RJ, Terasaki PI, Honig R, Peterson P: The absence of B-cell antigen B2 from leukaemia cells and lymphoblastoid cell lines. Lancet i:1365-1367, 1976
51. Kourilsky FM, Dausset J, Feingold N, Dupey JM, Bernard J: Leukocyte groups and acute leukemia. J Natl Cancer Inst 41:81-87, 1968
52. Casper JT, Duquesnoy RJ, Borella L: Transient appearance of HLA-DRW-positive leukocytes in peripheral blood after cessation of antileukemia therapy. Transplant Proc 12:130-133, 1980
53. Hattori T, Uchiyama T, Takatsuki K, Uchino H: Presence of human B-lymphocyte antigens on adult T-cell leukemia cells. Clin Immunol Immunopathol 17:287-295, 1980
54. Hors J: HLA and susceptibility to malignancies in humans. Bull Cancer (Paris) 69:199-207, 1982

Chronic Lymphatic Leukemia

Population Association

A and B loci frequency data are available on 48 patients from Switzerland,[1–3] 83 from the United

States,[4–7] 44 from France,[8] 70 from the Soviet Union,[9,10] and 38 from Germany.[11] In the combined sample there was no significant difference between the patients and controls.

Richter et al.[11] reported a significant increase of B18 in 38 German patients (15.8% in the patients vs. 1.5% in 600 controls; $p < 0.001$). However, this was not confirmed in other studies.

In 1977 some DR locus antigens were also tested by de Mouzon et al.[12] on 24 French patients. In comparison with 261 normal controls no significant difference was found. However, in another report on 26 American Caucasian patients, Winchester et al.[13] found the frequency of DR5 to be 62% as compared with 21.4% in 28 controls ($p < 0.005$).

Family Data

See ref. 14.

See also refs. 15–19.

References

1. Jeannet M, Magnin C: HL-A antigens in haematological malignant diseases. Eur J Clin Invest 2:39-42, 1976
2. Jeannet M, Magnin C: HL-A antigens in malignant diseases. Transplant Proc 3:1301-1303, 1971
3. Jeannet M, Alberto P: HL-A antigens in chronic lymphocytic leukemia: Preliminary evidence for the existence of (leukemia specific) antigens. Schweiz Med Wochenschr 102:1170-1172, 1972
4. Walford RL, Zeller E, Combs L, Konrad P: HL-A specificities in acute and chronic leukemia. Transplant Proc 3:1297-1300, 1971
5. Miller WV: HL-A antigens and hematologic malignancy. Arch Intern Med 133:397-399, 1974
6. Pollack MS, Dubois D: Possible effects of non-HLA antibodies in common typing sera on HLA antigen frequency data in leukemia. Cancer 39:2348-2354, 1977
7. Dick FR, Fortuny I, Theologides A, Greally J, Wood N, Yunis E: HL-A and lymphoid tumors. Cancer Res 32:2608-2611, 1972
8. Fingold N: Critical analysis of relationships between HL-A system and susceptibility to disease. Transplant Proc 3:1317-1320, 1971
9. Zotikov EA, Tananov AG, Musatova VS: Leucocytic antigens in man (HL-A) and diseases of the blood. Sov Med 7:25-28, 1976
10. Tananov AT, Kutyina RM, Turbina NS, Abakumov EM, Polyanskaya AM, Isaev VG, et al: HLA antigens in patients with blood pathology. Prob Gematol Pereliv Krovi 26:8-12, 1981
11. Richter KV, Fischer G, Menzel GR, Langfeld M, Aigte H, Ruckwarth G, et al: HL-A Antigene und Disposition für hamatologische Maligne Erkrankungen. Haematologia 7:203-209, 1973
12. De Mouzon A, Tongio MM, Jeannet M, Betuel H, De Boissezon JF, De Moerloose PH, et al: IA like serology in leukemia. Tissue Antigens 10:211, 1977
13. Winchester R, Toguchi T, Szer I, Burmester G, Lo Galbo P, Cuttner J, et al: Association of susceptibility to certain hematopoietic malignancies with the presence of Ia allodeterminants distinct from the DR series. Immunol Rev 70:155-165, 1983
14. Hors J, Dausset J: Maladies malignes identiques au sein d'une meme famille. Nouv Presse Med 3:1237, 1974
15. Dickson A: A raised incidence of HL-A2 plus HL-A9 and other anomalies of the HL-A antigens of patients with leukemia. Acta Haematol 54:143-151, 1975
16. Degos L, Drolet Y, Dausett J: HL-A antigens in chronic myeloid leukemia (CML) and chronic lymphoid leukemia (CLL). Transplant Proc 3:1309-1310, 1971
17. Billing RJ, Terasaki PI, Honig R, Peterson P: The absence of B-cell antigen B2 from leukaemia cells and lymphoblastoid cell lines. Lancet i:1365-1367, 1976
18. Walford RL, Smith GS, Waters H: Histocompatibility systems and disease states with particular reference to cancer. Transplant Rev 7:78-111, 1971
19. Warren RP, Storb R, Nelson NJ, Sale GE, Thomas ED: Increased frequency of the group 5a antigen in patients with hematologic malignancies. Tissue Antigens 18:85-91, 1981

Leukemic Reticuloendotheliosis (Hairy Cell Leukemia)

Population Association

Winchester et al.[1] noted an increased frequency of DR5 in 14 patients (50% vs. 21.4% in 28 controls) (see also ref. 2).

Family Data

Wylin et al.[3] reported a pedigree of 11 siblings. The haplotype A1-B7 was present in 4 brothers, 3 of whom developed hairy cell leukemia within a 7-year period.

References

1. Winchester R, Toguchi T, Szer I, Burmester G, Lo Galbo P, Cuttner J, et al: Association of susceptibility to certain hematopoietic malignancies with the presence of Ia allodeterminants distinct from the DR series. Immunol Rev 70:155-165, 1983

2. Naeim F, Gatti RA, Gossett T, Johns S, Walford RL: HLA and "B-cell" alloantigens in "hairy" cell leukemia. Tissue Antigens 10:210, 1977
3. Wylin RF, Greene MH, Palutke M, Khilanani P, Tabaczka P, Swiderski G: Hairy cell leukemia in three siblings: An apparent HLA-linked disease. Cancer 49:538-542, 1982

Lymphoma (Unspecified)

Population Association

Takasugi et al.[1] first reported an increased frequency of B35 in 51 American Caucasian patients (35% in patients vs. 22% in 906 controls). In the second updated report on 150 patients Terasaki et al.[2] did not confirm this. However, in these data a decreased frequency of A3 was noted (18% in patients compared with 27% in 3896 controls; $p < 0.05$ without correction for the number of comparisons).

In 21 Swiss patients Jeannet and Magnin[3] reported an association with A28. The frequency in patients was 24% but only 7% in 305 controls ($p < 0.02$). The same authors in an earlier paper on 11 patients[4] reported an association with B18. Thus, validity of these inconsistent results is doubtful.

A third study by Dick et al.[5] on 39 lymphocytic lymphoma patients found a significant association with B12. The frequency of this antigen in the patients was 39% and only 22% in 383 controls (corrected $p < 0.05$).

In view of the heterogeneity of the patients and variable results in 3 studies these associations are either chance occurrences or artifacts.

See also refs. 6–10.

References

1. Takasugi M, Terasaki PI, Henderson B, Mickey MR, Menck H, Thompson RW: HL-A antigens in solid tumors. Cancer Res 33:648-650, 1973
2. Terasaki PI, Perdue ST, and Mickey MR: HLA frequencies in cancer: A second study. In Mulvihill JJ, Miller RW, Fraumeni JF Jr (eds): Genetics of Human Cancer. Raven Press, New York, 1977, p 321
3. Jeannet M, Magnin C: HL-A antigens in haematological malignant diseases. Eur J Clin Invest 2:39-42, 1976
4. Jeannet M, Magnin C: HL-A antigens in malignant diseases. Transplant Proc 3:1301-1303, 1971
5. Dick FR, Fortuny I, Theologides A, Greally J, Wood N, Yunis E: HL-A and lymphoid tumors. Cancer Res 32:2608-2611, 1972
6. Seigler HF, Kremer WB, Metzgar RS, Ward FE, Haung AT, Amos DB: HL-A antigenic loss in malignant tranformation. J Natl Cancer Inst 46:577-584, 1971
7. Editorial: Genes may indicate prognosis in lymphoma. JAMA 235:2808, 1976
8. Walford RL, Smith GS, Waters H: Histocompatibility systems and disease states with particular reference to cancer. Transplant Rev 7:78-111, 1971
9. Naeim F, Stoddard A, Smith GS, Walford RL: HL-A antigens on cells isolated from malignant and nonmalignant lymph nodes. Tissue Antigens 4:166-171, 1974
10. Kadin ME: Ia-like (HLA-DR) antigens in the diagnosis of lymphoma and undifferentiated tumors. Arch Pathol Lab Med 104:503-508, 1980

Follicular Lymphoma

Population Association

A significant increase of B12 in 56 Australian patients has been reported by Forbes and Morris[1,2] (Table 12.21).

References

1. Forbes JF, Morris PJ: Transplantation antigens and malignant lymphomas in man: Follicular lymphoma, reticulum cell sarcoma and lymphosarcoma. Tissue Antigens 1:265-269, 1971
2. Morris PJ, Forbes JF: HL-A in follicular lymphoma, reticulum cell sarcoma, lymphosarcoma, and infectious mononucleosis. Transplant Proc 3:1315-1316, 1971

TABLE 12.21. Follicular Lymphoma

	Patients		Controls				
Country/Population	n	%+	n	%+	RR	χ^2	Ref.
HLA-B12							
Australia	56	63	273	32	3.57	17.96	1

Burkitt's Lymphoma

Population Association

In 3 independent studies on African Black populations reported simultaneously in 1975, no association with A and B loci antigens was found. Dausset et al.[1] studied 42 patients and 84 controls from Kenya, Dick et al.[2] 33 patients and 37 controls also from Kenya (several tribal groups), and Bodmer et al.[3] 31 patients and 48 controls from Uganda (6 tribal groups). There were no significant differences between patients and controls in all 3 studies.

A combined analysis of the data from the above 3 studies was also done by Bodmer et al.[4] No association was evident in the pooled sample.

In a fourth study by Jones et al.[5] 78 patients and 70 controls from Ghana (several tribes) were typed for A, B, and C loci antigens. DR locus typings were done on only 61 patients and 62 controls. As in the 3 previous studies A, B, and C loci antigens did not show any significant association with the disease.

However, DR7 was found to be increased in the patients (Table 12.22). The χ^2 for comparison between patients and controls is 6.67 (Table 12.22) and thus at this stage can only be considered as interesting. New data would be necessary to confirm the association of DR7 with this disease. (The authors have calculated a probability of 0.0078 by Fisher's exact method. The corrected p value is given as 0.05 and this would be considered as significant.)

Family Data

See ref. 6.

See also ref. 7.

References

1. Dausset J, Singh S, Gourand JL, Degos L, Solal CH, Klein G: HL-A and Burkitt's disease. Tissue Antigens 5:48-51, 1975
2. Dick HM, Steel CM, Levin AG, Henderson N: Burkitt's lymphoma and HL-A antigens. Tissue Antigens 5:52-58, 1975
3. Bodmer JG, Bodmer WF, Ziegler J, Magrath IT: HL-A and Burkitt's tumour—A study in Uganda. Tissue Antigens 5:59-62, 1975
4. Bodmer JG, Bodmer WF, Pickbourne P, Degos L, Dausset J, Dick HM: Combined analysis of three studies of patients with Burkitt's lymphoma. Tissue Antigens 5:63-68, 1975
5. Jones EH, Biggar RJ, Nkrumah FK, Lawler SD: Study of the HLA system in Burkitt's lymphoma. Hum Immunol 3:207-210, 1980
6. Joncas JH, Rioux E, Wastiaux JP, Leyritz M, Robillard L, Menezes J: Nasopharyngeal carcinoma and Burkitt's lymphoma in a Canadian family. I. HLA typing, EBV antibodies and serum immunoglobulins. Can Med Assoc J 115:858-860, 1976
7. Kalil J, Fellous M, Tanigaki N, Rosa F, Pagniez C, Herzog C, et al: A new Epstein-Barr virus negative Burkitt's lymphoma derived cell-line. Tissue Antigens 20:47-62, 1982

Glioblastoma

Family Data

Sib-pair data for 7 French families reported by Hors and Dausset[1] did not show evidence of linkage with HLA.

Reference

1. Hors J, Dausset J: Maladies malignes identiques au sein d'une meme famille. Nouv Presse Med 3:1237, 1974

Neuroblastoma

Population Association

Majsky et al.[1-3] noted nonsignificant increases of B13 and BW21 in a small sample of 20 patients. However, this trend was not confirmed, especially for

TABLE 12.22. Burkitt's Lymphoma

Country/Population	Patients n	Patients %+	Controls n	Controls %+	RR	χ^2	Ref.
HLA-DR7							
Ghana	61	33	62	13	3.17	6.67	5

TABLE 12.23. Neuroblastoma

Country/Population	Patients n	Patients %+	Controls n	Controls %+	RR	χ^2	Ref.
HLA-B13							
U.S.A.	45	5	113	2	2.56	1.37	4
Czechoslovakia	20	25	301	9	3.53	5.93	1
	65	11	414	7	3.21	7.18	
	Heterogeneity χ^2 (1 df)					0.11	
HLA-BW21							
U.S.A.	45	2	113	5	0.55	0.50	4
Czechoslovakia	20	15	301	5	3.68	4.58	1
	65	6	414	5	1.92	1.73	
	Heterogeneity χ^2 (1 df)					3.35	

BW21, in a larger sample of 45 American patients of unknown ethnic groups.[4] The frequency data for B13 and BW21 from these 2 studies are given in Table 12.23.

See also refs. 5 and 6.

References

1. Majsky A, Abrahamova J, Koutecky J: HLA antigens and neuroblastoma. Tissue Antigens 12:156, 1978
2. Abrahamova J, Majsky A, Koutecky J: HLA system U wilmsova nadoru a neuroblastomu. Cesk Pediatr 4:268-270, 1979
3. Abrahamova J, Majsky A, Koutecky J: Neuroblastoma and the HLA system. Cas Lek Cesk 117:593-594, 1978
4. McAlack RF: Normal HLA phenotypes and neo-HLA-like antigens on cultured human neuroblastoma. Transplant Proc 12:107-113, 1980
5. Majsky A, Abrahamova J: Pritomnost HLA-A2 antigenu na lymfocytech: Ochrana pred vznikem nadoru? Cas Lek Cesk 119:47-50, 1980
6. Majsky A, Abrahamova J: Schutzen die HLA-A2-Gene vor der Entwicklung eines Tumors? Eine Hypothese. Folia Haematol (Leipz) 108:90-96, 1981

Retinoblastoma

Population Association

The data of Bertrams et al.[1,2] showed significant associations with BW35 and B12 (Table 12.24) in 122 German children.

Disease Heterogeneity

In the German study[1] 89 patients had hereditary and 26 the nonhereditary form of the disease. The frequencies of B12 and BW35 in the hereditary group were 10.1% and 25.8%, respectively. In the nonhereditary group, these 2 antigens were present in 3.8% and 23.1% of the patients, respectively. When compared with the control group (see frequencies in Table 12.24) the deviations were significant only in

TABLE 12.24. Retinoblastoma

Country/Population	Patients n	Patients %+	Controls n	Controls %+	RR	χ^2	Ref.
HLA-B12							
West Germany	122	10	255	25	0.34	10.82	1
HLA-BW35							
West Germany	122	25	255	11	2.68	11.98	1

the hereditary subgroup. However, this may be due to the small sample size.

Family Data

Both hereditary and sporadic forms of retinoblastoma have been reported. In the hereditary form the disease is an autosomal dominant gene with a penetrance of about 80% (refs. see 1).

Jones[3] reported A, B, and D loci typing in a large and informative family. In this family retinoblastoma had occurred in 3 generations but it showed incomplete penetrance and variable expression.

In this pedigree no association of either of the grandparental haplotypes with the segregating retinoblastoma gene in generations II and III was evident.

References

1. Bertrams J, Schildberg P, Hopping W, Bohme U, Albert E: HL-A antigens in retinoblastoma. Tissue Antigens 3:78-87, 1973
2. Schildberg P, Bertrams J, Hopping W, Kuwert E: Histokompatibilitats (HL-A)-Antigene beim Retinoblastom. Albrecht Von Graefes Arch Klin Ophthalmol 186:33-38, 1973
3. Jones JL: Immunogenetics of retinoblastoma. Trans Ophthalmol Soc UK 94:945 952, 1974

Uveal Melanoblastoma

Population Association

In 47 patients from the Soviet Union increased frequencies of A3 (51.06% in patients vs. 26.80% in 306 controls) and A29 (27.16% in patients vs. 7.84% in controls) have been reported by Egnatov et al.[1] (see also ref. 2.)

Disease Heterogeneity

The investigators[1] subdivided the total sample into groups with (n = 25) and without (n = 22) enucleation. The frequency of B7 in the group with enucleation was 48% as compared with 24.18% in 306 controls. Sixteen patients of the subgroup with enucleation had localized type melanoblastoma and B7 was present in 68.71% of these patients.[1]

References

1. Ignatov RK, Terenteva LS, Shulgina NS: A study of antigen distribution of HLA-system in melanoblastoma of the uvea. Oftalmol Zh 32:289-294, 1977
2. Dieckhues B, Junemann G, Kuchle HJ, Puttman T: HLA-Antigene bei Augenerkrankungen. Klin Monatsbl Augenheilkd 175:681-685, 1979

Melanoma

Population Association

A and B loci frequency data are available for Caucasian American,[1-6] Canadian,[7] Belgian,[8] English,[9] Norwegian,[10] French,[11] Danish,[12] and Italian[13] patient populations. In the combined data there was no indication of association with A and B loci antigens.

The largest sample of patients (n = 226) was studied by Terasaki et al.[2] and no association was found. Similar results were also observed by the same authors[1] in an earlier report on 69 patients.

Pellegris et al.[13] reported A, B, and C loci frequency data on 140 melanoma patients from Italy. B40 was 15.0% in the patients as compared with 4.09% in 904 controls ($p = 5.6 \times 10^{-7}$). The frequency of BW35 was 12.85% in the patients and 28.13% in 853 controls ($p = 1.6 \times 10^{-4}$). However, as stated earlier, no other study has reported a significant association with these 2 antigens.

D-locus typing was done on 44 Norwegian patients by Bergholtz et al.[10] and no significant association was found. HLA-DR locus antigens were studied in 236 American Caucasian patients by Nathanson et al.[14,15] No association was found. However, in the data of Barger et al.[16] on American Caucasian patients a significant association with DR4 was observed (Table 12.25).

Disease Heterogeneity

Lamm et al.[12] subdivided their 212 patients on the basis of sex and estimated probability of survival at 5 years. No association in any subgroup of patients was found. Similar results were reported by Nathanson et al.[14,15] for DR locus antigens in subgroups based on sex and stage of the disease (stages I, II, and III).

Barger et al.[16] subdivided their patients into low-risk (n = 67) and high-risk (n = 24) categories based on their clinically defined risk status at pre-

TABLE 12.25. Melanoma

	Patients		Controls				
Country/Population	n	%+	n	%+	RR	χ^2	Ref.
HLA-DR4							
U.S.A.	236	22	575	22	1.00	0.00	15
U.S.A.	91	39	106	16	3.30	12.71	16
	327	27	681	21	1.33	3.05	
	Heterogeneity χ^2 (1 df)					9.66	

sentation. The increased frequency of DR4 was significant only in the low-risk subgroup.

In the Italian study,[13] the increase of B40 and the decrease of BW35 was reported in subgroups of patients with or without the clinical evidence of melanoma. However, as noted earlier, the other reports have not confirmed the association of melanoma with BW35 and B40.

Family Data

A large kindred with multiple cases of malignant melanoma has been reported by Hawkins et al.[17] In this kindred, the susceptibility to the disease apparently was inherited as an autosomal dominant gene and segregated with the HLA complex. The lod score analysis showed a maximum lod score of 1.25 at a recombination frequency of 10%.

See also refs. 18–24.

References

1. Takasugi M, Terasaki PI, Henderson B, Mickey MR, Menck H, Thompson RW: HL-A antigens in solid tumors. Cancer Res 33:648-650, 1973
2. Terasaki PI, Perdue ST, Mickey MR: HLA frequencies in cancer: A second study. In Mulvihill JJ, Miller RW, Fraumeni JF Jr(eds): Genetics of Human Cancer. Raven Press, New York, 1977, p 321
3. Tarpley JL, Chretien PB, Rogentine N, Twomey PL, Dellon AL: Histocompatibility antigens and solid malignant neoplasms. Arch Surg 110:269-271, 1975
4. Clark DA, Necheles T, Nathanson L, Silverman E: Apparent HL-A5 deficiency in malignant melanoma. Transplantation 15:326-328, 1973
5. Clark DA, Necheles TF, Nathanson L, Whitten D, Silverman E, Flowers A: Apparent HL-A5 deficiency in human malignant melanoma: The HLA-A5 masking activity in sera of patients with progressing disease. Isr J Med Sci 10:836-846, 1974
6. Pandey JP, Johnson AH, Fudenberg HH, Amos DB, Gutterman JU, Hersh EM: HLA antigens and immunoglobulin allotypes in patients with malignant melanoma. Hum Immunol 2:185-190, 1981
7. Singal DP, Bent PB, McCulloch PB, Blajchman MA, MacLaren RGC: HL-A antigens in malignant melanoma. Transplantation 18:186, 1974
8. VanWijck R, Bouillenne C: HL-A antigen and susceptibility to malignant melanoma. Transplant 16:371, 1973
9. Cordon AL: HL-A and malignant melanoma. Lancet i:938, 1973
10. Bergholtz B, Brennhovd I, Klepp O, Kaakinen A, Thorsby E: HLA antigens in malignant melanoma. Cancer 39:2342-2344, 1977
11. Bigel P, Heid E, Tongio MM, Mayer S: Melanomes malins et antigenes HL-A. Ann Dermatol Syphiligr (Paris) 102:63-65, 1975
12. Lamm LU, Kissmeyer-Nielsen F, Kjerbye KE, Mogensen B, Petersen NC: HL-A and ABO antigens and malignant melanoma. Cancer 33:1458-1461, 1974
13. Pellegris G, Illeni MT, Vaglini M, Rovini D, Cascinelli N, Masserini C: HLA antigens in maligant melanoma patients. Tumori 66:51-58, 1980
14. Nathanson SD, Park MS, Drew I, Morton DL, Terasaki PI: Serologically defined B-lymphocyte antigen expression in patients with malignant melanoma. Surg Forum 30:147-149, 1979
15. Nathanson SD, Park MS, Drew SI, Morton DL, Terasaki PI: First and second B-lymphocyte antigen expression in malignant melanoma. Transplant Proc 12:118-120, 1980
16. Barger BO, Acton RT, Soong SJ, Roseman J, Balch C: Increase of HLA-DR4 in melanoma patients from Alabama. Cancer Res 42:4276-4279, 1982
17. Hawkins BR, Dawkins RL, Hockey A, Houliston JB, Kirk RL: Evidence for linkage between HLA and malignant melanoma. Tissue Antigens 17:540-541, 1981

18. Ruiter DJ, Bhan AK, Harrist TJ, Sober AJ, Mihm Jr MC: Major histocompatibility antigens and mononuclear inflammatory infiltrate in benign nevomelanocytic proliferations and malignant melanoma. J Immunol 129:2808-2815, 1982
19. Mitchell KF, Ward FE, Koprowski H: DR antigens on melanoma cells: Analysis with monoclonal antibodies. Hum Immunol 4:15-26, 1982
20. Nathanson SD, Pellegrino MA, Ferrone S: Serum HLA-A and B alloantigens in patients with malignant melanoma. Transplant Proc 13:1939-1941, 1981
21. Hors J: HLA and susceptibility to malignancies in humans. Bull Cancer (Paris) 69:199-207, 1982
22. Pollack MS, Livingston PO, Fogh J, Carey TE, Oettgen HF, Dupont B: Genetically appropriate expression of HLA and DR (IA) alloantigens on human melanoma cell lines. Tissue Antigens 15:249-256, 1980
23. Liao SK, Kwong PC, Dent PB, Jerry LM: Changes in HLA-DR antigen expression on cultured human melanoma cells during theophylline treatment. Tissue Antigens 20:147-151, 1982
24. Pellegrino MA, Ferrone S, Reisfeld RA, Irie RF, Golub SH: Expression of histocompatibiliy (HLA) antigens on tumour cells and normal cells from patients with melanoma. Cancer 40:36-41, 1977

Malignant Choroidal Melanoma

Population Association

The antigen AW32 has been reported[1] to be significantly increased in 81 German patients (Table 12.26).

Reference

1. Bertrams J, Spitznas M, Rommelfanger M: Missing evidence for HLA antigen association with Eales' disease, chorioretinitis, central serous retinopathy, and malignant choroidal melanoma. Invest Ophthalmol Vis Sci 17:918-920, 1978

Lymphosarcoma

Population Association

Takasugi et al.[1] noted an increased frequency of A28 in 39 American Caucasian patients (26% in patients vs. 12% in 906 controls). Later, in an updated version of this study Terasaki et al.[2] reported this antigen to be elevated in the patients (Table 12.27).

Another report on 50 Australian patients and 273 controls by Forbes and Morris[3,4] did not show any significant deviations in 8 A and B loci antigens. A28, however, was not typed in this study. Similar results were also obtained by Miller[5] in a small sample of 19 American Caucasian patients. However, he noted an increase of B13 in the patient group (37% vs. 3% in 100 controls).

References

1. Takasugi M, Terasaki PI, Henderson B, Mickey MR, Menck H, Thompson RW: HL-A antigens in solid tumors. Cancer Res 33:648-650, 1973
2. Terasaki PI, Perdue ST, Mickey MR: HLA frequencies in cancer: A second study. In Mulvihill JJ, Miller RW, Fraumeni JF Jr, (eds): Genetics of

TABLE 12.26. Malignant Choroidal Melanoma

	Patients		Controls				
Country/Population	n	%+	n	%+	RR	χ^2	Ref.
HLA-AW32							
West Germany	81	11	1000	3	4.12	13.58	1

TABLE 12.27. Lymphosarcoma

	Patients		Controls				
Country/Population	n	%+	n	%+	RR	χ^2	Ref.
HLA-A28							
U.S.A.	63	16	3896	8	2.27	6.01	2

Human Cancer. Raven Press, New York, 1977, p 321
3. Forbes JF, Morris PJ: Transplantation antigens and malignant lymphomas in man: Follicular lymphoma, reticulum cell sarcoma and lymphosarcoma. Tissue Antigens 1:265-269, 1971
4. Morris PJ, Forbes JF: HL-A in follicular lymphoma, reticulum cell sarcoma, lymphosarcoma, and infectious mononucleosis. Transplant Proc 3:1315-1316, 1971
5. Miller WV: HL-A antigens and hematologic malignancy. Arch Intern Med 133:397-399, 1974

Reticulosarcoma

Population Association

Forbes and Morris[1,2] reported the frequencies of 8 A and B loci antigens in 28 Australian patients. In comparison with 273 controls there was no significant deviation.

See also ref. 3.

References

1. Forbes JF, Morris PJ: Transplantation antigens and malignant lymphomas in man: Follicular lymphoma, reticulum cell sarcoma and lymphosarcoma. Tissue Antigens 1:265-269, 1971
2. Morris PJ, Forbes JF: HL-A in follicular lymphoma, reticulum cell sarcoma, lymphosarcoma, and infectious mononucleosis. Transplant Proc 3:1315-1316, 1971
3. Fieldsteel AH, Dawson PJ, Kurahara C: Tumor-specific transplantation antigens in reticulum cell sarcomas and lymphomas induced by the Friend virus complex. Cancer Res 33:551-558, 1973

Liposarcoma

Population Association

A and B loci antigens were typed in 12 American Caucasian patients by Tarpley et al.[1] When compared with 389 controls, no significant deviations were observed.

Reference

1. Tarpley JL, Chretien PB, Rogentine N, Twomey PL, Dellon AL: Histocompatibility antigens and solid malignant neoplasms. Arch Surg 110:269-271, 1975

Ewing's Sarcoma

Population Association

Chan et al.[1] reported A and B loci antigen frequencies in 38 American Caucasian patients and 262 controls. The authors noted interesting increases in AW19 and B8 in these patients. None was statistically significant.

Two American Black patients were also typed. Both were AW19 (AW31).

Disease Heterogeneity

Patients were also categorized by their age at diagnosis into preadolescent (12 years or younger) and adolescent groups. There was no HLA difference between the 2 groups.

Reference

1. Chan KW, Rosen G, Pollack MS: Distribution of HLA antigens in patients with Ewing's sarcoma. Tissue Antigens 16:314-316, 1980

Osteosarcoma

Population Association

In 15 American Caucasian[1] and 53 Italian patients[2] no significant associations with A and B loci antigens have been found.

Also, there was no correlation between HLA and survival (measured by the time since diagnosis).

Disease Heterogeneity

In the Italian study[2] there was a positive correlation between A3 and metastases after 1 year from diagnosis.

References

1. Tarpley JL, Chretien PB, Rogentine N, Twomey PL, Dellon AL: Histocompatibility antigens and solid malignant neoplasms. Arch Surg 110:269-271, 1975
2. Tabacchi P, Chiricolo M, Cenci M, Barboni F, Mannfrini M, Bacci G, et al: Frequency and prognostic value of HLA antigens in osteosarcoma patients. Tissue Antigens 20:251-253, 1982

Kaposi's Sarcoma

Population Association

Brenner et al.[1] reported an increased frequency of AW19 in 19 Israeli patients (Table 12.28).

In another study of 27 American Caucasian patients, Pollack et al.[2] have found a significant association with DR5 antigen (Table 12.28).

Disease Heterogeneity

In the study by Pollack et al.[2] the patients were divided into "classic" disease affecting older patients and "aggressive homosexual form" of the disease. The association with DR5 was evident in both subgroups. The frequency data in Table 12.28 are the total of both these groups. The authors[2] have also noted an increased frequency of BW35 in 19 patients with the homosexual form of the disease (42.1% vs. 22.9% in 388 controls).

References

1. Brenner S, Krakowski A, Schewach-Millet M, Ronen M, Orgad S, Gazit E: Increased frequency of HLA-Aw19 in Kaposi's sarcoma. Tissue Antigens 19:392-394, 1982
2. Pollack MS, Safai B, Myskowski PL, Gold JWM, Pandey J, Dupont B: Frequencies of HLA and Gm immunogenetic markers in Kaposi's sarcoma. Tissue Antigens 21:1-8, 1983

Trophoblastic Neoplasms

Population Association

HLA-A and -B loci antigen frequency data are available on 53 patients from England,[1] 27 patients from Austria,[2] and 111 from the United States.[3] The antigen frequencies in the patients were not significantly different from those in controls.

Family Data

Mogensen and Kissmeyer-Nielsen[4] studied HLA-A and -B loci compatibility between mother and fetus in 44 cases of gestational carcinoma. Their data showed that the patients had a more favorable prognosis when the tumor was HLA-incompatible with the patients. However, in the data of Lawler et al.,[1,5] Lewis and Terasaki,[6] and Rudolph and Thomas[7] there was no correlation between presence of metastases and HLA compatibility. (See also ref. 3.)

Klouda et al.[8] also analyzed the mating frequencies for the A and B loci antigens in 75 patients and their husbands. The mating frequencies were found to be random and thus the risk of a woman getting a trophoblastic neoplasm appeared not to be influenced by her choice of mate as far as the A and B loci were concerned.

See also refs. 9–16.

References

1. Lawler SD, Klouda PT, Bagshawe KD: The HL-A system in trophoblastic neoplasia. Lancet ii:834-837, 1971
2. Tatra G, Wolf E: Untersuchungen uber Histokompatibilitatsantigene und Trophoblasttumore. Arch Gynaekol 213:341-351, 1973
3. Mittal KK, Kachru RB, Brewer JI: The HL-A and ABO antigens in trophoblastic disease. Tissue Antigens 6:57-69, 1975
4. Mogensen B, Kissmeyer-Nielsen F: Invasive mole, gestational choriocarcinoma and transplantation antigens. Ser Haemat 5:22-43, 1972
5. Lawler SD: HLA and trophoblastic tumours. Br Med Bull 34:305-308, 1978
6. Lewis JL Jr, Terasaki PI: HL-A leukocyte antigen studies in women with gestational trophoblastic neoplasms. Am J Obstet Gynecol 111:547-554, 1971
7. Rudolph RH,Thomas ED: Histocompatibility studies in patients with trophoblastic tumors. Am J Obstet Gynecol 108:1126-1129, 1976
8. Klouda PT, Lawler SD, Bagshawe KD: HL-A mat-

TABLE 12.28. Kaposi's Sarcoma

Country/Population	Patients n	Patients %+	Controls n	Controls %+	RR	χ^2	Ref.
HLA-AW19							
Jews (unspecified)	19	68	90	27	5.44	10.73	1
HLA-DR5							
U.S.A.	27	59	176	21	5.29	15.82	2

ings in trophoblastic neoplasia. Tissue Antigens 2:280-284, 1972
9. Bagshawe KD, Rawlings G, Pike MC, Lawler SD: ABO blood-groups in trophoblastic neoplasia. Lancet i:553-557, 1971
10. Amiel JL, Droz JP: Immunologie des tumeurs placentaires. J Gynecol Obstet Biol Reprod (Paris) 6:23-28, 1977
11. Shaw ARE, Dasgupta MK, Kovithavongs T, Johny KV, Leriche JC, Dossetor JB: Humoral and cellular immunity to paternal antigens in trophoblastic neoplasia. Int J Cancer 24:586-593, 1979
12. Jones EA, Bodmer WF: Lack of expression of HLA antigens on choriocarcinoma cell lines. Tissue Antigens 16:195-202, 1980
13. Tursz T, Lipinski M, Guillard M, Dutheil M, Bodmer JG, Amiel JL, et al.: Characterization of antibodies reacting with husband's lymphocytes in sera from patients with trophoblastic malignancies. Tissue Antigens 17:376-385, 1981
14. Pattillo RA: Histocompatibility antigens in pregnancy, abortions, infertility, preeclampsia and trophoblast neoplasms. Am J Reproduct Immunol 1:29-34, 1980
15. Yamashita K, Wake N, Araki T, Ichinoe K, Kuroda M: A further HLA study of hydatidiform moles. Gynecol Oncol 11:23-28, 1981
16. Honda J, Sato E, Ihara S, Munakata S, Sugawara N, Fukushima T: Pathogenetic study of complete and partial hydatidiform mole by HLA. Nippon Sanka Fujinka Gakkai Zasshi 34:83-88, 1982

Choriocarcinoma

Population Association

No frequency data are available. However, see refs. 1–5.

References

1. Lawler SD, Klouda PT, Bagshawe KD: The relationship between HLA antibodies and the causal pregnancy in choriocarcinoma. Br J Obstet Gynaecol 83:651-655, 1976
2. Trowsdale J, Travers P, Bodmer WF, Patillo RA: Expression of HLA-A, -B, and -C and beta 2 microglobulin antigens in human choriocarcinoma cell lines. J Exp Med 152:11s-17s, 1980
3. Mittal KK, Kachru RB, Brewer JI: The HL-A and ABO antigens in trophoblastic disease. Tissue Antigens 6:57-69, 1975
4. Tanimoto M, Takahashi T, Nishizuka Y: The expression of HLA on two cultured choriocarcinoma cell lines. Gann 73:27-34, 1983
5. Travers PJ, Arklie JL, Trowsdale J, Patillo RA, Bodmer WF: Lack of expression of HLA-ABC antigens in choriocarcinoma and other human tumor cell lines. Natl Cancer Inst Monogr 60:175-180, 1982

Waldstrom's Macroglobulinemia

Population Association

In a sample of 15 French patients studied by Youinou et al.[1,2] no significant associations with HLA-A and B loci antigens were observed.

References

1. Saleun JP, Youinou P, Le Goff P, Lemenn G, Morin JF: HLA antigen and monoclonal gammapathy. Tissue Antigens 13:233-235, 1979
2. Youinou P: Genetic propensity to benignity in monoclonal-gammopathy. Acta Haematol 62:173-175, 1979

Thymoma

Population Association

In 47 Dutch patients A and B loci antigen frequencies were not significantly different from those in 533 controls.[1]

Disease Heterogeneity

In the above study[1] 24 patients also had myasthenia gravis. There was no HLA difference between this group and 23 patients without myasthenia gravis. Also, antimuscle and antinuclear antibody titers in both groups of patients were not related to any HLA antigens.

Reference

1. Oosterhuis HJ, Feltkamp TEW, Van Rossum AL, Van Den Berg-Loonen PM, Nijenhuis LE: HL-A antigens, autoantibody production, and associated diseases in thymoma patients, with and without myasthenia gravis. Ann NY Acad Sci 274:468-474, 1976

Colorectal Adenoma

Population Association

The only data available are from a Japanese study[1] on 43 patients typed for A and B loci antigens in-

TABLE 12.29. Colorectal Adenoma

	Patients		Controls				
Country/Population	n	%+	n	%+	RR	χ^2	Ref.
HLA-B5							
Japan	43	16	120	40	0.30	7.66	1
HLA-B40							
Japan	43	56	120	35	2.34	5.72	1

dicating interesting deviations in B5 and B40 (Table 12.29).

Disease Heterogeneity

The total sample was subdivided, according to the location of the lesions, into colon (n = 13) or rectal adenoma (n = 30). In the colon group the frequency of BW35 was 30.1% as compared with 10% in 120 controls ($p < 0.005$). Only 13.3% of the 30 patients with the rectal adenoma were positive for BW35.

B5 and BW40 frequencies in the rectum group were 13.3% and 60%, respectively, and were significantly different from those in controls ($p < 0.01$). (Control frequencies are given in Table 12.29). There was no difference between the colon group and controls.

Also see ref. 2.

References

1. Hiwatashi N, Kikuchi T, Masamune O, Ouchi E, Watanabe H, Goto Y: HLA antigens in colorectal cancers and adenomas. Tohoku J Exp Med 131:257-260, 1980
2. Alcalay M, Bontoux D, Maire P, Matuchansky C, Alcalay D, Tanzer J: HLA-B27 and colorectal cancer. N Engl J Med 307:443-444, 1982

Multiple Myeloma

Population Association

A and B loci frequency data reported in several studies on Caucasians from Europe and the United States were variable. Although there was no antigen association in these studies, B5 appeared to be significantly increased in the combined sample (Table 12.30). However, there was also evidence of heterogeneity in the data.

It is interesting to note that in 40 German patients studied by Bertrams et al.[1] the frequency of B12 was 35%, which was significantly higher than 9.1% in 143 controls ($p < 0.0005$). This result was not confirmed in other studies, however. Smith et al.[2] also studied 12 American Black patients. The frequency of B5 in the patients was 0% and 9% in 914 controls. This difference was not significant.

Leech et al.[3] have observed a significant increase of CW5 in 22 American Black patients (4/22 vs. 2/138 in controls).

Disease Heterogeneity

Smith et al.[2] subdivided their patients on the basis of class of myeloma protein and by light chain type. The authors noted an increased frequency of A9 among IgA myelomas (n = 6) and a decreased frequency of BW22 in patients with κ chains (n = 11). A2 was also increased in the last subgroup. It should be noted that these observations are based on a very small sample of patients in each subgroup.

See also refs. 13 and 14.

References

1. Bertrams J, Kuwert E, Bohme U, Reis HE, Gallmeier WM, Wetter O, et al: HL-A antigens in Hodgkin's disease and multiple myeloma. Tissue Antigens 2:41-46, 1972
2. Smith G, Walford RL, Fishkin B, Carter PK, Tanaka K: HL-A phenotypes, immunoglobulins and κ and λ chains in multiple myeloma. Tissue Antigens 4:374-377, 1974
3. Leech SH, Bryan CF, Elston RC, Rainey J, Bickers JN, Pelias MZ: Genetic studies in multiple myeloma. Cancer 51:1408-1411, 1983
4. Miller WV: HL-A antigens and hematologic malignancy. Arch Intern Med 133:397-399, 1974
5. Tananov AT, Kutyina RM, Turbina NS, Abakumov EM, Polyanskaya AM, Isaev VG, et al: HLA antigens in patients with blood pathology. Prob Gematol Pereliv Krovi 26:8-12, 1981

TABLE 12.30. Multiple Myeloma

	Patients		Controls				
Country/Population	n	%+	n	%+	RR	χ^2	Ref.
HLA-B5							
U.S.A.	32	16	914	9	2.06	2.47	3
U.S.A.	11	64	100	2	66.61	26.34	4
	43	28	1014	8	4.77	15.12	
	Heterogeneity χ^2 (1 df)					13.69	
USSR	67	16	600	14	1.21	0.31	5
BENELUX	23	15	285	12	1.43	0.41	6
BENELUX	30	23	533	9	3.14	6.87	7
	53	20	818	10	2.32	6.03	
	Heterogeneity χ^2 (1 df)					1.25	
England	63	16	83	4	4.16	5.76	8
France	60	25	172	14	2.06	3.98	9
France	33	6	200	8	0.88	0.04	10
	93	18	372	11	1.69	2.73	
	Heterogeneity χ^2 (1 df)					1.28	
West Germany	40	3	255	11	0.34	2.19	1
Austria	68	16	3000	17	0.96	0.01	11
Switzerland	14	36	305	22	2.07	1.85	12
	441	18	6447	14	1.72	15.17	
	Heterogeneity χ^2 (10 df)					35.05	

6. Van Camp BGK, Cole J, Peetermans ME: HLA antigens and homogeneous immunoglobulins. Clin Immun Immunopathol 7:315-318, 1977
7. Festen JJM, Marrink J, Kaars Sijpesteijn JA, Van Loghem E, Nijenhuis LE, Mandema E: A study on the association between myelomatosis and immunoglobulin allotypes, HLA, and blood groups. Immunogenetics 3:201-203, 1976
8. Mason DY, Cullen P: HL-A antigen frequencies in myeloma. Tissue Antigens 5:238-245, 1975
9. Cassuto JP, Piereschi J, Maiolini R, Dujardin O, Ribeil R, Masseyeff R: Marqueurs HLA dans les myelomes et les dysglobulinemies monoclonales benignes. Nouv Presse Med 10:252-253, 1981
10. Saleun JP, Youinou P, Le Goff P, Lemenn G, Morin JF: HLA antigen and monoclonal gammapathy. Tissue Antigens 13:233-235, 1979
11. Ludwig H, Mayr W: Genetic aspects of susceptibility to multiple myeloma. Blood 59:1286-1291, 1982
12. Jeannet M, Magnin C: HL-A antigens in haematological malignant diseases. Eur J Clin Invest 2:39-42, 1976
13. Smith G, Walford RL, Fishkin B: Antibody specificity for HL-A in human myeloma sera and immune rabbit sera. Tissue Antigens 4:595-600, 1974
14. Youinou P: Genetic propensity to benignity in monoclonal gammopathy. Acta Haematol 62:173-175, 1979

Mycosis Fungoides

Population Association

In 19 patients with plaque style mycosis fungoides (stage II)[1,2] AW19 was significantly increased (Table 12.31). The 2 splits of AW19 (AW31 and AW32) were increased and the other 2, A29 and AW10, did not show any significant difference between the 2 groups. (AW33, a rare antigen in Caucasian populations, was not tested in this study.)

In a study of epidermal expression of HLA-DR antigens, Tjernlund[3] found that the number of cells expressing the DR antigens in the involved epidermis of mycosis fungoides patients increased with the severity of the disease. In stage IV virtually all cells expressed this antigen on the cell surface. This was an interesting result in view of a proposed hypothesis of "antigen persistence" as a possible cause of mycosis fungoides.[3]

TABLE 12.31. Mycosis Fungoides

Country/Population	Patients n	Patients %+	Controls n	Controls %+	RR	χ^2	Ref.
HLA-AW19							
England	19	42	342	15	4.14	9.29	1
HLA-AW31							
England	19	16	342	4	4.99	6.84	1
HLA-AW32							
England	19	16	342	4	4.99	6.84	1

References

1. Dick HM, Mackie R: Distribution of HLA antigens in patients with mycosis fungoides. Dermatologica 155:275-282, 1977
2. Mackie R, Dick HM, De Sousa MB: HLA and mycosis fungoides. Lancet i:1179, 1976
3. Tjernlund UM: Epidermal expression of HLA-DR antigens in mycosis fungoides. Arch Dermatol Res 261:81-86, 1978

Hodgkin's Disease

Population Association

In 1967, Amiel[1] reported a significant association of Hodgkin's disease with antigen 4c. In the patients there were 106 positive (43.62%) and 137 negative reactions and only 62 positive (43.48%) and 202 negative reactions in the healthy controls ($\chi^2 = 23.99$ for 1 degree of freedom). It is now known that 4c consisted of B5, B18, and BW35. Since then a large number of studies have reported variable and inconsistent results. The association subsequently reported in many of these studies could not be confirmed and also was not observed in earlier studies. However, analysis of pooled data on more than 1450 patients showed a significant association with A1, B5, B8 and B18 antigens (Table 10.32). There is also some evidence of heterogeneity in a pooled sample. The data in the table show that in most of the studies these antigens were not significant even at the probability level of 5%. It should be noted that in Caucasian populations there is strong linkage disequilibrium between A1 and B8. The combined estimates of relative risks for these 2 antigens are almost the same (1.35 and 1.26, respectively). The linkage disequilibrium between A1-B5 and A1-B18 is not very strong. The combined relative risk values for B5 and B8 are 1.63 and 1.76, respectively, and they are very similar to those for A1 and B8 antigens.

In 16 Japanese[2] and 109 English[3] patients, there was no evidence of any significant association with the DR locus antigens.

Disease Heterogeneity

Nodular Sclerosis

Patients with nodular sclerosis were studied in several reports. The interesting results presented by these authors are given in the following table:

Country	Patient Sample Size	Reported Deviations	Study
Sweden	19	B18—increased	Hornmark-Stenstam et al.[4]
Sweden	22	B12—increased	Bjorkholm et al.[5]
Australia	33	B7—increased	Forbes and Morris[6]
Canada	58	A1—increased	Falk and Osoba[7]
U.S.A.	67	B7—increased	Bowers et al.[8]
U.S.A.	8	B7—increased	Dick et al.[9]
U.S.A.	39	none	Graff et al.[10]

As in the case of the total patients reported by these authors, there is no common association. All antigen frequencies are not given in 5 of these studies and thus a combined analysis cannot be done. However, it is clear that this subgroup of patients cannot be distinguished on the basis of HLA typing.

Mixed Cellularity

Forbes and Morris[6] noted an increased frequency of B7 in this subgroup of patients (n = 57). Graff et al.[10], however, reported increased frequencies of A1, B5, B8 and a decreased frequency of B18 in 39 patients. In a third study by Bjorkholm et al.,[5] a decreased frequency of B5 was noted in a mixed sample consisting of 26 mixed cellularity types and

10 lymphocyte depletion types. Falk and Osoba[7] reported a significant increase of A1 and B8 in 33 Canadian patients.

Lymphocyte Predominance

Frequency data on 25 patients studied by Forbes and Morris[6] showed no significant HLA association. However, in 12 patients Graff et al.[10] demonstrated an increased frequency of B5. In a mixed sample (7 patients with lymphocyte predominance and 29 with nodular sclerosis) an increased frequency of B12 was also noted by Bjorkholm et al.[5] Increased frequencies of A1 and B8 were found by Falk and Osoba[7] in 16 patients from Canada.

Lymphocyte Depletion

In 2 studies[6,10] involving a total of only 14 patients no unusual HLA association was noted (see also ref. 5).

Sex

Forbes and Morris[6] calculated an increased frequency of B7 in female patients with nodular sclerosis and mixed cellularity type of disease. Furthermore, A11 and B7 were determined to be significantly increased in the total sample of 51 females as compared with 76 males. Bjorkholm et al.[5] and Falk and Oshoba[7], however, did not find any HLA and sex association.

Clinical Stage of the Disease

Graff et al.[10] subdivided their 39 mixed cellularity and 39 nodular sclerosis patients into 4 clinical stages (I-IV). B5 was found to be more frequent in patients with stages III or IV nodular sclerosis. Neither this nor any other HLA antigen deviation was found in 65 patients studied by Bjorkholm et al.[5] The number of T lymphocytes in blood and the spontaneous DNA synthesis and DNA synthesis induced by concanavalin A, pokeweed mitogen, and phytohemagglutinin were also measured by Bjorkholm[5] in 60 patients. A significant increase of A28 was found in patients with advanced disease ($p < 0.001$) and also in patients responding poorly to PPD ($p < 0.001$) and PWM ($p < 0.01$).

Duration of the Disease

Falk and Osoba[7,11] first reported an increased frequency of B8 (and or combinations of A1, A2, and B5) in patients having the disease for more than 5 years. In the second report,[12] these authors reported 5-year actuarial survival curves from date of diagnosis showing a significant higher survival rate for AW19-B5-positive patients as compared with AW19-B5-negative patients. Thus, except for the presence of B5 in both reports, there is no consistency in the data (see also ref. 13). In another report from Sweden, Hornmark-Stenstam et al.[4] reported a significant increase ($p < 0.05$) of A28 in 10 patients with very long symptom-free survival (mean 23 years). A28 was present in 30% (3/10) of the patients as compared with 7% (87/1263) in the control group.

Graff et al.[10] found no relationship between disease duration and any particular HLA type of the patients.

Age at Onset

Bjorkholm et al.[5] classified their sample into 2 subgroups: age at onset < 40 years and > 40 years. The frequency of B12 in 27 patients with age at onset < 40 years was 48% as compared with 19% in 100 controls ($p < 0.01$). In the subgroup with age at onset more than 40 years (n = 38) B8 was 42% and only 24% in 100 controls ($p < 0.05$).

Antibody Response to Influenza A Hong Kong Virus

A group of 29 patients and 27 healthy volunteers were vaccinated by Sybesma et al.[14,15] with influenza A Hong Kong Virus. Six patients did not respond with a fourfold or greater increase in titer as measured by hemagglutination inhibition assay. All healthy volunteers showed an adequate antibody response. The frequency of B12 was 13% in patients with adequate antibody response and 62% in those without antibody formation ($p < 0.02$).

Family Data

Bowers et al.[8] reported a family of 5 siblings in which the 2 affected sisters were HLA- and MLC (D locus)-identical. The third healthy sister had identical A and B loci antigens but was MLC-nonreactive. Similar A and B loci results were reported by Nunez-Roldan et al.[16] in another family of 7 siblings. All three affected siblings were HLA-(A and B loci)-identical.

Hors et al.[17] genotyped 13 multiple-case families and found a nonsignificant excess of HLA-identical siblings. When this and data from Greene et al.,[18] Nunez-Roldan et al.,[16] Bowers et al.,[8] and 2 other studies (see studies cited in ref. 17) were pooled the increased frequency of HLA identity among the affected siblings reached a significant level at $p < 0.05$.[17]

TABLE 12.32. Hodgkin's Disease

Country/Population	Patients n	Patients %+	Controls n	Controls %+	RR	χ^2	Ref.
HLA-A1							
Canada	112	41	122	25	2.07	6.71	7
U.S.A.	44	29	181	27	1.12	0.10	25
U.S.A.	8	50	100	3	27.86	16.77	26
U.S.A.	67	38	245	28	1.58	2.58	8
U.S.A.	103	41	459	29	1.70	5.70	10
U.S.A.	33	30	383	27	1.19	0.20	9
U.S.A.	411	32	3896	31	1.05	0.19	27
U.S.A.	72	45	80	20	3.21	10.55	28
	738	35	5344	30	1.30	9.64	
	Heterogeneity χ^2 (6 df)					26.44	
Australia	127	34	273	32	1.10	0.17	6
BENELUX	35	54	26	46	1.36	0.38	29
England	109	38	125	26	1.74	3.86	3
England	27	59	80	38	2.30	3.59	30
	136	42	205	31	1.88	7.16	
	Heterogeneity χ^2 (1 df)					0.29	
France	88	24	140	26	0.91	0.10	31
West Germany	20	35	600	29	1.36	0.46	32
West Germany	82	37	255	36	1.05	0.03	33
	102	37	855	31	1.12	0.25	
	Heterogeneity χ^2 (1 df)					0.25	
Switzerland	33	36	305	27	1.54	1.35	34
Denmark	50	50	477	28	2.57	10.17	35
Norway	39	31	891	28	1.18	0.23	36
Sweden	40	40	1263	29	1.65	2.43	4
Sweden	65	40	100	34	1.29	0.63	5
	105	40	1363	29	1.46	2.77	
	Heterogeneity χ^2 (1 df)					0.28	
	1565	37	10001	29	1.37	26.19	
	Heterogeneity χ^2 (19 df)					40.01	
HLA-B5							
Canada	112	22	122	10	2.49	6.13	7
U.S.A.	44	11	87	11	1.04	0.01	25
U.S.A.	103	20	459	6	3.92	19.52	10
U.S.A.	67	15	245	10	1.62	1.55	8
U.S.A.	48	19	155	5	4.37	8.89	37
U.S.A.	8	25	100	1	25.51	10.64	26
U.S.A.	33	15	383	11	1.53	0.79	9
U.S.A.	411	14	3896	10	1.47	6.62	27
U.S.A.	72	15	80	11	1.41	0.55	28
	786	15	5405	9	1.83	28.70	
	Heterogeneity χ^2 (7 df)					19.86	

TABLE 12.32. *(continued)*

	Patients		Controls				
Country/Population	n	%+	n	%+	RR	χ^2	Ref.
HLA-B5							
Australia	127	13	127	9	1.49	1.03	6
BENELUX	35	12	26	12	0.97	0.00	29
England	27	63	80	19	6.94	16.80	30
France	88	16	140	17	0.94	0.03	31
West Germany	20	25	600	14	2.17	2.47	32
West Germany	82	4	255	11	0.38	3.28	33
	102	8	855	13	0.97	0.01	
	Heterogeneity χ^2 (1 df)					5.75	
Switzerland	33	12	305	22	0.53	1.57	34
Denmark	50	10	477	12	0.88	0.08	35
Norway	39	15	891	8	2.16	3.10	36
Sweden	65	6	100	11	0.56	1.10	5
	1464	15	8528	10	1.63	30.96	
	Heterogeneity χ^2 (18 df)					53.19	
HLA-B8							
Canada	112	29	122	16	2.12	5.61	7
U.S.A.	44	11	178	16	0.70	0.55	25
U.S.A.	103	20	459	16	1.33	1.09	10
U.S.A.	411	20	3896	21	0.94	0.20	27
U.S.A.	33	21	383	20	1.11	0.06	9
U.S.A.	48	25	155	9	3.35	8.24	37
U.S.A.	67	26	245	20	1.42	1.24	8
U.S.A.	72	26	80	14	2.12	3.40	28
U.S.A.	8	13	100	2	8.13	4.58	26
	786	21	5496	20	1.17	2.56	
	Heterogeneity χ^2 (7 df)					16.79	
Australia	127	24	127	23	1.06	0.04	6
BENELUX	35	26	26	8	3.44	3.05	29
England	27	37	80	28	1.52	0.85	30
England	109	29	125	21	1.53	2.00	3
	136	31	205	24	1.53	2.85	
	Heterogeneity χ^2 (1 df)					0.00	
France	88	11	140	14	0.78	0.39	31
West Germany	20	15	600	21	0.75	0.26	32
West Germany	82	26	255	26	1.01	0.00	33
	102	24	855	22	0.95	0.04	
	Heterogeneity χ^2 (1 df)					0.22	
Switzerland	33	24	305	18	1.49	0.92	34
Denmark	50	44	477	22	2.79	11.68	35
Norway	39	26	891	26	1.03	0.01	36
Sweden	65	31	100	24	1.42	1.01	5
	1573	24	8744	21	1.27	11.64	
	Heterogeneity χ^2 (19 df)					33.54	

TABLE 12.32. *(continued)*

Country/Population	Patients n	Patients %+	Controls n	Controls %+	RR	χ^2	Ref.
HLA-B18							
U.S.A.	103	5	459	2	2.67	3.54	10
U.S.A.	44	7	87	9	0.83	0.09	25
U.S.A.	411	9	3896	8	1.15	0.60	27
U.S.A.	72	13	80	8	1.68	1.03	28
U.S.A.	67	6	245	6	1.08	0.02	8
	697	8	4767	7	1.24	2.11	
	Heterogeneity χ^2 (4 df)					3.17	
West Germany	82	29	143	9	4.04	14.23	33
West Germany	20	15	600	2	9.42	13.09	32
	102	26	743	3	5.05	25.95	
	Heterogeneity χ^2 (1 df)					1.37	
Switzerland	33	6	305	7	1.02	0.00	34
Sweden	65	6	100	4	1.53	0.42	5
Sweden	40	20	1263	5	4.93	16.13	4
	105	11	1363	5	3.60	14.23	
	Heterogeneity χ^2 (1 df)					2.32	
	937	11	7178	6	1.76	20.79	
	Heterogeneity χ^2 (9 df)					28.37	

An analysis, by the methods of sib-pairs and lod scores, of 33 multiple-case families was presented in a review paper by Hors and Dausset.[19] There was a highly significant distortion of segregation of HLA haplotypes in pairs of affected siblings ($p < 0.00025$). The lod score analysis provided maximum lod scores of 2.12 (at 8% recombination) and 2.18 (at 14% recombination) with a 60% and 10% penetrance, respectively, in dominant and recessive models. The precise mode of inheritance of the "disease susceptibility gene" could not be determined in this data.

Berberich et al.[20] have also shown an analysis of 16 families (12 reported in other studies) in which HLA haplotype concordance among patients was greater than that expected by chance alone ($p < 0.0015$).

Thus, in the available family data there is some evidence for linkage between HLA and Hodgkin's disease (see also refs. 6 and 21–24).

See also refs. 38–53.

References

1. Amiel JL: Study of the leucocyte phenotypes in Hodgkin's disease. In Curtoni ES, Mattiuz PL, Tosi RM (eds): Histocompatibility Testing 1967. Munksgaard, Copenhagen, 1967, pp 79-81
2. Sakurami T, Ueno Y, Iwaki Y, Park MS, Terasaki PI, Saji H: HLA-DR specificities among Japanese with several autoimmune disease. Tissue Antigens 19:129-133, 1982
3. Welsh KI, Amlot P, Batchelor JR: Do alleles in linkage disequilibrium compensate for each other's disadvantageous effects? Tissue Antigens 17:91-96, 1981
4. Hornmark-Stenstam B, Landberg T, Low B: HLA antigens in Hodgkin's disease of very long survival. Acta Radiol Oncol 17:283-288, 1978
5. Bjorkholm M, Holm G, Johansson B, Mellstedt H, Moller E: A prospective study of HL-A antigen phenotypes and lymphocyte abnormalities in Hodgkin's disease. Tissue Antigens 6:247-256, 1975
6. Forbes JF, Morris PJ: Analysis of HL-A antigens in patients with Hodgkin's disease and their families. J Clin Invest 51:1156-1163, 1972
7. Falk J, Osoba D: HL-A antigens and survival in Hodgkin's disease. Lancet ii:1118-1120, 1971
8. Bowers TK, Moldow CF, Bloomfield CD, Yunis EJ: Familial Hodgkin's disease and the major histocompatibility complex. Vox Sang 33:273-277, 1977
9. Dick FR, Fortuny I, Theologides A, Greally J,

Wood N, Yunis E: HL-A and lymphoid tumors. Cancer Res 32:2608-2611, 1972
10. Graff KS, Simon RM, Yankee RA, Devita VT, Rogentine CN: HL-A antigens in Hodgkin's disease: Histopathologic and clinical correlations. J Natl Cancer Inst 52:1087-1090, 1974
11. Falk J, Osoba D: The association of the human histocompatibility system with Hodgkin's disease. J Immunogenet 1:53-61, 1974
12. Falk J, Osoba D: The HLA system and survival in malignant disease: Hodgkin's disease and carcinoma of the breast. Prog Clin Biol Res 16:205-219, 1977
13. Osoba D, Falk JA, Sousan P, Ciampi A, Till JE: The prognostic value of HLA phenotypes in Hodgkin's disease. Cancer 46:1825-1832, 1980
14. Sybesma JPHB, Holtzer JD, Borst-Eilers E, Moes M, Zegers BJM: Antibody response in Hodgkin's disease and other lymphomas related to HL-A antigens, immunoglobulin levels and therapy. Vox Sang 25:254-262, 1973
15. Sybesma JPHB: Antibody response related to HL-A antigens in Hodgkin's disease and other lymphomas. Lancet ii:884, 1972
16. Nunez-Roldan A, Martinez-Guibelalde F, Gomez-Garcia P, Gomez-Pereira C, Nunez-Ollero G, Torres-Gomez A: Possible HLA role in a family with Hodgkin's disease. Tissue Antigens 13:377-378, 1979
17. Hors J, Steinberg G, Andrieu JM, Jacquillat C, Minev M, Messerschmitt T, et al.: HLA genotypes in familial Hodgkin's disease: Excess of HLA identical affected sibs. Eur J Cancer 16:809-815, 1980
18. Greene MH, McKeen EA, Li FP, Blattner WA, Fraumeni JF Jr: HLA antigens in familial Hodgkin's disease. Int J Cancer 23:777-780, 1979
19. Hors J, Dausset J: HLA and susceptibility to Hodgkin's disease. Immunol Rev 70:167-192, 1983
20. Berberich FR, Berberich MS, King MC, Engleman EG, Grumet FC: Hodgkin's disease susceptibility: Linkage to the HLA locus demonstrated by a new concordance method. Hum Immunol 6:207-217, 1983
21. Marshall WH, Barnard JM, Buehler SK, Crumley J, Larsen B: HLA in familial Hodgkin's disease: Results and a new hypothesis. Int J Cancer 19:450-455, 1977
22. Hors J, Dausset J: Maladies malignes identiques au sein d'une meme famille. Nouv Presse Med 3:1237, 1974
23. Torres A, Martinez F, Gomez P, Gomez C, Garcia JM, Nunez-Roldan A: Simultaneous Hodgkin's disease in three siblings with identical HLA-genotype. Cancer 46:838-843, 1980
24. McBride A, Fennelly JJ: Immunological depletion contributing to familial Hodgkin's disease. Eur J Cancer 13:549-554, 1977
25. Coukell A, Bodmer JG, Bodmer WF: HL-A types of 44 Hodgkin's patients. Transplant Proc 3:1291-1295, 1971
26. Miller WV: HL-A antigens and hematologic malignancy. Arch Intern Med 133:397-399, 1974
27. Terasaki PI, Perdue ST, Mickey MR: HLA frequencies in cancer: A second study. In Mulvihill JJ, Miller RW, Fraumeni JF Jr (eds): Genetics of Human Cancer. Raven Press, New York, 1977, p 321
28. Henderson BE, Dworsky R, Menck H, Alena B, Henle W: Case-control study of Hodgkin's disease. J Natl Cancer Inst 51:1443-1447, 1973
29. Sybesma JPHB, Borst-Eilers E, Holtzer JD, Moes M, Pielage E, De Planque BA: HL-A antigens in Hodgkin's disease and other lymphomas. Vox Sang 22:319-324, 1972
30. Zervas JD, Delamore IW, Israels MCG: Leukocyte phenotyes in Hodgkin's disease. Lancet ii:634-635, 1970
31. Moulinier MJ, Hoerni-Simon G, Merle MC, Mothey MC: Antigenes d'histocompitibilite et hematosarcomes. Bordeaux Med 5:1285-1289, 1972
32. Richter KV, Fischer G, Menzel GR, Langfeld M, Aigte H, Ruckwarth G, et al.: HL-A Antigene und Disposition fur hamatologische maligne Erkrankungen. Haematologia 7:203-209, 1973
33. Bertrams J, Kuwert E, Bohme U, Reis HE, Gallmeier WM, Wetter O, et al.: HL-A antigens in Hodgkin's disease and multiple myeloma. Tissue Antigens 2:41-46, 1972
34. Jeannet M, Magnin C: HL-A antigens in haematological malignant diseases. Eur J Clin Invest 2:39-42, 1976
35. Kissmeyer-Nielsen F, Bjorn Jensen K, Ferrara GB, Kjerbye KE, Svejgaard A: HL-A phenotypes in Hodgkin's disease preliminary report. Transplant Proc 3:1287-1289, 1971
36. Thorsby E, E'ngeset A, Lie SO: HL-A antigens and susceptibility to disease. Tissue Antigens 1:147-152, 1971
37. Perlin E, O'Donnell M: Another observation of increased frequency of HL-A5 and HL-A8 in Hodgkin's disease. Am J Clin Pathol 64:277-278, 1975
38. Harris R, Lawler SD, Oliver RTD: The HLA system in acute leukaemia and Hodgkin's disease. Br Med Bull 34:301-304, 1978
39. Takasugi M, Terasaki PI, Henderson B, Mickey MR, Menck H, Thompson RW: HL-A antigens in solid tumors. Cancer Res 33:648-650, 1973
40. Jeannet M, Magnin C: HL-A antigens in malignant diseases. Transplant Proc 3:1301-1303, 1971
41. Fingold N: Critical analysis of relationships between HL-A system and susceptibility to disease. Transplant Proc 3:1317-1320, 1971
42. Bertrams J, Kuwert E, Gallmeier WM, Reis HE, Schmidt CG: Transient lymphocyte HL-A antigen "loss" in a case of irradiated M. Hodgkin. Tissue Antigens 1:105-108, 1971

43. Forbes JF, Morris PJ: Leucocyte antigens in Hodgkin's disease. Lancet ii:849-851, 1970
44. Bodmer WF: Genetic factors in Hodgkin's disease: Association with a disease-susceptibility locus (DSA) in the HL-A region. Natl Cancer Inst Monogr 36:127-134, 1973
45. Morris PJ, Ting A, Forbes JF: Further studies of HL-A. Transplant Proc 3:109-111, 1971
46. Walford RL, Smith GS, Waters H: Histocompatibility systems and disease states with particular reference to cancer. Transplant Rev 7:78-111, 1971
47. Kourilsky FM: Symposium international sur les relations entre les antigenes de tumeurs et les systemes d'histocompatibilite. Bull Cancer 58:315-324, 1977
48. Kadin ME: Ia-like (HLA-DR) antigens in the diagnosis of lymphoma and undifferentiated tumors. Arch Pathol Lab Med 104:503-508, 1980
49. Pedersen-Bjergaard J, Philip P, Mortensen BT, Ersboll J, Jensen G, Panduro J, et al: Acute nonlymphocytic leukemia, preleukemia, and acute myeloproliferative syndrome secondary to treatment of other malignant disease. Blood 57:712-723, 1981
50. Warren RP, Storb R, Nelson NJ, Sale GE, Thomas ED: Increased frequency of the group 5a antigen in patients with hematologic malignancies. Tissue Antigens 18:85-91, 1981
51. Winchester R, Toguchi T, Szer I, Burmester G, Lo Galbo P, Cuttner J, et al: Association of susceptibility to certain hematopoietic malignancies with the presence of Ia allodeterminants distinct from the DR series. Immunol Rev 70:155-165, 1983
52. Hors J: HLA and susceptibility to malignancies in humans. Bull Cancer (Paris) 69:199-207, 1982
53. Naeim F, Stoddard A, Smith GS, Walford RL: HL-A antigens on cells isolated from malignant and nonmalignant lymph nodes. Tissue Antigens 4:166-171, 1974

Glioma

Population Association

A, B, and DR antigen frequencies of 80 Swiss patients[1] show an interesting increase in BW35 and DR1 (Table 12.33).

See also ref. 2.

References

1. De Moerloose PH, Jeannet M, Martin-Achard A, De Tribolet N, Seiler R, Guanella N: HLA and glioma. Tissue Antigens 12: 146-148, 1978
2. Hirschberg H, Endresen L, Wikeby P: HLA antigens on glioma cells from short term cultures. Tissue Antigens 19:146-153, 1982

Pheochromocytoma

Population Association

May et al.[1] reported no association with A and B loci antigens in 9 American Caucasian patients.

Family Data

The aforementioned study of May et al.[1] also had data on 3 multiple-case families. There was no evidence of linkage with HLA complex in these 3 pedigrees.

Reference

1. May AG, Moss A, Gutierrez OH, Burday SZ, Campbell RG: Clinical study of pheochromocytoma. Am J Surg 141:346-352, 1981

Sipple's Syndrome

Family Data

Five nuclear families within a large kindred with Sipple's syndrome (multiple endocrine neoplasia type 2) were analyzed by the method of lod score for linkage by Simpson and Falk.[1] The total lod score for a recombination frequency of 10% was < -2.0. Thus linkage with the HLA complex was excluded at this recombination value. The lod scores for recombination of $> 10\%$ were also negative but > -2.0.

Reference

1. Simpson NE, Falk J: Exclusion of linkage between the loci for multiple endocrine neoplasia type-2 (MEN-2) and HLA. Hum Genet 60:157, 1982

Wilms' Tumor

Population Association

Nonsignificantly increased frequency of A9 was first reported by Majsky et al.[1–7] in 46 patients from Czechoslovakia. This was not confirmed in another study on 30 German patients by Evers et al.[8] In the

TABLE 12.33. Glioma

	Patients		Controls				
Country/Population	n	%+	n	%+	RR	χ^2	Ref.
HLA-BW35							
Switzerland	80	35	176	19	2.29	7.67	1
HLA-DR1							
Switzerland	80	34	100	16	2.66	7.69	1

TABLE 12.34. Wilms' Tumor

	Patients		Controls				
Country/Population	n	%+	n	%+	RR	χ^2	Ref.
HLA-A9							
Czechoslovakia	46	37	301	19	2.52	7.74	1
West Germany	30	30	800	21	1.66	1.67	8
	76	34	1101	20	2.11	8.75	
	Heterogeneity χ^2 (1 df)					0.66	

combined sample the increase of A9 is marginally significant (Table 12.34), however.

It should be noted that in the German study[8] B40 was present in 26.7% of the patients as compared with 11% in 800 controls. The frequency of the antigen in the patients reported by Majsky et al.[3] was very similar to that of controls.

Disease Heterogeneity

In the aforementioned study,[2] there were 8 patients with IgA levels > 200 IU/ml. In this subgroup the frequency of A1 was 62.5% as compared with 28.24% in 301 controls ($p < 0.05$).

References

1. Majsky A, Abrahamova J, Koutecky J: Wilms' tumor and HLA antigens. Tissue Antigens 11:74, 1978
2. Abrahamova J, Majsky A, Fucikova T, Koutecky J: IGA-Immunglobuline und Antigen HLA-A1 beim Wilms-Tumor Bedeutung für die Prognose der Erkrankung. Onkologie 1:177-179, 1978
3. Abrahamova J, Majsky A, Koutecky J: HLA system U wilmsova nadoru a neuroblastomu. Cesk Pediatr 4:268-270, 1979
4. Abrahamova J, Majsky A, Koutecky J: Wilm's tumour and the HL-A locus. Cas Lek Cesk 116: 1059-1061, 1977
5. Abrahamova J, Majsky A, Fucikova T, Koutecky J, Strejcek J: Production of immunoglobins IgA and HLA antigen A: Significance for Wilms' tumour progonosis. Cas Lek Cesk 117:667-669, 1978
6. Majsky A, Abrahamova J: Pritomnost HLA-A2 antigenu na lymfocytech: Ochrana pred vznikem nadoru? Cas Lek Cesk 119:47-50, 1980
7. Majsky A, Abrahamova J: Schutzen die HLA-A2-Gene vor der Entwicklung eines Tumors? Eine Hypothese. Folia Haematol (Leipz) 108:90-96, 1981
8. Evers KG, Gutjahr P, Zschiedrich S, Haase W, Knoop U: Lack of association between HLA specificities and Wilms' tumour. Eur J Pediatr 136:47-49, 1981

Chapter 13

Allergy

Allergy to Insulin

Population Association

Bertrams and Gruneklee[1] typed 44 unrelated German insulin-dependent diabetics with cutaneous allergic reactions to insulin and 112 diabetics without insulin allergy. HLA-B7 was significantly increased in patients with insulin allergy (34.1% vs. 13.4% in patients without allergy, $p < 0.01$). This result was in contrast with the general decrease of this antigen in diabetic patients (see Insulin-Dependent Diabetes).

B21 was also increased in the patients with allergy. Its frequency was 17.6% in 34 patients with allergy as compared with 4.5% in 112 without allergy ($p < 0.005$). When compared with normal controls this antigen also showed a significant association with allergy to insulin in the diabetics (Table 13.1).

Disease Heterogeneity

In the above study,[1] when allergic patients were subdivided according to allergy to insulin or to conserving substances, the frequencies of B7 and BW21 were increased in both groups of patients. Thus, there was no difference between the 2 types of allergies.

Reference

1. Bertrams J, Gruneklee D: Association between HLA-B7 and allergic reactions to insulin in insulin-dependent diabetes mellitus. Tissue Antigens 10:273-277, 1977

Allergy to Cow's Milk

Population Association

Thirty-nine French children with intolerance to cow's milk were typed for A and B loci antigens.[1] The antigen frequencies were not significantly different from those in 591 normal controls.

See also ref. 2.

References

1. Mougenot JF, Hors J, Schmid M, Cathelineau M, Navarro J, Polonovski C: Les antigenes HLA dans la maladie coeliaque et l'intolerance digestive aux proteines du lait de vache chez l'enfant. Gastroenterol Clin Biol 1:507-514, 1977
2. Singal DP, Perets A, Dolovich J: HLA antigens and serum antibodies to bovine serum albumin. Transplant Proc 11:1864-1865, 1979

Allergy to Dust

Population Association

Seignalet et al.[1] studied the frequencies of A and B loci antigens in 60 French children with dust allergy. When compared with a group of 300 controls, AW19 and B5 were increased in the patients but this difference was not statistically significant. In another French study on 52 patients allergic to house dust[2] and 341 controls, a nonsignificant increase in BW21 was reported (17% in patients vs. 7% in controls). In this report, the frequency data on AW19 and B5

13.1. Allergy to Insulin

	Patients		Controls				
Country/Population	n	%+	n	%+	RR	χ^2	Ref.
HLA-BW21							
West Germany	44	18	1000	4	5.46	17.51	1

were not available. However, in the study by Seignalet et al.,[1] BW21 was present in 5% of the 60 patients as compared with 7% of the 300 controls. Thus, there is no evidence in these 2 sets of data of any HLA association with this disease. Marsh et al.[3] noted an association with B8 and DW2 antigens (no frequency data are given).

Family Data

Yoo et al.[4] published a pedigree in which 2 of the 12 siblings and the father were allergic to dust (as well as ragweed). Both affected siblings had the haplotype A31-B16. However, 6 siblings with this haplotype did not show symptoms of dust allergy.

References

1. Seignalet J, Levallois C, Lapinski H, Jean R: Les antigenes HLA dans l'allergie a la poussiere chez l'enfant. Arch Fr Pediatr 33:955-960, 1976
2. Perrin-Fayolle M, Betuel H, Biot N, Grosclaude M: HLA antigens in patients allergic to pollen and to house dust. Monogr Allergy 11:74, 1977
3. Marsh DG, Meyers DA, Freidhoff LR, Hussain R, Hsu SH, Bias W: Association of HLA phenotypes A1, B8, DW3 and A3, B7, DW2 with allergy. Int Arch Allergy Appl Immunol 66:48-50, 1981
4. Yoo TJ, Kuo CY, Thompson JS: Family study of HLA antigen and IR gene linkage in ragweed and dust allergy. Monogr Allergy 11:89-96, 1977

Allergy to Nickel

Population Association

HLA-A and -B loci antigen frequencies are available on 103 patients from Sweden,[1,2] 36 from Finland,[3] 60 from Belgium,[4] 29 from England,[5] and 51 from Denmark.[6] In all of these studies there was no evidence of any significant associations.

In the Finnish study[3] patients were also typed for C and D loci antigens. Furthermore, in the Danish study[6] 27 pairs of monozygotic female twins and 34 pairs of dizygotic female twins were also studied. No evidence of association was found.

Disease Heterogeneity

Subdivisions of 36 patients[7] into groups of atopic (n = 9) and nonatopic (n = 27) also did not reveal any significant difference between the groups.

Family Data

Silvennoinen-Kassinen and Tiilikainen[7] also HLA-typed (A, B, C, and D loci) the families of 10 probands with nickel allergy. Three of these were multiple-case families. In one family with 5 siblings, all 3 affected siblings had haplotype A9-B12-DW4 in common. The 2 unaffected siblings did not have this haplotype. In 5 of the affected siblings, both haplotypes were identical.

In the other 5 families, the affected individuals were mother-daughter pairs and thus were not informative.

In the report of Kapoor-Pillarisetti et al.[5] 3 multiple-case families were also investigated. All affected inviduals in these 3 families were positive for B21.

References

1. Liden S, Beckman L, Cedergren B, Groyh O, Gouansson K, Wahlby L: Lack of association between allergic contact dermatitis and HLA antigens of the A and B series. Acta Dermatol Venereol (Stockh) 61:155-157, 1981
2. Liden S, Beckman L, Cedergren B, Goransson K, Nyquist H: HLA antigens in allergic contact dermatitis. Acta Dermatol Venereol (Stockh) 79(Suppl):54-56, 1978
3. Silvennoinen-Kassinen S, Tiilikainen A, Karvonen J: No significant association between HLA and nickel contact sensitivity. Tissue Antigens 14:459-461, 1979
4. Dumont-Frutyier M, Van Neste D, De Bruyere M, Tenstedt D, Lachapelle JM: Nickel contact sensitivity in women and HLA antigens. Arch Dermatol Res 269:205-208, 1980

5. Kapoor-Pillarisetti A, Mowbray JF, Brostoff J, Coronin EA: HLA dependence of sensitivity to nickel and chromium. Tissue Antigens 17:261-264, 1981
6. Hansen HE, Menne T, Larsen SO: HLA antigens in nickel sensitive females. Based on a twin and a patient population. Tissue Antigens 19:306-310, 1982
7. Silvennoinen-Kassinen, Tiilikainen A: No significant HLA haplotype association in nickel contact sensitivity: A family study. Tissue Antigens 15:455-457, 1980

Allergy to Chromium

Population Association

HLA-A and -B loci antigen frequency data in 3 studies from Sweden[1-3] and one from England[4] do not show any indication of association with this allergy.

References

1. Roupe G, Rydberg L, Swanbeck G: HLA-antigens and contact hypersensitivity. J Invest Dermatol 72:131-132, 1979
2. Liden S, Beckman L, Cedergren B, Groyh O, Goransson K, Wahlby L: Lack of association between allergic contact dermatitis and HLA antigens of the A and B series. Acta Dermatol Venereol (Stockh) 61:155-157, 1981
3. Liden S, Beckman L, Cedergren B, Goransson K, Nyquist H: HLA antigens in allergic contact dermatitis. Acta Dermatol Venereol (Stockh) 79(Suppl):54-56, 1978
4. Kapoor-Pillarisetti A, Mowbray JF, Brostoff J, Coronin EA: HLA dependence of sensitivity to nickel and chromium. Tissue Antigens 17:261-264, 1981

Allergy to Rye

Population Association

Marsh et al.[1,2] compared 136 American Caucasian allergic and 64 individuals nonallergic to rye group I allergen (rye I, molecular weight 27,000 daltons). The frequency of B8 was significantly increased in the allergic group (Table 13.2).

Family Data

The same group of authors[3] also studied the segregation of HLA haplotypes and immune responsiveness to rye I in 76 members of 13 large families. Specific immune response was studied quantitatively by measurement of IgE-mediated skin sensitivity, serum IgG antibody, and antigen-induced lymphocyte proliferation *in vitro*. There was no evidence for association between a specific HLA haplotype and a specific response measured by any one or more of the above indices of immune function (See also ref. 4).

References

1. Marsh DG, Chase GA, Goodfriend L, Bias W: 'Mapping' of postulated IR genes within HLA by studies in allergic populations. Monogr Allergy 11:106-115, 1977
2. Marsh DG, Meyers DA, Freidhoff LR, Hussain R, Hsu SH, Bias W: Association of HLA phenotypes A1, -B8, -DW3 and A3, -B7, -DW2 with allergy. Int Arch Allergy Appl Immunol 66:48-50, 1981
3. Black PL, Marsh DG, Jarrett E, Delespesse GJ, Bias WB: Family studies of association between HLA and specific immune responses to highly purified pollen allergens. Immunogenetics 3:349-368, 1976
4. Marsh DG, Hsu SH, Hussain R, Meyers DA, Freidhoff LR, Bias WB: Genetics of human immune response to allergens. J Allergy Clin Immunol 65:322-332, 1980

Allergy to Ragweed

Population Association

In 1973 Marsh et al.[1] presented HLA-A and -B loci frequency data on 18 individuals sensitive to ragweed (*Ambrosia elalior*) pollen allergen Ra5 (molecular weight 52,000 ± 200 daltons). Thirteen of 18 patients (72.22%) were positive for 1 of the antigens of the B7 cross-reacting group. In the group of 77 individuals not sensitive to Ra5 antigens the fre-

TABLE 13.2. Allergy to Rye

	Patients		Controls				
Country/Population	n	%+	n	%+	RR	χ^2	Ref.
HLA-B8							
U.S.A.	136	32	64	9	4.44	11.23	1

quency of these antigens was only 33.77% (26/77). Thus, there was a significant ($p < 0.006$) increase of these antigens in the sensitive individuals. The frequency of B7 alone was not significantly increased in the patients.

In a second paper[2] on a larger group of patients (2 studies), the association with B7 and the B7 cross-reacting group of antigens was found to be significant (Table 13.3). The three reports by Marsh et al.[3-5] reported a stronger association with DW2 in 35 Ra5-sensitive patients (Table 13.3).

Marsh et al.[6] published data on allergic subjects with varying sensitivity to the minor ragweed allergen Ra3 (molecular weight 12,100 daltons). Using regression analysis on a series of subsets of Ra3 responders and nonresponders, 2 disease phenotypes, "responder" and "nonresponder," were defined.

In these data there was a significant positive association between Ra3 response and total serum IgE and the presence of the A2 cross-reacting group (A2 and A28). Also there was a significant negative association with the A3 cross-reacting group (A3 and A11). (See also refs. 4, 5, 7-9.)

It should be noted that Blumenthal et al.[10] studied 165 American Caucasians with ragweed rhinitis and asthma. No highly significant associations between HLA and Ra3 and Ra5 skin-test response, serum IgE levels, and some other parameters were found.

Disease Heterogeneity

Bruce et al.[11] reported no significant HLA difference between 41 ragweed allergic seasonal asthmatics and 41 ragweed allergic nonasthmatics. The 2 groups did not differ in either the distribution of leukocyte sensitivities to ragweed antigen E or in the distributions of skin test sensitivities to ragweed antigens Ra3 and Ra5. Interestingly, the frequency of B7 in the asthmatic group was 24.4% and that in the nonasthmatic group was 22%.

Family Data

Levine et al.[12] first reported a correlation between HLA haplotypes and clinical ragweed pollenosis and IgE antibody specific for antigen E (the major purified protein antigen from ragweed pollen extract) in 7 families. Another report by Blumenthal et al.[13] on 57 members of a large 3-generation family showed a significant association between the haplotype A2-B12 and antigen E skin sensitivity.

Mendell et al.[14] analyzed segregation and lod scores of the large pedigree data published by Blumenthal et al.[13] and 1 additional family. On the basis of segregation analysis the dominant hypothesis was determined to be about 6 times more likely than the recessive hypothesis. The maximum lod score for both pedigrees was 1.72 at a recombination frequency of 20%. Thus, there was some evidence supporting the existence of a locus for ragweed sensitivity loosely linked with the HLA complex. (See also ref. 15.) The existence of linkage between clinical ragweed hypersensitivity and HLA haplotype has also been reported in one family studied by Yoo et al.[16,17] The authors, however, did not give results of any formal linkage analysis.

A study by Black et al.[18] on 13 large families did not support the data reported in the previous section. The association between specific familial HLA haplotypes and immune responsiveness to 3 different highly purified pollen antigens (ragweed antigens E, Ra3, and Ra5) were investigated in 76 individuals of 13 large families. Specific immune response was studied quantitatively by measurement of IgE-mediated skin sensitivity, serum IgG antibody, and antigen-induced lymphocyte proliferation *in vitro*. There was no evidence in these families for an association between specific response measured by 1 or more of the above indices of immune function.

Thus, in the total family data, there was no strong evidence to support the linkage between ragweed allergy and HLA complex.

See also refs. 19 and 20.

Table 13.3. Allergy to Ragweed

	Patients		Controls				
Country/Population	n	%+	n	%+	RR	χ^2	Ref.
HLA-B7							
U.S.A.	65	40	125	17	3.22	11.71	2
HLA-DW2							
U.S.A.	35	69	35	17	9.95	17.52	3

References

1. Marsh DG, Bias WB, Hsu SH: Association of the HL-A7 cross-reacting group with a specific reaginic antibody response in allergic man. Science 179:691-693, 1973
2. Goodfriend L, Santilli J Jr, Schacter B, Bias WB, Marsh DG: HLA-B7 cross-reacting group and human IgE-mediated sensitivity to ragweed allergen Ra5. Monogr Allergy 11:80-82, 1977
3. Bias WB, Hsu SH, Meyers DA, Goodfriend L, Marsh DG: HLA associations with chemically defined ragweed pollen components. Transplant Proc 11:1853-1857, 1979
4. Marsh DG, Hsu SH, Roebber M, Ehrlich-Kautzky E, Freidhoff LR, Meyers DA, et al: HLA-Dw2: A genetic marker for human immune response to short ragweed pollen allergen Ra5; I. J Exp Med 155:1439-1451, 1982
5. Marsh DG, Meyers DA, Freidhoff LR, Ehrlich-Kautzky E, Roebber M, Norman PS, et al: HLA-Dw2: A genetic marker for human immune response to short ragweed pollen allergen Ra5; II. J Exp Med 155:1452-1463, 1982
6. Marsh DG, Chase GA, Freidhoff LR, Meyers DA, Bias WB: Association of HLA antigens and total serum immunoglobulin E level with allergic response and failure to respond to ragweed allergen Ra3. Proc Natl Acad Sci USA 76:2903-2907, 1979
7. Marsh DG, Chase GA, Goodfriend L, Bias W: 'Mapping' of postulated IR genes within HLA by studies in allergic populations. Monogr Allergy 11:106-115, 1977
8. Marsh DG, Hsu SH, Hussain R, Meyers DA, Freidhoff LR, Bias WB: Genetics of human immune response to allergens. J Allergy Clin Immunol 65:322-332, 1980
9. Mendell NR, Amos DB, Blumenthal MN, Gleich GJ, Yunis ED: Ra3 skin test response and HLA-A2, antigen E, and IgE: Evidence of interactions between antigen E and HLA. Hum Immunol 4:63-70, 1982
10. Blumenthal MN, Yunis E, Gleich G, Mendell N, Stoy P, Walsh G, et al: Lack of association of the immune response to ragweed antigen E, Ra3 and Ra5 with the HLA system. J Immunogenet 8:379-386, 1981
11. Bruce CA, Bias WB, Norman PS, Lichtenstein LM, Marsh DG: Studies of HLA antigen frequencies, IgE levels, and specific allergic sensitivities in patients having ragweed hayfever, with and without asthma. Clin Exp Immunol 25:67-72, 1976
12. Levine BB, Stember RH, Fotino M: Ragweed hay fever: Genetic control and linkage to HL-A haplotypes. Science 178: 1201-1203, 1972
13. Blumenthal MN, Amos DB, Noreen H, Mendell NR, Yunis EJ: Genetic mapping of IR locus in man: Linkage to second locus of HL-A. Science 184:1301-1303, 1974
14. Mendell NR, Blumenthal M, Amos DB, Yunis EJ, Elston RC: Ragweed sensitivity. Segregation analysis and linkage to HLA-B. Cytogenet Cell Genet 22:330-334, 1978
15. Blumenthal M, Mendell NR, Yunis E, Amos DB, Muscoplat C, Elston RC: HLA and ragweed allergy. Monogr Allergy 11:83-88, 1977
16. Yoo TJ, Kuo CY, Thompson JS: Family study of HLA antigen and IR gene linkage in ragweed and dust allergy. Monogr Allergy 11:89-96, 1977
17. Yoo TJ, Flink RJ, Thompson JS: The relationship between HL-A antigens and lymphocyte response in ragweed allergy. J Allergy Clin Immunol 57:25-28, 1976
18. Black PL, Marsh DG, Jarrett E, Delespesse GJ, Bias WB: Family studies of association between HLA and specific immune responses to highly purified pollen allergens. Immunogenetics 3:349-368, 1976
19. Seignalet J, Robinet-Levy M, Michel FB, Guilhou JJ, Lapinski H: HL-A et IgE seriques elevees. Nouv Presse Med 3:2263, 1977
20. Bias WB, Marsh DG: HL-A linked antigen E immune response genes: An unproved hypothesis. Science 188:375-377, 1975

Allergy to Aspergillus (Allergic Bronchopulmonary Aspergillosis)

Population Association

In 2 studies involving 22 American Caucasian patients[1] and 36 English patients[2] who had precipitins to *Aspergillus fumigatus*, no associations with A and B loci antigens were found. The patients in the British study[2] were also typed for C and DR loci antigens.

Family Data

See ref. 1.

References

1. Flaherty DK, Surfus JE, Geller M, Rosenberg M, Patterson R, Reed CE: HLA antigen frequencies in allergic bronchopulmonary aspergillosis. Clin Allergy 8:73-76, 1978
2. Morris MJ, Faux JA, Ting A, Morris PJ, Lane DJ: HLA-A, B and C and HLA-DR antigens in intrinsic and allergic asthma. Clin Allergy 10:173-179, 1980

Allergy to *Alternaria Tenuis*

Population Association

Flaherty et al.[1] typed A, B, and C antigens in 100 American Caucasians allergic to *Alternaria tenuis*. When the antigen frequencies were compared with 100 age- and sex-matched controls, no significant deviations were found.

Disease Heterogeneity

In the above study[1] there were associations with age at onset, total serum IgE levels, and *Alternaria*-specific IgE antibody.

Reference

1. Flaherty DK, Geller M, Surfus JE, Leo GM, Reed CE, Rankin J: HLA antigen frequencies and natural history in *Alternaria*-sensitive and perennial nonallergic asthmatics. J Allergy Clin Immunol 66:408-416, 1980

Allergy to Formalin

Population Association

Liden et al.,[1] in their first report on 11 Swedish patients, noted a decrease of A2 and an increase of B7 antigens. These results, however, were not confirmed in their second report[2] on 27 patients.

References

1. Liden S, Beckman L, Cedergren B, Goransson K, Nyquist H: HLA antigens in allergic contact dermatitis. Acta Dermatol Venereol (Stockh) 79(Suppl):54-56, 1978
2. Liden S, Beckman L, Cedergren B, Groyh O, Goransson K, Wahlby L: Lack of association between allergic contact dermatitis and HLA antigens of the A and B series. Acta Dermatol Venereol (Stockh) 61:155-157, 1981

Allergy to Balsam of Peru

Population Association

In 24 Swedish patients Liden et al.[1] observed an increased frequency of B7 (54.2% in the patients vs. 27.4% in 339 controls). In the second report by the same group of authors[2] the frequency of B7 in 24 patients was 46% as compared with 30.7% in 368 controls. These differences are not highly significant, however.

References

1. Liden S, Beckman L, Cedergren B, Goransson K, Nyquist H: HLA antigens in allergic contact dermatitis. Acta Dermatol Venereol (Stockh) 79(Suppl):54-56, 1978
2. Liden S, Beckman L, Cedergren B, Groyh O, Goransson K, Wahlby L: Lack of association between allergic contact dermatitis and HLA antigens of the A and B series. Acta Dermatol Venereol (Stockh) 61:155-157, 1981

Allergy to Colophony

Population Association

In 14 Swedish patients Liden et al.[1] noted an increased frequency of B27 antigen (35.7% in the patients vs. 15.6% in 339 controls; $p < 0.05$).

Reference

1. Liden S, Beckman L, Cedergren B, Goransson K, Nyquist H: HLA antigens in allergic contact dermatitis. Acta Dermatol Venereol (Stockh) 79(Suppl);54-56, 1978

Allergy to Wool Alcohols

Population Association

Liden et al.[1] compared A and B loci antigen frequencies in 14 Swedish patients and 339 controls. The antigen B7 was present in 57.1% of the patients as compared with 27.4% in the controls ($p < 0.05$).

Reference

1. Liden S, Beckman L, Cedergren B, Goransson K, Nyquist H: HLA antigens in allergic contact dermatitis. Acta Dermatol Venereol (Stockh) 79(Suppl):54-56, 1978

Allergy to Para Group Compounds

Population Association

In one report from Italy Valsecchi et al.[1] typed A, B, and C loci antigens in 40 patients (28 males and

12 females) with allergic contact dermatitis from the para group compounds (aniline, benzocaine, paraphenylenediamine, parahydroxybenzoates, promethazine hydrochloride, and sulfamide). The frequencies in the patients were compared with those in 321 healthy control subjects.

No significant association was found.

Reference

1. Valsecchi R, Bontempelli M, Vicari O, Scudeller G, Cainelli T: HLA antigens and contact sensitivity. Arch Dermatol 118:533-534, 1982

Allergy to Cat Dander

Population Association

In a brief report Marsh et al.[1] noted an association with B8 in American Caucasian patients. Neither the frequency data nor the sample size is given, however.

Reference

1. Marsh DG, Meyers DA, Freidhoff LR, Hussain R, Hsu SH, Bias W: Association of HLA phenotypes A1, B8, DW3 and A3, B7, DW2 with allergy. Int Arch Allergy Appl Immunol 66:48-50, 1981

Pigeon Breeder's Lung

Population Association

The data of Rittner et al.[1,2] showed an increased frequency of B8. However, in another study on American Caucasian patients[3] this increase was not confirmed. In the combined sample there was no indication of an association with B8.

In the American study 25 and 32 patients were typed for C and DR loci antigens, respectively. Again the frequencies did not differ from those in the control group.

See also ref. 4.

References

1. Rittner C, Sennekamp J, Vogel F: HLA-B8 in pigeon-fancier's lung. Lancet ii:1303, 1975
2. Sennekamp J, Rittner CH, Vogel F, Tauberecht I: Verteilung der HLA-Antigene bei Patienten mit Taubenzuechterlunge. Schweiz Med Wochenschr 108:315-317, 1978
3. Rodey GE, Fink J, Koethe S, Schlueter D, Witkowski J, Bettonville P, et al: A study of HLA-A, B, C, and DR specificities in pigeon breeder's disease. Am Rev Respir Dis 119:755-759, 1979
4. De La Vega VD, Bialostosky D, Lupi E, Castro G, Barrios R, Reyes PA: Familial pigeon breeder's disease: Possible association to HLA-Bw40 antigen. Rev Invest Clin 32:401-407, 1980

Farmer's Lung

Population Association

An association with B8 in 20 American Caucasian patients was first reported by Flaherty et al.[1] However, these authors could not confirm this association in their second report on 100 patients.[2] Similar nonsignificant results were also found in a Finnish study on 37 patients by Terho et al.[3]

Family Data

De Ridder and Berrens[4] published data on a family of 7 individuals. Laboratory diagnosis was done by examining serum for precipitins against extracts of moldy hay and *Mycropolyspora faeni* culture filtrate antigens and for autologous serum complement consumption by *M. faeni* culture filtrate antigens. There was no evidence of segregation of either manifest disease or serologic reactivity to *M. faeni* culture filtrate antigens with a specific HLA haplotype.

References

1. Flaherty DK, Iha T, Chmelik F, Dickie H, Reed CE: HL-A8 in farmer's lung. Lancet ii:507, 1975
2. Flaherty DK, Braun SR, Marx JJ, Blank JL, Emanuel DA, Rankin J: Serologically detectable HLA-A, B, and C loci antigens in farmer's lung disease. Am Rev Respir Dis 122:437-443, 1980
3. Terho EO, Koskimies S, Heinonen OP, Mantyjarvi R: HLA and farmer's lung. Eur J Respir Dis 63:361-362, 1981
4. De Ridder G, Berrens L: Family study of farmer's lung. Lancet i:832-833, 1978

Silicosis

Population Association

Gualde et al.[1] studied 75 French (Caucasians) patients who were exposed to silica particles for 10–40 years. Thirty-eight patients were gold, wolfram, and uranium miners, 35 were porcelain workers, and 2 were quarrymen. HLA-A and -B loci antigen frequencies were compared with 2 groups of controls:

100 healthy nonexposed and 46 healthy individuals who had been exposed to silica particles. Although no significant deviations in any of the antigens were observed, the frequency of B7 was 6.66% in patients compared with 20% in 160 healthy controls.

Disease Heterogeneity

There was no association between HLA and patient subgroups on the basis of age, length of exposure, clinical signs, or radiologic extent of disease. However, 5 of 14 patients (35.71%) who had pulmonary tuberculosis had B8 (compared with 13.12% in 160 controls).

Reference

1. Gualde N, De Leobardy J, Serizay B, Malinvaud G: HL-A and silicosis. Am Rev Respir Dis 116:334-336, 1977

Asbestosis

Population Association

Merchant et al.[1] first reported an increase in the frequency of B27 in a patient group (Table 13.4). This observation, however, was not confirmed in 2 other studies from England[2,3] and one from Finland.[4] In the pooled data the association with B27 is only marginally significant primarily because of the data of Merchant et al.[1] (Table 13.4).

See also refs. 5–8.

References

1. Merchant JA, Klouda PT, Soutar CA, Parkes W, Lawler SD, Turner-Warwick M: The HL-A system in asbestos workers. Br Med J 1:189-191, 1975
2. Evans CC, Lewinsohn HC, Evans JM: Frequency of HLA antigens in asbestos workers with and without pulmonary fibrosis. Br Med J 1:603-605, 1977
3. Darke C, Wagner MMF, McMillan GHG: HLA-A and B antigen frequencies in an asbestos exposed population with normal and abnormal chest radiographs. Tissue Antigens 13:228-232, 1979
4. Huuskonen MS, Tiilikainen A, Alanko K: HLA-B18 antigens and protection from pulmonary fibrosis in asbestos workers. Br J Dis Chest 73:253-259, 1979
5. Evans CC, Evans JM: HL-A type and asbestosis. Tubercle 56:171, 1975
6. Turner-Warwick M: HLA phenotypes in asbestos workers. Br J Dis Chest 73:243-244, 1979
7. Gregor A, Singh S, Turner-Warwick M, Lawler S, Parkes WR: The role of histocompatibility (HLA) antigens in asbestosis. Br J Dis Chest 73:245-252, 1979
8. Turner-Warwick M: HLA and asbestos-related lung disease. Br J Dis Chest 71:219-220, 1977

Cedar Pollinosis

Population Association

Terao and Sato[1] reported significant associations with A10 and B15 in a study involving 35 Japanese patients (Table 13.5).

Family Data

Sasazuki et al.[2] have given HLA haplotype data on 17 affected sib-pairs. Nine sib-pairs shared 2 haplotypes, 7 shared 1 haplotype, and 1 pair did not share any haplotype. This observed ratio was significantly different from the expected ratio of 1:2:1 for sharing 2, 1, and 0 haplotypes, respectively ($p < 0.02$). This analysis also showed that the distortion

TABLE 13.4. Asbestosis

	Patients		Controls				
Country/Population	n	%+	n	%+	RR	χ^2	Ref.
HLA-B27							
England	78	14	298	9	1.68	1.95	3
England	37	5	616	7	0.87	0.05	2
England	56	18	153	5	4.08	8.45	1
	171	13	1067	7	1.96	6.33	
	Heterogeneity χ^2 (2 df)					4.12	
Finland	64	14	900	14	1.04	0.01	4
	235	14	1967	10	1.56	4.34	
	Heterogeneity χ^2 (3 df)					6.12	

TABLE 13.5. Cedar Pollinosis

	Patients		Controls				
Country/Population	n	%+	n	%+	RR	χ^2	Ref.
HLA-A10							
Japan	35	69	128	12	15.49	38.70	1
HLA-B15							
Japan	35	37	128	12	4.25	11.34	1

in the affected sib-pairs ratio can be explained by a recessive "disease suspectibility locus" segregating with the HLA complex.

Refererences

1. Terao A, Sato Y: HLA specificities of cedar pollinosis. Nippon Jibiinkoka Gakkai Kaiho 81:101-105, 1978
2. Sasazuki T, Nishimura Y, Muto M, Ohta N: HLA-linked genes controlling immune response and disease susceptibility. Immunol Rev 70:51-75, 1983

Grass Pollinosis

Population Association

Jeannet et al.[1] found no signficant deviations in the frequencies of any particular antigen in 48 Swiss individuals with grass pollinosis (strong positive skin tests to crude timothy pollen extracts) who were typed for A and B loci antigens. In this study 16 persons were also sensitive to additional allergens, such as molds, wool, etc. In this subgroup A1 and B8 were increased. A preliminary analysis of DR antigens on 16 patients and 10 healthy individuals also did not reveal any significant association.

In another Swiss study[2] on 35 patients, a significant association with DW3 (D locus) has been reported. The frequency of DW3 was 43% in the patients and 13% in the unspecified number of controls.

Family Data

Black et al.[3] investigated immune responsiveness to 4 different highly purified pollen antigens (ragweed antigens E, Ra3, Ra5, and rye grass group 1) in 76 members of 13 large families. Specific immune response was studied quantitatively by measurement of IgE-mediated skin sensitivity, serum IgG antibody, and antigen-induced lymphocyte proliferation *in vitro*. There was no evidence for association between a specific HLA haplotype and specific response measured by any 1 or more of the indices of immune function.

Similar negative results have been reported by Pillier-Loriette et al.[4, 5] in 12 French families (62 individuals) in which hypersensitivity to cocksfoot (*Dactylis glomerata*) was studied. There was no distortion in joint segregation of HLA haplotypes and sensitivity to this particular antigen.

Jeannet et al.[1] also studied sensitivity to Timothy pollen in 11 Swiss families. Again susceptibility to grass pollinosis and IgE levels was not found linked to HLA.

References

1. Jeannet M, Girard JP, Varonier HS, Mirimanoff P, Joye P: HLA antigens in grass pollinosis. Monogr Allergy 11:69-73, 1977
2. De Moerloose PH, Chardonnens X, Vassalli P, Jeannet M: Antigenes HLA-D des lymphocytes B et susceptibilite a certaines Amaladies. Schweiz Med Wochenschr 107:1461, 1977
3. Black PL, Marsh DG, Jarrett E, Delespesse GJ, Bias WB: Family studies of association between HLA and specific immune responses to highly purified pollen allergens. Immunogenetics 3:349-368, 1976
4. Pillier-Loriette C, Marcelli-Barge A, Dausset J, Treich I, Gervais P, Rafford M, et al: Search for correlation between familial allergy to dactyl (pollen hypersensitivity) and HLA antigens. Tissue Antigens 8:87-90, 1976
5. Pillier-Loriette C, Marcelli-Barge A, Dausset J, Treich I, Gervais P, Raffard M: Search for a correlation between familial allergy to cocksfoot pollen and HLA antigens. Monogr Allergy 11:61-68, 1977

Flax Byssinosis

This disease occurs in workers who prepare flax for spinning and in those handling the spun yarn when it dries.

TABLE 13.6. Flax Byssinosis

	Patients		Controls				
Country/Population	n	%+	n	%+	RR	χ^2	Ref.
HLA-B27							
Ireland	40	23	200	6	4.67	11.23	1

Population Association

There is only 1 report by Middleton et al.[1] in which B27 was found to be significantly increased in the patients (Table 13.6).

Reference

1. Middleton D, Logan JS, Magennis BP, Nelson SD: HLA antigen frequencies in flax byssinosis patients. Br J Ind Med 36:123-126, 1979

Coalworker's Pneumoconiosis

Population Association

In 3 independent studies on 227 American[1] and 311 English patients,[2,3] there was no association with A and B loci antigens.

Disease Heterogeneity

In both the American and British studies, there were 3 groups of individuals: normal, with pneumoconiosis, and with massive fibrosis. The antigen frequencies did not differ significantly in these 3 groups. However, in the English study,[2] the frequency of BW21 was 1.1% in the total pneumoconiosis group (n = 256) compared with 8.2% in 134 normal coalworkers (corrected $p < 0.032$). This antigen was not typed in the American study.[1]

Soutar et al.[3] subdivided their 100 patients as 40 with "simple pneumoconiosis" and 60 with "complicated pneumoconiosis." There was no HLA antigen difference between these 2 subgroups.

References

1. Heise ER, Mentnech MS, Olenchock SA, Kutz SA, Morgan WKC, Merchant JA, et al: HLA-A1 and coalworkers' pneumoconiosis. Am Rev Respir Dis 119:903-908, 1979
2. Wagner MMF, Darke C: HLA-A and B antigen frequencies in Welsh coalworkers with pneumoconiosis and Caplan's syndrome. Tissue Antigens 14:165-168, 1979
3. Soutar CA, Coutts I, Parkes WR, Dodi IA, Gauld S, Castro JE, et al: Histocompatibility antigens in coal miners with pneumoconiosis. Br J Ind Med 40:34-38, 1983

Avian Hypersensitivity

Population Association

B40 was found to be associated in 1 Australian study[1] (Table 13.7). However, in Berrill's and Van Rood's data[2] on 24 patients no association with A, B, and C loci antigens was observed. They found an increase in the frequency of DW6 (Table 13.7).

Family Data

Allen et al.[1,3] published data on families with more than 1 affected member. There was no indication of linkage of this disease with HLA.

TABLE 13.7. Avian Hypersensitivity

	Patients		Controls				
Country/Population	n	%+	n	%+	RR	χ^2	Ref.
HLA-B40							
Australia	20	35	861	10	4.97	12.30	1
HLA-DW6							
England	24	42	100	17	3.50	6.99	2

References

1. Allen DH, Basten A, Woolcock AJ, Guinan J: HLA and bird breeder's hypersensitivity pneumonitis. Monogr Allergy 11:45-54, 1977
2. Berrill WT, Van Rood JJ: HLA-DW6 and avian hypersensitivity. Lancet ii:248-249, 1977
3. Allen DH, Basten A, Williams GV, Woolcock AJ: Familial hypersensitivity pneumonitis. Am J Med 59:505-514, 1975

Cryptogenic Fibrosing Alveolitis

Population Association

Caucasian patients from England,[1,2] the United States,[3] and Finland[4] were studied for A, B, C, and D antigens. In the first English report,[1] B12 was found to be significantly increased. However, this was not confirmed in a second study by Turton et al.[2] on 50 English patients. In their data B8 was increased in the patients.

In the Finnish[4] study there was a significant association with B15 and an increased frequency of DW6 in the patient group.

In the American report,[3] there was no association with any of the A and B loci antigens.

In the pooled data the increased frequencies of B8 and B12 were not significant. Table 13.8 gives all the available data on B15 and DW6 for this disease. The association with B15 remains significant in the combined sample.

Disease Heterogeneity

The 50 patients studied by Turton et al.[2] were subdivided into groups according to sex and age at onset. B8 was present in 67% of the 18 female patients and in 60% of the 20 patients with onset of disease before age 50. These values were significantly different when compared with a 23% frequency in 167 controls.

References

1. Evans CC, Evans JM: HL-A in farmer's lung. Lancet ii:975-976, 1975
2. Turton CWG, Morris LM, Lawler SD, Warwick MT: HLA in cryptogenic fibrosing alveolitis. Lancet i:507-508, 1978
3. Strimlan CV, Taswell HF, Deremee RA, Kueppers F: HL-A antigens and fibrosing alveolitis. Am Rev Respir Dis 116:1120-1121, 1977
4. Varpela E, Tiilikainen A, Varpela M, Tukiainen P: High prevalences of HLA-B15 and HLA-DW6 in patients with cryptogenic fibrosing alveolitis. Tissue Antigens 14:68-71, 1979

Idiopathic Pulmonary Fibrosis

Idiopathic pulmonary fibrosis is a progressive disease characterized by exertional breathlessness, an interstitial pattern on chest roentgenogram, and decreased lung volumes.

Population Association

In a sample of 33 American Caucasian patients[1] and 329 healthy controls, all typed for A and B loci antigens, there was no significant difference in the frequency of any of the antigens.

Reference

1. Fulmer JD, Sposovska MS, Von Gal ER, Crystal RG, Mittal KK: Distribution of HLA antigens in idiopathic pulmonary fibrosis. Am Rev Respir Dis 118:141-147, 1978

TABLE 13.8. Cryptogenic Fibrosing Alveolitis

	Patients		Controls				
Country/Population	n	%+	n	%+	RR	χ^2	Ref.
HLA-B15							
U.S.A.	32	19	567	12	1.81	1.82	3
Finland	38	45	900	20	3.28	13.11	4
	70	33	1467	17	2.66	13.77	
	Heterogeneity χ^2 (1 df)					1.16	
HLA-DW6							
Finland	27	52	77	23	3.55	7.70	4

IgE Levels in Healthy Individuals

Population Association

Perelmutter and Potvin[1] measured IgE levels in 58 Canadian military recruits. Twenty-five recruits in whom measurements were 153-2128 U/ml were classified as "high" IgE group. In the remaining 33 recruits the values ranged from 24 to 142 U/ml and they were classified as "low" IgE group. In the low group the CW2 was 55.5% compared with only 15% in the high group. No other interesting deviations for A and B loci antigens were observed.

Reference

1. Perelmutter L, Potvin L: A study on the IgE levels of military recruits and association with HLA antigens. Ann Allergy 40:319-321, 1978

Hay Fever

Population Association

Significant associations with AW19 and B8 have been observed in a German study[1] of 110 unrelated patients suffering from hay fever (Table 13.9). However, in another report by Turner et al.[2] from London on 40 similar patients, no significant deviations of any single antigen were observed (frequency data were not given). These authors reported a decreased frequency of A1 + B8 (10% in the patients vs. 17% in 1036 controls, $p < 0.05$) and an increased frequency of A3 + B7 (20% in the patients vs. 11.5% in the controls, $p < 0.05$). See also ref. 3.

References

1. Schunter F, Schieferstein G, Tchorz P, Fischer H, Schneider W: Histocompatibility antigens in hay fever. Z Immun Forsch 150:105-113, 1975
2. Turner MW, Brostoff J, Wells RS, Stokes CR, Soothill JF: HLA in eczema and hay fever. Clin Exp Immunol 27:43-47, 1977
3. Turner MW, Brostoff J, Wells RS, Soothill JF: Histocompatibility antigens in atopy with special reference to eczema and hay fever. Monogr Allergy 11:19-23, 1977

Schonlein-Henoch Nephritis

Population Association

Nyulassy et al.[1] reported significantly increased frequencies of B18 and BW35 antigens in 29 patients. However, this was not confirmed in the study of Kruger et al.[2] on 41 German patients (Table 13.10). In another study on 13 French patients,[3] an increase in the frequency of DR5 has also been noted (Table 13.10). (In this report, data on A, B, and C antigens were not given.)

References

1. Nyulassy S, Buc M, Sasinka M, Pavlovic M, Slugen I, Hirschova V, et al: The HLA system in glomerulonephritis. Clin Immunol Immunopathol 7:319-323, 1977
2. Kruger J, Opferkuch W, Evers KG, Bosecker L, Haase W: Lack of association between the HLA-A10 (A25), B18 and C2 haplotype and anaphylactoid purpura (AP). Tissue Antigens 15:68-74, 1980
3. De Mouzon-Cambon A, Ohayon E, Bouissou F, Barthe P: HLA-DR typing in children with glomerular diseases. Lancet ii:868, 1980

Sensitivity to the Odor of Androstenone

Population Association

Pollack et al.[1] compared the A, B, C, and DR loci antigen frequencies in 61 "mating pairs" analyzed

TABLE 13.9. Hay Fever

	Patients		Controls				
Country/Population	n	%+	n	%+	RR	χ^2	Ref.
HLA-AW19							
West Germany	110	33	353	18	2.25	11.07	1
HLA-B8							
West Germany	110	8	353	23	0.30	11.06	1

TABLE 13.10. Schonlein-Henoch Nephritis

	Patients		Controls				
Country/Population	n	%+	n	%+	RR	χ^2	Ref.
HLA-B18							
Czechoslovakia	29	21	312	5	5.19	11.01	1
West Germany	41	5	250	5	1.18	0.07	2
	70	12	562	5	3.03	7.84	
	Heterogeneity χ^2 (1 df)					3.23	
HLA-BW35							
Czechoslovakia	29	28	312	9	4.01	9.99	1
West Germany	41	20	250	17	1.26	0.33	2
	70	23	562	13	2.16	6.60	
	Heterogeneity χ^2 (1 df)					3.71	

for pyridine and androstenone sensitivity. These mating pairs included the 17 parents analyzed in a family study and 44 couples known to have been married or living together for a minimum of 3 years.

The antigen frequencies for the separate male and female members of this population did not differ significantly from each other or from a combined population of 388 unrelated New York metropolitan area controls.

Family Data

Lod score analysis of 17 families was also done by Pollack et al.[1] In each of these families all individuals were tested for the sensitivity to androstenone. The total lod score was < -2.00 at all recombination fractions $< 15\%$. Thus there was no evidence in favor of close linkage with the HLA complex.

See also ref. 2.

References

1. Pollack MS, Wysocki CJ, Beauchamp GK, Braun D Jr, Callaway C, Dupont B: Absence of HLA association or linkage for variations in sensitivity to the odor of androstenone. Immunogenetics 15:579-589, 1982
2. Boyse EA, Beauchamp GK, Yamazaki K: The sensory perception of genotypic polymorphism of the major histocompatibility complex and other genes: Some physiological and phylogenetic implications. Hum Immunol 6:117-183, 1983

Chapter 14

Urogenital Diseases

Herpes Gestationis

Population Association

Shornick et al.[1] observed a significantly increased frequency of DR3 in 26 American Caucasian patients (Table 14.1). Similarly, in a small sample of 8 Spanish patients studied by Ferrando et al.[2] 6 (75%) were positive for DR3. The frequency of this antigen in the control population of unknown size was 14.8%.

Family Data

Reunala et al.[3] described a case history of a Finnish female with herpes gestationis. She had a high titer of antibody against B8. Her child and her husband were positive for B8.

References

1. Shornick JK, Stastny P, Gilliam JN: High frequency of histocompatibility antigens HLA-DR3 and DR4 in herpes gestationis. J Clin Invest 68:553-555, 1981
2. Ferrando J, Arriaga F, Bordas X, Ercilla G, Vives J, Mascaro JM: Association of HLA-DR3 and Herpes gestationis. Acta Dermatol Venereol (Stockh) 61:462, 1981
3. Reunala T, Karvonen J, Tiilikainen A, Salo OP: Herpes gestationis. Br J Dermatol 96:563-568, 1977
4. Eberst E, Tongio MM, Eberst B, Mayer S, Basset A: Herpes gestationis and anti-HLA immunization. Br J Dermatol 104:553-559, 1981

Habitual Abortion

Population Association

In 3 reports from the Soviet Union[1] and Yugoslavia,[2,3] where frequencies of A and B antigens have been studied in women with recurrent abnormal pregnancies, a significant association with A9 was observed. B5 was also increased in the patients though it was not highly significant (Table 14.2).

Studies from Italy[4,5] on 35 females with at least 2 consecutive abortions found an increased frequency of BW35 (51.4%). This antigen was present in 30.3% of the 642 normal individuals ($p < 0.05$). The frequencies of other antigens are not available in this report.

Gerencer et al.[2,3] also studied 64 women with recurrent abnormal pregnancies of known etiology and in this group frequencies were similar to those in 158 controls.

Lauritsen et al.[6] compared A and B loci antigen frequencies in 215 Danish women with spontaneous abortions (8 women with 2 abortions) and their husbands with 1197 controls. Except for a slight increase of A1 in the patients there was no significant difference between the 2 groups. These authors also studied several red blood cell groups in the same group of patients, with similar results.

Schacter et al.[7] reported a significantly higher frequency of sharing of A and B antigens in 13 couples with recurrent fetal loss at 1 gestational age as compared with 17 couples with 3 or more normal pregnancies. Furthermore, the number of antigens shared by husbands and wives was significantly higher

TABLE 14.1. Herpes Gestationis

	Patients		Controls				
Country/Population	n	%+	n	%+	RR	χ^2	Ref.
HLA-DR3							
U.S.A.	23	61	126	22	5.37	13.35	1
HLA-DR4							
France	42	67	158	39	3.11	10.07	4

in 16 couples with 1 spontaneous abortion and in 23 couples with recurrent spontaneous abortions as compared with normal controls. The authors have hypothesized the existence of a human T-like locus linked to HLA with alleles in linkage disequilibrium with the alleles of HLA loci.

In another study from Israel[8] on 23 couples with repeated abortions, 13 with 1 abortion, and 18 with normal pregnancies, the percentages of couples sharing common HLA antigens was 77%, 70%, and 38%, respectively. Thus, there was a significant difference ($p < 0.05$) between controls and the group with repeated abortions. (See also ref. 9.)

Similar results, showing a significantly greater degree of HLA compatibility between 45 women with at least 3 spontaneous abortions and their husbands, compared with 79 control couples from Yugoslavia, have been reported by Gerencer et al.[2,3]

Tsuji et al.[10] studied 20 Japanese couples with habitual abortions (more than 2) and 13 couples with normal pregnancies (more than 2 children). The "average major incompatibility" in the experimental group was 15.4% as compared with 5.4% in the control group. These results appeared to be in contradiction with the 3 aforementioned studies. However, the authors did not give details for calculating average incompatibility or the meaning of major (and "minor") incompatibility as used in the report.

It is interesting to note here the hypothesis[11] that the evolution of histocompatibility polymorphisms results from the selective attrition of immunologically compatible fetuses in favor of immunologically stimulated incompatible fetuses. This condition would tend to select for histocompatible matings and will produce a selective advantage for populations that bear multiple alleles at their histocompatibility loci (for details see the studies cited in refs. 11 and 12).

See also refs. 13–18.

References

1. Muravieva LI, Volkova LS, Chen RI: Study of the human leucocyte antigen system in married couples in disturbed reproduction. Akush Ginekol (Mosk) 8:41-43, 1979
2. Gerencer M, Kastelan A, Drazancic A, Kerhin-Brkljacic V, Madharic M: The HLA antigens in

TABLE 14.2. Habitual Abortion

	Patients		Controls				
Country/Population	n	%+	n	%+	RR	χ^2	Ref.
HLA-A9							
USSR	65	41	40	18	3.02	5.74	1
Yugoslavia	71	49	158	25	2.86	12.57	2
	136	45	198	24	2.91	18.29	
	Heterogeneity χ^2 (1 df)					0.01	
HLA-B5							
USSR	65	31	40	15	2.42	3.24	1
Yugoslavia	71	28	158	17	1.90	3.72	2
	136	29	198	17	2.05	6.80	
	Heterogeneity χ^2 (1 df)					0.17	

women with recurrent abnormal pregnancies of unknown etiology. Tissue Antigens 12:223-227, 1978
3. Gerencer M, Drazancic A, Kuvacic I, Tomaskovic Z, Kastelan A, et al.: HLA antigen studies in women with recurrent gestational disorders. Fertil Steril 31:401-404, 1979
4. Carapella-De Luca E, Purpura M, Coghi I, Nicotra M, Bottini E: Blood groups and histocompatibility antigens in habitual abortion. Haematologia 13:105-111, 1980
5. Purpura M, Coghi I, Nicotra M, Carapella E, Bottini E: HLA Bw35 antigen and human reproduction. J Med Genet 17:157-158, 1980
6. Lauritsen JG, Jorgensen J, Kissmeyer-Nielsen F: Significance of HLA and blood-group incompatibility in spontaneous abortion. Clin Genet 9:575-582, 1976
7. Schacter B, Gyves M, Muir A, Tasin M: HLA-A,B compatibility in parents of offspring with neural-tube defects or couples experiencing involuntary fetal wastage. Lancet i:796-799, 1979
8. Komlos L, Zamir R, Joshua H, Halbrecht I: Common HLA antigens in couples with repeated abortions. Clin Immunol Immunopathol 7:330-335, 1977
9. Beer AE, Quebbeman JF, Ayers JWT, Haines RF: Major histocompatibility complex antigens, maternal and paternal immune responses, and chronic habitual abortions in humans. Am J Obstet Gynecol 141:987-999, 1981
10. Tsuji K, Miyamoto H, Motoaki I. HL-A and its clinical application. Keio J Med 21:159-169, 1972
11. Lappe M: HLA homozygosity and neural-tube defects. Lancet i:1342, 1979
12. Hull P: HLA incompatibility, genetic diversity, and survival. Lancet ii:933-934, 1981
13. Komlos L, Halbrecht I: Repeated abortions and histocompatibility antigens - can HLA antigen restricted gene dose effects influence the feto-maternal relationship? Med Hypotheses 5:901-908, 1979
14. Eberst B, Schumacher JC, Tongio MA, Walch R, Ritter J, Gandar R: Immunisation foeto-maternelle anti-HLA et pathologie gravidique et/ou neo-natale. J Gyn Obstet Biol Reprod (Paris) 7:57-62, 1978
15. Smith RT: The immunobiology of abortion. N Engl J Med 295:1249-1250, 1976
16. Gelabert A, Balasch J, Ercilla G, Vanrell JA, Vives J, Gonzalez-Merlo J, et al.: Abortion may sensitize the mother to HLA antigens. Tissue Antigens 17:353-356, 1981
17. Beer AE, Quebbeman JF, Ayers JWT, Haines RF: Discussion. Am J Obstet Gynecol 143:177-178, 1982
18. Pattillo RA: Histocompatibility antigens in pregnancy, abortions, infertility, preeclampsia and trophoblast neoplasms. Am J Reprod Immunol 1:29-34, 1980

Eclampsia

Population Association

In 23 eclamptic primigravidas (American Caucasians, Blacks, and Latin Americans) typed for A and B loci specificities no association was found.[1] See also ref. 2.

References

1. Scott JR, Beer AE, Stastny P: Immunogenetic factors in preeclampsia and eclampsia: Erythrocyte, histocompatibility, and y-dependent antigens. JAMA 235:402-404, 1976
2. Anichkova SI, Vasilieva ZF, Grigorieva VV: Study of compatibility in married couples according to the HLA antigen system in normal and complicated by late toxemia pregnancy. Akush Ginekol 8:20-23, 1981

Preeclampsia

Population Association

The population data from the United States[1] (sample was a mixture of Caucasians, Blacks, and Latin Americans), England,[2–4] and France[5] showed that no specific A or B loci antigens were associated with preeclampsia. In the French study[5] 24 patients were also typed for DR locus antigens. Though DR4 was slightly increased in the patients (37.5% in patients vs. 13% in 15 controls) no antigen was significantly associated with the disease. Eight of the 16 women with a family history of hypertension were positive for DR4 as compared with only 1 of the 8 without family history.

In 2 studies from England,[2,3] preeclampsia patients had no antibody to paternal HLA antigens. However, contradictory results have also been found in other studies (see studies cited in ref. 2).

Jenkins et al.[3] reported a greater incidence of matching of HLA antigens in 38 preeclampsia women and their husbands compared with 33 control pairs. Eleven out of 13 A and B loci antigens were more commonly matched in patients and their husbands than in the control pairs. Eighteen out of 20 antigens were found to be more often matched in preeclampsia pairs than expected from random pairs. This increased frequency of matching may be related to the risk of developing the disease. It should also be noted that the difference between the 2 groups was not significant for any single antigen.

Redman et al.[4] reported a significant excess of

patients with only 1 detectable antigen at the B locus (5/24 patients vs. 0/20 controls, $p = 0.025$). This difference was confirmed in a second group of 56 prospectively studied patients (13/56 patients vs. 5/59 controls, $p = 0.027$). The patients with only 1 detectable antigen were presumed to be homozygous for that particular antigen, because the frequency of unknown alleles at the B locus was very low. In this study there was a significant linear trend of maternal homozygosity at the B locus with increasing severity of the disorder, as measured by fetal survival and the time of delivery. The authors have hypothesized that homozygosity of A and B genes may be a marker of homozygosity at adjacent loci for immune response genes that produce deficient or absent immune response contributing to the development of preeclampsia.

Simon et al.[5] also reported HLA-B (6/26) and HLA-A and -B (4/26) homozygosities in French patients. The 16 women with normal pregnancies did not show any homozygosity. Also, there was a linear trend of increasing histocompatibility with increasing severity of preeclampsia.

Disease Heterogeneity

It should be noted that in 2 other studies[1,3] there was no evidence of homozygosity at HLA-A and -B loci. The data of Redman et al.[4] showed that such homozygosity contained very early onset preeclampsia and thus may have represented a different population of patients. The French study[5] does not have such detailed clinical information on the patients.

See also refs. 6 and 7.

References

1. Scott JR, Beer AE, Stastny P: Immunogenetic factors in preeclampsia and eclampsia: Erythrocyte, histocompatibility, and y-dependent antigens. JAMA 235:402-404, 1976
2. Jenkins DM, Need J, Rajah SM: Deficiency of specific HLA antibodies in severe pregnancy pre-eclampsia/eclampsia. Clin Exp Immunol 27:485-486, 1977
3. Jenkins DM, Need JA, Scott JS, Morris H, Pepper M: Human leucocyte antigens and mixed lymphocyte reaction in severe pre-eclampsia. Br Med J 1:542-544, 1978
4. Redman CWG, Bodmer JG, Bodmer WF, Beilin LJ, Bonnar J: HLA antigens in severe pre-eclampsia. Lancet ii:397-399, 1978
5. Simon P, Fauchet R, Menault M, Bombail D, Lefiblec B, Panguy E, et al.: HLA A, B, and DR antigens in pre-eclampsia: Preliminary results. Kidney Int 17:705-706, 1980
6. Pattillo RA: Histocompatibility antigens in pregnancy, abortions, infertility, preeclampsia and trophoblast neoplasms. Am J Reprod Immunol 1:29-34, 1980
7. Anichkova SI, Vasilieva ZF, Grigorieva VV: Study of compatibility in married couples according to the HLA antigen system in normal and complicated by late toxemia pregnancy. Akush Ginekol 8:20-23, 1981

Infertility (Unexplained)

Population Association

Kamidono et al.[1] reported a significant increase of BW35 in 30 Japanese couples with unexplained infertility (Table 14.3).

Family Data

Eight Swedish couples with a primary sterility of > 5 years duration and their parents were typed for A and B loci antigens.[2] There was no apparent cause of infertility in these couples. Linkage disequilibrium (Δ) values between the alleles of A and B loci were calculated for infertile couples and 95 fertile individuals. About half of the genotypes in the fertile group showed positive Δ values in both haplotypes compared with 12% in the infertile group. On the other hand, about half of the genotypes in the infertile group had negative Δ values compared with 5% in the fertile group. These differences were statistically significant.

It should be stressed that this result was based on only 16 individuals and there is no other study to

TABLE 14.3. Infertility (Unexplained)

	Patients		Controls				
Country/Population	n	%+	n	%+	RR	χ^2	Ref.
HLA-BW35							
Japan	60	32	70	9	4.50	10.03	1

support the idea that haplotypes with negative linkage disequilibria are significantly more frequent in infertile groups. It is difficult to draw any conclusion from this result.

In another study no HLA antibodies were found in 367 German women with undesired fertility.[3]

See also refs. 4 and 5.

References

1. Kamidono S, Matsumoto O, Ishigami J, Nakao Y, Tsuji K: Infertility and HLA antigen: Male infertility and infertile couples. Andrologia 12:317-322, 1980
2. Lindblom JB, Friberg J, Hogman CF, Gemzell C: HL-A haplotypes and unexplained infertility. Tissue Antigens 2:352-358, 1972
3. Malzer VG, Freistedt B, Berge H, Felker A, Hentschel W: Bereichert das HLA-System unsere Moglichkeiten im Rahmen der sterilitats-Diagnostik? Zentralbl Gynakol 101:72-74, 1979
4. Purpura M, Coghi I, Nicotra M, Carapella E, Bottini E: HLA Bw35 antigen and human reproduction. J Med Genet 17:157-158, 1980
5. Pattillo RA: Histocompatibility antigens in pregnancy, abortions, infertility, preeclampsia and trophoblast neoplasms. Am J Reprod Immunol 1:29-34, 1980

Peyronie's Disease

Peyronie's disease is characterized by the development of a fibrous plaque in the dorsum of the penis. This fibrosis results in dorsal curvature of the penis, making intercourse painful and preventing intromission in many cases.

Population Association

Willscher et al.[1] typed A and B loci antigens in 8 American Caucasian patients with idiopathic Peyronie's disease. Four were positive for B7, 2 for B27, and 1 had BW22. Thus, 7 patients (88%) were positive for 1 of the antigens of the B7 cross-reacting group (B7, BW22, B27, and BW42). The total frequency of these antigens in the general American Caucasian population is about 36%. Using this value for comparison, the authors reported a significant increase of this group of antigens in the patients. However, Leffell et al.[2] were unable to detect any significant deviations in the frequencies of A, B, and C loci antigens in 28 American Caucasian patients.

Family Data

Nyberg et al.[3] reported the HLA typings of 3 multiple case families. There was no strong evidence of linkage of this disorder with the HLA complex.

References

1. Willscher MK, Cwazka WF, Novicki DE: The association of histocompatibility antigens of the B7 cross-reacting group with Peyronie's disease. J Urol 122:34-35, 1979
2. Leffell MS, Devine CJ, Horton CE, Somers KD, Dawson D, Vande Berg JS, et al: Non-association of Peyronie's disease with HLA B7 cross-reactive antigens. J Urol 127:1223-1224,1982
3. Nyberg LM, Bias WB, Hochberg MC, Walsh P: Identification of an inherited form of Peyronie's disease with autosomal dominant inheritance and association with Dupuytren's contracture and HLA-B7 cross-reacting antigens. J Urol 128:48-51, 1982

Balanitis

Population Association

Seventeen Finnish patients with circinate erosive balanitis were typed for A and B loci antigens by Lassus et al.[1] There was a significant association with B27 (Table 14.4).

Disease Heterogeneity

HLA-B27 was present in 7 of the 8 patients with circinate balanitis and some signs of Reiter's disease. In the group of 9 patients without any indication of Reiter's disease, 9 were positive for B27. This high

TABLE 14.4. Balanitis

	Patients		Controls				
Country/Population	n	%+	n	%+	RR	χ^2	Ref.
HLA-B27							
Finland	17	88	326	14	37.05	31.32	1

frequency of B27 in both groups is comparable to that in patients with Reiter's disease (see Reiter's Disease).

Reference

1. Lassus A, Tiilikainen A, Stubb S, Reunala T, Johansson E: Circinate erosive balanitis and HL-A 27. Acta Dermatov 55:199-201, 1975

Azoospermia

Population Association

In a study of 50 Japanese patients Kamidono et al.[1] found a significant increase of BW35 antigen (Table 14.5). However, another report on 65 male patients from Germany by Mueller-Eckhardt et al.[2] did not reveal any significant association with A, B, C, and DR loci antigens.

Family Data

Mueller-Eckhardt et al.[2] published data on a small family in which 3 brothers were affected by idiopathic azoospermia. No single HLA haplotype was shared by all of the siblings. Also, the father of these siblings was unaffected.

References

1. Kamidono S, Matsumoto O, Ishigami J, Nakao Y, Tsuji K: Infertility and HLA antigen: Male infertility and infertile couples. Andrologia 12:317-322, 1980
2. Mueller-Eckhardt G, Krause W, Schierke G, Mueller-Eckhardt C: Male infertility due to idiopathic disorders of spermatogenesis: No association with HLA. Tissue Antigens 20:270-273, 1982

Ureteropelvic Junction Stenosis

Family Data

Sengar et al.[1, 2] published data on HLA typing of a French Canadian family with 5 affected and 8 unaffected siblings. All 5 affected siblings had inherited the AW30-BW22 haplotype from their father, who was not affected by the disorder. One other unaffected sibling also had this haplotype.

References

1. Sengar DPS, Rashid A, Wolfish NM: Familial urinary tract anomalies: Association with the major histocompatibility complex in man. J Urol 121:194-197, 1979
2. Sengar DPS, Rashid A, Wolfish NM: Histocompatibility antigens and urinary abnormalities. Br Med J 1:1146, 1978

Vesicoureteral Reflux

Population Association

Bailey and Wallace[1] typed 19 patients from New Zealand who presented with chronic renal failure due to reflux nephropathy and 46 patients with renal failure due to other causes. B12 was present in 47.37% of the patients with reflux nephropathy compared with 17.39% in the other group. This difference, however, was not highly significant. In the report of Torres et al.[2] 44 American Caucasian patients were compared with 526 controls. The frequency of B12 in the patient group was 40.9% and that in controls was 26.0% ($p = 0.005$).

In another report on 36 unrelated Caucasians (predominantly French Canadian, aged 3–16 years) with a history of recurring urinary tract infections due to *E. coli*, Sengar et al.[3] reported a reduced frequency of A2 (25% in patients vs. 48% in 188 normal controls) and increased frequencies of A10 (22% vs. 9%) and BW16 (14% vs. 3%). However, when the patients were divided into 2 groups—16 with reflux and 20 without reflux—the frequencies of these 3 antigens were not significantly different between the 2 groups.

Family Data

Data are available on 4 small families from Canada.[3,4] In these families the affected sib-pairs were

TABLE 14.5. Azoospermia

Country/Population	Patients n	Patients %+	Controls n	Controls %+	RR	χ^2	Ref.
HLA-BW35							
Japan	50	38	70	9	5.84	13.34	1

HLA-identical and in the fourth family 1 sibling (out of 4) was affected. In each of these 4 families 1 parent was also affected by the disease. Thus, in the data, there was some evidence in favor of linkage between HLA and this disorder.

References

1. Bailey RR, Wallace M: HLA-B12 as a genetic marker for vesicoureteric reflux. Br Med J 1:48-49, 1978
2. Torres VE, Moore SB, Kurtz SB, Offord KP, Kelalis PP: In search of a marker for genetic susceptibility to reflux nephropathy. Clin Nephrol 14:217-222, 1980
3. Sengar DPS, Rashid A, Wolfish NM: Histocompatibility antigens and urinary abnormalities. Br Med J 1:1146, 1978
4. Sengar DPS, Rashid A, Wolfish NM: Familial urinary tract anomalies: Association with the major histocompatibility complex in man. J Urol 121:194-197, 1979

Mesangial IgA Glomerulonephritis (Berger's Disease)

Population Association

HLA-A and -B loci antigen frequency data available from several studies (Table 14.6) show a significant association with BW35 and also a marginally significant association with B12. However, there is evidence of heterogeneity in the data.

A highly significant increase of DR4 and a decrease of DR3 was first reported by Fauchet et al.[1] These results, like those for B12, were also not confirmed in 3 other studies on Caucasian populations (from France[2,3] and England[4]) (Table 14.6).

Brettle et al.[4] found a significant association with CW1. The frequencies of this antigen were not available in other studies.

A report from Japan by Komori et al.[5] on 40 patients showed a highly significant increase (Table 14.6) of a D locus antigen—DEn (defined by MLC reactions). This antigen is related to DR locus antigen DRW6 in the Caucasian population. Furthermore, there was a significant linkage disequilibrium between B12 and DEn in the Japanese population.[5] Yet, the increase of B12 in the patients was not significant.

In 3 independent studies from Japan DR4 was also found to be significantly increased in the patients (Table 14.6).

Thirty-four unrelated Chinese patients from Singapore were typed for A and B loci antigens by Chan et al.[6] No significant difference between the patients and 330 normal controls was found.

Family Data

Sabatier et al.[7] reported 2 affected siblings with a rapidly progressive course of the disease who were also HLA-identical. Another report by Katz et al.[8] included a small pedigree in which the 2 affected siblings also had identical haplotypes.

See also refs. 9, 10, 22, and 23.

References

1. Fauchet R, Gueguen M, Genetet B, Pogamp PL, Ramee MP, Chevet D, et al: HLA-DR antigen and IgA nephropathy (Berger's disease). N Engl J Med 302:1033-1034, 1980
2. Bignon JD, Houssin A, Soulillou JP, Denis J, Guimbretiere J, Guenel J: HLA antigens and Berger's disease. Tissue Antigens 16:108-111, 1980
3. Le Petit JC, Cases MH, Berthoux FC, Van Loghem E, Goguen J, Seger J, et al: Genetic investigation in mesangial IgA nephropathy. Tissue Antigens 19:108-114, 1982
4. Brettle R, Peters DK, Batchelor JR: Mesangial IgA glomerulonephritis and HLA antigens. N Engl J Med 299:200, 1978
5. Komori K, Nose Y, Inouye H, Tsuji K, Nomoto Y, Sakai H: Study on HLA system in IgA nephropathy. Tissue Antigens 14:32-36, 1979
6. Chan Sh, Ku G, Sinniah R: HLA and Chinese IgA mesangial glomerulonephritis. Tissue Antigens 17:351-352, 1981
7. Sabatier JC, Genin C, Assenat H, Colon S, Ducret F, Berthoux FC: Mesangial IgA glomerulonephritis in HLA-identical brothers. Clin Nephrol 11:35-38, 1979
8. Katz A, Karanicolas S, Falk JA: Family study in IgA nephritis: The possible role of HLA antigens. Transplantation 29:505-506, 1980
9. Houssin A, Bignon JD, Soulillou JP, Guimbretiere J, Guenel J: HLA phenotypes in Berger's disease. Kidney Int 17:702-703, 1980
10. Pogamp PL, Fauchet R, Ramee MP: HLA-DRW4 antigen and IgA-nephropathy (Berger's disease). Eur J Clin Invest 10:29, 1980
11. Richman AV, Mahoney JJ, Fuller TJ: Higher prevalence of HLA-B12 in patients with IgA nephropathy. Ann Intern Med 90:201, 1979
12. Nagy J, Hamori A, Ambrus M, Hernadi E: More on IgA glomerulonephritis and HLA antigens. N Engl J Med 300:92, 1979
13. Noel LH, Descamps B, Jungers P, Bach JF, Bussom M, Suet C, et al: HLA antigens in three types

TABLE 14.6. Mesangial IgA Glomerulonephritis (Berger's Disease)

Country/Population	Patients n	Patients %+	Controls n	Controls %+	RR	χ^2	Ref.
HLA-B12							
U.S.A.	17	59	100	20	5.54	10.61	11
Hungary	24	33	60	25	1.49	0.63	12
England	17	53	200	33	2.27	2.86	4
France	29	31	591	29	1.13	0.10	13
France	78	28	104	31	0.87	0.18	3
France	73	40	587	32	1.42	1.97	2
	180	33	1282	31	1.17	0.80	
	Heterogeneity χ^2 (2 df)					1.45	
Italy	23	26	236	22	1.30	0.31	14
Spain	27	33	330	31	1.12	0.08	15
Ireland	25	40	453	36	1.20	0.21	16
Finland	33	12	114	14	0.90	0.03	17
	346	33	2775	30	1.35	5.68	
	Heterogeneity χ^2 (9 df)					11.30	
HLA-BW35							
U.S.A.	17	18	100	16	1.26	0.14	11
Hungary	24	4	60	15	0.34	1.77	12
England	17	18	200	13	1.62	0.66	4
France	43	40	105	13	4.37	12.69	18
France	40	28	356	14	2.43	5.71	1
France	73	18	587	15	1.27	0.59	2
France	78	26	104	13	2.32	4.91	3
France	29	48	591	19	3.93	13.38	13
	263	29	1743	16	2.44	29.44	
	Heterogeneity χ^2 (4 df)					7.82	
Italy	23	9	236	23	0.40	2.14	14
Spain	27	33	330	22	1.79	1.97	15
Ireland	25	8	453	12	0.77	0.17	16
Finland	33	33	114	23	1.66	1.48	17
	429	25	3236	17	1.83	22.24	
	Heterogeneity χ^2 (11 df)					23.35	
HLA-DW-En							
Japan	37	46	115	18	3.83	11.27	5
HLA-DR4							
Japan	80	66	884	41	2.77	17.65	19
Japan	42	67	158	39	3.11	10.07	20
Japan	24	67	64	30	4.53	9.43	21
	146	66	1106	40	3.06	36.34	
	Heterogeneity χ^2 (2 df)					0.81	

of glomerulonephritis. Clin Immunol Immunopathol 10:19-23, 1978

14. Savi M, Neri TM, Silvestri MG, Allegri L, Migone L: HLA antigens and IgA mesangial glomerulonephritis. Clin Nephrol 12:45-46, 1979
15. Arnaiz-Villena A, Gonzalo A, Mampaso F, Teruel JL, Ortunno J: HLA and IgA nephropathy in Spanish population. Tissue Antigens 17:549-550, 1981
16. O'Neill S, Walker F, Spencer S, O'Dwyer WF: HLA status in IgA nephropathy. Irish J Med Sci 150:113-115, 1981
17. Mustonen J, Pasternack A, Helin H, Rilva A, Pent-

tinen K, Wager O, et al: Circulating immune complexes, the concentration of serum IgA and the distribution of HLA antigens in IgA nephropathy. Nephron 29:170-175, 1981
18. Berthoux FC, Gagne A, Sabatier JC, Ducret F, Le Petit SC, Marcellin M, et al: HLA-BW35 and mesangial IgA glomerulonephritis. N Engl J Med 298:1034-1035, 1978
19. Hiki Y, Kobayashi Y, Tateno S, Sada M, Kashiwagi N: Strong association of HLA-DR4 with benign IgA nephropathy. Nephron 32:222-226, 1982
20. Kashiwabara H, Shishido H, Tomura S, Tuchida H, Miyajima T: Strong association between IgA nephropathy and HLA-DR4 antigen. Kidney Int 22:377-382, 1982
21. Kashwabara H, Shishido H, Yokoyama T, Miyajima T: HLA in IgA nephropathy. Tissue Antigens 16:411-412, 1980
22. Fauchet R, Le Pogamp P, Genetet B, Chevet D, Gueguen M, Simon P, et al: HLA-DR4 antigen and IgA nephropathy. Tissue Antigens 16:405-410, 1980
23. Kasahara M, Hamada K, Okuyama T, Ishikawa N, Ogasawara K, Ikeda H, et al: Role of HLA in IgA nephropathy. Clin Immunol Immunopathol 25:189-195, 1982

Chronic Glomerulonephritis

Population Association

Patel et al.[1] and Mickey et al.[2] originally reported an increased frequency of A2 in American Caucasian glomerulonephritis patients. In 3 later studies on 183 Danish,[3] 41 Czechoslovakian,[4] and 47 French[5] and 50 Polish[6] patients, neither A2 nor any other antigen was found to be associated with this disease. It should be noted that the group of 47 French patients consisted of 14 with IgA mesangial nephropathies (Berger's disease), 14 with Henoch-Schonlein nephritis, 10 with poststreptococcal glomerulonephritis, and 11 with miscellaneous glomerulonephritis based on histologic and clinical criteria.

In the French study[5] the patients were also typed for DR1, 2, 3, 4, 5, and 7 and there was no significant difference between this group and the control group of 90 individuals.

References

1. Patel R, Mickey MR, Terasaki PI: Leukocyte antigens and disease: I. Association of HL-A2 and chronic glomerulonephritis. Br Med J 2:424-426, 1969
2. Mickey MR, Kreisler M, Terasaki PI: Leukocyte antigens and disease. II. Alterations in frequencies of haplotypes associated with chronic glomerulonephritis. In Terasaki PI (ed): Histocompatibility Testing 1970. Munksgaard, Copenhagen, 1970, pp 237-242
3. Jensen H, Ryder LP, Staub Nielsen L, Clausen E, Jorgensen F, Elif Jorgensen H: HLA antigens and glomerulonephritis. Tissue Antigens 6:368-369, 1975
4. Nyulassy S, Buc M, Sasinka M, Pavlovic M, Slugen I, Hirschova V, et al.: The HLA system in glomerulonephritis. Clin Immunol Immunopathol 7:319-323, 1977
5. De Mouzon-Cambon A, Ohayon E, Bouissou F, Barthe P: HLA-DR typing in children with glomerular diseases. Lancet ii:868, 1980
6. Stefanova S, Andreev IG: HLA system and renal diseases. Ind J Exp Biol 18:282-284, 1980

Acute Poststreptococcal Glomerulonephritis

Population Association

Read et al.[1] typed 39 East Indian patients from Trinidad. This population, originally from a relatively restricted area of India, had lived in Trinidad for 6 generations. Controls were also selected from the same populations. HLA-A and -B antigen frequencies were similar in patients and controls.

In 46 Japanese patients a strong association with B12 and DEn, a new D locus antigen, has been

TABLE 14.7. Acute Poststreptococcal Glomerulonephritis

	Patients		Controls				
Country/Population	n	%+	n	%+	RR	χ^2	Ref.
HLA-B12							
Japan	46	35	150	13	3.58	11.03	2
HLA-DW-En							
Japan	28	36	69	6	8.09	12.39	2
HLA-DR4							
Venezuela	42	50	82	21	3.68	10.56	4

reported by Sasazuki et al.[2,3] The strong linkage disequilibrium between DEn and B12 in the Japanese[3] and higher relative risk for DEn suggest that the primary association was probably with DEn.

Layrisse et al.[4] also reported a significant association with DR4 in 42 patients from Venezuela (Table 14.7).

Family Data

In the study of Read et al.[1] 30 families with 1 or more children with the disease were also typed. There was no evidence for linkage with HLA. Layrisse et al.[4] also studied segregation and linkage in 18 Venezuelan families. The lod score analysis of these pedigrees did not provide conclusive evidence either to accept or reject the hypothesis of linkage with HLA.

See also ref. 5.

References

1. Read SE, Reid H, Poon-King T, Fischetti VA, Zabriskie JB, Rapaport FT: HLA and predisposition to the nonsuppurative sequelae of group A streptococcal infections. Transplant Proc 9:543-546, 1977
2. Sasazuki T, Hayase R, Iwamoto I, Tsuchida H: HLA and acute poststreptococcal glomerulonephritis. N Engl J Med 301:1184-1185, 1979
3. Sasazuki T, Kaneoka H, Ohta N, Hayase R, Iwamoto I: Common HLA haplotypes and their association with diseases in the Japanese population. Transplant Proc 11:1871-1873, 1979
4. Layrisse Z, Rodriguez-Iturbe B, Garcia-Ramirez R, Rodriguez A, Tiwari J: Family studies of the HLA system in acute post-streptococcal glomerulonephritis. Hum Immunol 7:177-185, 1983
5. Rodriguez-Iturbe B, Moreno-Fuenmayor H, Rubio L, Garcia R, Layrisse Z: Mendelian recessive ratios in acute poststreptococcal glomerulonephritis. Experientia (in press)

Idiopathic Membranous Nephropathy

Population Association

Klouda et al.[1] typed A, B, and DR loci antigens in 30 men and 18 women who satisfied the criteria for the diagnosis of idiopatic membranous nephropathy. B18 and DR3 were significantly increased in the patients. In the combined analysis of the data published in later studies (Table 14.8) the association with these antigens is also highly significant.

In another report[2] the same group of patients[1] was also typed for properdin factor B (Bf) allotypes. The rare allotype BfF1 also was found to be significantly associated with this disease. There are significant linkage disequilibria between B18 and DR3, DR3 and BfF1, and probably between B18-DR3-BfF1 (see ref. 2 and refs. therein). These 3 alleles may be on the same chromosome.

See also ref. 3.

References

1. Klouda PT, Acheson EJ, Goldby FS, Lawler W, Manos J, Dyer PA, et al.: Strong association between idiopathic membranous nephropathy and HLA-DRW3. Lancet ii:770-771, 1979
2. Dyer PA, Klouda PT, Harris R, Mallick NP: Properdin factor B alleles in patients with idiopathic membranous nephropathy. Tissue Antigens 15:505-507, 1980
3. Davies MG, Davies PG: Dermatitis herpetiformis, glomerulonephritis, and HLA-DRW3. Lancet ii:911, 1979
4. Le Petit JC, Laurent B, Berthoux FC: HLA-DR3 and idiopathic membranous nephritis (IMN) association. Tissue Antigens 20:227-228, 1982
5. Garavoy MR: Idiopathic membranous glomerulonephritis: An HLA-associated disease. In Terasaki PI (ed): Histocompatibility Testing 1980. UCLA Tissue Typing Laboratory, Los Angeles, 1981, pp 673-680
6. Muller GA, Muller C, Liebau G, Kompf J, Ising H, Wernet P: Strong association of idiopathic membranous nephropathy (IMN) with HLA-DR3 and MT-2 without involvement of HLA-B18 and no association to BfF1. Tissue Antigens 17:332-337, 1981

Balkan Endemic Nephropathy

Balkan endemic nephropathy is a familial disease with endemic distribution, limited to one area of northwest Bulgaria and in the adjacent regions of Yugoslavia and Romania. The initial stage of the disease is characterized by early manifested anemia and renal compensation. In the second stage there is renal decompensation, azothemia, and coma. The skin of a typical patient is of grayish-copper color.

Population Association

Minev et al.[1] studied 180 patients from 15 villages situated near Vratza in the center of the endemic region of Bulgaria (Table 14.9). The frequency of B18 was significantly increased in this sample. Sim-

TABLE 14.8. Idiopathic Membranous Nephropathy

Country/Population	Patients n	Patients %+	Controls n	Controls %+	RR	χ^2	Ref.
HLA-BfF1							
England	37	22	59	2	10.22	8.73	2
France	17	18	90	3	6.76	6.14	4
	54	21	149	3	8.28	14.73	
	Heterogeneity χ^2 (1 df)					0.14	
HLA-B8							
Caucasians (unspecified)	163	31	3416	16	2.37	24.49	5
England	48	46	230	28	2.19	6.02	1
France	28	53	104	14	6.71	17.32	4
West Germany	21	57	122	20	5.16	11.88	6
	260	38	3872	17	2.74	52.93	
	Heterogeneity χ^2 (3 df)					6.79	
HLA-B18							
Caucasians (unspecified)	163	20	3416	10	2.27	16.60	5
England	48	23	230	6	4.67	13.08	1
France	28	21	104	18	1.26	0.21	4
	239	21	3750	10	2.38	25.71	
	Heterogeneity χ^2 (2 df)					4.17	
HLA-DR3							
Caucasians (unspecified)	176	60	3184	21	5.63	118.06	5
England	48	75	230	20	11.59	45.94	1
France	26	65	74	20	7.07	16.30	4
West Germany	21	76	122	23	9.82	19.37	6
	271	64	3610	21	6.57	195.64	
	Heterogeneity χ^2 (3 df)					4.04	

TABLE 14.9. Balkan Endemic Nephropathy

Country/Population	Patients n	Patients %+	Controls n	Controls %+	RR	χ^2	Ref.
HLA-B18							
Bulgaria	180	19	1264	11	1.91	9.73	1
Bulgaria	30	20	50	16	1.33	0.25	2
	210	19	1314	11	1.83	9.61	
	Heterogeneity χ^2 (1 df)					0.37	

ilar results have also been reported in another study from Bulgaria by Stefanova and Andreev[2] (Table 14.9). However, it should be noted that in 65 patients from Zagreb, Yugoslavia, studied by Kastelan (unpublished results, quoted by Minev et al. in ref. 1) the frequency of BW35 was determined to be increased. (There was no information on B18 in this group of patients.)

Disease Heterogeneity

There was no difference in the frequency of B18 between 63 male and 114 female patients in the study of Minev et al.[1]

References

1. Minev M, Mikhaylov T, Kastelan A, Nyulassy S, Menzel G: HLA system and Balkan endemic nephropathy. Tissue Antigens 11:50-54, 1978
2. Stefanova S, Andreev IG: HLA system and renal diseases. Indian J Exp Biol 18:282-284, 1980

Nephrotic Syndrome

Population Association

HLA-A, -B, and -C loci antigens were studied in 25 Czechoslovakian,[1] 54 Spanish,[2] and 86 German[3,4] patients. In 3 of these reports no significant associations were found. However, in 1 of the German studies by Noss et al.[3] significant increase of B8 and B13 in the patients were observed.

DR locus antigens were typed in French[2, 5] and Spanish[6] studies. In both reports DR7 was significantly increased in the patient group (Table 14.10).

Disease Heterogeneity

De Mouzon-Cambon et al.[2] found that the increase of DR7 was more pronounced in the subgroup of patients with atopy.

References

1. Nyulassy S, Buc M, Sasinka M, Pavlovic M, Slugen I, Hirschova V, et al: The HLA system in glomerulonephritis. Clin Immunol Immunopathol 7:319-323, 1977
2. De Mouzon-Cambon A, Bouissou F, Dutau G, Barthe Ph, Parra MT, Sevin A, et al: HLA-DR7 in children with idiopathic nephrotic syndrome. Correlation with atopy. Tissue Antigens 17:518-524, 1981
3. Noss G, Bachmann HJ, Olbing H: Association of minimal change nephrotic syndrome (MCNS) with HLA-B8 and B13. Clin Nephrol 15:172-174, 1981
4. Dippell J, Wonne R: Atopie, HLA-System und steroidsensibles nephrotisches Syndrom im Kindesalter. Monatschr Kinderheilkd 129:684-687, 1981
5. De Mouzon-Cambon A, Ohayon E, Bouissou F, Barthe P: HLA-DR typing in children with glomerular diseases. Lancet ii:868, 1980
6. Nunez-Roldan A, Vellechenous E, Fernandez-Andrade C, Martin-Govantes J: Increased HLA-DR7 and decreased DR2 in steroid-responsive nephrotic syndrome. N Engl J Med 306:366-367, 1982

Steroid-Responsive Nephrotic Syndrome of Childhood

Population Association

The analysis of pooled data from England,[1,2] Ireland,[3] and Australia[4] showed significant increases of B8, B12, and B18 and a decrease of B7 in the patients (Table 14.11). However, as the χ^2 values indicate, there was considerable heterogeneity in the data.

The 42 Australian patients were also typed for 7 DR locus antigens and DR7 was found to be significantly associated with this syndrome (Table 14.11). Since there is linkage disequilibrium between B12 and DR7, the incidence of DR7 in B12-positive and -negative patients was compared to see if this association was secondary to that with B12 reported by Thomson et al.[1] The DR7 frequency was significantly increased in both B12-positive and -negative groups. On the basis of relative risk values it seems that the association of this syndrome with DR7 was

TABLE 14.10. Nephrotic Syndrome

Country/Population	Patients n	Patients %+	Controls n	Controls %+	RR	χ^2	Ref.
HLA-DR7							
France	54	67	90	31	4.41	16.89	5
Spain	50	72	181	38	4.10	17.01	6
	104	69	271	36	4.24	33.88	
	Heterogeneity χ^2 (1 df)					0.02	

stronger than that with B locus antigens (Table 14.11). However, the DR data were based on only 1 study.

Disease Heterogeneity

Thomson et al.[1] subgrouped their 71 patients into those with atopic symptoms (particularly hayfever), positive prick tests with grass pollen antigens, and high mean serum concentrations of IgE antibody to Timothy grass pollen. The frequency of B12 was significantly increased in these groups (compared with the patients without these clinical features). In the Australian study,[4] 19 patients presented with an atopic history and 16 (84%) had DR7 and 7 (37%) were positive for B12. Of the nonatopic patients, 14 (60%) and 8 (35%) had DR7 and B12, respectively. Thus, there was no significant difference in the frequencies of B12 and DR7 between atopic and nonatopic groups.

Antigen frequencies were also compared in patients who relapsed after treatment with cyclophosphamide. Thomson et al.[1] observed a significantly high frequency of B12 in the group with relapses compared with those without. No such association was evident in the Australian[4] and Irish[3] studies. Thus, there was no consistency in the data with respect to clinical features of this syndrome.

References

1. Thomson PD, Barret TM, Stokes CR, Turner MW, Soothill JF: HLA antigens and atopic features in ste-

TABLE 14.11. Steroid-Responsive Nephrotic Syndrome of Childhood

	Patients		Controls				
Country/Population	n	%+	n	%+	RR	χ^2	Ref.
HLA-B7							
Australia	45	11	308	24	0.42	3.51	4
England	71	7	1036	26	0.23	11.27	1
Ireland	54	9	253	31	0.24	9.78	3
	170	9	1597	26	0.28	23.46	
	Heterogeneity χ^2 (2 df)					1.10	
HLA-B8							
Australia	45	36	308	25	1.70	2.60	4
England	71	42	1036	25	2.18	9.90	1
Ireland	54	65	253	35	3.40	15.73	3
	170	48	1597	27	2.33	25.76	
	Heterogeneity χ^2 (2 df)					2.48	
HLA-B12							
Australia	45	33	308	30	1.16	0.21	4
England	71	54	1036	24	3.70	28.39	1
Ireland	54	41	253	37	1.19	0.33	3
	170	44	1597	27	1.98	17.01	
	Heterogeneity χ^2 (2 df)					11.92	
HLA-B18							
Australia	45	11	308	6	2.05	2.09	4
England	71	9	1036	3	3.37	8.07	1
Ireland	54	18	253	6	3.47	8.53	3
	170	12	1597	4	2.98	17.93	
	Heterogeneity χ^2 (2 df)					0.77	
HLA-DR7							
Australia	42	71	121	30	5.54	19.95	4

roid-responsive nephrotic syndrome of childhood. Lancet ii:765-768, 1976
2. Thomson PD, Barrat TM, Stokes CR, Soothill JF, Turner MW: HLA typing and atopic features in steroid sensitive nephrotic syndrome of childhood. Monogr Allergy 11:60, 1977
3. O'Regan D, O'Callaghan U, Dundon S, Reen DJ: HLA antigens and steroid responsive nephrotic syndrome of childhood. Tissue Antigens 16:147-151, 1980
4. Alfiler CA, Roy LP, Doran T, Sheldon A, Bashir H: HLA-DRW7 and steroid-responsive nephrotic syndrome of childhood. Clin Nephrol 14:71-74, 1980

Renal Patients Without Hepatitis B Surface Antigens

Population Association

Descamps et al. [1-3] compared the HLA types of 185 uremic hemodialyzed patients and 391 French controls. They found no difference in any of the antigen frequencies. Similar results were also reported for American Caucasian[4,5] and Canadian[6,7] patients.

References

1. Descamps B, Jungers P, Naret C, Degott C, Zingraff J, Bach JF: HLA-A1, B8-phenotype association and HBS antigenemia evolution in 440 hemodialyzed patients. Digestion 15:271-277, 1977
2. Bach JF, Zingraff J, Descamps B, Naret C, Jungers P: HL-A1, 8 phenotype and HBS antigenaemia in haemodialysis patients. Lancet ii:707, 1975
3. Jungers MP, Descamps B, Zingraff J, Naret C, Bach JF: Sur une correlation entre les antigenes d'histocompatibilite HL-A1 et 8 et une meilleure defense de l'uremique chronique contre le virus de l'hepatite B. C R Acad Sci (Paris) 281:675-678, 1975
4. Patterson MJ, Hourani MR, Mayor GH: HLA antigens and hepatitis B virus. N Engl J Med 297:1124, 1977
5. Hillis WD, Hillis A, Bias WB, Walker WG: Associations of hepatitis B surface antigenemia with HLA locus B specificities. N Engl J Med 296:1310-1314, 1977
6. Sengar DPS, Rashid A, Jindal SL, Christie CJ: HLA antigens in HBSAG infection. Vox Sang 36:353-355, 1979
7. Sengar DPS, McLeish WA, Sutherland M, Couture RA, Rashid A: Hepatitis B antigen (HBAG) infection in a hemodialysis unit. I. HL-A8 and immune response to HBAG. Can Med Assoc J 112:968-971, 1975

Renal Patients Transiently Carrying Hepatitis B Surface Antigens

Population Association

The data of Descamps et al. [1-3] showed a slight increase in the frequency of B8 (24.3% in 70 patients vs. 14% in 391 controls) in French hemodialyzed patients who were able to eliminate HBsAg. Similar results in 55 HBsAg-positive American Caucasian patients were reported by Patterson et al.[4] However, these authors did not report frequency data on control populations. Another study[5] on American patients (mixed races) showed B15, B17, and BW35 to be associated with transient or persistent (or both) antigenemia.

See also ref. 6.

References

1. Descamps B, Jungers P, Naret C, Degott C, Zingraff, Bach JF: HLA-A1, B8-phenotype association and HBS antigenemia evolution in 440 hemodialyzed patients. Digestion 15:271-277, 1977
2. Bach JF, Zingraff J, Descamps B, Naret C, Jungers P: HL-A1, 8 phenotype and HBS antigenaemia in haemodialysis patients. Lancet ii:707, 1975
3. Jungers MP, Descamps B, Zingraff J, Naret C, Bach JF: Sur une correlation entre les antigenes d'histocompatibilite HL-A1 et 8 et une meilleure defense de l'uremique chronique contre le virus de l'hepatite B. C R Acad Sci (Paris) 281:675-678, 1975
4. Patterson MJ, Hourani MR, Mayor GH: HLA antigens and hepatitis B virus. N Engl J Med 297:1124, 1977
5. Hillis WD, Hillis A, Bias WB, Walker WG: Associations of hepatitis B surface antigenemia with HLA locus B specificities. N Engl J Med 296:1310-1314, 1977
6. Adorno D, Valeri M, Piazzi A, Bonini S, Papola F, Casciani CU: Lymphocytotoxic HLA antibodies and HB infection in transfused hemodialysis patients waiting for kidney transplantation. Transplant Proc 11:1269-1270, 1979

Renal Patients Persistently Carrying Hepatitis B Surface Antigens

Population Association

No association in 185 patients was reported by Descamps et al.[1-3] Associations with B8[4] and B15, B17, and BW35[5] have been reported in American Caucasian patients. In the latter study,[5] the data on control populations were not given. Sengar et al.[6,7] also studied 148 Caucasian hemodialysis patients and 352 controls from Canada. In 42 HBsAg-positive and 58 anti-HBsAg-positive patients, a negative association of B8 and positive association of B5 with the development of anti-HBsAg was reported. BW35 was also negatively associated with HBsAg antigenemia.

None of these associations is highly significant. See also ref. 8.

References

1. Descamps B, Jungers P, Naret C, Degott C, Zingraff J, Bach JF: HLA-A1, B8-phenotype association and HBS antigenemia evolution in 440 hemodialyzed patients. Digestion 15:271-277, 1977
2. Bach JF, Zingraff J, Descamps B, Naret C, Jungers P: HL-A1, 8 phenotype and HBS antigenaemia in haemodialysis patients. Lancet ii:707, 1975
3. Jungers MP, Descamps B, Zingraff J, Naret C, Bach JF: Sur une correlation entre les antigenes d'histocompatibilite HL-A1 et 8 et une meilleure defense de l'uremique chronique contre le virus de l'hepatite B. C R Acad Sci (Paris) 281:675-678, 1975
4. Patterson MJ, Hourani MR, Mayor GH: HLA antigens and hepatitis B virus. N Engl J Med 297:1124, 1977
5. Hillis WD, Hillis A, Bias WB, Walker WG: Associations of hepatitis B surface antigenemia with HLA locus B specificities. N Engl J Med 296:1310-1314, 1977
6. Sengar DPS, Rashid A, Jindal SL, Christie CJ: HLA antigens in HBsAg infection. Vox Sang 36:353-355, 1979
7. Sengar DPS, McLeish WA, Sutherland M, Couture RA, Rashid A: Hepatitis B antigen (HBAG) infection in a hemodialysis unit. I. HL-A8 and immune response to HBAG. Can Med Assoc J 112:968-971, 1975
8. Adorno D, Valeri M, Piazzi A, Bonini S, Papola F, Casciani CU: Lymphocytotoxic HLA antibodies and HB infection in transfused hemodialysis patients waiting for kidney transplantation. Transplant Proc 11:1269-1270, 1979

Transplant Patients Carrying Hepatitis B Surface Antigens

Population Association

Opelz and Terasaki[1] studied 112 Caucasian patients from several North American transplant centers. The patients were considered HBsAg-positive regardless of whether they had received cadaver or related donor grafts or whether they were positive prior to or post-transplantation. There was no significant difference in the HLA antigen frequencies in these patients as compared with 629 normal controls or 344 HBsAg-negative patients.

When 38 patients (from the total 112) who had been found to be HBsAg-positive prior to their first transplant were considered as a separate group, the frequency of A2 was 87%. This was significantly higher than the 48% in healthy controls ($\chi^2 = 19.75$) or 54% in HBsAg-negative patients ($\chi^2 = 13.48$).

Reference

1. Opelz G, Terasaki PI: Graft survival rates and HLA antigen frequencies in renal cadaver transplant recipients with hepatitis B antigenemia. Transplantation 25:159-160, 1978

Polycystic Kidneys

Population Association

Macurova et al.[1] studied 81 patients from Czechoslovakia for A and B loci antigens and found no

TABLE 14.12. Renal Patients Transiently Carrying Hepatitis B Surface Antigens

	Patients		Controls				
Country/Population	n	%+	n	%+	RR	χ^2	Ref.
HLA-B8							
France	47	30	391	14	2.66	8.24	2
France	70	24	391	14	1.96	4.77	1
	117	26	782	14	2.25	12.57	
	Heterogeneity χ^2 (1 df)					0.44	

significant deviations in the frequencies. The control population consisted of > 1200 individuals.

Family Data

In the Czechoslovakian report, data were also available on 4 families with 2 or more affected members. Two families were not informative. They had 3 individuals each (2 parents and 1 offspring) and the patients were parent-offspring combinations. In the third family, both siblings were affected but they did not share any haplotype. The fourth family had 5 affected individuals. The 3 affected siblings had the A10-B18 haplotype. Two affected siblings also had offspring (1 each) and they were affected by the disease. One offspring had A10-B18 but the other did not have this haplotype. Thus, there is no evidence of linkage in these data.

Four multiplex families affected with adult polycystic kidney disease were also studied by Dyer et al.[2] The disease did not segregate with specific haplotypes within the families. Also, the disease was not associated with any of the A or B loci antigens either within or among the 4 reported families.

References

1. Macurova H, Prat V, Ivaskova E: HLA antigens in polycystic kidneys. Cas Lek Cesk 118:1296-1298, 1979
2. Dyer PA, Watters EA, Klouda PT, Harris R, Mallick NP: Absence of linkage between adult polycystic kidney disease and the major histocompatibility system. Tissue Antigens 20:108-111, 1982

Retroperitoneal Fibrosis

Population Association

Willscher et al.[1] published a case report of an American Black patient who was positive for B27. These authors also quoted another report by Olsson (see study cited in ref. 1) in which a young American Black patient was positive for B27. However, in a third report by Norton,[2] a Black patient was typed for B27 and found to be negative. (See also ref. 3).

See also ref. 4.

References

1. Willscher MK, Novicki DE, Cwazka WF: Association of HLA-B27 antigen with retroperitoneal fibrosis. J Urol 120:631-633, 1978
2. Norton JH: Idiopathic retroperitoneal fibrosis. J Urol 121:689-690, 1979
3. Vital Durand D, Rouhier D, Brette R: Could the HLA-B27 antigen be a predisposing factor in the development of fibrotic changes? J Urol 124:162, 1980
4. Fernandez-Herlihy L: Idiopathic retroperitoneal fibrosis and HLA-B27. J Urol 124:752, 1980

Uremia

Population Association

Chen et al.[1] typed A and B loci antigens in 65 Chinese uremic patients from Taiwan. In 24 patients the cause of uremia was chronic glomerulonephritis and in 14 patients it was due to arteriolar nephrosclerosis. The remaining patients had diabetic nephropathy (n = 7), chronic pyelonephritis (n = 5), acute tubular necrosis (n = 5), polycystic kidneys (n = 4), renal tuberculosis (n = 2), obstructive uropathy (n = 2), systemic lupus erythematosus (n = 1), and gouty nephropathy (n = 1).

In this report the frequency of B8 was 3.7% in all the patients vs. 0.6% in 69 controls. In view of the highly heterogeneous nature of the patient group, the validity of this result (or the method of analysis) is not clear.

See also ref. 2.

References

1. Chen WY, Hsieh BS, Yen TS, Hsia S: Histocompatibility antigen of patients with renal insufficiency tested by immune adherence. J Formosn Med Assoc 73:359-364, 1974
2. Fehrman I, Ringden O: Lymphocytes from multitransfused uremic patients have poor MLC reactivity. Tissue Antigens 17:386-395, 1981

Essential Mixed Cryoglobulinemia

Population Association

Migliorini et al.[1] tested 36 Italian patients and 169 controls for A, B, C, and DR loci antigens. The authors observed increased but statistically nonsignificant frequencies of DR3, DRW8, and CW6.

Disease Heterogeneity

Patients were grouped according to several clinical features and serologic abnormalities. There was no difference between the groups with and without signs of hepatitis B virus exposure, Raynaud's phenomenon, Sjögren's syndrome, neuropathy, and lung involvement. However, the frequency of DRW8 was increased in the patients with renal involvement (57.1% vs. 11.5%, corrected $p < 0.01$).

Reference

1. Migliorini P, Bombardieri S, Castellani A, Ferrara GB: HLA antigens in essential mixed cryoglobulinemia (EMC). Eur J Clin Invest 10:26, 1980

Benign Hematuria

Family Data

HLA data on 4 families with more than 2 affected members in each has been reported by Sengar et al.[1] The affected siblings in each of the families shared both haplotypes. No formal linkage analysis has been presented by the author. However, in these data there is some evidence of linkage with the HLA complex.

Reference

1. Sengar DPS, Rashid A, Couture RA, Schieman L, Acharya C, Wolfish NM: HLA and familial benign hematuria. Transplantation 31:310-311, 1981

Chronic Prostatitis

Population Association

Twenty-nine Norwegian patients were typed for A, B, and C loci antigens by Moller et al.[1,2] No significant deviation of antigen frequencies was found.

References

1. Moller P, Vinje O, Fryjordet A: HLA antigens and sacro-iliitis in chronic prostatitis. Scand J Rheumatol 9:138-140, 1980
2. Moller P, Berg K, Vinje O: HLA phenotypes and joint affection in psoriasis, acute anterior uveitis and chronic prostatitis. Clin Genet 19:266-270, 1981

Pustular Bacterid of Andrews

Population Association

Djawari and Deinlein[1] reported A and B loci antigen frequencies in 20 German patients. No highly significant deviations were found. However, the authors noted an increase of B14 in the patients (30% in the patients vs. 3.1% in 32 controls).

Reference

1. Djawari VD, Deinlein E: Zur Immunologie des Bakterid Andrews II: HLA-Typisierung. Dermatol Monatsschr 166:305-308, 1980

CHAPTER 15

Cardiovascular Diseases

Rheumatic Fever

Population Association

In 109 Finnish patients with acute or previous definite rheumatic fever a significant association with BW35 was reported by Leirisalo et al.[1] However, this was not confirmed in a second report by the same authors.[2] In another study on 49 Mexican-American patients and 100 controls, Murray et al.[3] found no significant deviation in any of the A and B loci antigens. (BW35 was present in 26% of the patients and in 30% of the controls.)

Yoshinoya and Pope[4] reported a significantly more pronounced immune response, as measured by circulating immune complexes, in patients positive for B5 (35 of the 72 patients in this study were included in Murray's study[3]).

Disease Heterogeneity

Leirisalo et al.[1] noted a slight increase in the frequency of B18 in 37 patients with acute carditis (19% in patients vs. 5% in 326 controls). There was no other HLA difference with respect to acute arthritis, chronic joint sequelae, and erythema nodosum.

In the Mexican-American sample,[3] there were only 9 patients with carditis and the distribution of HLA antigens in this subgroup was similar to that in controls.

Family Data

In a study of 30 East Indian families from Trinidad in which 1 or more members had rheumatic fever, Read et al.[5] reported a significantly lower frequency of B5 ($p < 0.001$) in the mothers of rheumatics compared with 30 mothers with healthy offspring. No pedigree information was given for these families. (These families were selected from a large group of East Indian families originally from a relatively restricted area of India. There was some inbreeding in this community.)

References

1. Leirisalo M, Laitinen O, Tiilikainen A: HLA phenotypes in patients with rheumatic fever, rheumatic heart disease, and *Yersinia* arthritis. J Rheumatol 4(Suppl 3):78-83, 1977
2. Leirisalo M, Koivuranta P, Laitinen O: Rheumatic fever and its sequels in childern. A follow-up study with HLA analysis. J Rheumatol 7:506-514, 1980
3. Murray GC, Nontiel MM, Persellin RH: A study of HLA antigens in adults with acute rheumatic fever. Arthritis Rheum 21:652-656, 1978
4. Yoshinoya S, Pope RM: Detection of immune complexes in acute rheumatic fever and their relationship to HLA-B5. J Clin Invest 65:136-145, 1980
5. Read SE, Reid H, Poon-King T, Fischetti VA, Zabriskie JB, Rapaport FT: HLA and predisposition to the nonsuppurative sequelae of group A streptococcal infections. Transplant Proc 9:543-546, 1977

Rheumatic Heart Disease

Population Association

The first report by Ward et al.[1,2] on 133 patients from England did not show any association with A and B loci antigens. In subsequent studies similar results were reported in 86 Finnish[3] and 94 British[4] patients (see also Swint et al. in ref. 5). In the British study a significant association with B15 was observed when the frequencies were compared with a control group of 1036 blood donors (Table 15.1). However, when the patients were compared with 2 other control groups of kidney donors (n = 371 and 100), there was no significant difference between patients and controls. The association of B15 when compared with the 1036 blood donors was attributed to its unusually low frequency in the controls. The frequencies of this antigen in the 2 groups of kidney donors were 9.2% and 12%. The authors considered these frequencies to be better estimates of B15 in the total population.

Reports on 48 Mexican (Mestizo) patients[6] and 74 Japanese patients[5, 7] also did not show any significant association with HLA. None of these studies contained data on D/DR antigens.

Disease Heterogeneity

Ward et al.[1] divided their patients into groups of those with no rheumatic history and those who had had rheumatic fever or chorea. A significant increase in AW30/31 (12.1% in 58 patients vs. 4.7% in 1000 controls) and AW29 (15.5% in patients vs. 5.7% in controls) was observed in the group with no history of rheumatic fever. Patients with no rheumatic history but with AW29 or AW30/31 had significantly less additional aortic valve disease and often needed surgery at an early age after a relatively short duration of symptoms.[2]

Naito et al.[7] subdivided their 54 patients into 3 subgroups: mitral stenosis (n = 34), mitral regurgitation (n = 6), and aortic valve disease (n = 10). The frequency of A10 in the aortic valve disease group was 50% compared with 15% in 84 controls ($p < 0.01$). Similarly, the frequency of B15 was also increased in the patient group (50% vs. 7% in 84 controls, $p < 0.01$).

References

1. Ward C, Gelsthorpe K, Doughty RW, Hardisty CA: HLA antigens and acquired valvular heart disease. Tissue Antigens 7:227-231, 1976
2. Ward C, Gelsthorpe K, Doughty RW: A relation between HLA antigens and clinical features in patients with acquired valvular heart disease. Br Med J 1:1499-1501, 1976
3. Leirisalo M, Laitinen O, Tiilikainen A: HLA phenotypes in patients with rheumatic fever, rheumatic heart disease, and *Yersinia* arthritis. J Rheumatol 4(Suppl 3):78-83, 1977
4. Joysey VC, Roger JH, Ashworth F, Bullman W, Hazleman BL, Lachman SM, Watson PG: Parallel studies of HLA antigens in patients with rheumatic heart disease and scleritis. J Rheumatol 4(Suppl 3):84-88, 1977
5. Matsumori A, Hirose K, Wakabayashi A, Kawai C, Nabeya N, Subusani T, et al: HLA in hypertrophic cardiomyopathy and rheumatic heart disease. Jpn Circ J 43:445-449, 1979
6. Gorodezky C, Ulloa-L S, Escobar-Gutierrez A: HLA antigens and rheumatic heart disease in Mexico. J Rheumatol 3(Suppl):112, 1977 (Abstr)
7. Naito S, Arakawa K, Kanaya H, Doi H, Sasaki Y, Sakai T, et al: HLA and cardiovascular disease. Jpn Circ J 42:1196-1199, 1978

Rheumatic Fever and Rheumatic Heart Disease

Population Association

Falk et al.[1] reported a decreased frequency of A3 in 76 Canadian patients with rheumatic fever and/or rheumatic heart disease (Table 15.2). In another study of Caucasian patients (a mixture of patients with rheumatic fever and rheumatic heart disease, some of whom had no history of rheumatic fever) from New Zealand[2] there was no significant difference between the patients and controls (Table 15.2). In this study, however, there was a significant increase in the frequency of B17 in the patient group.

The New Zealand study[2] had data on 50 Maori patients and 75 disease-free controls. There were minor nonsignificant differences in the frequencies of A3, A10, and B8.

References

1. Falk JA, Fleischman JL, Zabriskie JB, Falk RE: A study of HL-A antigen phenotype in rheumatic fever

TABLE 15.1. Rheumatic Heart Disease

	Patients		Controls				
Country/Population	n	%+	n	%+	RR	χ^2	Ref.
HLA-B15							
England	94	17	1036	5	3.95	20.64	4

TABLE 15.2. Rheumatic Fever and Rheumatic Heart Disease

	Patients		Controls				
Country/Population	n	%+	n	%+	RR	χ^2	Ref.
HLA-A3							
Canada	76	15	177	28	0.47	4.69	1
New Zealand	50	14	514	27	0.47	3.72	2
	126	15	691	27	0.47	8.41	
	Heterogeneity χ^2 (1 df)					0.00	
HLA-B17							
New Zealand	50	22	514	6	4.49	15.92	2

and rheumatic heart disease patients. Tissue Antigens 3:173-178, 1973
2. Caughey DE, Douglas R, Wilson W, Hassall IB: HL-A antigens in Europeans and Maoris with rheumatic fever and rheumatic heart disease. J Rheumatol 2:319-322, 1975

Ischemic Heart Disease

Population Association

Mathews[1] analyzed the death rate and the population frequency of B8 from several countries (8 Caucasian and 2 non-Caucasian populations). Death rates were found to be correlated with B8 and also with the A1-B8 haplotype in both Caucasian and Caucasian plus non-Caucasian populations. On the basis of these results, he suggested that 1 or more genes predisposing to heart disease are closely linked to the HLA complex. However, there was no association between myocardial infarction and HLA (see Myocardial Infarction).

Reference

1. Mathews JD: Ischaemic heart-disease: Possible genetic markers. Lancet ii:681-682, 1975

Essential Hypertension

Population Association

Data from 4 different Caucasian populations [1–4] do not provide convincing evidence for associations with A, B, and C loci antigens.

In the first report on 21 Swedish patients with insulin-dependent diabetes and essential hypertension, increased frequencies of B8 and B15 were reported by Low et al.[1] (B8 and B15 are associated with insulin-dependent diabetes). In another report on 107 patients from England[2] B12 was increased in the patient group. In 2 other reports[3, 4] where frequency data were available, there was no evidence of any significant association.

Patel and Johnson[5] studied the distribution of A and B loci antigens in 100 American Black hypertensives and 100 normal individuals. There was no significant association with any of the 25 antigens tested in this report.

Disease Heterogeneity

In the Danish study[3,6] there was no association evident in the total sample. The authors, however, have subdivided the patients into 6 different subgroups: with a family history of hypertension among first degree relatives (including borderline hypertensives), with 1 or more tissue antibodies (nucleus, smooth muscle, glomerulus, parietal cell, and mitochondrium) above a titer of 20, with significantly elevated serum levels of immunoglobulins (IgA, IgG, or IgM), and with elevated IgG only.

The frequency of B15 was 29.7% in 64 patients with a family history of hypertension (including borderline hypertensives) compared with 19% in 562 controls. This difference was significant after correcting the probability values for the number of comparisons. In 47 patients with established and tested hypertension and also with a family history the frequency of B15 was even higher—38.3%. No other subgroup showed any significant HLA association.

References

1. Low B, Schersten B, Sartor G, Thulin T, Mitelman F: HL-A8 and W15 in diabetes mellitus and essential hypertension. Lancet i:695, 1975
2. Gelsthorpe K, Doughty RW, Bing RF, O'Malley BC, Smith AJ, Talbot S: HL-A antigens in essential hypertension. Lancet i:1039-1040, 1975
3. Kristensen BO, Andersen PL, Lamm LU, Kissmeyer-Nielsen F: HLA antigens in essential hypertension. Tissue Antigens 10:70-74, 1977
4. Gualde N, Michel JP, Safar ME: Immunogenetics and hypertension. Lancet ii:897, 1978
5. Patel R, Johnson J: Histocompatibility antigens in Black patients with essential hypertension. Circulation 64:1042-1044, 1981

Hypertrophic Cardiomyopathy

Population Association

The population data on 10 American Caucasian and 32 American Black patients studied by Darsee et al.[1] showed a significant association with B12 in the Caucasian and with B5 in the Black nonhypertensive patients (Table 15.3). (*Note:* This paper was retracted by Nutter et al.[10] in 1983.) On the other hand, in 28 nonhypertensive patients from Switzerland,[2] there was no significant difference in the frequency of B12. In the combined data there was no significant difference between the patients and controls. There was highly significant heterogeneity in the pooled data. The observed difference between the 2 studies may have resulted from the different diagnostic criteria, population differences, serologic problems, or small samples.

Becque et al.[3] tested 25 French patients for DR locus antigens. No significant difference between the patients and 85 controls was found.

In 30 Japanese patients[4,5] typed for A and B loci antigens, there was no indication of association with any antigens.

In the report of Matsumori et al.[6] 30 Japanese patients were typed for DR locus antigens. When frequencies were compared with 144 controls no significant associations were found (see also ref. 7).

Disease Heterogeneity

The data of Darsee et al.[1] were subdivided into nonhypertensive and hypertensive groups. There was no association with B12 in the group of 12 hypertensive Caucasians and 16 Black patients.

Matsumori et al.[6] have subdivided their patients into obstructive type (n = 15) and nonobstructive type (n = 18). In the patients with the obstructive type of disease the frequency of DR4 was 73.3% as compared with 33.3% in nonobstructive type and 32.6% in 144 controls ($p = 0.0046$).

Family Data

Darsee et al.[1] also published 6 pedigrees (3 Caucasian and 3 Black) with more than 1 affected member (asymmetric septal hypertrophy) and calculated the lod scores for each. The maximum lod score was 7.688 at a 0.0% recombination frequency, indicating very strong evidence of close linkage with HLA.

Matsumori et al.[4,5] also published 2 Japanese pedigrees with 3 affected members in each pedigree. These families showed some evidence of linkage with HLA (no quantitative analysis is available).

See also refs. 8 and 9.

TABLE 15.3. Hypertrophic Cardiomyopathy

	Patients		Controls				
Country/Population	n	%+	n	%+	RR	χ^2	Ref.
HLA-B5							
U.S.A.—Black	32	94	70	33	25.38	23.93	1
HLA-B12							
U.S.A.	10	90	70	23	20.76	13.59	1
Switzerland	28	25	123	30	0.81	0.22	2
	38	42	193	27	1.73	1.90	
	Heterogeneity χ^2 (1 df)					11.91	

References

1. Darsee JR, Heymsfield SB, Nutter DO: Hypertrophic cardiomyopathy and human leukocyte antigen linkage. N Engl J Med 300:877-882, 1979
2. Bloch A, Crittin J, Barras C, Jeannet M: Hypertrophic cardiomyopathy and HLA. N Engl J Med 302:1033, 1980
3. Becque O, Herve P, Bassand JP, Bernard Y, Maurat JP: HLA-DR antigen linkage in hypertrophic cardiomyopathy. Am Heart J 102:806-808, 1981
4. Matsumori A, Hirose K, Wakabayashi A, Kawai C, Nabeya N, Subusani T, et al: HLA in hypertrophic cardiomyopathy and rheumatic heart disease. Jpn Circ J 43:445-449, 1979
5. Matsumori A, Hirose K, Wakabayashi A, Kawai C, Nabeya N, Sakurani T, et al: HL-A and hypertrophic cardiomyopathy. Am Heart J 97:428-431, 1979
6. Matsumori A, Kawai C, Wakabayashi A, Terasaki PI, Park MS, Sakurami T, et al: HLA-DRW4 antigen linkage in patients with hypertrophic obstructive cardiomyopathy. Am Heart J 101:14-16, 1981
7. Sakurami T, Ueno Y, Iwaki Y, Park MS, Terasaki PI, Saji H: HLA-DR specificities among Japanese with several autoimmune disease. Tissue Antigens 19:129-133, 1982
8. Motulsky AG: The HLA complex and disease: Some interpretations and new data in cardiomyopathy. N Engl J Med 300:918-919, 1979
9. MacArthur C, McKenna W: HL-A and hypertrophic cardiomyopathy. Am Heart J 99:542-543, 1980
10. Nutter DO, Heymsfield SB, Glenn JF: Retraction: (Darsee JR, Heymsfield SB, Nutter DO. Hypertrophic cardiomyopathy and human leukocyte antigen linkage: Differentiation of two forms of hypertrophic cardiomyopathy. N Engl J Med 300:877-882, 1979). N Engl J Med 308:1400, 1983

Alcoholic Cardiomyopathy

Population Association

The only report available is a study on 49 American Black patients and 226 controls.[1] All individuals were typed for 33 antigens of the A and B loci. There was a nonsignificant increase in the frequency of AW30 (37% vs. 21%) in the patient group.

Reference

1. Kachru RB, Proskey AJ, Telischi M: Histocompatibility antigens and alcoholic cardiomyopathy. Tissue Antigens 15:398-399, 1980

Buerger's Disease

Population Association

McLoughlin et al.[1] found a significant association with A9 and B5 in 18 English patients. However, this was not confirmed (Table 15.4) in another report on 46 patients from Switzerland.[2] In the Swiss study by De Moerloose[2] there was a significant decrease of B12 in the patients. The frequency data for A9, B12, B5, and B7 from these 2 studies and a combined analysis of these antigens are given in the Table 15.4. The only significant associations were with B5 and B12.

B12 was also associated with this disease in Japanese patients (Table 15.4). In the combined analysis of Japanese data from 2 studies[3, 4] there were marginally significant increases in BW52 and BW54.

De Moerloose et al.[2] also typed their patients for 7 DR antigens. The frequency of DR2 was increased in the patients (Table 15.4).

Disease Heterogeneity

In the Swiss study[2] no significant differences in the frequencies were observed between "probable" and "definite" subgroups of the disease. Similar results were also obtained for subgroups based on age at onset of the disease.

See also refs. 4 and 6.

References

1. McLoughlin GA, Helsby CR, Evans CC, Chapman DM: Association of HLA-A9 and HLA-B5 with Buerger's disease. Br Med J 2:1165-1166, 1976
2. De Moerloose PH, Jeannet M, Mirimanoff P, Bouvier CA: Evidence for an HLA-linked resistance gene in Buerger's disease. Tissue Antigens 14:169-173, 1979
3. Ohtawa T: HLA antigens in arterial occlusive diseases in Japan. Jpn J Surg 6:1-8, 1976
4. Yasuda K, Yokota A, Tanube T: Buerger's disease aortitis syndrome and HL-A. Nippon Rinsho 36:3171-3175, 1978
5. Hoshino K, Inouye H, Unokuchi T, Ito M, Tamaoki N, Tsuji K: HLA and disease in Japanese. In Dausset J, Svejgaard A (eds): HLA and Disease. De L'institut National De La Sante Et De La Recherche Medicale, Paris 1976, p 249
6. Ohtawa T, Juji T, Kawano N, Mishima Y, Tohyama H, Ishikawa K: HL-A antigens in thromboangiitis obliterans. JAMA 230:1128, 1974

TABLE 15.4. Buerger's Disease

Country/Population	Patients n	Patients %+	Controls n	Controls %+	RR	χ^2	Ref.
HLA-A9							
England	18	50	616	14	6.11	15.36	1
Switzerland	46	22	176	22	1.03	0.00	2
	64	30	792	16	2.14	6.58	
	Heterogeneity χ^2 (1 df)					8.78	
HLA-B5							
England	18	83	616	6	67.10	52.48	1
Switzerland	46	15	176	16	0.97	0.01	2
	64	34	792	8	4.52	18.55	
	Heterogeneity χ^2 (1 df)					33.94	
HLA-B7							
England	18	17	616	25	0.69	0.43	1
Switzerland	46	44	176	22	2.77	8.91	2
	64	36	792	24	1.91	4.89	
	Heterogeneity χ^2 (1 df)					4.45	
HLA-B12							
Japan	39	0	60	22	0.04	8.78	4
Japan	48	2	113	16	0.16	5.74	3
	87	1	173	18	0.10	13.56	
	Heterogeneity χ^2 (1 df)					0.96	
England	10	0	616	30	0.11	4.40	1
Switzerland	46	2	176	28	0.08	11.23	2
	56	2	792	30	0.09	15.56	
	Heterogeneity χ^2 (1 df)					0.07	
HLA-BW52							
Japan	39	46	60	18	3.76	8.66	4
HLA-BW54							
Japan	39	10	60	12	0.86	0.07	4
Japan	48	35	113	10	4.73	13.53	3
	87	24	173	11	2.72	8.29	
	Heterogeneity χ^2 (1 df)					5.31	
HLA-DR2							
Switzerland	46	59	100	34	2.75	7.92	2

Atherosclerosis

Population Association

There was no evidence for association with A and B loci antigens in 91 patients from England.[1] However, in 47 Japanese patients with arteriosclerosis obliterans, the frequency of CW1 was significantly decreased (Table 15.5).

References

1. Mcloughlin GA, Helsby CR, Evans CC, Chapman DM: Association of HLA-A9 and HLA-B5 with Buerger's disease. Br Med J 2:1165-1166, 1976

TABLE 15.5. Atherosclerosis

	Patients		Controls				
Country/Population	n	%+	n	%+	RR	χ^2	Ref.
HLA-CW1							
Japan	47	9	113	36	0.19	10.73	2

2. Ohtawa T: HLA antigens in arterial occlusive diseases in Japan. Jpn J Surg 6:1-8, 1976

Aortic Valve Disorders

Population Association

Hollingworth et al.[1] examined HLA-A and -B loci antigen frequencies in 20 patients with lone aortic regurgitation without overt spondylitis. All these patients had no past history suggestive of rheumatic fever. There was no significant disturbance in antigen frequencies.

Similar negative results were also reported by Tan et al.[2,3] in 20 patients (from New Zealand) with aortic incompetence.

See also ref. 4.

References

1. Hollingworth P, Hall PJ, Knight SC, Newman R: Lone aortic regurgitation, sacroiliitis, and HLA B27. Br Heart J 42:229-230, 1979
2. Tan PLJ, Butler MJ, Woodfield DG, Jacobson C, Grigor RR, Caughey DE: HLA antigens in isolated aortic incompetence. J Rheumatol 7:757-759, 1980
3. Tan PLJ, Butler M, Woodfield DG, Jacobson C, Grigor R, Caughey DE: HLA antigens in isolated aortic incompetence. NZ Med J 25:473, 1980
4. Calin A, Fries JF, Stinson EB, Payne R: Normal frequency of HL-A B27 in aortic insufficiency. N Engl J Med 294:397, 1976

Myocardial Infarction

Population Association

In 2 studies from England[1,2] in which a total of 150 men were typed for A and B loci antigens there were no significant deviations in the antigen frequencies.

Disease Heterogeneity

The group of 50 patients studied by Logan et al.[2] were subdivided into 3 subgroups: with a history of cigarette smoking, hypertension and/or hyperlipidemia, and with ischemic heart disease in a first-degree relative. There was no significant association with HLA in any of the subgroups of patients.

References

1. Scott BB, McGuffin P, Rajah SM, Strober JB, Losowsky MS: Histocompatibility antigens and myocardial infarction. Tissue Antigens 7:187-188, 1976
2. Logan RL, Oliver MF, McTavish J, Darg C, White AG: Histocompatibility antigens and myocardial infarction. Tissue Antigens 10:361-363, 1977

Mitral Valve Prolapse

Population Association

Braun et al.[1] observed a significant increase in BW35 in American Caucasian patients (Table 15.6). However, this was not confirmed in 22 Swiss patients studied by Jeannet et al.[2] In the pooled data the increased frequency of BW35 was only marginally significant.

The Swiss patients were also typed for 7 DR antigens and there was no difference in the frequencies between patient and control groups.

In the first report, Kachru et al.[3] reported a significant association with BW35 in 40 American black patients. In Table 15.6 we have given the frequency data for BW35 from another report by the same authors.[4] This report contained a larger sample of patients (the controls were the same in both reports).

TABLE 15.6. Mitral Valve Prolapse

	Patients		Controls				
Country/Population	n	%+	n	%+	RR	χ^2	Ref.
HLA-BW35							
U.S.A.—Black	42	74	194	39	4.32	15.66	4
U.S.A.	31	45	485	20	3.28	10.45	1
Switzerland	22	18	176	19	1.01	0.00	2
	53	34	661	20	2.26	7.21	
	Heterogeneity χ^2 (1 df)					3.24	

References

1. Braun WE, Ronan J, Schacter B, Gardin J, Isner J, Grecek D: HLA antigens in mitral valve prolapse. Transplant Proc 9:1869-1871, 1977
2. Jeannet M, Bloch A: HLA types in mitral valve prolapse. N Engl J Med 301:108, 1979
3. Kachru RB, Telischi M, Cruz JB, Patel R, Towne WD: HLA and ABO blood groups in Blacks with mitral-valve prolapse. N Engl J Med 299:1467, 1978
4. Kachru RB, Telischi M, Cruz JB, Patel R, Towne WD: The HLA antigens and ABO blood groups in an American Black population with mitral valve prolapse. Tissue Antigens 14:256-260, 1979

Aortitis Syndrome

Population Association

Hoshino et al.[1] reported an increased frequency of B5 in 31 Japanese patients.

Reference

1. Hoshino K, Inouye H, Unokuchi T, Ito M, Tamaoki N, Tsuji K: HLA and disease in Japanese. In Dausset J, Svejgaard A (eds): HLA and Disease. De L'institut National De La Sante Et De La Recherche Medicale, Paris 1976, p 249

Congenital Heart Malformation

Population Association

A significant association with A2 in 63 children born with heart malformations has been reported by Buc et al.[1] (Table 15.7).

Friedman and Paul[2] reported no frequency deviations in a sample of 10 American Caucasian patients (probands from 10 multiple-case families, see below). The data on antigen frequencies in patients and controls were not available in the report.

Hasegawa et al.[3] reported frequency data on 19 Japanese patients and 72 controls with no significant difference between the 2 groups. The 19 patients in this report were from 13 families studied for congenital heart malformations. There were 9 families with a single affected member in each and 4 multiple-case families with a total of 10 patients. Since all the patients were not unrelated the population analysis was not valid and the results did not provide any useful information.

Family Data

Hasegawa et al.[3] published data on 4 multiple-case families from Japan. Although no formal linkage analysis was given, there was no evidence of close linkage with HLA in this data.

TABLE 15.7. Congenital Heart Malformation

	Patients		Controls				
Country/Population	n	%+	n	%+	RR	χ^2	Ref.
HLA-A2							
Czechoslovakia	63	75	314	44	3.74	18.63	1

Friedman and Paul[2] studied 10 American Caucasian families in which 2 or more siblings had cardiac malformations. An analysis of the data by the sib-pair method showed no indication of linkage with HLA. Similar results were also reported by Barberis et al.[4] in a family in which 3 sisters and 1 brother were affected by atrial septal defect.

Mohl and Mayr[5] reported one 3-generation family with 4 and 9 children in the second and third generations, respectively, and two 2-generation families with 5 and 2 children, with a total of 10 patients affected by atrial septal defect of the secundum type. In this data a lod score of 3.612 was obtained for a 0% recombination between HLA and this disorder. These are the only data that showed significant evidence for linkage. The data from 15 other families mentioned before did not support these results. The family in an Italian study with no evidence of linkage had patients affected by atrial septal defect.[4] One reason for this discrepancy may be the heterogeneity of the disease.

References

1. Buc M, Nyulassy S, Stefanovic J, Jakubcova I, Benedekova M: HL-A2 and congenital heart malformations. Tissue Antigens 5:128-130, 1975
2. Friedman JM, Paul MH: Studies of the HLA complex in families of children with congenital heart disease. Tissue Antigens 11:479-483, 1978
3. Hasegawa T, Iwaki Y, Kusajima K, Ajiki H, Wada J, Hayashi T: Congenital heart disease found in same family and HLA antigens. Hokkaido J Med Sci 52:254-258, 1977
4. Barberis L, Reali G, Lijoi A, Passerone GC, Barbanti M, Ciccone MO, et al: Pervieta interatriale e familiarita. Minerva Cardioangiol 26:137-143, 1978
5. Mohl W, Mayr WR: Atrial septal defect of the secundum type and HLA. Tissue Antigens 10:121-122, 1977

Coronary Artery Disease

Population Association

HLA-A and B antigen frequencies were compared in 19 American Caucasian patients and 1157 controls by Stone et al.[1] The authors noted a nonsignificant increase of BW38 (21% in the patients vs. 4% in the controls, $p < 0.01$).

Reference

1. Stone PH, Sherrid MV, Cohn KE: Correlation of HLA types in premature coronary artery disease: An attempt to define independent genetic risk factors. Chest 79:381-385, 1981

Complete Heart Block

Population Association

Rodriguez et al.[1] typed A, B, C, and DR antigens in 8 Spanish mothers who had borne children with complete heart block. Four mothers were found to be positive for DR3 (50%) as compared with the 17% frequency of this antigen in Spanish controls on unknown size.

Reference

1. Rodriguez JJV, Seoane JG, Aguado AG, Sobrino JA, Barbado FJA, Villena AA: Complete heart block and the HLA system. Ann Intern Med 96:126, 1982

Polyarteritis Nodosa

Population Association

Elkon et al.[1] found no significant deviation of A, B, C, and DR antigens in 15 British patients and 113 controls.

Reference

1. Elkon KB, Sutherland DC, Rees AJ, Hughes GRV, Batchelor JR: HLA antigen frequencies in systemic vasculitis: Increase in HLA-DR2 in Wegener's granulomatosis. Arthritis Rheum 26:102-105, 1983

Churg-Strauss Vasculitis

Population Association

Fourteen British patients were typed for A, B, C, and DR antigens by Elkon et al.[1] No significant associations were found in this small sample.

Reference

1. Elkon KB, Sutherland DC, Rees AJ, Hughes GRV, Batchelor JR: HLA antigen frequencies in systemic

vasculitis: Increase in HLA-DR2 in Wegener's granulomatosis. Arthritis Rheum 26:102-105, 1983

Thrombophlebitis of Leg

Family Data

Perraudin et al.[1] published data on a small family of 3 siblings. All 3 had identical HLA haplotypes. However, only two siblings were affected by the disease. Both parents were normal.

Reference

1. Perraudin ML, Rousseau A, Desboid JC, Herrault A, Leveque B: Venous thrombosis, circulating anticoagulant and systemic lupus erythematosus. Two case reports in two HLA identical sisters. Semin Hop Paris 57:45-46, 1981

Venous Thromboembolism

Population Association

In two studies from Czechoslovakia, Riedel et al.[1–3] found significant associations with BW35, CW4, CW5, and CW6 antigens (Table 15.8). The frequency data in Table 15.8 are based on the total of the 2 studies.

References

1. Riedel M, Ivaskova E, Sajdlova H: HLA and venous thromboembolism. Tissue Antigens 18:280-281, 1981
2. Ivaskova E, Riedel M, Sajdlova H, Kupkova L: The susceptibility to venous thromoembolism associated with HLA-Cw4. Vnitr Lek 28:476-485, 1982
3. Riedel M, Ivaskova E, Sajdlova H: HLA antigens A B, and C in venous thromboembolic disease. Cas Lek Cesk 120:29-30, 1981

Varicose Veins of Lower Extremities

Population Association

In a report on 138 patients from Czechoslovakia, Riedel et al.[1] found significant deviations of AW19, B7, CW5, and CW6 antigens (Table 15.9).

Disease Heterogeneity

Subgroupings of the patients on the basis of sex and age at the onset of varices did not show any relationship with the HLA antigens.

Reference

1. Riedel M, Ivaskova E, Prerovsky I: Primary varicose veins and HLA. Blood Vessels 20:99-104, 1983

Varicocele

Population Association

In their first study, Sengar et al.[1] reported a significant association with B5 and BW51 antigens in 50 Canadian patients. However, the second study by the

TABLE 15.8. Venous Thromboembolism

	Patients		Controls				
Country/Population	n	%+	n	%+	RR	χ^2	Ref.
HLA-BW35							
Czechoslovakia	154	27	1200	16	1.95	11.63	1
HLA-CW4							
Czechoslovakia	154	34	1200	15	2.93	32.94	1
HLA-CW5							
Czechoslovakia	154	1	1200	10	0.12	11.02	1
HLA-CW6							
Czechoslovakia	154	7	1200	27	0.21	25.05	1

TABLE 15.9. Varicose Veins of Lower Extremities

	Patients		Controls				
Country/Population	n	%+	n	%+	RR	χ^2	Ref.
HLA-AW19							
Czechoslovakia	138	9	1200	25	0.31	16.05	1
HLA-B7							
Czechoslovakia	138	36	1212	23	1.89	11.37	1
HLA-CW5							
Czechoslovakia	138	1	244	10	0.12	9.45	1
HLA-CW6							
Czechoslovakia	138	7	130	27	0.21	17.30	1

TABLE 15.10. Raynaud's Phenomenon

	Patients		Controls				
Country/Population	n	%+	n	%+	RR	χ^2	Ref.
HLA-A2							
BENELUX	79	72	4000	53	2.25	10.68	1

same authors on 48 new patients could not confirm these associations.[2]

References

1. Sengar DPS, Mervart H, Hudson RW: Histocompatibility antigens in varicocele. Tissue Antigens 19:230-232, 1982
2. Sengar DPS, Mervart H, Hudson RW: Histocompatibility antigens in varicocele: A prospective study. Tissue Antigens 21:345-347, 1983

Idiopathic Portal Hypertension

Population Association

Satoh et al.[1] compared A and B loci antigen in 31 Japanese patients and 174 controls. There was no significant difference between the two groups.

Reference

1. Satoh H, Iwasaki Y, Ohkubo A, Beppu T, Futagawa S, Sugiura M, et al: Human leukocyte antigen (HLA) in patients with idiopathic portal hypertension (IPH). Tohoku J Exp Med 131:393-397, 1980

Raynaud's Phenomenon

Population Association

van der Meulen et al.[1] studied A and B loci antigens in 79 Dutch patients with isolated Raynaud's phenomenon or with a history of isolated Raynaud's phenomenon. In this sample a significant association with A2 antigen was reported.

Disease Heterogeneity

Twenty-two of the above 79 Dutch patients also had connective tissue disease (5 with systemic lupus erythematosus and 17 with scleroderma). In this subgroup the frequency of B8 was significantly increased (59.09% in the patients vs. 25.35% in the controls, corrected $p = 0.005$).

In the group of 57 patients without connective tissue diseases the frequency of A2 was also increased (78.95% in the patients vs. 53% in the controls, corrected $p < 0.02$).

Reference

1. van der Meulen J, van der Voort-Beelen JM, D'Amaro J, The TH: HLA-B8 in Raynaud's phenomenon. Tissue Antigens 15:81-85, 1980

CHAPTER 16

Connective Tissue Diseases

Systemic Lupus Erythematosus

Population Association

An analysis of combined data on A and B loci antigens from all the available studies showed that B5 and B8 frequencies were significantly increased in Caucasian patients (Table 16.1). However, it should be noted that only Szegedi et al.'s data[1] showed a significant association with B5. B8 was found to be associated with this disease in several independent studies.

An increased frequency of A1 in American Black patients observed by Goldberg et al.[2] was not confirmed by Nies et al.[3] and in both of these studies B8 was also not determined to be associated with systemic lupus erythematosus (SLE).

The data of Nies et al.[3] showed a marginally significant increase of B40 in 40 Mexican-American patients (Table 16.1).

In a study from Iran by Davatchi et al.[4] there was a highly significant increase of B13 and B17 in a small sample of 21 patients. These 2 antigens are associated with psoriasis in Caucasian patients.

Kohno,[5] Sakurami et al.,[6] and Kameda et al.[7] typed Japanese patients for A and B loci antigens. There were no significant deviations when compared with the controls.

DR Locus

The frequency data from several independent studies given in the Table 16.1 showed that DR2 and DR3 were also associated with SLE. However, the estimate of relative risk in the combined sample was still higher for B8.

DR2 and DR3 were not found to be associated with SLE in American Black patients.

Kameda et al.[7] reported a highly significant decrease of DR4 in 45 Japanese patients. These results, however, were not confirmed in the data of Sakurami et al.[6] Thus in the pooled data this antigen is not associated with the disease. There is also evidence of a significant heterogeneity in these data.

Chan et al.[8] studied A and B loci antigens in 75 unrelated Chinese patients from Singapore. In the total sample there was no evidence of any significant association.

Disease Heterogeneity

Age at Onset

Szegedi et al.[1] reported a lower age at onset in B5-positive (mean age 27 years) and B8-positive (mean age 28 years) as compared with B5-negative (45 years) and B8-negative (22 years) patients. The average age at onset for the total sample of 86 female patients was 34.7 years (see also ref. 9).

In the report of Scherak et al.[10] the mean age at onset in 13 B8-positive patients was 45.3 years as compared with 31.3 years in 14 B8-negative patients ($p < 0.01$). However, in 2 other reports by Kampf et al.[11] and Goldberg et al.[2] there was no HLA association with age at onset.

In another report by Scherak et al.[12] SLE patients with DR3 were found to have significantly later onset of their disease than DR3-negative patients.

Antibody to Native DNA

In 30 SLE patients with high antibody titer to native DNA (2 mg DNA/ml serum) Griffing et al.[13] found

TABLE 16.1. Systemic Lupus Erythematosus

	Patients		Controls				
Country/Population	n	%+	n	%+	RR	χ^2	Ref.
HLA-B5							
U.S.A.—Black	40	23	120	5	5.46	10.25	3
U.S.A.	42	24	886	11	2.63	7.07	3
U.S.A.	25	16	82	11	1.62	0.64	26
U.S.A.	106	13	1024	12	1.13	0.16	15
	173	16	1992	12	1.58	4.60	
	Heterogeneity χ^2 (2 df)					3.28	
Australia	53	9	180	9	1.06	0.01	27
Australia	44	16	700	7	2.65	5.51	28
Australia	44	2	1037	8	0.36	1.82	21
	141	9	1917	8	1.43	1.47	
	Heterogeneity χ^2 (2 df)					5.87	
Bulgaria	20	40	50	34	1.30	0.25	29
Czechoslovakia	45	11	350	13	0.89	0.06	30
Hungary	90	33	50	19	2.04	3.01	9
Hungary	100	34	450	15	2.92	18.94	1
	190	34	500	15	2.66	21.38	
	Heterogeneity χ^2 (1 df)					0.57	
West Germany	27	15	283	13	1.28	0.23	11
West Germany	42	17	2100	17	1.05	0.02	31
	69	16	2383	17	1.13	0.16	
	Heterogeneity χ^2 (1 df)					0.09	
Austria	27	11	450	17	0.69	0.46	10
Switzerland	39	15	176	16	0.98	0.00	20
Finland	49	12	900	12	1.07	0.02	19
	753	19	8718	13	1.52	15.41	
	Heterogeneity χ^2 (14 df)					22.80	
HLA-B8							
U.S.A.	49	35	49	12	3.73	6.84	2
U.S.A.	106	39	1024	17	3.13	28.43	15
U.S.A.	25	36	82	16	2.93	4.75	26
U.S.A.	42	19	886	21	0.92	0.04	3
	222	34	2041	19	2.52	31.45	
	Heterogeneity χ^2 (3 df)					8.61	
Australia	44	45	700	24	2.60	9.53	28
Australia	44	36	1037	31	1.27	0.57	21
Australia	53	55	180	26	3.44	15.01	27
	141	46	1917	28	2.24	19.78	
	Heterogeneity χ^2 (2 df)					5.34	
Bulgaria	20	35	50	14	3.22	3.98	29
Czechoslovakia	45	38	350	22	2.19	5.76	30
Hungary	90	32	50	19	1.95	2.63	9
Hungary	100	38	450	19	2.61	16.55	1
	190	35	500	19	2.43	18.79	
	Heterogeneity χ^2 (1 df)					0.39	

TABLE 16.1. *(continued)*

Country/Population	Patients n	Patients %+	Controls n	Controls %+	RR	χ^2	Ref.
HLA-B8							
England	53	43	188	22	2.67	9.20	16
West Germany	42	48	2100	16	4.85	26.36	31
West Germany	27	59	283	21	5.31	17.11	11
	69	52	2383	17	5.01	43.43	
	Heterogeneity χ^2 (1 df)					0.03	
Austria	27	48	450	18	4.20	13.45	10
Switzerland	39	36	176	17	2.75	7.11	20
Finland	49	47	900	20	3.55	18.74	19
	855	40	8955	20	2.77	161.23	
	Heterogeneity χ^2 (16 df)					24.82	
HLA-B13							
Iran	21	29	400	7	5.59	12.28	4
HLA-B17							
Iran	21	19	400	3	7.97	12.84	4
HLA-B40							
Mexico	40	28	283	12	2.89	7.61	3
HLA-DW3							
Finland	20	60	900	24	4.65	12.17	19
HLA-DR2							
U.S.A.	24	50	40	25	2.90	4.10	32
U.S.A.	63	38	1145	25	1.85	5.44	15
U.S.A.	30	53	258	26	3.18	9.22	338
	117	44	1443	25	2.30	17.17	
	Heterogeneity χ^2 (2 df)					1.60	
Australia	35	29	140	28	1.07	0.03	27
England	48	38	148	22	2.17	4.90	16
England	20	40	113	19	2.85	4.50	34
	68	39	261	21	2.38	9.20	
	Heterogeneity χ^2 (1 df)					0.20	
Austria	28	21	125	20	1.11	0.05	35
Austria	28	21	125	20	1.11	0.05	12
	56	21	250	20	1.11	0.09	
	Heterogeneity χ^2 (1 df)					0.00	
Switzerland	40	20	123	28	0.67	0.91	22
	316	34	2217	24	1.70	16.10	
	Heterogeneity χ^2 (8 df)					13.10	
HLA-DR3							
U.S.A.	63	37	1145	22	2.10	7.75	15
U.S.A.	24	54	40	20	4.46	7.55	32
U.S.A.	30	37	258	17	2.89	7.06	33
	117	40	1443	21	2.54	20.67	
	Heterogeneity χ^2 (2 df)					1.69	

TABLE 16.1. *(continued)*

Country/Population	Patients n	Patients %+	Controls n	Controls %+	RR	χ^2	Ref.
HLA-DR3							
Australia	35	54	140	30	2.71	6.99	27
England	48	44	148	28	2.02	4.31	16
England	20	30	113	30	1.04	0.01	34
	68	40	261	29	1.64	3.11	
	Heterogeneity χ^2 (1 df)					1.21	
Austria	28	39	125	16	3.34	7.42	12
Austria	28	39	125	16	3.34	7.42	35
	56	39	250	16	3.34	14.84	
	Heterogeneity χ^2 (1 df)					0.00	
Switzerland	40	43	123	11	5.95	18.21	22
	316	42	2217	21	2.65	56.51	
	Heterogeneity χ^2 (8 df)					10.20	
HLA-DR4							
Japan	45	20	36	58	0.19	11.74	7
Japan	18	56	144	33	2.54	3.72	6
	63	30	180	38	0.70	1.11	
	Heterogeneity χ^2 (1 df)					14.35	

20 (67%) DR3-positive. This frequency was significantly higher ($p < 0.0001$) than that in a population of SLE patients who did not have high antibody titer native to DNA. The authors do not give data on the latter population (see also ref. 14).

Schur et al.[15] reported a significant association with anti-DNA antibody and DR7.

However, the data of Scherak et al.[10] on 20 patients, of Kampf et al.[11] on 27 patients, and of Black et al.[16] on 67 patients did not show any antibody titer difference between B8-positive and -negative patients. The report of Black et al.[16] also had data on DR locus antigens with similar results.

Duration of the Disease

No association with any HLA antigens was found.[10]

Prognosis

No association with HLA antigens was found.[11]

Antinuclear Antibody

No association between antinuclear antibody titers and HLA antigens was found.[2,10,11,15,17–20]

Severity

Rigby et al.[21] classified their 44 patients as mild (n = 30) or severe (n = 14) on the basis of renal biopsy changes and the degree of proteinuria. Individual antigen frequencies were not significantly different between the 2 subgroups and controls. The authors noted increased frequencies of A2 plus B7 in the mild group (37% vs. 13.5% in 1037 controls) and A1 plus B8 in the severe group (57% vs. 18.4% in controls). The biologic meaning of such an association with antigen combinations is not clear, however (see also ref. 17).

In two other reports[12,20] no association between severity of SLE and any of the DR locus antigens was found.

The Singapore Chinese patients studied by Chan et al.[8] were subdivided into "mild" and "severe" groups. The frequency of B13 in 30 patients with "mild" SLE was 40% as compared with 17.9% in 330 normals and 13.3% in 45 patients with "severe" disease. Thus in this sample B13 was found to be associated with mild disease.

C3 in Serum

No association with HLA and complement level in serum was found.[2,11]

Family History
No association with HLA antigens was found.[3]

Lymphocytotoxic Alloantibodies
Celada et al.[20,22] did not find the presence of lymphocytotoxic alloantibodies or autoantibodies against T and B lymphocytes to be associated with DR3. In this report DR3 was significantly increased in the patients (Table 16.1).

Cutaneous Reactions to Drugs
Johansson et al.[23] studied cutaneous reactions to acetylsalicylic acid, sulfonamides, and penicillin in 42 Finnish patients typed for A and B loci antigens. Twenty-two patients reacted to these drugs. However, there was no HLA difference between this group and a group of 20 patients who did not react.

Another classification was made on the basis of acetylation phenotype by means of a sulfamethazine test. Twenty-nine patients were slow acetylators and 13 were rapid acetylators. Again there was no HLA difference between the 2 groups.

Organ System Involvement
No association between any HLA antigens and involvement of lung, central nervous system, skin, kidneys, or hematopoietic system was found.[2,3,10,11]

Antibody to Cytoplasmic Antigen R_0
Maddison and Bell[18,24] reported an association between DR3 and antibody to cytoplasmic antigen R_0 in SLE patients.

Family Data

Cleland et al.[25] published data on 4 pedigrees with multiple cases of SLE in each family. Linkage analysis by the lod score method showed a maximum lod score of 2.6 at a recombination frequency of 5%. These data are highly suggestive of linkage between HLA and a SLE susceptibility gene (see also ref. 18).

See also refs. 36–57.

References

1. Szegedi G: Immunological investigations in systemic lupus erythematosus. Panminerva Med 20:9-22, 1978
2. Goldberg MA, Arnett FC, Bias WB, Shulman LE: Histocompatibility antigens in systemic lupus erythematosus. Arthritis Rheum 19:129-132, 1976
3. Nies KM, Brown JC, Dubois EL, Guismorio FG, Friou GJ, Terasaki PI: Histocompatibility (HLA) antigens and lymphocytotoxic antibodies in systemic lupus erythematosus (SLE). Arthritis Rheum 17:397-402, 1974
4. Davatchi F, Nikbin B, Ala F: Histocompatibility antigens (HLA) in rheumatic disases in Iran. J Rheumatol 4 (Suppl 3):36-38, 1977
5. Kohno M: SLE and HLA antigens. Nippon Rinsho 36:3143-3146,1978
6. Sakurami T, Ueno Y, Iwaki Y, Park MS, Terasaki PI, Saji H: HLA-DR specificities among Japanese with several autoimmune disease. Tissue Antigens 19:129-133, 1982
7. Kameda S, Naito S, Tanaka K, Kajiyama K, Kunihiro K, Nishigouri S, et al: HLA antigens of patients with systemic lupus erythematosus in Japan. Tissue Antigens 20:221-222, 1982
8. Chan SH, Feng PH, Srinivasan N, Wee GB, Chan HC: HLA and systemic lupus erythematosus. Hum Immunol 3:345-350, 1981
9. Stenszky V, Szegedi GY, Aszodi L, Petranyi GY: HL-A and systemic lupus erythematosus. Haematologia 7:211-217, 1973
10. Scherak O, Kolarz G, Mayr WR: HLA-B8 in Caucasian patients with systemic lupus erythematosus. Scand J Rheumatol 7:3-6, 1978
11. Kampf D, Malchus R, Alexander M, Hoppe I: HLA-antigens in systemic lupus erythematosus (SLE). Arch Dermatol Res 264:345-350, 1979
12. Scherak O, Smolen JS, Mayr WR: HLA-DRw3 and systemic lupus erythematosus. Arthritis Rheum 23:954-957, 1980
13. Griffing WL, Moore SB, Luthra HS, McKenna CH, Fathman CG: Associations of antibodies to native DNA with HLA-DRW3: A possible MHC linked immune response gene. Arthritis Rheum 23:684-685, 1980
14. Griffing WL, Moore SB, Luthra HS, McKenna CH, Fathman CG: Associations of antibodies native to DNA with HLA-DRw3. A possible major histocompatibility complex-linked human immune response gene. J Exp Med 152:319s-325s, 1980
15. Schur PH, Meyer I, Garovoy M, Carpenter CB: Associations between systemic lupus erythematosus and the major histocompatibility complex: Clinical and immunological considerations. Clin Immunol Immunopathol 24:263-275, 1982
16. Black CM, Welsh KI, Fiuelder A, Hughes GRV, Batchelor JR: HLA antigens and Bf allotypes in SLE: Evidence for the association being with specific haplotypes. Tissue Antigens 19:115-120, 1982
17. Hawkins BR, Dawkins RL, Richmond J, Rigby RJ: Immunogenetic factors in systemic lupus erythematosus. Arthritis Rheum 22:94, 1979
18. Bell DA, Maddison P: Serologic subsets in systemic lupus erythematosus: An examination of autoantibodies in relationship to clinical features of disease and HLA antigens. Arthritis Rheum 23:1268-1273, 1980

19. Johansson EA, Koskimies S, Tiilikainen A, Lassus A: HLA antigens in patients with chronic biologically false-positive seroreactions for syphilis and systemic lupus erythematosus. Arch Dermatol Res 272:55-60, 1982
20. Celada A, Barras C, Benzonana G, Jeannet M: Increased frequency of HLA-DRw3 in systemic lupus erythematosus. Tissue Antigens 15:282-288, 1980
21. Rigby RJ, Dawkins RL, Wetherall JD, Hawkins BR: HLA in systemic lupus erythematosus: Influence on severity. Tissue Antigens 12:25-31, 1978
22. Celada A, Barras C, Benzonana G, Jeannet M: Increased frequency of HLA-DRW3 in systemic lupus erythematosus. N Engl J Med 301:1398-1399, 1979
23. Johansson EA, Mustakallio KK, Mattila MM, Tiilikainen A: Cutaneous reactions to drugs, acetylation phenotype and HLA antigens in patients with and without systemic lupus erythematosus (SLE). Ann Clin Res 8:126-128, 1976
24. Maddison P, Bell DA: HLA antigens in relationship to serologic subsets of systemic lupus erythematosus. Arthritis Rheum 23:714-715, 1980
25. Cleland LG, Bell DA, Willans M, Saurino BC: Familial lupus: Family studies of HLA and serologic findings. Arthritis Rheum 21:183-191, 1978
26. Grumet FC, Coukell A, Bodmer JG, Bodmer WF, McDevitt HO: Histocompatibility (HL-A) antigens associated with systemic lupus erythematosus. N Engl J Med 285:193-196, 1971
27. Whittingham S, Mathews JD, Schanfield MS, Tait BD, Mackay IR. HLA and Gm genes in systemic lupus erythematosus. Tissue Antigens 21:50-57, 1983
28. Morris PJ, Vaughan H, Tait BD, Mackay IR: Histocompatibility antigens (HLA): Association with immunopathic diseases and with response to microbial antigens. Aust NZ J Med 7:616-624, 1977
29. Stefanova S, Andreev IG: HLA system and renal diseases. Ind J Exp Biol 18:282-284, 1980
30. Dostal C, Ivanyi D, Macurova H, Hana I, Strejcek J: HLA antigens in systemic lupus erythematosus. Ann Rheum Dis 36:83-85, 1977
31. Lakomek HJ, Specker Ch, Kuntz BME, Goerz G: Assoziationen von HLA-Antigenen zum Systemischen Lupus Erythematodes under seiner Krankheitssymptomatik. Dtsch Med Wochenschr 107:766-770, 1982
32. Gibofsky A, Winchester RJ, Patarroyo M, Fotino M, Kunkel MG: Disease associations of the IA-like human alloantigens. J Exp Med 148:1728-1732, 1978
33. Gladman DD, Terasaki PI, Park MS, Iwaki Y, Louie S, Quismorio FP, et al: Increased frequency of HLA-DRW2 in SLE. Lancet ii:902, 1979
34. Batchelor JR, Welsh KI, Tinoco RM, Dollery CT, Hughes GRV, Bernstein R, et al: Hydralazine-induced systemic lupus erythematosus: Influence of HLA-DR and sex on susceptibility. Lancet i:1107-1109, 1980
35. Scherak O, Smolen JS, Mayr WR: Prevalence of HLA-DRW2 not increased in systemic lupus erythematosus. N Engl J Med 301:612, 1979
36. Fruman LS: Diabetes mellitus, islet-cell antibodies, and HLA-B8 in a patient with systemic lupus erythematosus. Am J Dis Child 131:1252-1254, 1977
37. Ivanyi D, Dostal C, Mrklas L: HLA-B8 in systemic lupus erythematosus. Tissue Antigens 8:91-93, 1976
38. Walford: HL-A and systemic lupus erythematosus. Transplant Proc 3:1313-1314, 1971
39. Waters H, Konrad P, Walford RL: The distribution of HL-A histocompatibility factors and genes in patients with systemic lupus erythematosus. Tissue Antigens 1:68-73, 1971
40. Brouet JC, Fridman WH, Clauvel JP, Sasportes M, Danon F, and Seligmann M: Deficit genetique de la deuxieme fraction du complement avec manifestation lupiques. Nouv Presse Med 6:3199-3203, 1977
41. Stastny P: The distribution of HL-A antigens in black patients with systemic lupus erythematosus (SLE). Arthritis Rheum 15:455-456, 1972
42. Arnett FC, Bias WB, Shulman LE: HL-A antigens in systemic lupus erythematosus (SLE). Athritis Rheum 15:428, 1972
43. Stastny P, Gilliam JN: HLA-A1, B8, DRW3 in patients with a distinct form of lupus erythematosus. Transplant Proc 11:1869-1870, 1979
44. Walford RL, Smith GS, Waters H: Histocompatibility systems and disease states with particular reference to cancer. Transplant Rev 7:78-111, 1971
45. Bitter T, Mottironi WD, Terasaki PI: HL-A antigens associated with lupus erythematosus. N Engl J Med 286:435-436, 1972
46. O'Regan S: HLA-B8 autoimmune polyendocrinopathy and systemic lupus erythematosus. Can Med Assoc J 121:1168-1169, 1979
47. Raum D, Glass D, Soter NA, Stillman JS, Carpenter CB, Schur PH: Lymphocytotoxic antibodies: HLA antigen associations, disease associations, and family studies. Arthritis Rheum 20:933-936, 1977
48. Messner RP, De Horatius R, Ferrone S: Lymphocytotoxic antibodies in systemic lupus erythematosus patients and their relatives: Reactivity with the HLA antigenic molecular complex. Arthritis Rheum 23:265-272, 1980
49. Ting A, Mackay LR, Morris PJ: HL-A in autoimmune diseases and infectious mononucleosis. Symp Ser Immunobiol Stand 18:276-281, 1973
50. Boyer J, Chouvet B, Gebuhrer L, Betuel H, Descos L, Thivolet J: Maladie coeliaque et lupus erythemateux dissemine:Association familiale et relation avec le systeme HLA-DR. Nouv Press Med 11:525-526, 1982
51. Nashel DJ, Leonard A, Mann DL, Guccion JG,

Katz AL, Sliwinski AJ: Ankylosing spondylitis and systemic lupus erythematosus. Arch Intern Med 142:1227-1228, 1982
52. Fielder AHL, Walport MJ, Batchelor JR, Dodi IA, Hughes GRV, Rynes RI, et al: Family study of the MHC in patients with SLE: Importance of null alleles of C4A and C4B in determining disease susceptibility. Br Med J 286:425-428, 1983
53. Calin A: Epidemiology of the rheumatic diseases, with a focus on HLA. Curr Ther Res 30:S15-S23, 1981
54. Sach JA: HLA systems and rheumatic diseases. Curr Top Pathol 71:235-262, 1982
55. Dawkins RL, Christiansen FT, Kay PH, Garlepp M, McCluskey J, Hollingsworth PN, et al: Disease associations with complotypes, supratypes and haplotypes. Immunol Rev 70:5-22, 1983
56. Johansson EA, Koskimies S: HLA antigens in patients with chronic biologically false positive seroreactions for syphilis and systemic lupus erythematosus. Scand J Rheumatol 42:11, 1982
57. Perraudin ML, Rousseau A, Desboid JC, Herrault A, Leveque B: Venous thrombosis, circulating anticoagulant and systemic lupus erythematosus. Two case reports in two HLA identical sisters. Semin Hop Paris 57:45-46, 1981

Hydralazine-Induced Systemic Lupus Erythematosus

Population Association

Batchelor et al.[1] studied 26 Caucasian patients who developed systemic lupus erythematosus (SLE) after using hydralazine for a minimum period of 6 months. All were typed for 8 DR locus antigens. As the data in Table 16.2 show there was a significant increase of DR4 in the patients.

These SLE patients were compared with 16 individuals who received hydralazine but did not develop SLE and with 20 patients with idiopathic SLE. The DR antigen frequencies in these 2 groups were similar to those in 113 healthy controls.

It should be noted that the analysis of combined data on idiopathic SLE showed an association with DR3. Thus, idiopathic SLE and hydralazine-induced SLE may be 2 separate entities.

Reference

1. Batchelor JR, Welsh KI, Tinoco RM, Dollery CT, Hughes GRV, Bernstein R, et al: Hydralazine-induced systemic lupus erythematosus: Influence of HLA-DR and sex on susceptibility. Lancet i:1107-1109, 1980

Sjögren's Syndrome (Sicca Syndrome)

Population Association

The first report on this disease by Sturrock et al.[1] did not show any association with A and B loci antigens. Later Gershwin et al.[2] found a significant increase of B8 in the patients. Subsequent reports by several authors have confirmed the association of B8 with this disorder (Table 16.3).

A stronger association with DW3 was later reported independently by Chused et al.[3] and Hinzova et al.[4] Fye et al.[5] and Manthorpe et al.[6] also found similar results. As the data in Table 16.3 indicate, the relative risk for DW3 was greater than that with B8. Statistical analyses of DW3 frequencies in B8-positive and B8-negative patients and controls done by Chused et al.[3] and Fye et al.[5] showed that the primary association of the disease was with DW3. The increased frequency of B8 in the patients was due to the linkage disequilibrium between B8 and DW3.

In a study of 14 Japanese patients Ohno[7] did not find any significant association with A or B locus antigens.

Moutsopoulos et al.[8] reported 100% positivity for 2 immunologically and genetically related B lymphocyte antigens in 24 patients. The frequencies of these 2 antigens in normal control populations were only 37% and 24%, respectively.

TABLE 16.2. Hydralazine-Induced Systemic Lupus Erythematosus

	Patients		Controls				
Country/Population	n	%+	n	%+	RR	χ^2	Ref.
HLA-DR4							
England	26	73	113	33	5.22	12.78	1

TABLE 16.3. Sjögren's Syndrome

Country/Population	Patients n	Patients %+	Controls n	Controls %+	RR	χ^2	Ref.
HLA-B8							
U.S.A.	24	58	1205	21	5.12	16.44	2
U.S.A.	46	46	485	22	3.02	12.76	9
U.S.A.	22	50	1205	21	3.76	10.20	11
	92	50	2895	21	3.70	38.32	
	Heterogeneity χ^2 (2 df)					1.08	
Czechoslovakia	36	53	350	22	3.97	15.55	12
England	21	38	597	31	1.39	0.58	1
Denmark	35	54	3304	25	3.50	14.25	6
	184	50	7146	24	3.30	64.21	
	Heterogeneity χ^2 (5 df)					5.58	
HLA-DW2							
Denmark	32	56	345	26	3.58	12.14	6
HLA-DW3							
U.S.A.	19	74	96	24	8.35	15.54	5
U.S.A.	25	68	91	24	6.42	15.39	3
	44	71	187	24	7.20	30.79	
	Heterogeneity χ^2 (1 df)					0.13	
Czechoslovakia	29	69	58	10	18.08	26.72	4
Denmark	32	50	334	26	2.84	8.16	6
	105	64	579	24	5.79	57.34	
	Heterogeneity χ^2 (3 df)					8.48	

Disease Heterogeneity

In the sample of 19 patients studied by Fye et al.,[5] there was a significant correlation between the severity of the clinical manifestations and the presence of DW3. The mean parotid salivary flow rate was lower in 14 patients positive for DW3 as compared with 5 negative patients. The mean focus scores of the DW3 and non-DW3 patients were not significantly different.

It should be noted that Gershwin et al.[2] and Clough et al.[9] also compared several clinical features (including the 2 mentioned earlier) in B8-positive and B8-negative patients. There was no significant difference between the 2 groups. (The clinical features and the frequency data are available in these reports in tabular forms.)

Powell et al.[10] and Manthorpe et al.[6] studied patients with Sjögren's syndrome and associated rheumatoid arthritis. In the report of Powell et al.[10] BW44 and DR4 and in that of Manthorpe[6] DW4 were found to be significantly increased in the patients. On the basis of these results the authors have argued that the combination of these two diseases may be a genetically distinct entity.

See also refs. 13–16.

References

1. Sturrock RD, Canesi BA, Dick HM, Dick WC: HL-A antigens and the sicca syndrome. Ann Rheum Dis 33:165-166, 1974
2. Gershwin ME, Terasaki PI, Graw R, Chused TM: Increased frequency of HL-A8 in Sjögren's syndrome. Tissue Antigens 6:342-346, 1975
3. Chused TM, Kassan SS, Opelz G, Moutsopoulos HM, Terasaki PI: Sjögren's syndrome associated with HLA-DW3. N Engl J Med 296:895-897, 1977
4. Hinzova E, Ivanyi D, Sula K, Horejs J, Dostal C, Drizhal I: HLA-DW3 in Sjögren's syndrome. Tissue Antigens 9:8-10, 1977
5. Fye KH, Terasaki PI, Michalski JP, Daniels TE, Opelz G, Talal N: Relationship of HLA-DW3 and

HLA-B8 to Sjögren's syndrome. Arthritis Rheum 21:337-342, 1978
6. Manthorpe R, Morling N, Platz P, Ryder LP, Svejgaard A, Thomsen M: HLA-D antigen frequencies in Sjögren's syndrome. Scand J Rheumatol 10:124-128, 1981
7. Ohno S: Immunogenetic studies on various ocular diseases. Nippon Ganka Gakkai Zasshi 83:1875-1908, 1980
8. Moutsopoulos HM, Chused TM, Johnson AH, Knudsen B, Mann DL: B lymphocyte antigens in sicca syndrome. Science 199:1441-1442, 1978
9. Clough JD, Aponte CJ, Braun WE: HLA-B8 and clinical features of Sjögren's syndrome. Clin Immunol Immunopathol 7:324-329, 1977
10. Powell TR, Michalski JP, McCombs CC, Danilovs JA, Terasaki PI, Park MS, et al.: HLA-Bw44 and HLA-DRw4 in male Sjögren's syndrome patients with associated rheumatoid arthritis. Clin Immunol Immunopathol 17:463-468, 1980
11. Fye KH, Terasaki PI, Moutsopoulos H, Daniels TE, Michalski JP, Talal N: Association of Sjögren's syndrome with HLA-B8. Arthritis Rheum 19:883-886, 1976
12. Ivanyi D, Drizhal I, Erbenova E, Horej SJ, Salavec M, Macurova H, et al: HL-A in Sjögren's syndrome. Tissue Antigens 7:45-51, 1976
13. Alspaugh MA, Tan EM: Antibodies to cellular antigens in Sjögren's syndromes. J Clin Invest 55:1067-1073, 1975
14. Hochberg MC: Autoimmune disease and histocompatibility antigen. Ann Intern Med 86:660, 1977
15. McCombs CC, Michalski JP: Decreased suboptimal phytohemagglutinin associated with HLA-B8 in clinically normal individuals. Arthritis Rheum 23:717-718, 1980
16. Manthorpe R, Teppo AM, Bendixen G, Wegelius O: Antibodies to SS-B in chronic inflammatory connective tissue diseases. Relationship with HLA-Dw2 and Dw3 antigens in primary Sjögren's syndrome Arthritis. Rheum 25:662-667, 1982

Scleroderma

Population Association

The study of Clements et al.[1] is the only one in which a clearly significant increase of A9 in the patients was observed. However, in the pooled data this antigen is significantly associated with the disease. An increase of B8 in the patients apparent in the data of Freudenberg et al[2] was also not confirmed in 6 other studies (Table 16.4). In the combined sample the association with B8 is only marginally significant.

It should be noted that in Clements et al.'s study[1] AW24 (1 split of A9) was present in 30% of the 40 patients compared with only 11% in 200 controls ($p < 0.09$). AW23, the other split of A9, was present in 8% of the patients and in 3% of the controls and, thus, there was no difference between the 2 groups.

DR locus antigens were also typed in several reports (Table 16.4). In the combined sample DR5 is significantly increased in the patients (primarily because of the data of Gladman et al.[3]).

Disease Heterogeneity

Clements et al.[1] grouped their patients on the basis of organ system involvement (31 pulmonary, 18 cardiac, 25 gastrointestinal, 34 diffuse). AW24 was increased in all these subgroups.

Hughes et al.[4] classified their patients according to the severity of the disease. In the sample of 19 patients with the severe form of the disease 12 (63.16%) were positive for B8. The frequency of this antigen was only 27.27% (9/33) in 33 patients with the mild form of the disease (corrected $p < 0.047$). Also, B8-positive patients had more extensive, rapidly progressing disease and higher mortality (for details see ref. 4).

Family Data

A large pedigree with 13 patients was studied by Crouzet et al.[5] There were no HLA-identical affected siblings and the segregation of the disease through 4 generations did not appear to be with a particular HLA haplotype. Thus, in the pedigree there was no evidence of linkage with HLA (see also ref. 6).

See also refs. 13–17.

References

1. Clements PJ, Opelz G, Terasaki PI, Mickey MR, Furst D: Association of HLA antigen A9 with progressive systemic sclerosis (scleroderma). Tissue Antigens 11:357-361, 1978
2. Freudenberg J, Holzmann H, Schneider S, Korting GW: HLA antigen frequencies in patients with progressive systemic sclerosis and morphea. Arch Dermatol Res 263:197-205, 1978
3. Gladman DD, Keystone EC, Baron M, Lee P, Cane D, Mervert H: Increased frequency of HLA-DR5 in scleroderma. Arthritis Rheum 24:854-856, 1981
4. Hughes P, Gelsthorpe K, Doughty RW, Rowell

TABLE 16.4. Scleroderma (Progressive Systemic Sclerosis)

Country/Population	Patients n	Patients %+	Controls n	Controls %+	RR	χ^2	Ref.
HLA-A9							
U.S.A.	237	4	200	3	1.31	0.29	7
U.S.A.	40	38	200	14	3.76	12.44	1
U.S.A.	106	18	208	14	1.36	0.93	8
	383	11	608	10	1.90	8.67	
	Heterogeneity χ^2 (2 df)					4.99	
Czechoslovakia	58	29	301	19	1.76	3.16	9
England	71	18	3000	17	1.10	0.11	4
France	49	24	152	21	1.21	0.25	5
West Germany	67	19	503	22	0.85	0.24	2
Spain	21	47	120	18	3.99	8.37	10
	649	17	4684	17	1.51	10.75	
	Heterogeneity χ^2 (7 df)					15.05	
HLA-B8							
U.S.A.	106	25	208	17	1.63	2.91	8
U.S.A.	40	18	200	22	0.81	0.24	1
U.S.A.	237	19	200	18	1.07	0.07	7
	383	21	608	19	1.19	1.00	
	Heterogeneity χ^2 (2 df)					2.21	
Czechoslovakia	58	7	301	17	0.41	3.40	9
USSR	53	18	89	12	1.61	1.05	11
England	71	35	3000	29	1.33	1.32	4
France	49	16	152	11	1.58	1.04	5
West Germany	67	33	503	20	1.99	6.08	2
Spain	21	14	120	6	2.73	2.30	10
	702	21	4773	25	1.32	6.28	
	Heterogeneity χ^2 (8 df)					12.12	
HLA-DR5							
Canada	34	53	180	18	5.06	17.74	3
U.S.A.	145	35	95	31	1.19	0.40	7
Czechoslovakia	45	38	115	21	2.30	4.92	12
	224	38	390	22	2.05	13.69	
	Heterogeneity χ^2 (2 df)					9.37	

NR, Rosenthal FD, Sneddon IB: The association of HLA-B8 with visceral disease in systemic sclerosis. Clin Exp Immunol 31:351:356, 1978

5. Crouzet J, Marbech MC, Camus JP, Godeau P, Herreman G, Richier D, et al: Recherche d'une association entre antigenes HL-A et sclerodermie systemique. Nouv Presse Med 4:2489-2492, 1975
6. Valenta LJ, Bull RW, Hackel E, Bottazzo GF: Correlation of the HLA-A1,B8 haplotypes with circulating autoantibodies in a family with increased incidence of autoimmune disease. Acta Endocrinol 100:143-149, 1982
7. Lynch CJ, Singh G, Whitside TL, Rodnan GP, Medsger TA Jr, Rabin B: Histocompatibility antigens in progressive systemic sclerosis (PSS; scleroderma). J Clin Immunol 2:314-318, 1982
8. Birnbaum NS, Rodnan GP, Rabin BS, Bassion S: Histocompatibility antigens in progressive systemic sclerosis (scleroderma). J Rheum 4:425-428, 1977
9. Majsky A, Kobikova M, Stava Z: HLA and scleroderma. Tissue Antigens 14:359-360, 1979
10. Ercilla MG, Arriaga F, Gratacos MR, Coll J, Lecha V, Vives J, et al.: HLA antigens and scleroderma. Arch Dermatol Res 271:381-385, 1981
11. Dolbin AG, Fedorova EG, Zaretskaya YM: Antigens of the HLA system in patients with focal

TABLE 16.5. Mixed Connective Tissue Disease

	Patients		Controls				
Country/Population	n	%+	n	%+	RR	χ^2	Ref.
HLA-B7							
Japan	24	33	220	12	3.66	7.94	1
HLA-DW1							
Japan	21	33	171	14	3.08	5.28	1

sclerodermia and atrophodermia pazini-pierini. Vestn Dermatol Venerol 7:16-19, 1978
12. Niks M, Rovensky J, Nyulassy S, Buc M, Stefanovic J, Zitnan D: Lack of association of HLA-DR antigens with progressive systemic sclerosis (scleroderma). Tissue Antigens 19:238-239, 1982
13. Rabin BS, Rodnan GP, Bassion S, Gill TJ: HL-A antigens in progressive systemic sclerosis (scleroderma). Arthritis Rheum 18:381-382, 1975
14. Giordano M, Magri D, Valentini G, Tirri G, De Biasi R: HLA-SD antigens in progressive systemic sclerosis. Arch Dermatol Res 266:213, 1979
15. Lynch CJ, Singh G, Rabin BS, Rodnan GP: Histocompatibility antigens in progressive systemic sclerosis. Arthritis Rheum 23:713, 1980
16. DiBartolemeo AG, Rabin BS, Rodnan GP: HLA-D antigens in progressive systemic sclerosis (scleroderma). Immunol Commun 10:733-740, 1981
17. Whiteside TL, Medsger TA Jr, Rodnan GP: HLA-DR antigens in progresive systemic sclerosis (scleroderma). J Rheumatol 10:128-131, 1983

Mixed Connective Tissue Disease

Population Association

Sasazuki et al.[1] reported the increased frequencies of B7 and DW1 in Japanese patients (Table 16.5). The patients were diagnosed on the basis of common features of systemic lupus erythematosus, polymyositis, and progressive systemic sclerosis. Antinuclear acidic protein antibody was also present in these patients.

In this small sample the association of the disease with DW1 did not appear to be stronger than that with B7.

Reference

1. Sasazuki T, Kaneoka H, Ohta N, Hayase R, Iwamoto I: Common HLA haplotypes and their association with diseases in the Japanese population. Transplant Proc 11:1871-1873, 1979

Polymyositis

Population Association

Cumming et al.[1,2] revealed a significant association with B14 in a group of 11 English patients with polymyositis. All these patients were in clinical "group III" as defined by Walton and Adams and satisfied the stringent diagnostic criteria of Bohan and Peter (for these references see 1). The frequency of B14 was 40% in patients and 8% in the control group of unknown size.[2] In other clinical groups of patients there was no significant difference in the antigen frequencies.

In another report from Scotland,[3] 14 cases of adult polymyositis were HLA-typed and B8 was found in 9 (the report does not give any information about a control population).

DR locus antigens were studied by Hirsch et al.[4, 5] in 12 American Caucasian and 9 American Black patients and DR3 was increased in the Caucasians (Table 16.6). Seven of the 9 (78%) Black

TABLE 16.6. Polymyositis

	Patients		Controls				
Country/Population	n	%+	n	%+	RR	χ^2	Ref.
HLA-DR3							
U.S.A.	12	67	273	24	6.03	9.73	4

patients were positive for DRW6 as compared with 42 of 110 (38%) controls.

References

1. Cumming WJK, Hudgson P, Lattimer D, Sussman M, Wilcox CB: HLA and serum complement in polymyositis. Lancet ii:978-979, 1977
2. Cumming WJK, Hudgson P, Wilcox CB: HLA antigens in adult polymyositis. N Engl J Med 299:1365, 1978
3. Behan WMH, Behan PO, Dick HA: HLA-B8 in polymyositis. N Engl J Med 298:1260-1261, 1978
4. Hirsch TJ, Enlow RW, Bias WB, Arnett FC: HLA-D related (DR) antigens in polymyositis: Evidence for clinical and immunogenetic heterogeneity. Arthritis Rheum 23:689, 1980
5. Hirsch TJ, Enlow RW, Bias WB, Arnett FC: HLA-D related (DR) antigens in various kinds of myositis. Hum Immunol 3:181-186, 1981

Dermatomyositis

Population Association

In 2 small samples of American Caucasians (n = 7) and American Blacks (n = 9), typed for A, B, C, and DR antigens, no significant association was observed by Hirsch et al.[1]

Reference

1. Hirsch TJ, Enlow RW, Bias WB, Arnett FC: HLA-D related (DR) antigens in various kinds of myositis. Hum Immunol 3:181-186, 1981

Hereditary Hemorrhagic Telangiectasia

Family Data

Kissel et al.[1] published data on a large 4-generation pedigree with 6 affected individuals. The haplotype A2-B17 was found in all the patients. Only 2 unaffected individuals of the third generation had this haplotype. The authors[1] suggest that the possibility of visceral angiomatosis in these 2 individuals cannot be excluded, for it was not possible to give complete angiographic examination.

Reference

1. Kissel P, Raffoux C, Faure G, Andre J, Netter P, Streiff F: HLA antigens and hereditary hemorrhagic telangiectasia. Int Arch Allergy Appl Immunol 54:281-284, 1977

Vasculitis (Venulitis)

Population Association

Glass et al.[1] studied A and B loci antigens in 31 American Caucasian patients with cutaneous necrotizing venulitis (vasculitis). When compared with 346 controls no significant deviations in the antigen frequencies were observed. The authors, however, noted an increase in the A11-BW35 haplotype in the patient group.

Disease Heterogeneity

Patients were also divided into 2 subgroups: simple vasculitis (n = 12) and complicated vasculitis (n = 19). No significant association was observed in any of the subgroups.

See also ref. 2.

References

1. Glass D, Soter NA, Gibson D, Carpenter CB, Schur PH: Association between HLA and cutaneous necrotizing venulitis. Arthritis Rheum 19:945-949, 1976
2. Friend P, Repine JE, Kim Y, et al.: Deficiency of the second component of complement (C2) with chronic vasculitis. Ann Intern Med 83:813-816, 1975

Wegener's Granulomatosis

Population Association

The population frequency data on A and B antigens are available in 3 different studies on the Caucasian populations.[1–3] In the combined data the association with B8 was highly significant (Table 16.7).

In the British study[3] there is also an interesting increase of DR2 in the patients (Table 16.7).

References

1. Strimlan CV, Taswell HF, Kueppers F, Deremee RA, McDonald TJ: HL-A antigens of patients with Wegener's granulomatosis. Tissue Antigens 11:129-131, 1978
2. Katz P, Alling DW, Haynes BF, Fauci AS: Association of Wegener's granulomatosis with HLA-B8. Clin Immunol Immunopathol 14:268-270, 1979
3. Elkon KB, Sutherland DC, Rees AJ, Hughes GRV, Batchelor JR: HLA antigen frequencies in systemic vasculitis: Increase in HLA-DR2 in Wegener's granulomatosis. Arthritis Rheum 26:102-105, 1983

TABLE 16.7. Wegener's Granulomatosis

	Patients		Controls				
Country/Population	n	%+	n	%+	RR	χ^2	Ref.
HLA-B8							
U.S.A.	31	29	701	24	1.33	0.54	1
U.S.A.	31	39	418	19	2.75	7.22	2
	62	34	1119	22	1.94	5.97	
	Heterogeneity χ^2 (1 df)					1.79	
England	17	47	153	22	3.13	5.25	3
	79	37	1272	22	2.16	10.50	
	Heterogeneity χ^2 (2 df)					2.51	
HLA-DR2							
England	17	35	20	7	5.61	4.29	3

Polymyalgia Rheumatica

Population Association

The associations of this disease with A10, B8, and BW38 were marginally significant in the combined data on Caucasian populations and all the available data are given in Table 16.8.

Sanford and Berney[1] typed 5 American Black patients and reported an increased incidence of AW30 and BW16 in comparison with American Caucasians.

Disease Heterogeneity

Hunder et al.[2] analyzed the frequencies in the subgroups of polymyalgia rheumatica patients with temporal arteritis (n = 25) and polymyalgia rheumatica patients without temporal arteritis (n = 18) and found no evidence of association in either of the subgroups.

See also refs. 7 and 8.

References

1. Sanford RG, Berney SN: Polymyalgia rheumatica and temporal arteritis in Blacks: Clinical features and HLA typing. J Rheumatol 4:435-442, 1977
2. Hunder GG, Taswell HF, Pineda AA, Elveback LR: HLA antigens in patients with giant cell arteritis and polymyalgia rheumatica. J Rheumatol 4:321-323, 1977
3. Terasaki PI, Healey LA, Wilske KR: Distribution of HLA haplotypes in polymyalgia rheumatica. N Engl J Med 295:905, 1976
4. Hazleman B, Goldstone A, Voak D: Association of polymyalgia rheumatica and giant-cell arteritis with HLA-B8. Br Med J 2:989-991, 1977
5. Rosenthal M, Muller W, Albert ED, Schattenkirchner M: HL-A antigens in polymyalgia rheumatica. N Engl J Med 292:595, 1975
6. Seignalet J, Janbon C, Sany J, Janbom F, Bidet JM, Brunel M, et al: HLA in temporal arteritis. Tissue Antigens 9:69, 1977
7. Sany J, Seignalet J, Serre H, Lapinski H: HLA in polymyalgia rheumatica. J Rheumatol (Suppl 3):112, 1977 (Abstr)
8. Von Knorring J: Association of autoimmune diseases with HLA-B8. Br Med J 2:1354-1355, 1977

Temporal Arteritis (Giant Cell Arteritis, Horton's Disease)

Population Association

Hazleman et al.[1] reported an association with B8 in 30 patients from England (Table 16.9). However, this was not evident in 3 studies on Caucasian populations from Europe and the United States. In the combined sample the association with B8 is only marginally significant. Similarly, Seignalet et al.[2,3] observed an association of this disease with B14 in French patients but this was not confirmed in other studies. Thus, the data on A and B loci antigens did not show any strong association with this disease in Caucasians.

Table 16.8. Polymyalgia Rheumatica

Country/Population	Patients n	Patients %+	Controls n	Controls %+	RR	χ^2	Ref.
HLA-A10							
U.S.A.	25	4	701	9	0.61	0.43	2
U.S.A.	56	0	3895	12	0.06	7.34	3
	81	1	4596	12	0.28	4.56	
	Heterogeneity χ^2 (1 df)					3.21	
England	27	26	216	10	3.24	6.23	4
Switzerland	15	40	1142	12	5.00	10.32	5
	123	11	5954	12	2.06	5.90	
	Heterogeneity χ^2 (3 df)					18.41	
HLA-B8							
U.S.A.	56	20	3895	21	0.97	0.01	2
U.S.A.	25	32	701	24	1.53	1.05	3
	81	24	4596	21	1.15	0.31	
	Heterogeneity χ^2 (1 df)					0.75	
England	27	59	216	27	3.82	10.88	4
Switzerland	15	40	1142	18	3.11	5.18	5
	123	33	5954	21	1.80	8.73	
	Heterogeneity χ^2 (3 df)					8.39	
HLA-BW38							
France	50	18	300	5	4.22	10.91	6

Disease Heterogeneity

Hunder et al.[4] subdivided the 43 American Caucasian patients into the categories of temporal arteritis with polymyalgia rheumatica (n = 25) and arteritis without polymyalgia rheumatica (n = 18). No association was evident in either of the subgroups.

See also refs. 8–11.

References

1. Hazleman B, Goldstone A, Voak D: Association of polymyalgia rheumatica and giant-cell arteritis with HLA-B8. Br Med J 2:989-991, 1977
2. Seignalet J, Janbon C, Sany J, Janbom F, Bidet JM, Brunel M, et al.: HLA in temporal arteritis. Tissue Antigens 9:69, 1977

Table 16.9. Temporal Arteritis (Giant Cell Arteritis, Horton's Disease)

Country/Population	Patients n	Patients %+	Controls n	Controls %+	RR	χ^2	Ref.
HLA-B8							
U.S.A.	43	28	701	24	1.26	0.46	4
England	30	50	216	27	2.69	6.61	1
France	26	19	100	15	1.39	0.38	5
Denmark	88	32	3164	23	1.59	4.09	6
Sweden	63	22	449	24	0.91	0.08	7
	250	30	4630	23	1.45	6.55	
	Heterogeneity χ^2 (4 df)					5.06	

3. Sany J, Seignalet J, Serre H, Lapinski H: HLA in polymyalgia rheumatica. J Rheumatol (Suppl 3):112, 1977 (Abstr)
4. Hunder GG, Taswell HF, Pineda AA, Elveback LR: HLA antigens in patients with giant cell arteritis and polymyalgia rheumatica. J Rheumatol 4:321-323, 1977
5. Chaouat O, Benlahrache C, Yannoutsos H, Hoffman H, Fruchart WC, Le Parc JM, et al.: Pseudo-polyarthrite rhizomelique et maladie de Horton. Nouv Presse Med 11:101-104, 1982
6. Kemp A, Marner K, Nissen SH, Heyn J, Kissmeyer-Nielsen F: HLA antigens in cases of giant cell arteritis. Acta Ophthalmol 58:1000-1004, 1980
7. Malmvall BE, Bengtsson BA, Rydberg L: HLA antigens in patients with giant arteritis, compared with two control groups of different ages. Scand J Rheumatol 9:65-68, 1980
8. Terasaki PI, Healey LA, Wilske KR: Distribution of HLA haplotypes in polymyalgia rheumatica. N Engl J Med 295:905, 1976
9. Sanford RG, Berney SN: Polymyalgia rheumatica and temporal arteritis in Blacks: Clinical features and HLA typing. J Rheumatol 4:435-442, 1977
10. Von Knorring J: Association of autoimmune diseases with HLA-B8. Br Med J 2:1354-1355, 1977
11. Adenis JP, Bonnetblanc JM, Gualde N, Queroy M, Rammaert B: Apport de l'immunoflorescence et de la recherche des phenotypes HLA dans l'etude de la maladie de horton. Bull Soc Opthtalmol Fr 79:907-911, 1979

Takayasu's Disease

Takayasu's disease is a form of vasculitis with the characteristic feature of "pulselessness." The flow of the blood is obstructed due to stenosis of the aortic arch and/or abdominal aorta and their main branches. Patients are predominantly young females and the disease most often occurs in Asian and South American countries.

Population Association

HLA data were available only from Japan and the results from several studies (Table 16.10) showed that B5 and BW52 were associated with this disease. C locus (CW1-CW5) typing was done by Ohtawa[1]

TABLE 16.10. Takayasu's Disease

	Patients		Controls				
Country/Population	n	%+	n	%+	RR	χ^2	Ref.
HLA-B5							
Japan	15	40	113	33	1.38	0.37	1
Japan	38	66	160	32	4.03	14.03	5
Japan	18	72	553	38	3.96	7.74	6
Japan	65	63	128	32	3.56	16.33	4
Japan	27	67	84	36	3.49	7.66	7
	163	63	1038	36	3.32	42.93	
	Heterogeneity χ^2 (4 df)					3.19	
HLA-BW52							
Japan	75	44	181	16	4.08	21.37	2
Japan	18	56	553	14	7.68	19.13	6
Japan	82	44	128	13	5.14	23.55	8
	175	45	862	14	5.01	62.74	
	Heterogeneity χ^2 (2 df)					1.30	
HLA-DHO							
Japan	75	40	181	18	3.02	13.48	2
HLA-DR2							
Japan	30	77	51	35	5.85	12.46	9
Japan	9	89	44	34	10.91	8.05	6
Japan	52	46	884	36	1.52	2.19	10
	91	60	979	36	2.39	13.66	
	Heterogeneity χ^2 (2 df)					9.04	

on 15 patients and there was no difference between patients and controls.

Sasazuki et al.[2,3] determined D locus antigens in 75 patients (71 females and 4 males) by the mixed lymphocyte culture test. A significant association with a newly defined antigen, DHO, was observed in this sample (Table 16.10). However, the association with BW52 was stronger (as measured by the relative risk) than that with DHO and there was strong linkage disequilibrium between BW52 and DHO in the Japanese population.[2] Thus, the association of DHO with Takayasu's disease may be secondary to that with BW52.

DR locus antigens have also been typed in 3 studies (Table 16.10) and the frequency of DR2 appeared to be significantly increased in the patients. However, it should be noted that the estimate of relative risk for DR2 is lower than that for BW52.

Family Data

Data on 6 families have been published by Numano et al.[4] In 3 families, mother and daughters were affected. In 1 family the 2 affected sisters were identical twins and in the other the affected brother and sister were HLA-identical (2 other brothers were healthy). In the sixth family, out of 10 siblings 1 brother and 1 sister (deceased) were affected. These families were not very informative for linkage analysis.

See also ref. 11.

References

1. Ohtawa T: HLA antigens in arterial occlusive diseases in Japan. Jpn J Surg 6:1-8, 1976
2. Sasazuki T, Ohta N, Isohisa I, Mumano F, Maezawa H: Association between Takayasu disease and HLA-DHO. Tissue Antigens 14:177-178, 1979
3. Sasazuki T, Kaneoka H, Ohta N, Hayase R, Iwamoto I: Common HLA haplotypes and their association with diseases in the Japanese population. Transplant Proc 11:1871-1873, 1979
4. Numano F, Isohisa I, Maezawa H, Juji T: HL-A antigens in Takayasu's disease. Am Heart J 98:153-159, 1979
5. Naito S, Arakawa K, Saito S, Toyoda K, Takeshita A: Takayasu's disease: Association with HLA-B5. Tissue Antigens 12:143-145, 1978
6. Ohno S: Immunogenetic studies on various ocular diseases. Nippon Ganka Gakkai Zasshi 83:1875-1908, 1980
7. Naito S, Arakawa K, Kanaya H, Doi H, Sasaki Y, Sakai T, et al: HLA and cardiovascular disease. Jpn Circ J 42:1196-1199, 1978
8. Isohisa I, Numano F, Maezawa H, Sasazuki T: HLA-BW52 in Takayasu disease. Tissue Antigens 12:246-248, 1978
9. Moriuchi J, Wakisaka A, Aizawa M, Yasuda K, Yokota A, Tanabe T, et al: HLA-linked susceptibility gene of Takayasu disease. Hum Immunol 4:87-91, 1982
10. Numano F, Isohisa I, Egami M, Ohta N, Sasazuki T: HLA-DR MT and MB antigens in Takayasu disease. Tissue Antigens 21:208-212, 1983
11. Numano F, Ohta N, Sasazuki T: HLA and clinical manifestations in Takayasu disease. Jpn Circ J 46:184-189, 1982

Eosinophilic Fasciitis

Population Association

HLA-A and -B antigen frequencies in 21 American Caucasian patients studied by Lynch et al.[1] did not show any significant deviations.

Reference

1. Lynch CJ, Rodnan GP, Singh G, Scibold JR: HLA-A and B antigens in eosinophilic fasciitis. J Rheumatol 8:352-353, 1981

CREST Syndrome

Population Association

A study of A, B, C, and DR antigens in 14 American Caucasian patients with CREST syndrome (calcinosis, Raynaud's phenomenon, esophageal dysfunction, sclerodactyly, and telangiectasia) and 45 healthy controls was reported by Germain et al.[1] The authors noted an increased frequency of DR3 (57.1% in the patients vs. 17.7% in the controls). However, the difference would not be significant if the probability is multiplied by the number of antigens compared in this study.

Reference

1. Germain BF, Espinoza LR, Bergen LL, Vagesh M, Vasey FB: Increased prevalence of DRw3 in the CREST syndrome. Arthritis Rheum 24:857-859, 1981

CHAPTER 17

Pulmonary Diseases

Asthma

Population Association

Intrinsic (Nonallergic) Asthma

Brostoff et al.[1] reported that 81% of the 26 English patients studied were homozygous for W6, thus suggesting that intrinsic asthma may be a recessive disease. This was confirmed in a later study on 39 American Caucasian patients by Flaherty et al.[2] In their first study on 39 patients, Morris et al.[3] found a significant decrease in B12 but these authors were unable to confirm this in their second study in which the patients were also typed for DR locus antigens.[4]

Similar nonsignificant results were also obtained for A, B, and C loci antigens by Turton et al.[5] (see also refs. 6, 7) and Flaherty et al.[8] Thus, existing data provide no evidence for association.

Extrinsic (Allergic) Asthma

Data are available on American Caucasian,[8-10] English,[3-5,11] Danish,[12] and Indian[13] populations. There was no evidence of any HLA association in any of these studies. Two reports[4,10] also contained data on DR locus antigens. Some authors have suggested an increased frequency of haplotype A1-B8 but in the combined data there was no evidence in support of the A1-B8 haplotype association.

Family Data

Families with more than 1 member with extrinsic asthma have been HLA-typed by several authors.[5,10,11,13,14] These data do not show linkage with the HLA complex. A formal linkage analysis, however, was not done in any of these studies. We have calculated lod scores for all the families published by Rachelefsky et al.[10] There was no evidence in support of close linkage with HLA in this sample (see also ref. 15).

See also refs. 16-18.

References

1. Brostoff J, Mowbray JF, Kapoor A, Hollowell SJ, Rudolf M, Saunders KB: 80% of patients with intrinsic asthma are homozygous for HLA W6. Lancet ii:872-876, 1976
2. Flaherty DK, Geller M, Bach FH, Reed CE: Frequency of W4 and W6 antigens in perennial, nonallergic asthmatics. J Allergy Clin Immunol 60:236-237, 1977
3. Morris MJ, Vaughan H, Lane DJ, Morris PJ: HLA in asthma. Monogr Allergy 11:30-34, 1977
4. Morris MJ, Faux JA, Ting A, Morris PJ, Lane DJ: HLA-A, B and C and HLA-DR antigens in intrinsic and allergic asthma. Clin Allergy 10:173-179, 1980
5. Turton CWG, Morris L, Buckingham JA, Lawler SD, Turner-Warwick M: Histocompatibility antigens in asthma: Population and family studies. Thorax 34:670-676, 1979
6. Thorsby E, Lie SO: Relationship between the HL-A system and susceptibility to disease. Transplant Proc 3:1305-1307, 1971
7. Thorsby E, Engeset A, Lie SO: HL-A antigens and susceptibility to disease. Tissue Antigens 1:147-152, 1971
8. Flaherty DK, Geller M, Surfus JE, Leo GM, Reed CE, Rankin J: HLA antigen frequencies and natural history in Alternaria-sensitive and perennial nonallergic asthmatics. J Allergy Clin Immunol 66:408-416, 1980

9. Bruce CA, Bias WB, Norman PS, Lichtenstein LM, Marsh DG: Studies of HLA antigen frequencies, IgE levels, and specific allergic sensitivities in patients having ragweed hayfever, with and without asthma. Clin Exp Immunol 25:67-72, 1976
10. Rachelefsky G, Terasaki PI, Park MS, Katz R, Siegal S, Saito S: Strong association between B-lymphocyte group-2 specificity and asthma. Lancet ii:1042-1044, 1976
11. Gwynn CM, Mackintosh P: HLA haplotypes and hayfever: A possible protective role. Clin Allergy 9:425-427, 1979
12. Ostergaard PA, Eriksen J: Association between HLA-A1, B8 in children with extrinsic asthma and IgA deficiency. Eur J Pediatr 131:263-270, 1979
13. Dasgupta A, Misri N, Bala S: Population and family studies to demonstrate IR genes: HLA haplotype in atopic allergy. Monogr Allergy 11:75-79, 1977
14. Wagatsuma Y, Yakura H, Nakayama E, Wabisaba A, Aizawa M, Miyata M, et al: Inheritance of asthma in families and its linkage to HLA haplotypes. Acta Allergol (Kbh) 31:455-462, 1976
15. Brady RE, Glovsky MM, Opelz G, Terasaki PI, Malish DM: The association of an HLA 'asthma-associated' haplotype and immediate hypersensitivity in familial asthma. J Immunogenet 8:509-517, 1981
16. Perrin-Fayolle M, Betuel H, Biot N, Grosclaude M: Systeme HLA et atopie. Enquete systematique et familiale chez une population d'asthmatiques. Acta Allergol (Kbh) 32:222, 1977
17. Rachelefsky GS, Terasaki PI, Katz RM, Siegel SC: B lymphocyte and histocompatibility antigens in extrinsic asthma. Monogr Allergy 11:35, 1977
18. Serova LD, Uslontev BM, Mishina LV, Shabalin VN: Distribution of HLA antigens in patients with bronchial asthma. Klin Med (Mosk) 58:74-78, 1980

Emphysema

Population Association

A and B loci typing was done in 9 French patients with panlobular emphysema.[1] The authors reported no significant difference between the patients and the controls (number unknown).

Reference

1. Lochon B, Vercaigne D, Lochon C, Fiyrbuer N Martin JP, Derenne JP, et al.: Emphyseme pan-lobulaire: Relations avec le taux d'alpha 1-antitrypsine serique, le phenotype pi et le systeme HLA. Nouv Presse Med 7:1167-1170, 1978

Goodpasture's Syndrome

Population Association

Rees et al.[1] studied the frequencies of A, B, C, and DR loci antigens in 17 Caucasian patients with nephritis due to antibodies to glomerular basement membrane. The frequncies of A, B, and C loci antigens were normal. However, there was a significant association with DR2 (Table 17.1) giving a relative risk of 12.83. An increased frequency of DR2 in 8 Australian patients has also been reported by Perl et al.[2]

References

1. Rees AJ, Peters DK, Compston DAS, Batchelor JR: Strong association between HLA-DRW2 and antibody-mediated Goodpasture's syndrome. Lancet i:966-968, 1978
2. Perl SI, Pussell BA, Charlesworth JA, MacDonald GJ, Wolnizer M: Goodpasture's (anti-GBM) disease and HLA-DRW2. N Engl J Med 305:463-464, 1981

Sarcoidosis

Population Association

Caucasians

Patients with sarcoidosis have been HLA typed in Sweden,[1] Germany,[2,3] Denmark,[4] England,[5,6] United States,[7] and Turkey.[8] Only the Swedish data[1] showed an increased frequency of B7 in the patient group. However, when data from other populations were pooled, there was no evidence of an association with B7.

In 23 Turkish patients, a "significant" increase in B5 ($p < 0.01$) and A9 ($p < 0.05$) was reported by Akokan et al.[8]; no frequency data are given.

Japanese

In a study of 117 patients, Hoshino et al.[9] reported an increased frequency of B13 ($p < 0.05$). This abstract, however, does not give frequency data on patients and controls.

American Black

In 28 patients from South Carolina, B7 and BW35 were increased.[10] However, this was not confirmed

TABLE 17.1. Goodpasture's Syndrome

Country/Population	Patients n	Patients %+	Controls n	Controls %+	RR	χ^2	Ref.
HLA-DR2							
Australia	8	88	225	25	15.40	11.37	2
England	17	88	100	32	12.83	14.92	1
	25	88	325	27	13.80	26.25	
	Heterogeneity χ^2 (1 df)					0.03	

in a group of 32 patients from Los Angeles[11] and 41 from North Carolina.[12]

Disease Heterogeneity

In the Danish study,[4] there was no HLA association in the total sample of 80 patients. However, in 47 patients with negative sensitivity to tuberculin when tested for the first time after the diagnosis was made, there was a significant increase of B7 (46.8% vs. 26.8% in 1967 controls, $p = 0.003$). In the group with positive sensitivity to tuberculin (maintaining or developing a positive reaction after diagnosis), the frequency of B7 was 0 and this, compared with controls, was also significant ($p = 0.0002$). The difference between the positive and negative groups (with respect to frequency of B7) was highly significant ($p = 3 \times 10^{-6}$). There was no significant association between B7 and age at onset or duration of the disease. Neville[5] and Brewerton et al.[13] subdivided sarcoidosis patients into groups with anterior uveitis, erythema nodosum, arthritis, etc. In 11 patients with arthritis,[5] the frequency of B8 was 82%. This was a significant increase when compared with only 27% in 1300 controls ($p = 0.0004$).

Smith et al.[6] reported an association of B8 with spontaneous resolution in sarcoidosis. In 21 patients with "sarcoidosis resolved" the frequency of B8 was 57% as compared with 23% in 38 controls ($p < 0.001$).

Family Data

In 2 Swedish families typed for HLA (also mixed lymphocyte reactivity [MLR]) by Moller et al.,[14] there was no segregation of disease either with the haplotypes of A and B loci or the alleles of the D locus (MLR).

References

1. Hedfors E, Moller E: HL-A antigens in sarcoidosis. Tissue Antigens 3:95-98, 1973
2. Kueppers F, Brackertz D, Mueller-Eckhardt CH: HL-A antigens in sarcoidosis and rheumatoid arthritis. Lancet ii:1425, 1972
3. Kueppers F, Mueller-Eckhardt CH, Heinrich D, Schwab B, Brackertz D: HL-A antigens of patients with sarcoidosis. Tissue Antigens 4:56-58, 1974
4. Persson IB, Ryder LP, Staub Nielsen L, Svejgaard A: The HL-A7 histocompatibility antigen in sarcoidosis in relation to tuberculin sensitivity. Tissue Antigens 6:50-53, 1975
5. Neville E: HLA antigens and disease. Mt Sinai J Med NY 44:772-777, 1977
6. Smith MJ, Turton CWG, Mitchell DN, Turner-Warwick M, Morris LM, Lawler SD: Association of HLA B8 with spontaneous resolution in sarcoidosis. Thorax 36:296-298, 1981
7. Olenchock SA, Heise ER, Marx Jr JJ, Mentnech MS, Mull JC, Spurgeon DE, et al.: HLA-B8 in sarcoidosis. Ann Allergy 47:151-153, 1981
8. Akokan G, Celikoglu S, Goksel F, Demirci S: Antigens in Turkish patients with sarcoidosis. N Engl J Med 296:759, 1977
9. Hoshino K, Inouye H, Unokuchi T, Ito M, Tamaoki N, Tsuji K: HLA and disease in Japanese. In Dausset J, Svejgaard A (eds): HLA and Disease. De L'institut National De La Sante Et De La Recherche Medicale, Paris 1976, p 249
10. McIntyre JA, McKee KT, Loadholt CB, Mercurio S, Lim I: Increased HLA-B7 antigen frequency in South Carolina Blacks in association with sarcoidosis. Transplant Proc 9:173-176, 1977
11. Eisenberg H, Terasaki PI, Sharma OP, Mickey MR: HLA association studies in Black sarcoidosis patients. Tissue Antigens 11:484-486, 1978
12. Whitsett CF, Merritt JC, Mower P, Daffin L: HLA-A, B and DR antigens in North Carolina blacks and sarcoidosis. Tissue Antigens 21:348-350, 1983
13. Brewerton DA, Cockburn C, James DCO, James DG, Neville E: HLA antigens in sarcoidosis. Clin Exp Immunol 27:227-229, 1977
14. Moller E, Hedfors E, Wiman LG: HL-A genotypes

and MLR in familial sarcoidosis. Tissue Antigens 4:299-305, 1974

Kartagener's Syndrome

Kartagener's syndrome is a recessive hereditary disease with classic symptoms of situs inversus, bronchiectasis, and polyposis nasi.

Family Data

Rott et al.[1] described a family of 10 siblings in which 2 siblings were affected by this syndrome. The parents were first cousins and were not affected by the disease.

The 2 affected siblings had identical HLA haplotypes. None of the unaffected siblings had haplotypes identical to those of the affected ones.

Reference

1. Rott HD, Warnatz H, Pasch-Hilgers R, Weikl A: Kartagener's syndrome in sibs: Clinical and immunologic investigations. Hum Genet 43:1-11, 1978

Pulmonary Apical Fibrocystic Disease

Population Association

Kentala et al.[1] typed 7 Finnish patients for A and B loci antigens. One patient had Reiter's syndrome and a second had ankylosing spondylitis. Both of these patients had B27.

Family Data

Sharpe et al.[2] reported a pedigree with 6 affected individuals. In this pedigree, assuming a dominant disease gene with 50% penetrance, the hypothesis of linkage was almost 8 times more likely than the hypothesis of no linkage. The most probable recombination distance was 10%.[3]

References

1. Kentala E, Repo UK, Lehtipuu AL, Vuornos T: HLA-antigens and pulmonary upper lobe fibrocystic changes with and without ankylosing spondylitis. Scand J Respir Dis 59:8-12, 1978
2. Sharpe IK, Ahmad M, Braun W: Familial spontaneous pneumothorax and HLA antigens. Chest 2:264-268, 1980
3. Pierce JA, Suarez B, Reich T: More on familial spontaneous pneumothorax. Chest 2:263, 1980

CHAPTER 18

Infectious Diseases

Leprosy

Population Association

HLA association has been tested in patient populations from several countries and the results are variable and inconsistent. No specific antigen is significantly increased or decreased in all the populations. Also, the results of the studies on relatively homogeneous patient populations such as Japan[1–4] are not consistent. No single antigen was found to be associated in all these studies. Similar results were found in two reports from India[5,6]. (Indian population samples are more heterogeneous). Since complete frequency data are not available in some of the published studies, analysis of the pooled data is not possible for all the published reports.

A summary of all the interesting deviations is given in Table 18.1. It should be noted that the antigens given in this table were not found to be associated in other studies even on the patients from the same population.

B17 was increased in tuberculoid patient populations in 2 studies from Thailand. B8 was increased in all leprosy patients in 2 Japanese reports. In 2 other Japanese reports[3,4] B8 was not found to be associated with the disease (no frequency data are given).

Kriesler et al.[7] reported a significant increase of B14 in 30 patients from Spain (Table 18.1). Other associations were with B17 in Singapore Chinese[8] and with BW21 in Amhara Ethiopians.[9]

Rea and Terasaki[10] did not find any significant association in 38 Mexican patients typed for A, B, C, and DR loci antigens.

Nocera and Barocci[11] studied 32 Italian Caucasian patients. HLA-A, -B, and -C antigens were not significantly different from those in the group of 210 healthy individuals.

A list of all the reports on various patient populations is given in the bibliography. For detailed description the individual reports should be consulted.

Disease Heterogeneity

In most of the population studies listed in Table 18.1, the patients were classified into tuberculoid and lepromatous types. However, as the data in Tables 18.2 and 18.3 indicate, there was no consistent pattern of association in any specific group.

As an example, in the data of Miyanaga et al.[3] DR2 was found to be significantly increased in 54 tuberculoid leprosy patients. However, Izumi et al.[4] did not find significant association with DR2 in another independent study of Japanese patients (Table 18.2).

van Eden et al.[5] studied DR antigens in tuberculoid leprosy patients from Wardha District, Maharashtra (India). No significant deviations were found.

In another report by van Eden et al.[12] on patients from Surinam, DR3 was found to be increased in the polar tuberculoid patients.

For detailed descriptions and specific results the reader is referred to the individual report given in the bibliography.

Family Data

Family studies revealed some heterogeneity in this disease. De Vries et al.[13] studied 16 families with at

TABLE 18.1. Leprosy

Country/Population	Patients n	Patients %+	Controls n	Controls %+	RR	χ^2	Ref.
HLA-A9							
Japan	59	46	125	68	0.40	8.03	1
HLA-AW24							
Japan	59	25	125	63	0.20	21.58	1
HLA-B8							
Japan	59	10	125	1	8.48	7.42	1
Japan	60	10	184	1	9.31	9.60	2
	119	10	309	1	8.92	17.01	
	Heterogeneity χ^2 (1 df)					0.01	
HLA-B14							
Spain	30	23	149	4	6.97	11.82	7
HLA-B17							
Singapore—Chinese	77	30	238	14	2.63	9.99	8
HLA-BW21							
Ethiopia	39	26	36	0	26.46	9.33	9
HLA-BW39							
Japan	59	14	125	0	42.91	12.45	1
HLA-B40							
Thailand	36	31	150	9	4.50	11.48	20

least 2 affected siblings. The analysis of parental HLA haplotype segregation in affected siblings from sibships of different sizes was done by a method developed by these investigators. When siblings were affected with the same type of leprosy (mostly tuberculoid form), they observed a highly significant ($p < 0.005$) excess of identical HLA haplotypes. These results were confirmed in an independent study from India.[14-16]. Thirteen families with at least 2 affected siblings in the Wardha district of the state of Maharashtra (central India) were typed for HLA (A, B, C, and DR), GLO, and several other markers not located on chromosome 6. A significant excess ($p < 0.05$) of identical HLA-GLO haplotypes was observed in siblings who were affected with tuberculoid leprosy but had healthy parents.

The frequency of DR2 was significantly increased, suggesting a recessive inheritance of the disease. The segregation of other markers was as expected on the basis of Mendelian segregation ratios.

Fine et al.[17] also studied 72 families from south India (Karigiri in the state of Tamil Nadu) with at least 2 affected siblings. The analysis of the sib-pair data done by the aforementioned method of De Vries et al.[13] showed a significant excess of identical HLA haplotypes in the siblings who were affected with the tuberculoid form of the disease but had normal parents. Thus, 3 independent family studies suggest that a genetic determinant for tuberculoid leprosy is linked to the HLA locus or chromosome 6. The mode of inheritance appears to be recessive.

A formal linkage analysis of 109 published multiple case families was done by Serjeantson.[18] With the assumption of a 3-allele recessive model for susceptibility to leprosy, linkage was observed between a leprosy susceptibility locus and the HLA complex. The estimated recombination frequency was 20%. The significance of the linkage relationship was confined to families with at least 2 tuberculoid leprosy offspring and neither parent affected. When 1 parent was affected, with leprosy of any clinical type, the lod score was not significant to provide evidence for or against linkage between HLA complex and susceptibility to leprosy.

It is interesting to note that in a study on lymphoproliferative response to *Mycobacterium leprae* by Stoner et al.,[19] 7 siblings who were HLA-D iden-

TABLE 18.2. Tuberculoid Leprosy

Country/Population	Patients n	Patients %+	Controls n	Controls %+	RR	χ^2	Ref.
HLA-A2							
Thailand	26	27	183	51	0.37	5.01	21
HLA-B17							
Thailand	26	31	183	12	3.34	6.83	21
Singapore—Chinese	37	41	238	14	4.26	15.03	8
	63	37	421	13	3.87	21.69	
	Heterogeneity χ^2 (1 df)					0.17	
HLA-DR2							
Japan	28	54	55	16	5.86	12.16	4
Japan	54	65	167	39	2.86	10.76	3
	82	61	222	33	3.51	21.49	
	Heterogeneity χ^2 (1 df)					1.43	

tical to the lepromatous patients responded as well to *M. leprae* as did the 20 HLA-D nonidentical normal siblings. Thus, it may be that an HLA-linked genetic defect is not responsible for this absence of T cell reactivity in the lepromatous form of the disease. In this study there were 23 lepromatous patients and 27 normal siblings of these patients. In a sample of 27 normal siblings, the 7 siblings observed as HLA-identical to the lepromatous patients were very close to the 25% expected on the theoretical basis.

See also refs. 22–34.

References

1. Nakajima S, Kobayashi S, Nohara M, Sato S: HLA antigens and susceptibility to leprosy. Int J Lepr 45:273-277, 1977
2. Takata H, Sada M, Ozawa S, Sekiguchi S: HLA and mycobacterial infection: Increased frequency of B8 in Japanese leprosy. Tissue Antigens 11:61-64, 1978
3. Miyanaga K, Juji T, Maeda H, Nakajima S, Kobayashi S: Tuberculoid leprosy and HLA in Japanese. Tissue Antigens 18:331-334, 1981
4. Izumi S, Sugiyama K, Matsumoto Y, Ohkawa S: Analysis of the immunogenetic background of Japanese leprosy patients by HLA system. Vox Sang 42:243-247, 1982
5. van Eden W, Mehra NK, Vaidya MC, D'Amaro J, Schreuder GM Th, Van Rood JJ: HLA and sporadic tuberculoid leprosy: A population study in Maharashtra, India. Tissue Antigens 18:189-193, 1981
6. Bale UM, Mehta MM, Contractor NM, Bhatia HM, Koticha KK: HLA antigens in leprosy patients. Tissue Antigens 20:141-143, 1982
7. Kreisler M, Arnaiz A, Perez B, Fernandez Cruz E, Bootello A: HL-A antigens in leprosy. Tissue Antigens 4:197-201, 1974

TABLE 18.3. Lepromatous Leprosy

Country/Population	Patients n	Patients %+	Controls n	Controls %+	RR	χ^2	Ref.
HLA-AW19							
India	158	4	170	18	0.20	14.10	6
HLA-B7							
Thailand	70	10	183	2	5.11	7.37	21
HLA-B40							
India	158	43	170	19	3.18	21.39	6

8. Chan SH, Oon BB, Kamarudin A, Wee GB: HLA and leprosy in Chinese. Tissue Antigens 13:73-74, 1979
9. Thorsby E, Godal T, Myrvang B: HL-A antigens and susceptibility to diseases. II. Leprosy. Tissue Antigens 3:373-377, 1973
10. Rea TH, Terasaki PI: HLA-DR antigens in tuberculoid and lepromatous leprosy. Lepr Rev 51:117-123, 1980
11. Nocera A, Barocci S, Chiarla W: HLA antigens and leprosy. Int J Lepr 48:69-70, 1980
12. van Eden W, De Vries RRP, D'Amaro J, Schreuder I, Leiker DL, Van Rood JJ: HLA-DR-associated genetic control of the type of leprosy in a population from Surinam. Hum Immunol 4:343-350, 1982
13. De Vries RRP, Fat RFMLA, Nijenhuis LE, Van Rood JJ: HLA-linked genetic control of host response to mycobacterium leprae. Lancet ii:1328-1330, 1976
14. De Vries RRP, Mehra NK, Vaidya MC, Gupte MD, Khan PM, Van Rood JJ: HLA-linked control of susceptibility to tuberculoid leprosy and association with HLA-DR types. Tissue Antigens 16:294-304, 1980
15. van Eden W, De Vries RRP, Mehra NK, Vaidya MC, D'amaro J, Van Rood JJ: HLA segregation of tuberculoid leprosy: Confirmation of the DR2 marker. J Infect Diseases 141:693-701, 1980
16. De Vries RRP, Van Rood JJ, Lai A Fat FRM, Mehra NK: Is susceptibility to tuberculoid leprosy due to a recessive HLA-linked gene? In Amos DB, Schwartz RS, Janichi BW (eds): Immune Mechanisms and Disease. Academic Press, New York, 1979, pp 283-299
17. Fine PEM, Wolf E, Pritchard J, Watson B, Bradley DJ, Festenstein H, et al: HLA-linked genes and leprosy: A family study in Karigiri, South India. J Infect Dis 140:152-161, 1979
18. Serjeantson SW: HLA susceptibility to leprosy. Immunol Rev 70:89-112, 1983
19. Stoner GL, Touw J, Belehu A, Naafs B: In-vitro lymphoproliferative response to mycobacterium leprae of HLA-D-identical siblings of lepromatous leprosy patients. Lancet ii:543-547, 1978
20. Youngchaiyud U, Chandanayingyong C, Vibhatavanija T: The incidence of HLA antigens in leprosy. Vox Sang 32:342-345, 1977
21. Greiner J, Schleiermacher E, Smith T, Lenhard V, Vogel F: The HLA system and leprosy in Thailand. Hum Genet 42:201-213, 1978
22. Reis AP, Maia F, Reis VF, Andrade IM, Campos AAS: HL-A antigens in leprosy. Lancet ii:1384, 1974
23. Chiewsilp P, Athkambhira S, Chirachariyavej T, Bhamarapravati N, Entwistle C: The HLA antigens and leprosy in Thailand. Tissue Antigens 13:186-188, 1979
24. Smith GS, Walford RL, Shepard CC, Payne R, Prochazka GJ: Histocompatibility antigens in leprosy. Vox Sang 28:42-49, 1975
25. Dasgupta A, Mehra NK, Ghei SK, Vaidya MC: Histocompatibility antigens (HL-A) in leprosy. Tissue Antigens 5:85-87, 1975
26. Escobar-Gutierrez A, Gorodezky C, Salazar-Mallen M: Distribution of some of the HL-A system lymphocyte antigens in Mexicans. Vox Sang 25:151-155, 1973
27. Rea TH, Levan NE, Terasaki PI: Histocompatibility antigens in patients with leprosy. J Infect Dis 134:615-618, 1976
28. Massoud A, Nikbin B, Nazari GR, Syadat NA, Ala F: A study of cell-mediated immunity and histocompatibility antigens in leprosy patients in Iran. Int J Leprosy 46:149-153, 1978
29. Wolf E, Fine PEM, Pritchard J, Watson B, Bradley DJ, Festenstein H, et al.: HLA-A, B and C antigens in south Indian families with leprosy. Tissue Antigens 15:436-446, 1980
30. Lawrence DN, Bodmer JG, Bodmer WF: Distribution of HLA antigens in Ticuna Indians of Brazil: Results of typing a leprosy-affected family. Tissue Antigens 16:152-160, 1980
31. Garfield E: Leprosy: Down but not out. Curr Contents 23:5-12, 1980
32. Van Eden W, Elferink D, De Vries RRP: An approach to study in vitro the expression of HLA-encoded genetic factors predisposing to tuberculoid leprosy. J Immunogenet 10:107-114, 1983
33. De Vries RRP, van Eden W, Van Rood JJ: HLA-linked control of the course of *M. leprae* infections. Lepr Rev 52:109-119, 1981
34. Nath I, Van Rood JJ, Mehra NK, Vaidya MC: Natural suppressor cells in human leprosy: The role of HLA-D-identical peripheral lymphocytes and macrophages in the in vitro modulation of lymphoproliferative response. Clin Exp Immunol 42:203-210, 1980

Tuberculosis

Population Association

Caucasian

Selby et al.[1] observed a highly significant increase in the frequency of B8 (Table 18.4) in 46 Caucasian patients from Newfoundland, Canada. However, in a sample of 119 German patients, no deviations in the frequency of any antigen were observed (see studies cited in ref. 2).

Japanese
No associations with any of the HLA-A and -B loci antigens were found in 70 Japanese patients.[3]

Mexican American
One hundred Mexican American patients were typed by Cox et al.[2] for A, B, and C loci antigens. When compared with a sample of 50 controls no significant deviations were found.

American Black
Al-Arif et al.[4] typed 60 American Black tuberculosis patients for A and B loci antigens. B15 was significantly increased, giving a relative risk of 7.18 (Table 18.4).

Bf Locus
In the Newfoundland study, the patients were also typed for the alleles at the Bf locus. No deviations in the frequencies of any of the alleles were observed.[1]

Disease Heterogeneity

In the American Black patients,[4] clinical manifestations of tuberculosis were also compared in B15-positive and B15-negative patients. Of 12 patients positive for B15, all had cavitation and 9 (75%) had extrapulmonary involvement. In the 48 patients negative for B15, 15 (31%) had cavitation and 7 (15%) had extrapulmonary involvement. Thus, the patients with B15 had significantly more advanced disease with cavitation and more extrapulmonary involvement.

References

1. Selby R, Barnard JM, Buehler SK, Crumley J, Larsen B, Marshall WH: Tuberculosis associated with HLA-B8, BfS in a Newfoundland community study. Tissue Antigens 11:403-408, 1978
2. Cox RA, Arnold DR, Cook D, Lundberg DI: HLA phenotypes in Mexican Americans with tuberculosis. Am Rev Respir Dis 126:653-655, 1982
3. Takata H, Sada M, Ozawa S, Sekiguchi S: HLA and mycobacterial infection: Increased frequency of B8 in Japanese leprosy. Tissue Antigens 11:61-64, 1978
4. Al-Arif LI, Goldstein RA, Affronti LF, Janicki BW: HLA-BW15 and tuberculosis in a North American Black population. Am Rev Respir Dis 120:1275-1278, 1979

Syphilis

Population Association

In a study of 148 unrelated Chinese female prostitutes from Singapore, Chan et al.[1] divided the total sample into 4 groups: (1) 56 patients with repeated gonococcal infections (see below); (2) 31 patients with latent syphilis who had been treated and at the time of study had no symptoms or signs of infection; (3) 31 patients with combined (syphilis and gonorrhea) infections; and (4) 30 patients who had been exposed to gonorrhea and syphilis for at least 1 year but were resistant to infection.

When compared with 238 controls, the frequency of BW46 in group 3 was 38.7% vs. 22.7% in the controls. A2 was lower in group 4 (30% vs. 52.9% in controls). These differences, however, were not significant with correction for the number of comparisons.

The authors also noted the increased frequency of the AW19-B17 haplotype in group 3 (25.8% in patients vs. 6.7% in 238 controls, $\chi^2 = 12.29$).

Reference

1. Chan SH, Tan T, Kamarudin A, Wee GB, Rajan VS: HLA and sexually transmitted diseases in prostitutes. Br J Vener Dis 55:207-210, 1979

TABLE 18.4. Tuberculosis

	Patients		Controls				
Country/Population	n	%+	n	%+	RR	χ^2	Ref.
HLA-B8							
Canada	46	57	543	20	5.25	28.57	1
HLA-B15							
U.S.A.—Black	60	20	100	3	7.18	10.87	4

Gonorrhea

Population Association

The only data available are on 148 Chinese female prostitutes from Singapore[1] discussed in the preceding section (Syphilis).

There was no difference in the HLA frequencies in the group of 56 patients with only gonococcal infections. As mentioned in the section on Syphilis, the frequency of BW46 was higher in the 31 patients with combined infections (gonorrhea and syphilis) and A2 was lower in the group of 30 patients with resistance to both diseases. The AW19-B17 haplotype was increased in 31 patients with combined infections (group 3).

Reference

1. Chan SH, Tan T, Kamarudin A, Wee GB, Rajan VS: HLA and sexually transmitted diseases in prostitutes. Br J Vener Dis 55:207-210, 1979

Venereal Urethritis

Population Association

Keat et al.[1] studied 482 heterosexual men with new episodes of nonspecific urethritis. This diagnosis was determined if more than 10 polymorphs were found in at least 3 consecutive highpower fields (magnification × 600) on a urethral smear, provided that microscopy, culture, and serology excluded gonorrhea and syphillis.

The frequency of B27 in this group of patients was 6.2%, not significantly different from that found in the healthy population. The data on other antigens were not given.

Reference

1. Keat AC, Maini RN, Nkwazi GC, Pegrum GD, Ridgway GL, Scott JT: Role of *Chlamydia trachomatis* and HLA-B27 in sexually acquired reactive arthritis. Br Med J 1:605-607, 1978

Urethritis (Nonspecific and Nongonococcal)

Population Association

In England, Brewerton et al.[1] compared 33 nonspecific urethritis patients (6 with recurrent attacks and 27 seen during their first attack) and 33 controls. No difference in HLA frequencies was found.

Lange and Muller[2] also studied 16 patients with recurrent nongonococcal urethritis and 413 German controls and observed no difference.

Wahlby et al.[3] typed 79 women with urethritis for the antigens of A and B loci. When the frequencies were compared with 692 controls no significant difference was found.

References

1. Brewerton DA, Caffrey M, Nicholls A, Wlaters D, Oates JK, James DCO: Reiter's disease and HL-A27. Lancet ii:996-997, 1973
2. Lange CE, Muller N: HLA-B27 bei Morbus reiter unter besonderer berucksichtigung oligosymptomatischer Verlaufsformen. Z Hautkr 52:1153-1159, 1977
3. Wahlby L, Cedergren B, Lindqvist B, Segerbrand E: HLA and urethritis. Tissue Antigens 15:210-211, 1980

Presumed Ocular Histoplasmosis

Population Association

Two groups of American workers, Meredith et al.[1,2,3,4] and Godfrey et al.[5,6] published several reports (with overlapping data) showing a significant association with HLA-B7 (Table 18.5). DR typing of 1 group of patients[2,3] also indicated a significant association with DR2 (Table 18.5). It is interesting to note that in data from the Netherlands[7] on a sample of 20 patients with juvenile disciform maculopathy, which clinically cannot be differentiated from presumed ocular histoplasmosis, the association with B7 was observed (Table 18.5). These authors noted an increase in B15 (40% in patients vs. 15.7% in 4000 controls, $\chi^2 = 7.76$).

Disease Heterogeneity

Meredith et al.[4] studied 15 presumed ocular histoplasmosis patients with peripheral atrophic scars and found no significant difference in the frequency of B7 (compared with normal controls). The patients with macular or peripapillary hemorrhagic lesions showed a highly significant association with B7.

Godfrey et al.[5,6] found no significant difference between B7-positive and -negative patients with re-

TABLE 18.5. Presumed Ocular Histoplasmosis

Country/Population	Patients n	Patients %+	Controls n	Controls %+	RR	χ^2	Ref.
HLA-B7							
U.S.A.	26	77	3240	26	9.01	25.11	3
U.S.A.	64	53	295	21	4.21	25.51	6
	90	60	3535	26	5.27	48.51	
	Heterogeneity χ^2 (1 df)					2.12	
BENELUX	20	35	4000	29	1.36	0.48	7
	110	55	7535	27	3.89	41.77	
	Heterogeneity χ^2 (2 df)					9.33	
HLA-DR2							
U.S.A.	26	81	3240	28	10.19	25.04	3

spect to age at onset, sex, and serologic positivity for histoplasmosis.

References

1. Braley RE, Meredith TA, Aaberg TM, Koethe SM, Witkowski JA: The prevalence of HLA-B7 in presumed ocular histoplasmosis. Am J Ophthalmol 85:859-861, 1978
2. Duquesnoy RJ, Annen K, Meredith TA: Association of presumed ocular histoplasmosis with HLA-B7 and DRW2. Transplant Proc 11:1877-1878, 1979
3. Meredith TA, Smith RE, Duquesnoy RJ: Association of HLA-DRW2 antigen with presumed ocular histoplasmosis. Am J Ophthalmol 89:70-76, 1980
4. Meredith TA, Smith RE, Braley RE, Witkowski JA, Koethe SM: The prevalence of HLA-B7 in presumed ocular histoplasmosis in patients with peripheral atrophic scars. Am J Ophthalmol 86:325-328, 1978
5. Godfrey WA, Sabates R, Cross DE: Association of presumed ocular histoplasmosis with HLA-B7. Am J Ophthalmol 85:854-858, 1978
6. Godfrey WA, Cross DE, Ziemianski MC, Sabates R: HLA-B7 in presumed ocular histoplasmosis maculopathy. Transplant Proc 11:1874-1875, 1979
7. Craandijk A, Schreuder GMT: Association of juvenile disciform maculopathy with HLA B15. Br J Ophthalmol 63:678-679, 1979

Tetanus

Population Association

The only data available are for 154 patients from Bombay, India.[1] The patients and 118 normal controls were typed for 27 A and B loci specificities. The frequency of B7 was 12.99% and 25.42% in patients and controls, respectively ($p < 0.01$). However, this is not significant after correction for multiple comparisons.

Disease Heterogeneity

The Indian patients were also divided into groups with mild, moderate, and severe disease conditions. No significant association with any of these groups was found; the frequency of B7 was low in all 3 categories.

See also ref. 2.

References

1. Bale UM, Mehta MM, Contractor NM, Bhatia HM, Dastur FD: HLA antigens and E-rosettes in tetanus patients. Tissue Antigens 16:181-186, 1980
2. Repo H, Leirsalo M, Laitenen O: A contribution to immunopathogenesis of B27-associated diseases. Scand J Rheumatol 42:12, 1982

Mononucleosis

Population Association

In 1971 Morris and Forbes[1] reported an increased frequency of BW35 (W5) in 40 Australian patients. Later studies by Schiller and Davey[2,3] on 40 American Caucasian, by Ting et al.[4] on 110 Australian, by Rosdahl and Svejgaard,[5] and Ythier et al.[6] on 116 Danish patients did not confirm this association. However, in the combined data the association with BW35 appeared to be significant with a χ^2 of 9.18 (Table 18.6).

See also ref. 7.

References

1. Morris PJ, Forbes JF: HL-A in follicular lymphoma, reticulum cell sarcoma, lymphosarcoma, and infectious mononucleosis. Transplant Proc 3:1315-1316, 1971
2. Schiller J, Davey FR: HL-A antigens and infectious mononucleosis. Lancet ii:1500, 1973
3. Schiller J, Davey FR: Human leukocyte locus (HL-A) antigens and infectious mononucleosis. Am J Clin Pathol 62:325-328, 1974
4. Ting A, Mackay LR, Morris PJ: HL-A in autoimmune diseases and infectious mononucleosis. Symp Ser Immunobiol Standard 18:276-281, 1973
5. Rosdahl N, Svejgaard A: HLA types and ABO blood groups in patients with infectious mononucleosis. Tissue Antigens 13:223-227, 1979
6. Ythier A, Moreau JF, Peyrat MA, Bignon JD, Soulillou JP: HLA-AB and -DR types in patients with infectious mononucleosis (IM). Tissue Antigens 21:329-332, 1983
7. Edmond E, Steel CM, Ennis M, Cameron F, Dick H: HLA antigens in adults negative for antibody to Epstein-Barr virus (EBV). Tissue Antigens 18:252-257, 1981

Congenital Rubella

Population Association

Honeyman et al.[1] studied the HLA-A and -B types of 87 (53 adults and 34 children) congenital rubella subjects (Caucasians) from Australia. The frequency of A1 was somewhat increased (nonsignificant) in the total sample.

The correlation coefficients were also calculated between seropositivity to rubella virus in young adults (i.e., percentage of the population between 20 and 30 years showing serologic evidence of past rubella infection) and the gene frequency of various HLA-A and B loci alleles in that population. The authors analyzed data from several countries. There was a significant correlation between A1, A3, and B8 and the percentage of the population seropositive for rubella. The highest correlation coefficients were for A1 (0.71), B8 (0.60), and A1-B8 (0.68).

Disease Heterogeneity

The antigen frequency data were also analyzed separately for adults and children and for males and females within each subgroup. The frequency of A1 in 30 adult female subjects was 63.6% as compared with 32.0% in 983 controls (corrected $p < 0.02$). No other significant difference was found.

Reference

1. Honeyman MC, Dorman DC, Menser MA, Forrest JM, Guinan JJ, Clark P: HL-A antigens in congenital rubella and the role of antigens 1 and 8 in the epidemiology of natural rubella. Tissue Antigens 5:12-18, 1975

Aseptic Meningitis

Population Association

Fryden et al.[1] studied 26 Swedish patients who had aseptic meningitis with oligoclonal Ig in cerebrospinal fluid (CSF) but not in the serum. The patients and 135 controls were typed for A, B, and D loci antigens. They found no difference in frequencies, especially of A3, B7, and DW2, between patients and controls.

Reference

1. Fryden A, Moller E, Link H: No association between oligoclonal immunoglobulins in cerebrospinal fluid and HLA antigens in acute aseptic meningitis. Neurology 29:1422-1423, 1979

Paralytic Poliomyelitis

Population Association

The first reports by Morris and Pietsch in 1973[1,2] on 111 Australian patients and 395 controls showed a significant positive association with A3 and B7 antigens. In a later study on 62 German[3] patients, this association was not confirmed. Moreover, in these data the frequencies of A3 and B7 in the patients were lower than that in the controls.

In the German study,[3] patients were also typed for D locus specificities and again no association was found.

In 58 Arab children from the Gaza strip with paralytic poliomyelitis[4] and 113 controls, an in-

TABLE 18.6. Mononucleosis

	Patients		Controls				
Country/Population	n	%+	n	%+	RR	χ^2	Ref.
HLA-BW35							
U.S.A.	40	3	32	3	0.93	0.00	3
Australia	40	33	273	12	3.63	11.87	1
Australia	110	17	200	12	1.51	1.57	4
	150	21	473	12	2.21	10.31	
	Heterogeneity χ^2 (1 df)					3.13	
France	48	20	284	12	1.88	2.62	6
Denmark	68	15	3301	15	1.04	0.01	5
	306	17	4090	14	1.69	9.18	
	Heterogeneity χ^2 (4 df)					6.89	

creased frequency of B7 and decreased frequencies of A11, B12, and B13 were noted. None of these deviations, however, was statistically significant.

See also ref. 5.

Family Data

van Eden et al.[6] reported HLA data in 17 families. In sib pairs consisting of a patient with paralytic poliomyelitis and a nonparalytic control sibling, significantly less sharing of HLA haplotypes was observed than would be expected by chance alone ($p = 0.014$). The sharing of haplotypes between patients with nonparalytic poliomyelitis and healthy controls did not deviate significantly from the expected value. On the basis of these results the authors suggested the involvement of HLA-encoded genetic factors in the control of resistance to the paralytic form of poliomyelitis.

References

1. Morris P, Pietsch MC: A possible association between paralytic poliomyelitis and multiple sclerosis. Lancet ii:847-848, 1973
2. Pietsch MC, Morris PJ: An association of HL-A3 and HL-A7 with paralytic poliomyelitis. Tissue Antigens 4:50-55, 1974
3. Zander H, Grosse-Wilde H, Kuntz B, Scholz S, Albert ED: HLA-A, -B, and -D antigens in paralytic poliomyelitis. Tissue Antigens 13:310-313, 1979
4. Lasch EE, Joshua H, Gazit E, El-Massri M, Marcus O, Zamir R: Study of the HLA antigen in Arab children with paralytic poliomyelitis. Isr J Med Sci 15:12-13, 1979
5. Steigman AJ: HL-A types and paralytic poliomyelitis. Lancet ii:1383, 1973
6. van Eden W, Persijn GG, Bijkerk H, De Vries RRP, Schuurman RKB, Van Rood JJ: Differential resistance to paralytic poliomyelitis controlled by histocompatibility leukocyte antigens. J Infect Dis 147:422-426, 1983

Hemophilus Influenza Type B Infection

Population Association

In a study of 65 American Caucasian patients (30 with epiglottitis and 35 with meningitis) and 451 controls,[1] no striking association was reported. The frequency of B17 was 3.2% in controls and 12% in the total patient group (10% in epiglottitis and 6% in meningitis). AW28 was also increased in the patients (6.2% in controls vs. 17% in the total patient group; 20% in epiglottitis and 14% in meningitis).

In another study of 50 patients from New York by Tejani et al.[2,3] increased (nonsignificant) frequency of B12 has been reported.

Disease Heterogeneity

In the study on 65 American Caucasian patients,[1] epiglottitis (n = 30) and meningitis (n = 35) patients were also compared separately with the controls. There was no evidence of significant heterogeneity.

See also refs. 4–6.

References

1. Robbins JB, Schneerson R, Argaman M, Handzel ZT: Haemophilus influenzae type B: Disease and immunity in humans. Ann Intern Med 78:259-269, 1973
2. Tejani A, Fotino M, Khan R, Dobias B, Nangia B: HLA and hemophilus influenzae disease. Tissue Antigens 9:132, 1977
3. Tejani A, Mahadevan R, Dobias B, Nangia B, Weiner M: Occurrence of HLA types in *H. influenzae* type B disease. Tissue Antigens 17:205-211, 1981
4. Biddison WE, Payne SM, Shearer GM, Shaw S: Human cytotoxic T cell responses to trinitrophenyl hapten and influenza virus. Diversity of restriction antigens and specificity of HLA-linked genetic regulation. J Exp Med 152:204s-217s, 1980
5. Biddison WE, Kostyu DD, Strominger JL, Krangel MS: Delineation of immunologically and biochemically distinct HLA-A2 antigens. J Immunol 129:730-734, 1982
6. Aho K, Pyhala R, Visakorpi R: ABO associated genetic determinant in H1N1 influenza. Tissue Antigens 16:310-313, 1980

Recurrent Herpes Labialis

Population Association

In 1975, Russel and Schlaut[1] typed 90 Caucasian patients with recrudescent circumoral herpes (herpes simplex type 1). When the frequencies were compared with those of 606 controls, A1, A10, A29, and B8 were significantly increased. The same in-

TABLE 18.7. Recurrent Herpes Labialis

	Patients		Controls				
Country/Population	n	%+	n	%+	RR	χ^2	Ref.
HLA-A1							
Canada	260	50	606	25	2.99	50.05	2
Switzerland	21	19	52	25	0.75	0.23	3
Ireland	29	48	200	43	1.23	0.28	4
Norway	50	28	31	36	0.69	0.60	6
	360	45	889	29	2.23	35.68	
	Heterogeneity χ^2 (3 df)					15.48	
HLA-A10							
Canada	260	4	606	11	0.35	10.16	2
Switzerland	21	0	52	6	0.32	1.01	3
Ireland	29	10	200	10	1.13	0.04	4
Norway	50	6	31	16	0.36	2.22	6
	360	5	889	11	0.44	10.22	
	Heterogeneity χ^2 (3 df)					3.20	
HLA-A29							
Canada	260	14	606	5	3.08	19.51	2
Switzerland	21	5	52	10	0.63	0.30	3
Ireland	29	10	200	8	1.43	0.36	4
Norway	50	0	31	4	0.17	2.07	6
	360	11	889	6	2.26	13.46	
	Heterogeneity χ^2 (3 df)					8.77	
HLA-B8							
Canada	260	29	606	17	1.99	15.84	2
Switzerland	21	10	52	15	0.72	0.21	3
Ireland	29	38	200	35	1.15	0.13	4
Norway	50	24	31	27	0.85	0.11	6
	360	28	889	21	1.64	11.18	
	Heterogeneity χ^2 (3 df)					5.12	

vestigators later prospectively studied 210 new patients and found that the frequency of A1 was again increased.[2] The results of the significant associations in the combined sample from all the available studies are given in the Table 18.7.

It should be noted that a significant association with A9 observed in the data of Legendre et al.[3] was not found in the combined analysis. The results were also nonsignificant for B15 reported by Middleton et al.[4]

Family Data

England and Tait[5] published a 3-generation pedigree with 6 individuals with recurrent herpes simplex infection. The disease appeared to segregate with a particular haplotype. The complete HLA typing of the pedigree, however, is not given.

Berle[6] studied 5 families where 1 parent and 2 or more children were affected by recurrent herpes labialis. This data did not reveal strong evidence of linkage with HLA complex.

See also refs. 7–11.

References

1. Russell AS, Schlaut J: HL-A transplantation antigens in subjects susceptible to recrudescent herpes labialis. Tissue Antigens 6:257-261, 1975
2. Russell AS, Schlaut J: Association of HLA-A1 antigens and susceptibility to recurrent cold sores. Arch Dermatol 113:1721-1722, 1977
3. Legendre C, Russell AS, Jeannet M: HLA antigens in patients with recrudescent herpes simplex infections. Tissue Antigens 19:85-89, 1982
4. Middleton D, Hutchison TH, Lynd J: HLA antigen frequency in erythema multiforme and in recurrent herpes simplex. Tissue Antigens 21:264-267, 1983
5. England JF, Tait B: HLA and herpes simplex. Med J Aust 1:464, 1977
6. Berle EJ Jr: Recurrent herpes labialis and HLA. In Terasaki PI: Histocompatibility Testing 1980. UCLA Tissue Typing Laboratory, Los Angeles, 1981, p 718
7. Fabiani G, Ruffault A, Fauconnier B, Genetet B, Fauchet R, et al.: Association d'une infection herpetique latente avec les antigenes HLA-A2, B12, et BW35 chez des malades atteints d'insuffisance renale chronique. Nouv Presse Med 6:3437, 1977
8. Ruffault A, Fauconnier B, Fauchet R, Genetet B: Relations entre les antigenes HLA A2, A3 et B12, ainsi que l'association haplotypique presumee A2-B12 et une infection herpetique. Pathol Biol 27:293-296, 1979
9. Berle EJ, Thorsby E: The proliferative T cell response to herpes simplex virus (HSV) antigen is restricted by self HLA-D. Clin Exp Immunol 39:668-675, 1980
10. Blackwelder WC, Dolin R, Mittal KK, McNamara PM, Payne FJ: A population study of herpesvirus infections and HLA antigens. Am J Epidemiol 115:569-572, 1982
11. Stewart GJ, Kelsall BL, Charron DJ, Grumet FC, Merigan T: The role of HLA-DR determinants in monocyte-macrophage presentation of herpes simplex virus antigen to human T cells. Cell Immunol 61:11-21, 1981

Recurrent Corneal Herpes (Herpetic Keratitis)

Population Association

A first report by Zimmerman et al.[1] on 46 American Caucasian patients showed an increased frequency

TABLE 18.8. Recurrent Corneal Herpes (Herpetic Keratitis)

	Patients		Controls				
Country/Population	n	%+	n	%+	RR	χ^2	Ref.
HLA-B5							
U.S.A.	48	15	545	13	1.24	0.29	3
U.S.A.	46	26	282	11	2.88	7.93	1
	94	20	827	12	1.95	5.88	
	Heterogeneity χ^2 (1 df)					2.34	
Denmark	37	22	2865	10	2.64	6.44	3
	131	21	3692	11	2.16	11.90	
	Heterogeneity χ^2 (2 df)					2.76	

TABLE 18.9. Recurrent Herpes Progenitalis (HSV-2)

Country/Population	Patients n	Patients %+	Controls n	Controls %+	RR	χ^2	Ref.
HLA-DR7							
U.S.A.	87	37	218	22	2.08	7.22	1

of B5 (Table 18.8). However, in a later study on the same population by Meyers-Elliott et al.,[2] this deviation was not seen. In the combined data analyses, the difference was significant enough to be considered interesting for other followup studies. In a third paper on 37 patients and 2860 normal controls from Denmark,[3] the increased frequency of B5 was again significant (Table 18.8). In the pooled analysis of all 3 samples, there is a significant association with B5 and no evidence of heterogeneity in the data.

References

1. Zimmerman TJ, McNeill JI, Richman A, Kaufman HE, Waltman SR: HLA types and recurrent corneal herpes simplex infection. Invest Ophthalmol Vis Sci 16:756-757, 1977
2. Meyers-Elliott RH, Elliott JH, Maxwell WA, Pettit TH, O'Day DM, Terasaki PI, et al: HLA antigens in recurrent stromal herpes simplex virus keratitis. Am J Ophthalmol 89:54-57, 1980
3. Damgaard-Jensen L, Ehlers N, Kissmeyer-Nielsen F: HLA types in corneal disease. Acta Ophthalmol 57:982-985, 1979

Recurrent Herpes Progenitalis (HSV-2)

Population Association

Ahmed et al[1] reported an increased frequency of DR7 in 87 American Caucasian male patients (Table 18.9).

Reference

1. Ahmed AR, Strom H, Bierman S, Myers-Elliot R, Tiwari J, Terasaki PI: A study of HLA and DRw antigens in severe recurrent herpes progenitalis (HSV-2) infection. Am Acad Dermatol 6:898-901, 1982

Chronic Brucellosis

Population Association

Sixty-three male and 5 female Hungarian patients were studied by Hodinka et al.[1] There was an increased frequency of B27 (Table 18.10).

Disease Heterogeneity

There were 27 patients (39%) with a history of exudative arthritis, severe back pain, or clinical signs of arthritis or painful and limited spine movements with a tenderness of the dorsolumbar vertebrae and sacroiliac joints. This group also had radiologic evidence of sacroiliitis or osteochondritis of the dorsal vertebrae. The frequency of B27 in this group was 44% as compared with 12% in the remaining 41 patients who did not have the above symptoms ($p < 0.01$) (See also ref. 2).

References

1. Hodinka L, Gomor B, Meretey K, Zahumansky Z, Geher P, Telegdy L, et al: HLA-B27-associated spondylarthritis in chronic brucellosis. Lancet i:499, 1978

TABLE 18.10. Chronic Brucellosis

Country/Population	Patients n	Patients %+	Controls n	Controls %+	RR	χ^2	Ref.
HLA-B27							
Hungary	68	25	352	13	2.25	6.64	1

2. Hodinka L, Geher P, Meretey K, Gyodi EK, Petranyi GG, Bozsoky S: Lavamisole-induced neutropenia and agranulocytosis: Association of HLA B27 leukocyte agglutinating and lymphocytotoxic antibodies. Int Arch Allergy Appl Immunol 65:460-464, 1981

Infection by *Schistosoma Mansoni*

Population Association

Salam et al.[1] studied 51 Egyptian children from the northern part of the Nile Delta who were infected with *S. mansoni*. The authors did not use normal control frequencies for comparisons and thus the nature of HLA association in the total sample is not clear. However, when comparisons were made between the groups with and without hepatomegaly and splenomegaly, the frequencies of A1 and B5 were significantly increased in the groups with hepatomegaly and splenomegaly (Table 18.11).

Disease Heterogeneity

Most individuals infected with *S. mansoni* do not show any apparent disease symptoms. Hepatomegaly and splenomegaly occur in only a small proportion of the infected individuals. Thus, the significant increase of A1 and B5 in this subgroup of individuals is very interesting.

The authors further subdivided the patients into groups according to the degree of hepatomegaly. In 23 individuals negative for A1 and B5, only 3 (13%) had mild hepatomegaly and 20 (87%) showed no liver enlargement. Of 8 children positive for A1 (and negative for B5), 6 had mild and 1 had moderate/severe hepatomegaly. Similarly, there were 11 B5-positive and A1-negative children and, in this group, 9 had mild hepatomegaly. All 9 individuals positive for both A1 and B5 had moderate/severe hepatomegaly. Thus, there is some indication that severity of the hepatomegaly may be associated with A1 and/or B5. It should be stressed that the sample is small and thus the results need confirmation in other independent studies.

Reference

1. Salam EA, Ishaac S, Mahmoud AF: Histocompatibility-linked susceptibility for hepatosplenomegaly in human schistosomiasis mansoni. J Immunol 123:1829-1831, 1979

Vogt-Koyanagi-Harada Syndrome

Population Association

In a study of A, B, and D loci antigens in Japanese patients, Tagawa et al.[1-3] reported significant associations with BW54 and DW-Wa (a new D locus antigen). As the data in Table 18.12 indicate the association of the disease with antigen Wa was stronger than that with BW54. Tagawa's[2] data on some additional Japanese patients (a total of 65 for A and B antigens and 42 for Wa) confirmed these results.

Ohno[4] reported a significant association with DR4 antigen (Table 18.12).

Ohno et al.[5] HLA typed 9 patients (7 American Caucasians and 2 Orientals; no Japanese). These patients were also typed with antisera of Tagawa et al.[1-3] recognizing BW54. In this small sample there was no HLA association, especially with BW54. It may be that association is not the same in different ethnic groups (see also ref. 6).

Richard et al.[7] tested 8 German patients for the antigens of A and B loci. None of the patients in this sample was positive for B12.

Disease Heterogeneity

BW54 was not present in 7 American Caucasian and 2 non-Japanese Oriental patients (see ref. 5 and discussion in section on Population Association, above).

See also ref. 9.

References

1. Tagawa Y, Sugiura S, Yakura H, Wakasaba A, Aizawa M: HLA and Vogt-Koyanagi-Harada syndrome. N Engl J Med 295:173, 1976

2. Tagawa Y: Study on HLA antigens in Vogt-Koyanagi-Harada disease. Nippon Ganka Gakkai Zasshi 83:162-166, 1979

3. Tagawa Y, Sugiura S, Yakura H, Wakisaka A, Aizawa M, Itakura K: The association between major histocompatibility antigens (HLA) and Vogt-Koyanagi-Harada syndrome. Nippon Ganka Gakkai Zasshi 80:486-490, 1976

4. Ohno S: Immunogenetic studies on various ocular

TABLE 18.11. HLA-A1 and B5 in 51 Egyptian School Children with *Schistosoma Mansoni* Infection

	A1		B5	
	+	−	−	+
With hepatomegaly	16 (57%)	12 (43%)	18 (64%)	10 (36%)
Without hepatomegaly	1 (4%)	22 (96%)	2 (9%)	21 (91%)
χ^2	13.55		14.72	
With splenomegaly	11 (85%)	2 (15%)	10 (77%)	3 (23%)
Without splenomegaly	5 (13%)	33 (87%)	8 (21%)	30 (79%)
χ^2	19.77		10.91	

diseases. Nippon Ganka Gakkai Zasshi 83:1875-1908, 1980
5. Ohno S, Char DH, Kimura SJ, O'Connor GR: HLA and Vogt-Koyanagi-Harada syndrome. N Engl J Med 294:788, 1976
6. Crews SJ, Mackintosh P, Barry DR, Willshaw HE: HLA antigens and certain types of uveitis. Trans Ophthalmol Soc UK 99:156-159, 1979
7. Richard G, Dieckhues B, Junemann G: Immunological examinations in Vogt-Koyanagi-Harada disease. Albrect Von Graefes Arch Klin Exp Ophthalmol 217:325-330, 1981
8. Yakura H, Wakisaka A, Aizawa M, Itabura K, Tagawa Y, Sugiura S: HLA-D antigens of Japanese origin (LD-WA) and its association with Vogt-Koyanagi-Harada syndrome. Tissue Antigens 8:35-42, 1976
9. Sugiura S, Sanefuji M, Ohno S: Immunological studies on Behçet's and Harada's diseases. Mod Probl Ophthalmol 16:267-278, 1976

Healthy Hepatitis B Surface Antigen Carriers

Population Association

Caucasians

Giani et al.[1] reported a significant increase of B15 in healthy HBsAg carriers. Similar results were obtained by Jeannet and Farquet.[2] A combined analysis of these and 3 other reports[3-5] in which B15 frequency data are available is given in the Table 18.13. In the pooled data, B15 seemed to be associated with HBsAg carrier status. However, there was also indication of heterogeneity in this data.

It should be noted that in the data of Sampliner et al.[5] a significant decrease of B7 in the patients was observed (0% in 33 patients vs. 24.23% in 1391 controls, corrected $p \sim 0.006$).

Carbonara et al.[6] reported an association with B40 in 24 carriers from Sardinia (Table 18.13). This re-

TABLE 18.12. Vogt-Koyanagi-Harada Syndrome

	Patients		Controls				
Country/Population	n	%+	n	%+	RR	χ^2	Ref.
HLA-BW54							
Japan	72	36	130	14	3.41	12.59	4
Japan	35	43	76	13	4.88	11.59	1
	107	38	206	14	3.87	23.79	
	Heterogeneity χ^2 (1 df)					0.38	
HLA-DW-Wa							
Japan	42	67	81	16	10.16	28.62	4
Japan	33	67	81	16	10.11	25.07	8
	75	67	162	16	10.13	53.69	
	Heterogeneity χ^2 (1 df)					0.00	
HLA-DR4							
Japan	33	88	74	32	13.92	23.51	4

TABLE 18.13. Healthy Hepatitis B Surface Antigen Carriers

	Patients		Controls				
Country/Population	n	%+	n	%+	RR	χ^2	Ref.
HLA-B15							
U.S.A.	33	12	1391	8	1.73	1.23	5
Czechoslovakia	75	9	301	13	0.70	0.75	4
Hungary	83	11	175	8	1.44	0.73	3
Italy	24	33	824	8	5.80	16.53	1
Switzerland	98	19	500	8	2.72	11.14	2
	313	15	3191	8	2.04	16.17	
	Heterogeneity χ^2 (4 df)					14.20	
HLA-B40							
Sardinia	24	17	405	3	6.97	11.67	6

port does not give frequencies of other antigens, however. An analysis of the data subdivided by sex also showed a decrease of DR4 in females (0% in 14 females vs. 29.4% in 405 controls; $p = 0.0003$).

In 41 individuals from Chile,[7] 66 from France,[8] and 48 from Belgium,[9] no significant association with any HLA antigen was found (in these 3 studies, the frequency data for B15 were not available).

Mongoloids
No association in Japanese[10,11] and Thai[12] populations has been observed.

American Black
Sampliner et al.[5] typed 32 American Blacks for A and B loci antigens. When the antigen frequencies were compared with those in 346 controls, no significant deviations were found.

Family Data

Majsky et al.[4] studied 11 families with at least 2 HBsAg carriers in each family (42 HBsAg carriers in a total of 64 members). There was no evidence of linkage with HLA.

Kashiwagi et al.[10] and Sampliner et al.[5] found similar results in 11 Japanese families and 1 Caucasian family, respectively.

See also refs. 13–15.

References

1. Giani G, Chiaramonte M, Pasini CV, Fagiolo U, Naccarato R: Hepatitis B surface antigenemia and HLA antigens. N Engl J Med 300:1056-1057, 1979
2. Jeannet M, Farquet JJ: HL-A antigens in asymptomatic chronic HBAG carriers. Lancet ii:1383-1384, 1974
3. Gyodi E, Penke S, Novak E, Hollan R: HL-A specificities in individuals with persistence of hepatitis-associated antigenaemia. Haematologia 7:199-202, 1973
4. Majsky A, Horejsi J, Cerhova M, Korinkova P, Mimra J, Novak J, et al: The frequency of HBS antigen and its independence of the HLA system. Cas Lek Cesk 118:199-200, 1979
5. Sampliner RE, Bias WB, Carney E, Hillis A, Hillis WD: HLA antigens and HBV infection: Evaluation in the chronic carrier state and in a large family. Tissue Antigens 18:247-251, 1981
6. Carbonara A, Mayr W, Rizzetto M, Contu L, Curtoni ES, DeMarchi M, Farci P, Lavarini C, Olivetti E: Endemic HBV infection, tissue autoantibodies and HLA. Tissue Antigens 22:289-294, 1983
7. Dorlhiac P, Fuentes C, De La Fuente C, Velasco M: HLA, ABO and RH antigens in blood donors with and without surface antigen for hepatitis B (HBsAg). Rev Med Chil 106:755-757, 1978
8. Seignalet J, Robinet-Levy M, Lemaire JM: Les antigenes HL-A chez les porteurs sains de l'antigene Australia. Nouv Rev Fr Hematol 14:89-104, 1974
9. Vermylen C, Goethals TH, Van De Putte I: Healthy carrier state and Australia antigen liver disease. Lancet i:1119, 1972
10. Kashiwagi S, Natio S, Kaneoka H, Miyanaga O, Jimi S, Yamaguchi M, et al: A family study of HBsAg carrier and major histocompatibility antigens. Fukuoka Igaku Zasshi 69:156-161, 1978
11. Itoh C: Association of HLA with humoral immune responses. Tohoku J Exp Med 134:281-288, 1981
12. Chiewsilp P, Vinyan S, Bhamarapravati N: HB AG and HB AB in Thai blood donors. Trans R Soc Trop Med Hyg 68:339-340, 1974

13. Paronetto F, Popper H: Two immunologic reactions in the pathogenesis of hepatitis. N Engl J Med 294:606-607, 1976
14. Ziegenfuss JF: Susceptibility to disease states. Lancet i:705, 1971
15. Vladutiu AO: Hepatitis B virus, HLA types and interferon. N Engl J Med 297:399, 1977

Meningococcal Meningitis

Population Association

Zervas et al.[1] reported a significant association with B27 in 37 Greek children (19 males and 18 females) ranging in age from 2 months to 10 years (Table 18.14).

Reference

1. Zervas J, Valassi-Adam H, Constandopoulos C: Histocompatibility leukocyte antigens in children with meningococcal meningitis. J Infect Dis 143:854, 1981

Meningococcal Infection

Population Association

Pokrovsky et al.[1] studied A, B, and C loci antigens in 104 children (4 months to 13 years) with meningococcal infection and 600 healthy blood donors from the Soviet Union. The frequency of BW16 in the patients was significantly increased in the patients (Table 18.15).

In another study from Norway, Kristiansen and Thorsby[2] typed A, B, C, and DR antigens in 43 unrelated patients recovered from meningococcal disease. The diagnosis of meningococcal disease was based on typical clinical signs and positive culture of the meningococcus from blood and/or cerebrospinal fluid. In this study BW16 was not found to be significantly associated with the disease. However, in the combined analysis this association was statistically significant.

References

1. Pokrovsky VI, Petrunin YP, Shapkin VI, Tananov AT: Risk of meningococcal infection for children with different HLA phenotypes. Zh Mikrobiol Epidemiol Immunobiol 1:54-56, 1981
2. Kristiansen BE, Thorsby E: HLA histocompatibility antigens and meningococcal disease. NIPH Ann 3:75-79, 1982

Jakob-Creutzfeldt Disease

Family Data

Kovanen et al.[1] typed 25 members of a Finnish family with 7 cases of Jakob-Creutzfeldt disease and 3 cases

TABLE 18.14. Meningococcal Meningitis

	Patients		Controls				
Country/Population	n	%+	n	%+	RR	χ^2	Ref.
HLA-B27							
Greece	37	27	218	6	5.77	15.16	1

TABLE 18.15. Meningococcal Infection

	Patients		Controls				
Country/Population	n	%+	n	%+	RR	χ^2	Ref.
HLA-BW16							
USSR	104	20	600	6	3.94	21.69	1
Norway	43	3	37	0	3.18	0.90	2
	147	15	637	6	3.89	22.56	
	Heterogeneity χ^2 (1 df)					0.03	

of presenile dementia. The disease was not found to be segregating with any single haplotype.

Reference

1. Kovanen J, Tiilikainen A, Haltia M: Histocompatibility antigens in familial Creutzfeldt-Jakob disease. J Neurol Sci 45:317-321, 1980

Infection with Measles

Population Association

Coovadia et al.[1] typed 69 South African Black children with severe measles for A, B, and C loci antigens. The antigen AW32 was significantly increased in the patients (Table 18.16).

Disease Heterogeneity

Subgrouping of the patients on the basis of clinical outcome (good and poor) did not show any specific deviations in the frequencies of any of the HLA antigens.

Reference

1. Coovadia HM, Wesley A, Hammond MG, Kiepiela P: Measles, histocompatibility leukocyte antigen polymorphism, and natural selection in humans. J Infect Dis 144:142-147, 1981

Infection with Rubella Virus

Population Association

Kato et al.[1] investigated A and B antigen frequencies in 115 Japanese children born with congenital rubella syndrome. When compared with 110 controls, no significant deviations in the antigen frequencies were found. However the frequency of B15 in 93 mothers with this syndrome was 30.1% as compared with 12.7% in 110 controls (corrected $p = 0.05$).

Similar results have also been reported in another Japanese study by Ishii et al.[2]

See also ref. 3.

References

1. Kato S, Kimura M, Takakura I, Tsuji K, Ueda K: HLA-linked genetic control in natural rubella infection. Tissue Antigens 15:86-89, 1980
2. Ishii K, Nakazono N, Sawada H, Fukuda K, Wakisaka A, Moriuchi J, et al: Host factors and susceptibility to rubella virus infection: The association of HLA antigens. J Med Virol 7:287-297, 1981
3. Griffiths P, Clarke C, Richards M: Family outbreak of rubella with encephalopathy occurring in sibling with maternal HLA crossover. Lancet i:1143, 1980

Dengue Hemorrhagic Fever

Population Association

Eighty-seven unrelated Thai children who had been hospitalized with dengue shock syndrome and/or dengue hemorrhagic fever were typed for A and B loci antigens by Chiewsilp et al.[1] In comparison with 138 controls no significant deviations in the frequencies were found.

Reference

1. Chiewsilp P, Scott RM, Bhamarapravati N: Histocompatibility antigens and dengue hemorrhagic fever. Am J Trop Med Hyg 30:1100-1105, 1981

Mumps

Population Association

No frequency data are available. However, see ref. 1.

TABLE 18.16. Infection with Measles

	Patients		Controls				
Country/Population	n	%+	n	%+	RR	χ^2	Ref.
HLA-AW32							
South Africa—Black	69	10	1132	2	5.67	16.22	1

Reference

1. Kress HG, Kreth HW: HLA restriction of secondary mumps-specific cytotoxic T lymphocytes. J Immunol 129:844-849, 1982

Paracoccidioidomycosis

Population Association

De Restrepo et al.[1] studied A and B antigens in 41 Colombian patients with paracoccidioidomycosis. The diagnosis was based on direct microscopic observation of the causative agent in pathologic specimens and/or the isolation of *Paracoccidioides brasiliensis* in culture. The frequency of A9 was significantly increased in the patients (Table 18.17). Also, there was a marginally significant decrease of A1 in the patient group.

Disease Heterogeneity

Patients were also analyzed on the basis of clinical presentation. In 6 patients with the progressive pulmonary form of the disease 5 were positive (83.33%) for A9 as compared with only 19% in 158 controls ($p < 0.0005$). Thirty-five patients were classified as having disseminated pulmonary form of the disease. The frequency of A9 in this group was 51.43% and this was not significantly different from that of the control group.

Reference

1. De Restrepo FM, Restrepo M, Restrepo A: Blood groups and HLA antigens in paracoccidioidomycosis. Sabouraudia 21:35-49, 1983

Filariasis

Population Association

Ottesen et al.[1] typed A and B loci antigens in 110 patients and 128 controls from a South Pacific Island (Mauke) in the Cook Island group. All the patients had evidence of filariasis due to *Wuchereria bancrofti*.

No significant difference between patients and controls was found.

Family Data

In the aforementioned study[1] HLA data were also available on 3 families with more than 1 affected member. A linkage analysis by the method of lod score did not show any evidence of linkage of the disease with the HLA complex.

Reference

1. Ottesen EA, Mendell NR, MacQueen JM, Weller PF, Amos DB, Ward FE: Familial predisposition to filarial infection—not linked to HLA-A or -B locus specificities. Acta Trop 38:205-216, 1981

Scabies

Population Association

Falk and Thorsby[1] typed 60 Norwegian patients for A, B, and C loci antigens. A significant increase of A11 in the patients was found (Table 18.18).

Disease Heterogeneity

The total sample was divided into 16 atopic (those with either current atopic disease or a past history

TABLE 18.17. Paracoccidioidomycosis

	Patients		Controls				
Country/Population	n	%+	n	%+	RR	χ^2	Ref.
HLA-A1							
Colombia	41	10	158	32	0.26	7.23	1
HLA-A9							
Colombia	41	56	158	19	5.33	20.84	1

TABLE 18.18. Scabies

	Patients		Controls				
Country/Population	n	%+	n	%+	RR	χ^2	Ref.
HLA-A11							
Norway	60	28	1468	10	3.55	18.61	1

of such illness, including atopic dermatitis, allergic rhinitis, or extrinsic asthma), and 44 nonatopic patients. Only the nonatopic subgroup showed a significantly increased frequency (36.4%) of A11. This antigen was present in only 1 of the 16 (6.3%) atopic patients.

Reference

1. Falk ES, Thorsby E: HLA antigens in patients with scabies. Br J Dermatol 104:317-320, 1981

Amyloidosis

Family Data

De Pietro[1] reported a 3-generation family in which 3 patients had lichen amyloidosis. Two patients were father and daughter. The third was the son of the sister of the affected daughter. All 3 patients had 4c antigen in common.

Reference

1. De Pietro WP: Primary familial cutaneous amyloidosis. Arch Dermatol 117:639-642, 1981

Thalassemia Major

Population Association

Pollack et al.[1] reported A, B, C, and DR antigen frequencies in 75 unrelated American Caucasian patients (only 65 were typed for DR) from New York. There was no significant association with any of these antigens.

Reference

1. Pollack MS, Levine LS, Oberfield SE, Markenson AL: HLA-A, B, C, and DR antigen frequencies in relation to development of diabetes and variations in white cell antibody formation in highly transfused thalassemia patients. Transfusion 22:279-82,1982

CHAPTER 19

Musculoskeletal Diseases

Tendinous Calcifications

Population Association

Amor et al.[1] studied A and B loci antigens in 38 patients. The frequencies of A2 and BW35 appeared to be nonsignificantly increased in the patient group (Table 19.1).

Disease Heterogeneity

The aforementioned study[1] consisted of 28 cases with multiple and 10 cases with single tendinous calcifications. The frequency of A2 in the multiple-calcification group was 71% and was significantly different from that in the controls ($p < 0.005$). No other differences between the 3 groups were observed in this study.

Reference

1. Amor B, Kahan A, Cherot A, Delbarre F, Rabaud M, Aubouy G: Etude microscopique-antigene HLA-arthrite experimentale-pathogenie. Rev Rhum Mal Osteoartic 44:309-316, 1977

Iron-Overload-Associated Myopathy

Population Association

Bregman et al.[1] HLA-typed 10 patients on maintenance hemodialysis with proximal muscle weakness of variable duration. All patients had severe iron overload (serum ferritin level > 1000 mg/ml) and none had evidence of active liver disease or infection.

Nine of the 10 (90%) patients were positive for A3, B7, or B4 as compared with the expected frequency of 25% to 33% ($p < 0.001$).

See also ref. 2.

References

1. Bregman H, Gelfand MC, Winchester JF, Manz HJ, Knepshield JH, Schreiner GE: Iron-overload associated myopathy in patients on maintenance haemodialysis: A histocompatibility-linked disorder. Lancet ii:882-885, 1980
2. Gomez E, Ortega F, Morales JM, Gago E, Comas A, Alvarez J: Serum ferritin and HLA antigens in

TABLE 19.1. Tendinous Calcifications

	Patients		Controls				
Country/Population	n	%+	n	%+	RR	χ^2	Ref.
HLA-A2							
France	38	66	591	44	2.42	6.71	1
HLA-BW35							
France	38	34	591	19	2.23	5.31	1

patients on maintenance haemodialysis. Lancet i:836-837, 1981

Dupuytren's Contracture

Population Association

Tait and Mackay[1] typed A and B loci antigens in 100 patients and 748 controls from Melbourne, Australia. The antigen frequencies between these two groups did not differ significantly.

Family Data

See ref. 2.

References

1. Tait BD, Mackay IR: HLA phenotypes in Dupuytren's contracture. Tissue Antigens 19:240-241, 1982
2. Nyberg LM, Bias WB, Hochberg MC, Walsh P: Identification of an inherited form of Peyronie's disease with autosomal dominant inheritance and association with Dupuytren's contracture and HLA-B7 cross-reacting antigens. J Urol 128:48-51, 1982

CHAPTER 20

Psychiatric Diseases

Schizophrenia

Population Association

A and B loci antigen frequency data are available on Caucasian patients from France,[1,2,3,4] Italy,[5,6,7,8] Czechoslovakia,[9,10,11,12] Sweden,[13,14] England,[15,16] Germany,[17,18] Belgium,[19] and the United States.[20,21,22] The results are variable and inconsistent. A summary of all the significant deviations reported in the above studies is given in Table 20.1. In general, an association reported in 1 study has not been confirmed in the data from other countries or even from the same country (e.g., see data from Sweden). In the combined data, only the association with A28 was significant (Table 20.2). Even this association seemed primarily the result of the data from Czechoslovakia[10] where a highly significant increase of A28 in 19 patients was observed. None of the other reports confirmed this result (Table 20.2).

C locus typings are also available in 2 reports.[3,10] As in the case of A28 the Czechoslovakian study reported an increase of CW4 in the patients (Table 20.2) but this could not be confirmed in the data from France.[3]

Thus, available data on Caucasian patients from several countries do not show strong evidence in favor of an HLA association. The significant increased frequency of A28 and CW4 in the total data (Table 20.2) was the result of the sample from Czechoslovakia.[10] If patients in all these studies were clinically the same it is very difficult to assume that schizophrenia is associated with different antigens in the United States and various countries of Western Europe (Table 20.1). Most probably these associations are artifacts of HLA serology and problems associated with the diagnosis of this disorder.

Disease Heterogeneity

Paranoid

Several investigators have subgrouped their patients as paranoid. The diagnostic criteria for classification was variable. The results, again, were variable. The reported deviations have not been confirmed in other studies. In the pooled data the increase of A9 was significant (Table 20.3).

Ivanyi et al.[10] also reported a significant association with CW4 (40.0% in 159 patients vs. 15.3% in 438 controls, $p < 0.001$).

Hebephrenic

The frequency data on this subgroup of patients were given by Crowe et al.,[20] Mercier et al.,[1] Julien et al.,[2] Ivanyi et al.,[10] McGuffin et al.,[23] and Smeraldi et al.[6] There was no association with A and B loci antigens.

Simplex and Catatonic

Ivanyi et al.[10] reported data on 28 patients within these 2 subgroups (19 simplex and 9 catatonic). The frequency of A28 in the total sample was 28.5% as compared with 6.3% in 1200 controls, ($p < 0.001$).

Chronic

In 61 patients of this subgroup, Gattaz and Beckmann[17] showed B27 frequency of 23% compared with 7.8% in 472 controls ($p < 0.001$).

Poor Prognosis

The frequency of B27 was reported as 22% in 58 patients as compared with 7.8% in 472 controls by Gattaz and Beckmann.[17]

Early Onset
There was no association in 31 patients studied by Gattaz and Beckmann.[17]

Patients Exhibiting Schneider's First Rank Symptoms
Increased frequencies of A1 and A2 and a decreased frequency of B17 were reported by McGuffin[15] in 57 patients. None of these was significant after correcting the probability value, however.

Brain Atrophy
Gattaz et al.[18] measured the third ventricle of 40 patients by computed tomographic study. On the basis of a transverse measure the patients were divided into 2 groups with the third ventricle larger and smaller than the median measure of 4.5 mm. There was no HLA difference betweeen the 2 subgroups.

Clinical Response to Neuroleptics
Luchins et al.[22] studied 17 chronic schizophrenia patients with respect to clinical response to neuroleptics, serum neuroleptic-like concentrations as measured by dopamine receptor binding, and in vitro haloperidol binding. There was no evidence of HLA associations.

Family History
Perris et al.[14] subdivided their patients on the basis of family history of schizophrenia. There was no

TABLE 20.1. Reported HLA Associations in Schizophrenia

Studies		Patients		Controls		
	Antigens	n	%+	n	%+	*p* Value
USA						
Bennahum et al.[21]	A11	38	0	102	13	< 0.01
	B17	38	18	102	7	< 0.05
Crowe et al.[20]	None	45	—	1263	—	
Italy						
Smeraldi et al.[7]	A10	144	13	386	28	< 0.0001
England						
McGuffin et al.[15]	A29	80	1	9		0.018
	B17	80	1	9		0.015
	BW35	80	21	13		0.047
France						
Mercier et al.[1]	A9	30	33	591	24	< 0.05
	B5	30	27	591	13	< 0.05
Julien et al.[3]	A9	65	40	250	21	< 0.005
Singer et al.[4]	A10	99	3	184	12	< 0.05
	A29	95	14	184	5	< 0.05
Belgium						
Mendlewicz and Linkowski[19]	A1	64	14	113	28	< 0.05
	B7	64	12	113	26	< 0.05
	BW16	64	18	113	4	< 0.01
Czechoslovakia						
Ivanyi et al.[10]	A28	200	17	1200	6	< 0.001
	CW4	52	31	438	15	< 0.01
Sweden						
Eberhard et al.[13]	A9	47	34	1263	15	< 0.001
	AW19	47	30	1263	16	< 0.05
	B5	47	21	1263	8	< 0.01
Perris et al.[14]	A10	50	22	449	11	< 0.02
Germany						
Gattaz and Beckmann[17]	B27	100	16	472	8	0.017

TABLE 20.2. Schizophrenia

Country/Population	Patients n	Patients %+	Controls n	Controls %+	RR	χ^2	Ref.
HLA-A28							
U.S.A.	45	7	1263	6	1.34	0.31	20
Czechoslovakia	200	17	1200	6	3.23	27.90	10
BENELUX	32	6	1018	10	0.71	0.31	25
England	80	8	458	7	1.22	0.22	15
France	30	7	591	6	1.42	0.31	1
Sweden	50	4	449	10	0.46	1.60	14
Sweden	47	4	1263	7	0.69	0.36	13
	97	4	1712	8	0.56	1.75	
	Heterogeneity χ^2 (1 df)					0.22	
	484	11	6242	7	1.78	13.20	
	Heterogeneity χ^2 (6 df)					17.81	
HLA-CW4							
Czechoslovakia	52	31	438	15	2.57	8.65	10
BENELUX	32	28	1018	21	1.51	1.15	25
France	63	22	250	18	1.31	0.63	3
	147	26	1706	19	1.76	8.09	
	Heterogeneity χ^2 (2 df)					2.34	

significant HLA difference between 20 patients with positive and 30 with negative family histories.

Age

Eberhard et al.[13] subgrouped their patients on the basis of age and reported an increased frequency of A9 in older patients (age > 50 years).

Clinical Response to Treatment with Chlorpromazine

Smeraldi et al.[5] published data on 33 chronic schizophrenia patients who had taken chlorpromazine (200-300 mg/day) for at least 8 months during the preceding year. The correlation coefficient showed that there was a highly significant positive response to chlorpromazine in patients positive for A1 ($r = -0.4$; $p < 0.05$).

In a second group of 17 patients, clinical responses to chlorpromazine were evaluated quantitatively by using the Wittenborn psychiatric rating scale in A1-positive and -negative patients. Before the treatment there was no difference in the scores of the 2 groups. After the treatment the scores of the A1 positive patients were significantly lower, indicating a greater degree of response to the treatment.

In a study by Canoso et al.,[24] 97 patients (schizophrenic and schizoaffective disorders) chronically treated with chlorpromazine were typed for A, B, C, and DR loci antigens. The frequency of BW44 was found to be significantly increased among patients who developed autoantibodies (46%) as compared with that of normal Caucasians (19%; $p < 0.001$).

Response to Treatment with γ-Type Endorphins

De Jongh et al.[25] typed 32 Dutch patients for the A, B, C, and DR loci antigens. In 16 patients who responded moderately or markedly to treatment with γ-type endorphins an increase of B15 (31%) was found, as compared with 6% in 16 with no or slight response (17.0% in 1018 normal controls). The difference, in view of large numbers of antigens tested in this study, was not statistically significant, however.

Family Data

Goudemand et al.[26] published data on a 3-generation family in which the mother and her 2 sons were affected by schizophrenia. Both affected sons had the A9-BW21 haplotype transmitted by the mother. Two other siblings did not have this haplotype and were free of this disorder (see also ref. 27).

McGuffin et al.[28] have performed linkage analysis by the method of lod scores on 12 families with 2

TABLE 20.3. HLA-A9 in Paranoid Schizophrenia

Studies	Patients +	Patients −	Controls +	Controls −	RR	χ^2
USA						
Crowe et al.[20]	3	11	133	1130	2.317	0.773
Germany						
Gattaz and Beckmann[17]	19	42	99	373	1.704	2.680
France						
Julien et al.[2]	18	20	53	197	3.345	10.793
France						
Mercier et al.[1]	7	8	142	449	2.767	2.915
Czechoslovakia						
Ivanyi et al.[10]	47	112	274	926	1.418	3.158
Italy						
Smeraldi et al.[6]	18	24	106	280	1.981	3.647
England						
McGuffin et al.[23]	9	23	82	376	1.794	1.446
Netherlands						
De Jongh et al.[25]	2	18	198	820	0.460	0.600

or more members diagnosed as schizophrenic. Under the assumptions of dominant and recessive models of inheritance, close linkage between a major locus for schizophrenia and HLA was excluded at recombination frequencies of 15–20%. In the case of intermediate models, the results were less certain but linkage still appeared to be unlikely.

See also refs. 29–36.

References

1. Mercier P, Sutter JM, Julien RA, Kieffer N: Schizophrenie: Association de la forme paranoide aux antigenes HLA-A9 et B5. Encephale 3:49-53, 1977
2. Julien RA, Mercier P, Chouraqui P, Sutter JM: Schizophrenies et antigenes d'histocompatibilite. Encephale 4:99-113, 1978
3. Julien RA, Mercier P, Chouraqui P: Schizophrenies et systeme d'histocompatibilite tissulaire mise en evidence de l'augmentation des antigenes ag et CW4 dans la schizophrenie paranoide. Ann Med Psychol (Paris) 2:939-944, 1977
4. Singer L, Mayer S, Tongio MM, Hauptmann G, Roos M, Danion JM, et al: Antigenes HLA-A, B, C, antigene Bf et schizophrenie. J Hum Genet 29:555-563, 1981
5. Smeraldi E, Bellodi L, Sacchetti E, Cazzullo CL: The HLA system and the clinical response to treatment with chlorpromazine. Br J Psychiatry 129:486-489, 1976
6. Smeraldi E, Bellodi L, Cazzullo CL: Further studies on the major histocompatibility complex as a genetic marker for schizophrenia. Biol Psychiatry 11:655-661, 1976
7. Smeraldi E, Bellodi L, Scorza-Smeraldi R, Fabio G, Sacchetti E: HLA-SD antigens and schizophrenia: Statistical and genetical considerations. Tissue Antigens 8:191-196, 1976
8. Cazzullo CL, Smeraldi E, Penati G: The leucocyte antigenic system HL-A as a possible genetic marker of schizophrenia. Br J Psychiatry 125:25-27, 1974
9. Ivanyi P, Ivanyi D, Zemek P: HLA-CW4 in paranoid schizophrenia. Tissue Antigens 9:41-44, 1977
10. Ivanyi D, Zemek P, Ivanyi P: HLA antigens as possible markers of heterogeneity in schizophrenia. J Immunogenet 5:165-172, 1978
11. Zemek P: HL-A antigens and their possible relationship to schizophrenia. Cesk Psychiatr 73:184-187, 1977
12. Ivanyi D, Zemek P, Ivanyi P: HLA antigens in schizophrenia. Tissue Antigens 8:217-220, 1976
13. Eberhard G, Franzen G, Low B: Schizophrenia susceptibility and HL-A antigens. Neuropsychobiology 1:211-217, 1975
14. Perris C, Romain G, Wahlby L: HLA antigens in patients with schizophrenic syndromes. Neuropsychobiology 5:290-293, 1979
15. McGuffin P, Farmer AE, Rajah SM: Histocompatibility antigens and schizophrenia. Br J Psychiatry 132:149-151, 1978
16. McGuffin P: Is schizophrenia an HLA-associated disease? Psychol Med 9:721-728, 1979
17. Gattaz WF, Beckman H: HLA antigens and schizophrenia. Lancet i:98-99, 1980
18. Gattaz WF, Kasper S, Beckmann H: HLA-antigens, schizophrenia and brain atrophy. Br J Psychiatry 137:398-399, 1980
19. Mendlewicz J, Linkowski P: HLA antigens and schizophrenia. Lancet i:765, 1980

20. Crowe RR, Thompson JS, Flink R, Weinberger B: HLA antigens and schizophrenia. Arch Gen Psychiatry 136:231-233, 1979
21. Bennahum DA, Troup GM, Rada RT, Kellner R, Ryner T: HLA antigens in schizophrenia and manic depressive mental disorders. Clin Res 25:114a, 1977
22. Luchins DJ, Weinberger DR, Kleinman JE, Neckers L, Rosenblatt JE, Bigelow LB, et al: Human leukocyte antigen A2 and psychopathology in chronic schizophrenia. Am J Psychiatry 137:499-500, 1980
23. McGuffin P, Farmer AE, Yonace AH: HLA antigens and subtypes of schizophrenia. Psychiatry Res 5:115-122, 1981
24. Canoso RT, Lewis ME, Yunis EJ: Association of HLA-Bw44 with chlorpromazine-induced autoantibodies. Clin Immunol Immunopathol 25:278-282, 1982
25. De Jongh BM, Verhoeven WMA, Van Ree JM, De Wied D, Van Rood JJ: HLA, and the response to treatment with gamma type endorphins in schizophrenia. J Immunogenet 9:381-388, 1982
26. Goudemand M, Goudemand-Joubert C, Lelievre-Lalligier A, Julliot JP, Goudemand J: Coexistence intra-familiale d'une osteopathie condensante genotypique et d'une psychose: chronique. Nouv Presse Med 6:3434, 1977
27. Smeraldi E, Bellodi L: Possible linkage between primary affective disorder susceptibility locus and HLA haplotypes. Am J Psychiatry 138:1232-1234, 1981
28. McGuffin P, Festenstein H, Murray R: A family study of HLA antigens and other genetic markers in schizophrenia. Psychol Med 13:31-43, 1983
29. Comings DE: PC 1 Duarte, a common polymorphism of a human brain protein, and its relationship to depressive disease and multiple sclerosis. Nature 277:28-32, 1979
30. Morasiewicz J: The study of HLA antigens in endogenous psychosis. Psychiatr Pol 13:511-517, 1979
31. Torrey EF: Birth weights, perinatal insults, and HLA types: Return to "original din." Schizophrenia Bull 3:347-351, 1977
32. McGuffin P: What have transplant antigens got to do with psychosis? Br J Psychiatry 136:510-512, 1980
33. Mendlewicz J, Verbanvk P, Linkowski P, Govaerts A: HLA antigens in affective disorders and schizophrenia. J Affect Disord 3:17-24, 1981
34. Gattaz WF, Beckmann H, Mendlewicz J: HLA antigens and schizophrenia: A pool of two studies. Pscychiatry Res 5:123-128, 1981
35. Beckmann VH, Gattaz WF, Moises HW, Haas S, Ewald RW: HLA antigens and schizophrenia. Arzneimittelforsch 30:1211-1212, 1980
36. Gattaz WF, Beckmann H: HLA system in psychiatric research. Fortschr Neurol Psychiatr 49:145-151, 1981

Manic-Depressive Disorder

Population Association

Various authors have noted the increased and decreased frequencies of certain antigens in their individual studies. A summary of all such deviations is given in Table 20.4. Two interesting points can be noted in this summary. First, there was no com-

TABLE 20.4. Reported HLA Associations in Manic Depressive Disorder

Country/Population	n	Antigen Increased	*p*	Antigen Decreased	*p*	Reference
Sweden	168	A10	< 0.025	B7	< 0.050	15
U.S.A.	50	B5	< 0.050	B12	< 0.050	16
		B13	< 0.010			
	38	BW22	> 0.05	A9	0.01	17
		CW1	> 0.01	CW3	0.001	
	114	None		None		18
Belgium	118	B5	0.050	BW15	< 0.02	3
Czechoslovakia	125	CW4	0.050			19
Italy	91	A29	< 0.006	A10	< 0.05	4
		BW22	< 0.006	AW30	< 0.05	
	49	None		None		8
Denmark	107	B7	0.004			1, 2
		B16	0.0002			
Australia		None		None		20

TABLE 20.5. Manic-Depressive Disorder

	Patients		Controls				
Country/Population	n	%+	n	%+	RR	χ^2	Ref.
HLA-BW16							
BENELUX	118	9	113	5	1.81	1.38	3
Italy	91	11	646	7	1.70	2.21	4
Denmark	107	14	1967	5	3.16	15.81	2
	316	11	2726	5	2.34	17.23	
	Heterogeneity χ^2 (2 df)					2.16	

mon antigen (increased or decreased) in all these reports; second, except for the Danish study,[1,2] all these deviations were significant ($p \leq 0.05$) only prior to the correction for multiple comparisons. When this is considered none of the deviations was significant.

In the first Danish study by Shapiro et al.[1] on 47 manic-depressive patients, antigens A3, B7, and BW16 were increased and B8 was decreased. After correcting the probabilities, only the association with BW16 remained significant. In a second report,[2] the authors studied 107 patients and found significant associations with B7 and BW16.

When the available frequency data for B7 and BW16 are combined with those of the Danish study (Table 20.5) the association with B7 is no longer significant. However, BW16 does show a highly significant association ($\chi^2 = 17.23$) with no indication of heterogeneity in the data. In the studies from Belgium[3] and Italy[4], the frequency of BW16 was higher in the patient group but not significant (BW16 was not typed in other studies).

Disease Heterogeneity

Unipolar vs. Bipolar

In many of the studies, the total sample was divided into unipolar and bipolar patient groups and the results were as inconsistent as in the total sample (Tables 20.4, 20.6, and 20.7). No antigen seemed to be significantly associated with either unipolar or bipolar groups. Even in Shapiro's study[2] there was no significant difference between the 2 groups.

In 21 Ashkenazi Jewish bipolar patients, no significant HLA association was observed.[5]

Family History

Shapiro et al.[2] grouped their patients into those with and those without a positive family history of affective disorder. A significantly higher percentage of patients with a positive family history had B7 (55% vs. 19% in those without family history; corrected $p = 0.001$). This trend was reversed for BW16. Its frequency was decreased in patients without a family history of affective disorder (28% vs. 9% in

TABLE 20.6. Reported HLA Associations in Manic Depressive Disorder: Unipolar

Country/Population	n	Antigen Increased	p	Antigen Decreased	p	Reference
Sweden	50	A10	< 0.025	A1	< 0.025	15
U.S.A.	19	B5 B13				16
	5	—		—		17
Belgium	68			BW15	< 0.02	3
Czechoslovakia	24	BW40	< 0.03			19
Italy	41	A29 BW22		A10 AW30		4
Australia	—	—		—		20
Denmark	27	—		—		2

TABLE 20.7. Manic Depressive Disorder: Bipolar

Country/Population	n	Antigen Increased	p	Antigen Decreased	p	Reference
Sweden	38			B7	< 0.025	15
U.S.A.	31	B5 B13		B12		16
	92	B14	< 0.05	B27	< 0.05	5
	29	—		—		17
	49	—		—		18
Czechoslovakia	77	—		—		19
Italy	50	A29 BW22		A10 AW30		4
Australia	36	—		—		20
Denmark	51	—		—		2
Belgium	50	B5	0.060	BW15	< 0.02	3

patients with positive family history, corrected $p = 0.064$).

In the Italian data[4] there was no correlation of HLA antigens with positive or negative history for the disease. Thus, again with respect to this attribute the results were inconsistent.

Family History of Suicide

In the Danish study,[2] it was observed that 64% of the patients with a family history of suicide had B7 as compared with 33% of those without such a family history (corrected $p = 0.02$). The frequency of BW16 was lower in the group with a family history of suicide but when compared with that in the group without a family history, the difference was not statistically significant.

Sex

In the Danish study,[2] classification according to the sex of the probands did not show any association between HLA and this disease.

Lithium Therapy

Perris et al.[6] studied the HLA antigens of 82 patients who had been on lithium therapy for at least 6 months. There was a higher frequency of A3 in the subgroup of patients (n = 34) with relapse (11.2% vs. 4.0% in 48 patients who did not relapse; $\chi^2 = 6.84$). B18 was absent from the group without relapse.

An increase in the frequency of B5 was noted in the Italian patients[4] (n = 29) who did not relapse (48.8% vs. 13.6% in 22 patients who relapsed; uncorrected $p < 0.05$).

In 46 patients with cyclophrenia treated with lithium for a long period of time no association between HLA and prognosis of lithium treatment has been observed.[7]

Del Vecchio et al.[8] typed A, B, and C loci antigens in a sample of 49 Italian patients (22 bipolar affective psychotics, 18 unipolar depressive psychotics, and 9 cycloid psychotics) receiving prophylactic lithium for 1–4 years and maintained at lithium plasma levels of 0.6–1.2 mEq/liter. In 21 patients who did not show clinical response to lithium prophylaxis the frequency of A3 was 47.6%. This antigen was present in 17.8% of the 28 patients who showed response to lithium ($p < 0.05$).

Antinuclear Antibodies

Whalley et al.[9] studied antinuclear antibodies in 54 British patients on long-term lithium therapy. There was no significant HLA frequency difference between 11 patients with and 43 without these antibodies.

Family Data

Smeraldi et al.[10] studied the segregation pattern of HLA haplotypes in 21 families with 2 or more siblings with manic-depressive disorder. In 21 pairs of affected siblings, 52% shared both and 38% shared only 1 haplotype. Only 9% of the sib pairs did not share any haplotype. In this data when 2 or more siblings were affected, the frequency of haplotype repeats was significantly higher than expected on the basis of random zygotic assortment ($p = 0.046$). This distribution of haplotypes among the sib pairs discordant for the disease was random. When the observed frequencies of sib pairs sharing 2, 1, and 0 haplotypes were compared with the expected value of 42.8%, 49.1%, and 8.1%, respectively, under the assumption of a dominant disease susceptibility gene, the χ^2 was 1.02. If a recessive disease susceptibility gene was assumed then the expected number of sib pairs in the 3 categories would be 51%, 40.8%, and 8.2%, respectively. This would give a χ^2value of 0.09. Thus, although the recessive model fits better, the dominant model could not be excluded completely. In a later report, Smeraldi and Bellodi[11] analyzed 17 affected sib pairs sharing both haplotypes, 29 sharing 1 haplotype, and 9 sharing no haplotype. In these data there was an excess of sib pairs sharing both haplotypes.

Weitkamp et al.[12] studied the HLA haplotypes in 20 families containing at least 2 affected members, either siblings or a parent and offspring. Haplotype identity among pairs of affected siblings in families with 2 affected siblings and among pairs of older unaffected siblings in families with 1 or 2 affected siblings was increased over random expectation ($p < 0.005$). There was no increase in HLA haplotype identity among affected siblings in sibships with more than 2 affected members.

In 2 large pedigrees Kruger et al.[13] also found, by the method of lod score analysis, results strongly supportive of linkage with HLA. In these data, using the most favorable assumption, a lod score of 3.901 at a recombination frequency of 10% was found.

Targum et al.,[5] using the lod score method, did linkage analysis of "bipolar and related affective illness" to HLA-A and −B loci in 9 two-generation families. The sum of the lod scores was −2.0 (or less) for recombination frequencies of < 15%. Thus, the hypothesis of linkage could be rejected for < 15% recombination. For frequencies of recombination > 15%, the lod scores were > −2.0 and thus linkage could not be ruled out.

Johnson et al.[14] have also calculated lod scores in 4 multiple-case families typed for HLA and some other genetic markers. In these families the segregation of specific HLA alleles was not associated with affective illness. All the lod scores were negative. At 5% recombination the lod score was −1.91, suggesting the presence of close linkage with HLA as unlikely.

See also refs. 21–29.

References

1. Shapiro RW, Bock E, Rafaelsen OJ, Ryder LP, Svejgaard A: Histocompatibility antigens and manic-depressive disorders. Arch Gen Psychiatry 33:823-825, 1976
2. Shapiro RW, Ryder LP, Svejgaard A, Rafaelsen OJ: HLA antigens and manic-depressive disorders: Further evidence of an association. Psychol Med 7:387-396, 1977
3. Govaerts A, Mendlewicz J, Verbanck: Manic-depressive illness and HLA. Tissue Antigens 10:60-62, 1977
4. Smeraldi E, Negri F, Melica AM, Scorza-Smeraldi R, Fabio G, Bonara P, et al: HLA typing and affective disorders: A study in the Italian population. Neuropsychobiology 4:344-352, 1978
5. Targum SD, Gershon ES, Van Eerdewegh M, Rogentine N: Human leukocyte antigen system not closely linked to or associated with bipolar manic-depressive illness. Biol Psychiatry 14:615-636, 1979
6. Perris C, Strandman E, Wahlby L: HL-A antigens and the response to prophylactic lithium. Neuropsychobiology 5:114-118, 1979
7. Zemek P, Zeoacku II, Coymek K, et al.: Chief histocompatibility system in cyclophrenia and its relationship to lithium therapy. Zh Nevropatol Psikhiatr 77:1199-1200, 1977
8. Del Vecchio M, Farzati B, Minucci MMP, Guida L, Kemali D: Cell membrane predictors of response to lithium prophylaxis of affective disorders. Neuropsychobiology 7:243-247, 1981
9. Whalley LJ, Roberts DF, Wentzel J, Watson KC: Antinuclear antibodies and histocompatibility antigens in patients on long-term lithium therapy. J Affect Disord 3:123-130, 1981
10. Smeraldi E, Negri F, Melica AM, Scorza-Smeraldi R: HLA system and affective disorders: A sibship genetic study. Tissue Antigens 12:270-274, 1978
11. Smeraldi E, Bellodi L: Possible linkage between primary affective disorder susceptibility locus and HLA haplotypes. Am J Psychiatry 138:1232-1234, 1981
12. Weitkamp LR, Stanger HC, Persad E, Flood C, Guttormsen MS: Depressive disorders and HLA: A gene on chromosome 6 that can affect behavior. N Engl J Med 305:1301-1306, 1981
13. Kruger SD, Turner WJ, Kidd KK: The effects of requisite assumptions on linkage analysis of manic-depressive illness with HLA. Biol Psychiatry 17:1081-1099, 1982
14. Johnson GFS, Hunt GE, Robertson S, Doran TJ: A linkage study of manic-depressive disorder with HLA antigens, blood groups, serum proteins and red cell enzymes. J Affect Disord 3:43-58, 1981
15. Beckman L, Perris C, Strandman E, Wahlby L: HLA antigens and affective disorders. Hum Hered 28:96-99, 1978
16. Stember RH, Fieve RR: Histocompatibility antigens in affective disorders. Clin Immunol Immunopathol 7:10-14, 1977
17. Temple H, Dupont B, Shopsin B: HLA antigen and affective disorders: A report and critical assessment

of histocompatibility studies. Neuropsychobiology 5:50-58, 1979
18. James NM, Smouse PE, Carroll BJ, Haines RF: Affective illness and HLA frequencies: No compelling association. Neuropsychobiology 6:208-216, 1980
19. Majsky A, Zvolsky P, Dvorakova M: Primary affective disorders and HLA antigens. Tissue Antigens 11:190-191, 1978
20. Johnson GFS: HLA antigens and manic-depressive disorders. Biol Psychiatry 13:409-412, 1978
21. Majsky A, Dvorakova M, Zvolsky P: Modifikationen von HLA-Antigenen an Lymphozyten ALS Therapiefolge bei Kranken mit manisch-depressiver Psychose. Folia Haematol (Leipz) 105:509-517, 1978
22. Plantey F: Genotypes HLA chez les malades atteints d'affections psychiatriques. Nouv Presse Med 7:471, 1978
23. Zvolsky P, Dvorakova M, Majsky A, Soucek K: Histocompatibility antigens in primary affective disorders. Arch Psychiatr Nervenkr 225:159-162, 1978
24. McGuffin P: What have transplant antigens got to do with psychosis? Br J Psychiatry 136:510-512, 1980
25. Mendlewicz J, Verbanvk P, Linkowski P, Govaerts A: HLA antigens in affective disorders and schizophrenia. J Affec Disord 3:17-24, 1981
26. Rihmer Z, Arato M: ABO blood groups in manic-depressive patients. J Affect Disord 3:1-7, 1981
27. Matthysse S, Kidd KK: Evidence of HLA linkage in depressive disorders. N Engl J Med 305:1340-1341, 1981
28. Faber R: Depressive disorders and HLA. N Engl J Med 306:1238-1239, 1982
29. Gattaz WF, Beckmann H: HLA system in psychiatric research. Fortschr Neurol Psychiatr 49:145-151, 1981

Psychosis Proto-Infantilis

Population Association

In a sample of 15 French children studied by Golse et al.,[1] nonsignificantly increased frequencies of A9 and B5 were noted. In a second independent study of 30 French children and 74 controls by Goudemand et al.,[2-4] the increase in A9 and B5 was not confirmed. Instead, they noted an increase in the frequencies of AW32 and B18.

From these data it appears that this disorder does not show any association with the antigens of the A and B loci.

References

1. Golse B, Debray-Ritzen P, Dausset J, Lipinski M, Hors J: Etudes des groupes HLA dans les psychoses infantiles de developpement et hypothese d'une enzymopathie. C R Acad Sci (Paris) 284:1733-1735, 1977
2. Goudemand M, Goudemand-Joubert C, Parquet PHJ, Goudemand J: Les antigenes d'histocompatibilite (HLA A et B) dans les psychoses infantiles precoces. Nouv Presse Med 9:3278, 1980
3. Goudemand M, Goudemand J, Goudemand-Joubert C, Parquet PJ: Heredity and childhood psychoses: Histocompatibility antigens (HLA A and B) and early onset childhood psychoses. Acta Psychiatr Belg 81:57-71, 1981
4. Goudemand M, Goudemand J, Parquet PJ, Goudemand-Joubert C, Letallec-Duytschaever F, Fontan M: Antigenes d'histocompatibilite et psychoses infantiles (precoces et tardives). J Hum Genet 419-429, 1981

Chronic Alcoholism

Population Association

Ninety-four chronic alcoholics (with mean daily alcohol intake of 150 g of 20-year duration) from Japan were typed for A, B, and C loci antigens by Shigeta et al.[1] The frequency of CW3 was significantly increased in the patient group (Table 20.8).

Disease Heterogeneity

The frequency of CW3 was significantly increased in patients with hepatitis (64% in patients vs. 30% in controls) and those with liver cirrhosis (59% vs. 30% in controls).[1]

Reference

1. Shigeta Y, Ishii H, Takagi S, Yoshitake Y, Hirano T, Kohno H, et al: HLA antigens as immunogenetic markers of alcoholism in Japan. Drug Alcohol Depend 6:33-34, 1980

Alzheimer's Disease

Population Association

A significant increase in B15 was reported in 124 British patients by Renvoize et al.[1] But in 4 other independent studies on Caucasian populations (small samples), this association was not clearly evident

TABLE 20.8. Chronic Alcoholism

Country/Population	Patients n	Patients %+	Controls n	Controls %+	RR	χ^2	Ref.
HLA-CW3							
Japan	94	59	80	30	3.31	14.22	1

(Table 20.9). The pooled analysis of all 5 samples, however, showed a significant association with B15 and there was no evidence of significant heterogeneity in these data.

Walford and Hodge[2] found a significant increase of B7 in the patient group. Henschke et al.,[3] Wilcox et al.,[4] and Cohen et al.[5] also reported nonsignificant increase of B7 in 34, 10, and 17 patients, respectively. On the other hand, reports by Whalley et al.[6] on 14 patients, Sulkava et al.[7] on 32, Reisner et al.[8] on 52, and Reed et al.[9] on 44 patients showed a nonsignificant decrease of B7 in the patient samples. Thus in the combined analysis the association of B7 with this disease does not appear to be significant.

C locus antigens were tested by Henschke et al.[3] and Sulkava et al.[7] A nonsignificant increase in CW3[3] was reported. This was probably the result of the linkage disequilibrium of CW3 with B15 in Caucasians.

DR locus antigens were typed in the reports by Reed et al.[9] and Walford and Hodge[2]. No significant deviations were found.

Disease Heterogeneity

Renvoize et al.[1] also measured complement-fixation antibody titers to cytomegalovirus in the sera of 33 B15-positive and 81 B15-negative patients. Significantly more B15 positive patients had titers ≥ 1/64 ($p = 0.0013$). In the study by Whalley et al.,[6] the sera were also tested against several viral and bacterial antigens but no HLA association was observed.

Family Data

In 3 families, affected siblings had identical haplotypes and they did not share any haplotype with the unaffected siblings.[3] In a large pedigree reported by Walford and Hodge,[2] there was no strong evidence of linkage with HLA. In the population study of Reed et al.,[9] 1 of the patients had 1 affected sibling and another patient had 2 siblings with Alzheimer's disease. The affected sib pairs were HLA-identical in both families.

References

1. Renvoize EB, Hambling MH, Pepper MD, Rajah SM: Possible association of Alzheimer's disease with HLA-BW15 and cytomegalovirus infection. Lancet i:1238, 1979
2. Walford RL, Hodge SE: HLA distribution in Alzheimer's disease. In Terasaki PI (ed): Histocompa-

TABLE 20.9. Alzheimer's Disease

Country/Population	Patients n	Patients %+	Controls n	Controls %+	RR	χ^2	Ref.
HLA-B15							
Canada	34	15	239	10	1.68	1.12	3
England	50	14	550	12	1.26	0.32	10
England	124	28	458	14	2.39	13.38	1
England	14	29	64	17	2.06	1.33	6
	188	24	1072	13	2.03	13.15	
	Heterogeneity χ^2 (2 df)					1.88	
Finland	32	19	35	31	0.54	1.25	7
	254	22	1346	13	1.74	10.37	
	Heterogeneity χ^2 (4 df)					7.02	

tibility Testing 1980. UCLA Tissue Typing Laboratory, Los Angeles, 1981, pp 727-729
3. Henschke PJ, Bell DA, Cape RDT: Alzheimer's disease and HLA. Tissue Antigens 12:132-135, 1978
4. Wilcox CB, Caspary EA, Behan PO: Histocompatibility antigens in Alzheimer's disease. Eur Neurol 19:262-265, 1980
5. Cohen D, Eisdorfer C, Walford RL: Histocompatibility antigens (HLA) and patterns of cognitive loss in dementia of the Alzheimer type. Neurobiol Aging 2:277-280, 1981
6. Whalley LJ, Urbaniak SJ, Darg C, Peutherer JF, Christie JE: Histocompatibility antigens and antibodies to viral and other antigens in Alzheimer presenile dementia. Acta Psychiatr Scand 61:1-7, 1980
7. Sulkava R, Koskimies S, Wikstrom J, Palo J: HLA antigens in Alzheimer's disease. Tissue Antigens 16:191-194, 1980
8. Reisner E, Heyman A, Weinberg T, Dawson D, Ciftan E: Lack of association between Alzheimer's disease and histocompatibility antigens. Tissue Antigens 21:31-34, 1983
9. Reed E, Thompson D, Mayeaux R, Suciu-Foca N: HLA antigens in Alzheimer's disease. Tissue Antigens 21:164-167, 1983
10. Snowden PR, Woodrow JC, Copeland JRM: HLA antigens in senile dementia and multiple infarct dementia. Age Ageing 10:259-263, 1981

Multiple Infarct Dementia

Population Association

In 50 British patients typed for A and B loci antigens by Snowden et al.[1] no significant associaion has been found.

Reference

1. Snowden PR, Woodrow JC, Copeland JRM: HLA antigens in senile dementia and multiple infarct dementia. Age Ageing 10:259-263, 1981

Autism

Population Association

See ref. 1.

Reference

1. Stubbs G: Shared parental HLA antigens and autism. Lancet ii:534, 1981

Narcotic Dependence

Population Association

Maiskii et al.[1] reported significant associations with B5 and CW4 in 59 patients with a diagnosis of multiple drug dependence of stage II-III (Table 20.10).

Reference

1. Maiskii AI, Vedernikova N, Vedernikov AA, Shoshina SV, Borovkova NK, Naidenova NG, et al: Correlation between the principal histocompatibility system in mice and men and development of narcotic dependence. Byull Eksp Biol Med 90:596-598, 1980

Tourette Syndrome

Population Association

Comings et al.[1] studied the antigens of A and B loci in 12 American Caucasian patients. No significant deviations in the antigen frequencies were found.

Reference

1. Comings DE, Gursey BT, Hecht T, Blume K: HLA typing in Tourette syndrome. In Friedhoff AJ, Chase TN (eds): Gilles de la Tourette Syndrome. Raven Press, New York, 1982, pp 251-253

TABLE 20.10. Narcotic Dependence

	Patients		Controls				
Country/Population	n	%+	n	%+	RR	χ^2	Ref.
HLA-B5							
USSR	59	37	126	12	4.23	14.74	1
HLA-CW4							
USSR	59	42	126	20	2.87	9.65	1

CHAPTER 21

Hematologic Diseases

Aplastic Anemia

Population Association

In 200 patients studied by Albert et al.,[1] the frequencies of A2 and BW40 were found to be increased. Another report by Dausset et al.[2] on 68 French patients showed a significant increase in A2 (see also ref. 3). Similar results have also been reported by D'Amaro et al.[11] (Table 21.1).

Albert et al.[1] also reported an increase in the frequency of A2-BW40 and A3-B14 haplotypes.

Family Data

In the French study[2] the patients' siblings were more frequently homozygous for A2 ($p < 0.005$).

Thirty-four Swiss couples having a child with aplastic anemia were typed for A and B loci antigens by Werner-Favre and Jeannet.[5] An increased frequency of couples sharing 2 common HLA antigens was reported by these authors ($p \leq 0.05$).

See also refs. 6–9.

References

1. Albert E, Thomas ED, Nisperos B, Storb R: HLA antigens and haplotypes in 200 patients with aplastic anemia. Transplantation 22:528-531, 1976
2. Dausset J, Gluckman E, Lemarchand F, Nunez-Roldan A, Contu L, Hors J: Exces d'HLA-A2 et d'homozygotes HLA-A2 parmi les malades atteints d'aplasie medullaire et maladie de fanconi. Nouv Rev Fr Hematol Blood Cells 18:315-324, 1977
3. Gluckman E, Papon L, Hors J, Devergie A, Busson M, Gony J, et al: HLA markers in patients suffering from aplastic anaemia. Haematologia 14:165-172, 1981
4. D'Amaro J, Van Rood JJ, Rimm AA, Bortin MM: HLA association in Italian and non-Italian Caucasoid aplastic anaemia patients. Tissue Antigens 21:184-191, 1983
5. Werner-Favre CH, Jeannet M: HLA compatibility in couples with children suffering from acute leukemia or aplastic anemia. Tissue Antigens 13:307-309, 1979
6. Werner-Favre CH, Von Fliedner W, Jeannet M: Similitude des antigenes HLA chez les parents de patients atteints de leucemie aigue ou d'anemie aplastique. Schweiz Med Wochenschr 109:1399, 1979
7. Prusek W, Rudkowski Z, Zylka W, Lindner-Czygrinow I: Hematologic syndrome of severe anemia with hyperthrombocytemia and periodic leukopenia with co-existing incompatibility in the HL-A groups. Pediatr Pol 49:327-332, 1974
8. Van Leeuwen A, Goulmy E, Van Rood JJ: Major histocompatibility complex-restricted antibody reactivity mainly, but not exclusively, directed against cells from male donors. J Exp Med 150:1075-1083, 1979
9. Warren RP, Storb R, Thomas ED, Su PJ, Mickelson EM, Weiden PL: Autoimmune and alloimmune phenomena in patients with aplastic anemia: Cytotoxicity against autologous lymphocytes and lymphocytes from HLA identical siblings. Blood 56:683-689, 1980

Fanconi's Anemia

Family Data

In 14 families, Dausset et al.[1] (see also ref. 2) reported an excess of HLA homozygosity. Of the 18

TABLE 21.1. Aplastic Anemia

Country/Population	Patients n	Patients %+	Controls n	Controls %+	RR	χ^2	Ref.
HLA-A2							
Caucasians (unspecified)	187	60	1029	47	1.69	10.56	4
U.S.A.	200	61	1028	50	1.56	8.03	1
France	68	68	400	43	2.78	13.91	2
Italy	25	52	522	42	1.49	1.02	4
	480	61	2979	47	1.73	29.92	
	Heterogeneity χ^2 (3 df)					3.59	

patients, 4 were homozygous for A2 and 3 were homozygous for other antigens.

See also refs. 3 and 4.

References

1. Dausset J, Gluckman E, Lemarchand F, Nunez-Roldan A, Contu L, Hors J: Exces d'HLA-A2 et d'homozygotes HLA-A2 parmi les malades atteints d'aplasie medullaire et maladie de fanconi. Nouv Rev Fr Hematol Blood Cells 18:315-324, 1977
2. Hors J, Dausset J: Maladies malignes identiques au sein d'une meme famille. Nouv Presse Med 3:1237, 1974
3. Hansen JA, Good RA, Dupont B: HLA-D compatibility between parent and child. Transplantation 23:366-374, 1977
4. Hodge SE, Degos L, Walford RL: Four chromosomal instability syndromes: Bloom's syndrome, Fanconi's anemia, Werner's syndrome, and xeroderma pigmentosum. In Terasaki PI (ed): Histocompatibility Testing 1980. UCLA Tissue Typing Laboratory. Los Angeles, 1980, pp 730-731

Pernicious Anemia

Population Association

Available data (Table 21.2) on the association of A and B loci antigens suggest that in the pooled sample B7 showed a significant association with this disease. However, as can be seen from the Table 21.2, this association was significant in only 3 of the individual studies.[1–3] A3 was reported by Chanarin et al.[4] to be associated with this disease. However, in the combined analysis there was no evidence to support that conclusion.

Carmel et al.[5] typed A, B, C, and DR antigens in 38 American Black and 20 Latin American patients. When compared with the frequencies in 367 American Black and 332 Latin American controls no significant deviations were found.

Disease Heterogeneity

Association with the presence or absence of serum intrinsic factor antibody and thyroid antibody has been examined by several authors.[1,2,4,6–9] The data did not indicate such associations. Similar results have also been reported for age at onset,[9] sex,[6,9] and gastric parietal cell antibody.[1,6,9]

Ungar et al.[10] subdivided their 127 patients into 2 clinical subgroups. In 27 patients with concomitant endocrine disease, frequencies of B8 (44% vs. 27% in 586 controls), B18 (22% vs. 3% in controls), and BW15 (11% vs. 6% in controls) were increased. In the remaining 100 patients without endocrine disease, B7 (34% vs. 25%) and B12 (40% vs. 26%) were found to be increased. These 100 patients were further subdivided according to the functional severity of the gastric lesion as measured by Schilling test results. Sixty-two patients with Schilling values < 2% were categorized as having "gastric atrophy" and in this group the frequency of B12 was found to be 52%. This was significantly different from a frequency of 21% observed in 38 patients with "atrophic gastritis" (Schilling values 2–5%). Increased frequencies of B7 (62%) and B12 (62%), corresponding to the severity of the gastric atrophy, were also observed in 13 patients with vitamin B_{12} neuromyelopathy.

In another report by Ungar et al.[11] DR2 was significantly increased in the subgroup of 48 patients with anemia and no endocrine disease (56.2% vs. 25.8% in 120 controls).

TABLE 21.2. Pernicious Anemia

	Patients		Controls				
Country/Population	n	%+	n	%+	RR	χ^2	Ref.
HLA-B7							
U.S.A.	19	26	113	34	0.72	0.39	7
Czechoslovakia	27	8	301	27	0.28	4.29	3
England	29	52	400	27	2.91	8.06	1
England	127	31	586	25	1.35	2.04	10
England	66	27	86	22	1.31	0.53	8
England	33	27	537	28	0.98	0.00	4
England	53	29	100	32	0.88	0.13	7
England	52	43	300	31	1.68	2.98	6
England	42	43	216	26	2.15	5.03	2
	402	34	2225	27	1.48	10.68	
	Heterogeneity χ^2 (6 df)					8.09	
France	42	38	591	19	2.64	8.79	9
Denmark	106	32	3301	26	1.35	2.04	12
	596	33	6531	26	1.43	13.77	
	Heterogeneity χ^2 (10 df)					20.52	
HLA-DW2							
Denmark	93	41	293	26	1.98	7.62	12
HLA-DR2							
Australia	66	44	120	26	2.22	6.26	11
BENELUX	22	64	158	23	5.74	14.32	13
	88	49	278	24	3.02	17.71	
	Heterogeneity χ^2 (1 df)					2.86	

Thomsen et al.[17] subdivided their patients on the basis of presence of anemia or myelopathy at the time of diagnosis, presence of antibodies toward parietal cells or intrinsic factor, and the presence of organ-specific autoimmune disease in first-degree relatives. The frequency of DW2 in 34 patients with intrinsic factor antibody was 55.9% as compared with 34.5% in 55 patients without this antibody ($p < 0.05$). The other subgroups did not show any association with HLA.

Family Data

The typing of 4 families,[7] each with 2 or more patients, did not indicate close linkage between the disease and the HLA locus.

See also refs. 14 and 15.

References

1. Mawhinney H, Lawton JWM, White AG, Irvine WJ: HL-A3 and HL-A7 in pernicious anaemia and autoimmune atrophic gastritis. Clin Exp Immunol 22:47-53, 1975
2. Goldstone AH, Voak D, Cawley JC, Irvine WJ: HLA antigens in pernicious anaemia. Clin Exp Immunol 25:352-354, 1976
3. Majsky A, Fortynova J: HLA u perniciozni anemie a idiopaticke trombopenicke purpury. Cas Lek Cesk 119:275-277, 1980
4. Chanarin I, Knight S, O'Brien J, James D: HL-A groups in pernicious anaemia. Br J Haematol 33:539-541, 1976
5. Carmel R, Ozturk G, Johnson CS, Tunk KK, Terasaki PI: Profiles of Black and Latin-American patients having pernicious anemia. HLA antigens, lymphocytotoxic antibody, anti-parietal cell antibody, serum gastrin levels, and ABO blood groups. Am J Clin Pathol 75:291-296, 1981
6. Eastmond CJ, Woodrow JC: Lack of association between the HL-A system and pernicious anaemia. Br J Haematol 33:113-116, 1976
7. Wright JP, Callender STE, Grumet FC, Payne RO, Taylor KB: HLA antigens in Addisonian pernicious anaemia: Absence of an HLA and disease association. Br J Haematol 36:15-21, 1977

8. Horton MA, Oliver RTD: HLA antigen (A & B loci) frequency in Addisonian pernicious anaemia. Tissue Antigens 7:239-242, 1976
9. Zittoun R, Zittoun J, Seignalet J, Dausset J: HL-A and pernicious anemia. N Engl J Med 293:1324, 1975
10. Ungar B, Mathews JD, Tait BD, Cowling DC: HLA patterns in pernicious anaemia. Br Med J 1:798-800, 1977
11. Ungar B, Mathews JD, Tait BD, Cowling DC: HLA-DR patterns in pernicious anaemia. Br Med J 282:768-770, 1981
12. Thomsen M, Jorgensen F, Brandsborg M, Gimsing P, Nielsen JL, Ryder LP, et al.: Association of pernicious anemia and intrinsic factor antibody with HLA-D. Tissue Antigens 17:97-103, 1981
13. Van Den Berg-Loonen EM, Hilterman TCM, Bins M, Nijenhuis LE, Engelfriet CEP: Increased incidence of HLA-DR2 in patients with pernicious anemia. Tissue Antigens 19:158-160, 1982
14. Horton MA, Oliver RTD: HL-A and pernicious anemia. N Engl J Med 294:396-397, 1976
15. Horton MA. Oliver RTD: HLA phenotype A2;B12 in vitamin B_{12} neuromyelopathy. J Neurol Sci 32:79-89, 1977

Idiopathic Autoimmune Hemolytic Anemia

Population Association

An increase in the frequency of A3 (41.67%) in 38 French patients has been reported by Clauvel et al.[1] (The authors, however, did not give frequency data for the control groups.) The frequency of B8 in this sample of patients was 5.6%.

Da Costa et al.[2] also studied 12 British patients with this condition but reported no significant association with A and B antigens.

In the report of Abdel-Khalik et al.[3] B8 was found to be significantly increased in the patients. The frequency data from this and from the report by Da Costa et al.[2] are given in Table 21.3.

References

1. Clauvel JP, Marcelli-Barge A, Coggia IG, Poirier JC, Benajam A, Dausset J: HL-A antigens and idiopathic autoimmune hemolytic anemias. Transplant Proc 6:447-448, 1974
2. Da Costa JAG, White AG, Parker AC, Grigor GB: Increased incidence of HL-A 1 and 8 in patients showing IgG or complement coating on their red cells. J Clin Pathol 27:353-355, 1974
3. Abdel-Khalik A, Paton L, White AG, Urbaniak SJ: Human leucocyte antigens A, B, C, and DRW in idiopathic "warm" autoimmune haemolytic anaemia. Br Med J 280:760-761, 1980

Congenital Neutropenia

This disease is inherited as an autosomal recessive gene and is characterized by profound neutropenia, an apparent maturational arrest of neutrophils at the promyelocytic stage, and severe bacterial infection. The disease is fatal and death occurs during the first few years of life.

Population Association

Hansen et al.[1] typed A, B, and D loci antigens in 7 patients ranging in age from 2 months to 2 years. There was an increase in the frequency of B12 in the patient group (Table 21.4). The sample, however, was very small.

Family Data

The authors[1] also typed the family members of the 7 patients. There was a significant increase in the

TABLE 21.3. Idiopathic Autoimmune Hemolytic Anemia

	Patients		Controls				
Country/Population	n	%+	n	%+	RR	χ^2	Ref.
HLA-B8							
England	12	68	613	31	4.43	6.86	2
England	20	75	40	28	7.06	11.08	3
	32	72	653	31	5.55	17.62	
	Heterogeneity χ^2 (1 df)					0.32	

TABLE 21.4. Congenital Neutropenia

	Patients		Controls				
Country/Population	n	%+	n	%+	RR	χ^2	Ref.
HLA-B12							
U.S.A.	7	71	855	21	8.12	8.69	1

frequency of B12 homozygotes in the patients (42.8% vs. 1.2% in controls; $p = 0.0002$).

Reference

1. Hansen JA, Dupont B, L'esperance P, Good RA: Congenital neutropenia: Abnormal neutrophil differentiation associated with HLA. Immunogenetics 4:327-332, 1977

Chronic Familial Neutropenia

This disease is inherited as an autosomal dominant gene and is characterized by low total leukocyte count, absolute neutropenia, normal bone marrow, and no special tendency to infection.

Population Association

Weinberger et al.[1] studied A and B loci antigens in 49 Yemenite Jews. When compared with 107 controls, no significant deviations were observed.

Family Data

Weinberger's report[1] also contained data on 5 families typed for A and B antigens. There was no evidence of linkage of this disorder with HLA.

Reference

1. Weinberger A, Shoenfeld Y, Zamir R, Gazit E, Joshua H, Pinkhas J: HLA antigens in genetic neutropenia of Yemenite Jews. Vox Sang 36:105-108, 1979

Autoimmune Thrombocytopenic Purpura

Population Association

Karpatkin et al.[1] studied A, B, C, and DR antigens in 38 American Caucasian (55% Ashkenazi Jews) patients. Only 20 of these patients were typed for DR antigens. The frequency of DR2 was significantly increased. DR2 was present in 67% of the non-Jewish and in 79% of the Jewish patients. (See also refs. 2–4.)

References

1. Karpatkin S, Fotino M, Gibofsky A, Winchester RJ: Association of HLA-DRW2 with autoimmune thrombocytopenic purpura. J Clin Invest 63:1085-1088, 1979
2. Goebel KM, Hahn E, Havemann K: HLA matching in autoimmune thrombocytopenic purpura. Br J Haematol 35:341-342, 1977
3. Remuzzi G, Misiani R, Livio M, Dall'olio A, Donati MB, De Gaetano G: Possible role of HLA-B8 antigen as a genetic marker of autoimmune thrombocytopenia in a patient with myasthenia gravis. Thromb Haemost 38:593-594, 1977
4. Goebel KM, Hahn E, Gassel WD, Havemann K: Lymphozytenantigene bei autoimmun-Thrombozytopenien. Schweiz Med Wochenschr 106:1360-1361, 1976

TABLE 21.5. Autoimmune Thrombocytopenic Purpura

	Patients		Controls				
Country/Population	n	%+	n	%+	RR	χ^2	Ref.
HLA-DR2							
U.S.A.—Caucasian + Jews	20	75	66	23	9.22	15.91	1

Idiopathic Thrombocytopenic Purpura

Population Association

Available data for idiopathic thrombocytopenic purpura (ITP) are variable and inconsistent.

Evers et al.[1-3] and Westphal and Muller-Ruchholtz[4] reported a significant association with AW32 (27% in 26 patients vs. 1% in 250 controls, $\chi^2 = 25.82$). However, the frequency of AW32 in the authors' control groups was unusually low as compared with other German data.

Goebel et al.[5,6] and Exadaktylos et al.[7] found increased frequencies of B18 and B12 in a sample of 20 German patients (no data on other antigens are given).

Mueller-Eckhardt et al.[8] studied 79 patients (German and Austrian) with definite ITP for A, B, and C loci antigens. There was no significant difference in the frequencies when compared with a control sample of 350 Germans and 3000 Austrians. Similar results have also been reported by Veenhoven et al.[9] on 60 German patients.

Majsky and Fortynova[10,11] found no significant association with A and B loci antigens in 62 Czechoslovakian patients and 301 controls.

Mohanty et al.[12] also reported data on 20 patients and 60 controls from North India. There was no association with A and B loci antigens.

Thus, increased frequencies of AW32, B8, and B12 observed by Evers et al.[3] and Goebel et al.[5] could not be confirmed in other German and Austrian samples. From these data it appears that at present there is no evidence of association between ITP and HLA-A, -B, and -C antigens.

DR locus antigens were typed in a sample of 76 European Caucasian patients (39 from Vienna and 37 from Giessen) by Mayr et al.[13] No significant deviations, when compared with 266 controls, were found.

Sakurami et al.[14] also studied DR antigens in 9 Japanese patients. Again, no significant association was observed.

Family Data

In 1 family reported by Goebel et al.,[5,6] the B8-B12 phenotype was present in all 3 patients.

Stuart et al. (quoted in ref. 8, p 350) examined 3 children with chronic ITP and their families. A3-B7 was present in all 3 cases (see also ref. 15).

References

1. Evers KG, Thouet R, Haase W, Kruger J: HLA frequencies and haplotypes in children with idiopathic thrombocytopenic purpura (ITP). Eur J Pediatr 131:82-83, 1979
2. Evers KG, Haase W, Thouet R, Kruger J: Assoziation von HLA-AW32 und reversibler postinfektioser thrombozytopenischer Purpura des Kindesalters. Monatsschr Kinderheilkd 127:268-269, 1979
3. Evers KG, Thouet R, Haase W, Krueger: HLA frequencies and haplotypes in children with idiopathic thrombocytopenic purpura (ITP). Eur J Pediatr 129:267-272, 1978
4. Westphal E, Muller-Ruchholtz W: HLA frequencies and haplotypes in children with idiopathic thrombocytopenic purpura (ITP). Eur J Pediatr 131:81-83, 1979
5. Goebel KM, Hahn E, Havemann K: HLA matching in autoimmune thrombocytopenic purpura. Br J Haematol 35:341-342, 1977
6. Goebel KM, Hahn E, Gassel WD, Havemann K: Lymphozytenantigene bei autoimmun-Thrombozytopenien. Schweiz Med Wochenschr 106:1360-1361, 1976
7. Exadaktylos P, Tesar V, Heinrichs I, Rumler W. HLA-Phanotypen bei idiopathischer Thrombozytopenie im Kindesalter. Acta Biol Med Ger 39:1095-1097, 1980
8. Mueller-Eckhardt C, Mayr W, Lechner K, Mueller-Eckhardt G, Niessner H, Pralle H: HLA antigens in immunologic thrombocytogenic purpura (ITP). Scand J Haematol 23:348-352, 1979
9. Veenhoven WA, Kaars Sijpesteijn JAK, Van Der Schans GS: HLA antigens in idiopathic thrombocytopenic purpura. Acta Haematol 62:153-158, 1979
10. Majsky A, Fortynova: HLA and idiopathic thrombopenic purpura (ITP). Tissue Antigens 15:222-223, 1980
11. Majsky A, Fortynova J: HLA u perniciozni anemie a idiopaticke trombopenicke purpury. Cas Lek Cesk 119:275-277, 1980
12. Mohanty D, Quadri MI, Das KC, Sengupta S: HLA and idiopathic thrombocytopenic purpura (ITP). Br J Haematol 42:329-330, 1979
13. Mayr WR, Mueller-Eckhardt G, Kruger M, Mueller-Eckhardt C, Lechner K, Niessner H: HLA-DR in chronic idiopathic thrombocytopenic purpura (ITP). Tissue Antigens 18:56-57, 1981
14. Sakurami T, Ueno Y, Iwaki Y, Park MS, Terasaki PI, Saji H: HLA-DR specificities among Japanese with several autoimmune disease. Tissue Antigens 19:129-133, 1982

15. Hellman RM, Jackson DV, Buss DH: Thrombotic thrombocytopenic purpura and hemolytic-uremic syndrome in HLA-identical siblings. Ann Intern Med 93:283-284, 1980

Paroxysmal Nocturnal Hemoglobinuria

Population Association

Ten Cuban patients with paroxysmal nocturnal hemoglobinuria and 109 controls were typed for A and B loci antigens by Ustariz et al.[1] No significant association was observed.

Reference

1. Ustariz CR, Arce S, Hernandez P, Almaguer M, Perez S, Ballester JM: HLA antigens in paroxysmal nocturnal hemoglobinuria. Acta Haematol 63:52-54, 1980

Thalassemia Minor

Family Data

Parfrey et al.[1] studied the segregation of A, B, and C loci antigens and thalassemia minor in 2 British families. Lod score calculations presented by the authors did not indicate linkage between HLA and this disorder (see also ref. 2).

References

1. Parfrey PS, Turnbull AL, Wolf E, Sachs J, Festenstein H: Independent segregation of HLA-A, -B, and -C antigens from thalassemia minor. Tissue Antigens 13:373-376, 1979
2. Edwards CQ, Skolnick MH, Kushner JP: Coincidental nontransfusional iron overload and thalassemia minor: Association with HLA-linked hemochromatosis. Blood 58:844-848, 1981

Erythrocyte Glucose-6-Phosphate Dehydrogenase (G-6-PD) Deficiency

Population Association

The frequency of A2 in 76 patients from Sardinia[1] was significantly increased (36% in the patients vs. 15% in 157 controls). In another report from Bulgaria,[2] however, this increase was not observed. In the pooled data A2 was not significantly associated with the disease and also there was evidence of significant heterogeneity. In the Bulgarian sample Minev and Bulanov[2] observed no significant increase in the frequencies of A1, AW23, and BW35.

References

1. Carcassi U, Del Giacco GS, Pintus A, Perpignaho G, Locci F, Roy M, et al: HLA antigens and erythrocyte glucose-6-phosphate dehydrogenase (G-6-PD) deficiency in Sardinia. Int Arch Allergy Appl Immunol 54:285-287, 1977
2. Minev M, Bulanov AG: The HLA system and G6PD deficiency in the Bulgarian population. Tissue Antigens 15:467-470, 1980

Positive Direct Coomb's Test

Population Association

Da Costa et al.[1] observed significant associations with A1 and B8 in 56 patients with positive Coomb's tests (Table 21.6). The patients were diagnosed for a variety of medical conditions. However, they shared the common feature of Coomb's positivity of the red cells.

TABLE 21.6. Positive Direct Coomb's Test

	Patients		Controls				
Country/Population	n	%+	n	%+	RR	χ^2	Ref.
HLA-A1							
England	56	63	613	36	2.99	14.92	1
HLA-B8							
England	56	59	613	31	3.18	16.98	1

Reference

1. Da Costa JAG, White AG, Parker AC, Grigor GB: Increased incidence of HL-A 1 and 8 in patients showing IgG or complement coating on their red cells. J Clin Pathol 27:353-355, 1974

Hereditary Spherocytosis

Hereditary spherocytosis is an autosomal dominant disease characterized by splenomegaly, variable degrees of anemia, spherocytosis, and increased osmotic fragility of red corpuscles.

Family Data

In a report on 2 Canadian families typed for A and B loci antigens, Sengar et al.[1] suggested that this condition may be linked with HLA. The first family had 3 affected and 1 healthy sibling. All 3 affected siblings had received the A3-B14 haplotype from the affected father. In the second family the 2 affected siblings had the A9-B12 haplotype in common. One of the affected siblings had 3 offspring. Two of them had A9-B12 but only 1 was affected.

In another study of 19 families by de Jongh et al.[2,3] the linkage analysis was done by calculating lod scores for each of the families. All the lod score values for recombination fractions < 30% were < −2.00, indicating the absence of close linkage of this disease with the HLA complex.[2] The segregation analysis of these families indicated an autosomal dominant (100% penetrance) pattern of inheritance.

See also ref. 4.

References

1. Sengar DPS, Mcleish WA, Smiley RK, Luke B: HLA and hereditary spherocytosis. Vox Sang 33:278-279, 1977
2. De Jongh BM, Blacklock HA, Reekers P, Volkers WS, Khan PM, Bernini LF, et al: Absence of close linkage between hereditary spherocytosis (SPH) and 24 genetic marker systems including HLA and GM. Ann Hum Genet 47:55-65, 1983
3. De Jongh BM, Schreuder I, Hawkins B, and Van Rood JJ: Hereditary spherocytosis. In Terasaki PI (ed): Histocompatibility Testing 1980. UCLA Tissue Typing Laboratory, Los Angeles, 1981, pp 734-735
4. Edwards CQ, Skolnick MH, Dadone MM, Kushner JP: Iron overload in hereditary spherocytosis: Association with HLA-linked hemochromatosis. Am J Hematol 13:101-109, 1982

Agranulocytosis Following Treatment with Levamisole

Population Association

Teerenhovi et al.[1] compared 17 breast cancer patients, treated with levamisole (150–250 mg daily on 2 consecutive days every week) and showing a high frequency of agranulocytosis and severe granulocytopenia, with 900 Finnish blood donors. The frequency of B27 was 33% in the patients and 14% in the controls, showing no significant difference between the 2 groups.

Schmidt and Mueller-Eckhardt[2] reported 3 female German patients with definite rheumatoid arthritis who were treated with levamisole. Two patients had typical agranulocytosis and the third had granulocytopenia, severe thrombocytopenia, and acute renal failure. All 3 were positive for B27.

Hodinka et al.[3] also reported data on 37 Hungarian patients who were treated with levamisole for 6–12 months. Three of these patients developed agranulocytosis and 2 were found to be positive for B27.

References

1. Teerenhovi L, Heinonen E, Grohn P, Klefstrom P, Mehtonen M, Tiibikainen A: High frequency of agranulocytosis in breast-cancer patients treated with levamisole. Lancet ii:151-152, 1978
2. Schmidt KL, Mueller-Eckhardt C: Agranulocytosis, levamisole, and HLA-B27. Lancet ii:85, 1977
3. Hodinka L, Geher P, Meretey K, Gyodi EK, Petranyi GG, Bozsoky S: Lavamisole-induced neutropenia and agranulocytosis: Association of HLA B27 leukocyte agglutinating and lymphocytotoxic antibodies. Int Arch Allergy Appl Immunol 65:460-464, 1981

Von Willebrand's Disease

Population Association

In 28 French patients and 326 controls Goudemand et al.[1] observed no significant difference.

Family Data

The authors[1] also examined the families of 26 patients and reported no evidence of linkage between this disease and HLA.

Reference

1. Goudemand J, Mazurier C, Parquet-Gernez A, Goudemand M: Antigenes HLA et maladie de Willebrand. Pathol Biol (Paris) 25:241-243, 1977

Antibody to Factor VIII in Classic Hemophilia

Family Data

Ten brother-pairs, each consisting of 2 hemophiliacs, were typed for A, B, and D antigens by Frommel et al.[1] In 8 pairs both patients were immune to factor VIII and in 2 remaining pairs, 1 sibling was with and the other without factor VIII antibody. The 2 patients without antibody had been exposed to factor VIII for more than 75 cumulative days.

Seven sib-pairs shared 1 haplotype and 1 pair was HLA- and MLC-identical. The haplotypes of the 2 pairs with and without factor VIII antibody were not identical. The authors have calculated that the probability that this observed distribution was due to chance alone is $(0.75)^{10} = 0.056$.

The authors also cite 2 reports in which no significant increase in 1 or more HLA antigens was observed.

In a second report by Frommel et al.[2] 26 families in which 2 or more brothers had classic hemophilia were analyzed for linkage with HLA complex. The distribution of parental HLA haplotype among hemophilic brothers did not differ from random segregation whether analysis was done on the cohort of 53 patients or on the subgroups of concordant and nonconcordant brother pairs. On the basis of this analysis the authors have concluded that linkage with the HLA complex was very unlikely.

References

1. Frommel D, Muller JY, Prou-Wartelle O, Allain JP: Possible linkage between the major histocompatibility complex and the immune response to factor VIII in classic haemophilia. Vox Sang 33:270-272, 1977
2. Frommel D, Allain JP, Saint-Paul E, Bosser C, Noel B, and Mannucci PM, et al: HLA antigens and factor VIII antibody in classic hemophilia. European and study group of factor VIII antibody. Suppl Thromb Haemostas 46:687-689, 1981

Benign Monoclonal Gammopathy

Population Association

In 52 French patients[1, 2] the frequency of B15 was found to be significantly increased. In another French study by Cassuto et al.[3] this was not confirmed, however. The data from both studies are given in Table 21.7.

Disease Heterogeneity

In the aforementioned French study,[2] when the 52 benign monoclonal gammopathy patients were compared with 48 patients with unrelated malignant gammopathy (33 with multiple myeloma and 15 with Waldenstrom's macroglobulinemia), the frequency of BW40 was 25% in the benign monoclonal gammopathy group and 2% in the malignant group. This difference was significant even after correction for the number of antigens compared in the study.

References

1. Saleun JP, Youinou P, Le Goff P, Lemenn G, Morin JF: HLA antigen and monoclonal gammopathy. Tissue Antigens 13:233-235, 1979
2. Youinou P: Genetic propensity to benignity in monoclonal-gammopathy. Acta Haematol 62:173-175, 1979
3. Cassuto JP, Pierecchi J, Maiolini R, Dujardin O, Ribeil R, Masseyeff R: Marqueurs HLA dians les myelomes et les dysglobulinemies monoclonales benignes. Nouv Presse Med 10:252-253, 1981

TABLE 21.7. Benign Monoclonal Gammopathy

	Patients		Controls				
Country/Population	n	%+	n	%+	RR	χ^2	Ref.
HLA-B15							
France	52	25	200	5	6.20	17.29	1
France	51	10	172	8	1.34	0.34	3
	103	18	372	6	3.23	12.45	
	Heterogeneity χ^2 (1 df)					5.18	

TABLE 21.8. Polycythemia Vera

	Patients		Controls				
Country/Population	n	%+	n	%+	RR	χ^2	Ref.
HLA-B5							
U.S.A.	9	67	100	16	9.64	11.05	1
Hungary	46	29	490	10	3.72	14.20	2
	55	35	590	11	4.54	23.70	
	Heterogeneity χ^2 (1 df)					1.54	
HLA-BW21							
Jews (unspecified)	122	17	366	8	2.36	8.06	3

Polycythemia Vera

Population Association

Two independent studies from the United States[1] and Hungary[2] have reported significant associations with B5 (Table 21.8).

A third report on 122 Jewish patients (101 Ashkenazi and 21 non-Ashkenazi) from Israel[3] has shown a marginally significant increased frequency of BW21 (Table 21.8). The frequency of B5 did not differ between patients and controls (14% in 122 patients vs. 13% in 366 controls).

Disease Heterogeneity

When the Israeli patients[3] were subdivided according to the age at onset (20–40, 41–60, and 61–80 years) the antigen frequencies, including BW21, were similar in all 3 subgroups.

References

1. Miller WV: HL-A antigens and hematologic malignancy. Arch Intern Med 133:397-399, 1974
2. Nagy G, Stenszky V, Timar I, Murvay K: Tissue antigens and cytotoxic antibodies in polycythaemia rubra vera. Haematologia 9:279-282, 1975
3. Benjamin D, Zamir R, Gazit E, Pinkhas J, Yehoshua H: HLA antigens in polycythemia vera. Tissue Antigens 11:65-67, 1978

Glanzmann's Thrombasthenia Type I

Family Data

Tongio et al.[1] reported 2 multiple-case families of the Manouches Gypsy tribe from France. These data showed that the disease segregated independently of the HLA system.

Reference

1. Tongio MM, Lutz P, Hauptmann G, Rodier L, Levy JM, Mayer S, et al: Type I Glanzmann's thrombasthenia segregates independently of Ss and Duffy systems and the A,B,C, factor B, C2 and C4 loci of the HLA complex. Tissue Antigens 20:22-27, 1982.

CHAPTER 22

Complement and Immune Deficiencies

Complement Factor C1q Deficiency

Family Data

Arnaiz-Villena et al.[1] reported a family of 6 siblings in which 3 were C1q-deficient. The 3 affected siblings did not have a common haplotype. One of the normal siblings was HLA identical with his C1q-deficient brother.

Thus this family does not show evidence of linkage between C1q deficiency and the HLA complex.

Reference

1. Arnaiz-Villena A, Lopez-Larrea C, Leyva-Cobian F, Bootello GA: Genetic independence between HLA and first component (C1q) of complement. Transplantation 31:139-140, 1981

Complement Factor Clr Deficiency

Family Data

In 2 families reported by Day et al.[1] no evidence of linkage between the Clr gene and HLA has been found (see also refs. 2 and 3).

References

1. Day NK, Rubinstein P, DeBracco M, Moncada B, Hensen JA, Dupont B, et al: Hereditary Clr deficiency: Lack of linkage to the HL-A region in 2 families. In Kissmeyer-Nielsen F (ed): Histocompatibility Testing 1975. Munksgaard, Copenhagen, 1975, p 96
2. Jersild C, Rubinstein P, Day NK: The HLA system and inherited deficiencies of the complement system. Transplant Rev 32:43-71, 1976
3. Mittal KK, Wolski KP, Lim D, Gewurz A, Gewurz H, Schmid FR: Genetic independence between the HL-A system and deficits in the first and sixth components of complement. Tissue Antigens 7:97-104, 1976

Complement Factor C2 Deficiency

Population Association

In a study of 62 DW2-positive and 64 DW2-negative healthy individuals, Nerl et al. [1] reported that DW2-positive persons had a significantly higher incidence of low C2 (and also C4) levels. Sixty-three percent of the DW2-positive but only 37% of the DW2-negative individuals had low C2 levels. On the other hand, only 37% of the DW2-positive and 63% of the DW2-negative individuals had high C2 levels. The difference between the 2 groups was significant ($p = 0.004$).

Family Data

Fu et al.[2] were the first to report the close linkage between C2 deficiency and HLA. In the family the authors studied, the proband was homozygous both for C2 deficiency and the HLA haplotype A10-BW18. There were no recombinants in 7 children of 3 double back-cross matings. In a second report by the same group of authors[3,4] these results were confirmed. Since then data on 1 family by Wolski et al.,[5] 2 by Day et al.,[6,7] 9 by Gibson et al.,[8] 1 by Opelz and Glovsky,[9] 1 by Brouet et al.,[10] 1 by Lehner-Netsch et al.,[11] and 1 by Mahowald et al.,[12] have clearly established the close linkage of the C2 deficiency gene with HLA. The position of this gene is within the HLA complex near the B or D loci. Based on a probable recombination between C2 and HLA-D loci, Gibson et al.[8] have given the likely order of these loci on chromosome 6 as C2 complement, HLA-D, HLA-B, and HLA-A.

See also refs. 13–17.

References

1. Nerl CH, Grosse-Wilde, Valet G: Association of low C2 and C4 serum levels with the HLA-DW2 allele in healthy individuals. J Exp Med 148:704-713, 1978
2. Fu SM, Kunkel HG, Brusman HP, Allen FH Jr, Fotino M: Evidence for linkage between HL-A histocompatibility genes and those involved in the syntheses of the second component of complement. J Exp Med 140:1108-1111, 1974
3. Fu SM, Stern R, Kunkel HG, Dupont B, Hansen JA, Day NK, et al: Mixed lymphocyte culture determinants and C2 deficiency: LD-7A associated with C2 deficiency in four families. J Exp Med 142:495-506, 1975
4. Fu SM, Kunkel HG: Association of C2 deficiency and the HL-A haplotype 10, W18. Transplantation 20:179-180, 1975
5. Wolski KP, Schmid FR, Mittal KK: Genetic linkage between the HL-A system and a deficit of the second component (C2) of complement. Science 188:1020-1022, 1975
6. Day NK, L'Esperance P, Good RA, Michael AF, Hansen JA, Dupont B, et al: Hereditary C2 deficiency: Genetic studies and association with the HL-A system. J Exp Med 141:1464-1469, 1975
7. Day NK, Rubinstein P, Case D, Hansen JA, Good RA, Walker ME, et al: Linkage of gene for C2 deficiency and the major histocompatibility complex MHC in man: Family study of a further case. Vox Sang 31:96-102, 1976
8. Gibson DJ, Glass D, Carpenter CB, Schur PH: Hereditary C2 deficiency: Diagnosis and HLA gene complex associations. J Immunol 116:1065-1070, 1976
9. Opelz G, Glovsky MM: HLA antigen studies in a family with C2 deficiency. J Immunogenet 3:303-306, 1976
10. Brouet JC, Fridman WH, Clauvel JP, Sasportes M, Danon F, Seligmann M: Deficit genetique de la deuxieme fraction du complement avec manifestation lupiques. Nouv Presse Med 6:3199-3203, 1977
11. Lehner-Netsch G, Simard J, Prochazka E, Brun G, Delage JM: Double deficit en C2 et en C7, chez un meme sujet etude du complement et du systeme HLA. Union Med Can 107:928-932, 1978
12. Mahowald ML, Dalmasso AP, Petzel RA, Yunis EJ: Linkage relationship of C2 deficiency, HLA and glyoxalase I loci. Vox Sang 37:321-328, 1979
13. Jersild C, Rubinstein P, Day NK: The HLA system and inherited deficiencies of the complement system. Transplant Rev 32:43-71, 1976
14. Berrens L, Baart De La Faille H, Borst-Eilers E: HLA-linked C2 deficiency in a Dutch patient with systemic lupus erythematosus. J Clin Pathol 32:528-533, 1979
15. Suciu-Foca N, O'Neill G: Families with C2 and C4 functional deficiencies. In Terasaki PI (ed): Histocompatibility Testing 1980. UCLA Tissue Typing Laboratory, Los Angeles, 1981, pp 938-959
16. Mortensen P, Buskjaer L, Lamm LU: Studies on the C2-deficiency gene in man. Immunology 39:541-549, 1980
17. Awdeh ZL, Raum DD, Glass D, Agnello V, Schur PH, Johnston RB JR, et al: Complement-human histocompatibility antigen haplotypes in C2 deficiency. J Clin Invest 67:581-583, 1981

Complement Factor C3 Deficiency

Family Data

Lod score data on 23 families presented by Lamm et al.[1] have shown no evidence of linkage between HLA and C3 deficiency. In another family of 15 members[2] in which the proband had complete C3 deficiency and 6 other individuals had a 50% C3 deficiency (heterozygous), no evidence of linkage with HLA was found.

See also refs. 3 and 4.

References

1. Lamm LU, Thorsen I, Peterson GB, Jorgensen J, Hemmingsen K, Bech B, et al: Data on the HL-A linkage group. Ann Hum Genet 38:383-390, 1975
2. Osofsky SG, Thompson BH, Gewurz H, Schmid FR, Mittal KK: Evidence for lack of linkage between HLA and C3 deficiency in man. Immunogenetics 4:195-197, 1977
3. Sissons JGP, Williams DG, Peters DK, and Boulton-Jones JM: Skin lesions, angio-oedema, and hypocomplementaemia. Lancet ii:1350-1352, 1974
4. Jersild C, Rubinstein P, Day NK: The HLA system and inherited deficiencies of the complement system. Transplant Rev 32:43-71, 1976

Complement Factor C4 Deficency

Population Association

Nerl et al.[1] examined 64 DW2-positive and 72 DW2-negative unrelated healthy individuals for their C4 serum protein levels. A bimodal distribution was found in DW2-positive as well as in DW2-negative persons. Furthermore, DW2-positive individuals had a significantly higher incidence of low C4 serum levels. Thus, there is some evidence for the hypothesis of the existence of linkage disequilibrium between the C4 gene and the HLA-DW2 allele.

Family Data

The linkage of C4 with HLA was first shown in a family studied by Rittner et al.[2] Later studies by Ochs et al.,[3] Ballow et al.,[4,5] and O'Neill et al.[6,7] have provided further data and have confirmed this linkage (see also ref. 8).

See also refs. 9–12.

References

1. Nerl CH, Grosse-Wilde, Valet G: Association of low C2 and C4 serum levels with the HLA-DW2 allele in healthy individuals. J Exp Med 148:704-713, 1978
2. Rittner C, Hauptmann, Gross-Wilde H, Grosshans E, Tongio MM, Mayer S: Linkage between HL-A (major histocompatibility complex) and genes controlling the synthesis of the 4th component of complement. In Kissmeyer F (ed): Histocompatibility Testing 1975. Munksgaard, Copenhagen, 1975, pp. 945–954.
3. Ochs HD, Rosenfeld SI, Thomas ED, Giblett ER, Alber CA, Dupont B, et al: Linkage between the gene (or genes) controlling synthesis of the fourth component of complement and the major histocompatibility complex. N Engl J Med 296:470-475, 1977
4. Ballow M, Mclean RH, Einarson M, Martin S, Yunis EJ, Dupont B, et al: Hereditary C4 deficiency-genetic studies and linkage to HLA. Transplant Proc 11:1710-1712, 1979
5. Ballow M, McLean RH, Yunis EJ, Awdeh ZL, O'-Neill J, Einarson M, et al: C4 polymorphism and HLA linkage: Studies in a family with hereditary C4 deficiency. Clin Immunol Immunopathol 20:354-360, 1981
6. O'Neill GJ, Yang SY, Tegoli J, Berger R, Dupont B: Chido and Rogers blood groups are distinct antigenic components of human complement C4. Nature 273:668-670, 1978
7. O'Neill GJ, Berger R, Ballow M, Yunis EJ, Dupont B: Chido, Rogers, and C4 deficiency. Transplant Proc 11:1941-1943, 1979
8. Jersild C, Rubinstein P, Day NK: The HLA system and inherited deficiencies of the complement system. Transplant Rev 32:43-71, 1976
9. Suciu-Foca N, O'Neill G: Families with C2 and C4 functional deficiencies. In Terasaki PI (ed): Histocompatibility Testing 1980. UCLA Tissue Typing Laboratory, Los Angeles, 1981, pp 938-959
10. Pollack MS, Ochs HD, Dupont B: HLA typing of cultured amniotic cells for the prenatal diagnosis of complement C4 deficiency. Clin Genet 18:197-200, 1980
11. O'Neill GJ, Nerl C, Pollack MS: Analysis of active and inactive complement C4 complotypes associated with subtypes of HLA-B17 in different racial groups. Am J Hum Genet 35:309-317, 1983
12. Rittner CH, Zaschke S, Berghoff E, Mollenhauer E, Opferkuch W, Baur MP: Comparative studies of human C4 phenotypes, their population genetics, and association with HLA-B antigens. Immunobiology 158:119-128, 1980

Complement Factor C6 Deficiency

Family Data

Data on 1 small pedigree reported by Mittal et al.[1] suggested no linkage between C6 deficiency and HLA (see also ref. 2).

Lod score data for several families have been presented by Hobart et al.[3] These calculations showed that C6 was at least 18% recombination units from HLA in the male (lod score −2.7). (The authors assumed that the female recombination fraction was 1.7 times that of the male.)

Thus, the available data indicate that there is no evidence of close linkage between HLA and C6.

References

1. Mittal KK, Wolski KP, Lim D, Gewurz A, Gewurz H, Schmid FR: Genetic independence between the HL-A system and deficits in the first and sixth components of complement. Tissue Antigens 7:97-104, 1976
2. Jersild C, Rubinstein P, Day NK: The HLA system and inherited deficiencies of the complement system. Transplant Rev 32:43-71, 1976
3. Hobart MJ, Cook PJL, Lachmann PJ: Linkage studies with C6. J Immunogenet 4:423-428, 1977

Complement Factor C7 Deficiency

Family Data

Available data on 3 families[1–4] showed no evidence of linkage between C7 deficiency and HLA.

The pedigree studied by Rittner et al.[1] was also typed for Bf, GLO, and HLA-D antigens.

See also ref. 5.

References

1. Rittner CH, Opferkuch W, Wellek B, Grosse-Wilde H, Wernet P: Lack of linkage between gene(s) controlling the synthesis of the seventh component of complement and the HLA region on chromosome no. 6 in man. Hum Genet 34:137-142, 1976
2. Lint TF, Osofsky SG, Nemerow GR, Tausk K, Gewurz H: Inherited deficiency of the seventh component of complement (C7) in man: Description, relationship to HLA and partial characterization of an inhibitory activity. Clin Res 24:543a, 1976
3. Delage JM, Bergeron P, Simard J, Lehner-Netsch G, Prochazka E: Hereditary C7 deficiency: Diagnosis and HLA studies in a French-Canadian family. J Clin Invest 60:1061-1069, 1977
4. Lehner-Netsch G, Simard J, Prochazka E, Brun G, Delage JM: Double deficit en C2 et en C7, chez un meme sujet etude du complement et du systeme HLA. Union Med Can 107:928-932, 1978
5. Jersild C, Rubinstein P, Day NK: The HLA system and inherited deficiencies of the complement system. Transplant Rev 32:43-71, 1976

Complement Factor C8 Deficiency

Family Data

HLA typing of an American Black family with C8 deficiency (see ref. 1) indicated close linkage with HLA. However, in another study by Giraldo et al.[2] of a 23-member pedigree from Tunisia with C8 deficiency (with a high incidence of xeroderma pigmentosum) no close linkage between HLA and a "C8-defective" chromosome was found. These authors also quoted a report on another small family (3 members) in which no linkage with HLA was observed.

See also ref. 3.

References

1. Jersild C, Rubinstein P, Day NK: The HLA system and inherited deficiencies of the complement system. Transplant Rev 32:43-71, 1976
2. Giraldo G, Degos L, Beth E, Sasportes M, Marelli A, Gharbi R, et al: C8 deficiency in a family with xeroderma pigmentosum: Lack of linkage to the HL-A region. Clin Immunol Immunopathol 8:377-384, 1977
3. Densen P, Brown EJ, O'Neill GJ, Tedesco F, Clark RA, Frank MM, et al: Inherited deficiency of C8 in a patient with recurrent meningococcal infections. Further evidence for a dysfunctional C8 molecule and nonlinkage to the HLA system. J Clin Immunol 3:90-99, 1983

IgA Deficiency

Population Association

Ambrus et al.[1] studied 26 Hungarian patients with selective IgA deficiency determined by 1) immunoglobulin measured by single radial immunodiffusion, 2) lymphocyte DNA synthesis after nitrogen stimulation, 3) rosette-binding tests for E and EAC rosettes, and 4) immunofluorescent studies of circulating B lymphocytes. A comparison of A and B loci antigen frequencies with 60 controls showed

TABLE 22.1. IgA Deficiency

Country/Population	Patients n	Patients %+	Controls n	Controls %+	RR	χ^2	Ref.
HLA-B8							
Canada	62	44	608	23	2.63	12.92	2
Hungary	26	46	60	15	4.65	8.97	1
Denmark	32	44	3301	25	2.37	6.19	4
Sweden	19	74	272	25	7.99	17.00	3
	139	48	4241	25	3.19	40.00	
	Heterogeneity χ^2 (3 df)					5.08	
HLA-DR3							
Sweden	21	81	272	25	11.64	21.89	3

increased frequencies of A1 and B8 in the patients. This increase of B8 frequency was also found in the studies of Oen et al.,[2] Hammarstrom and Smith,[3] Jersild et al.,[4] and also in 2 patients by Perez-Jimenez.[5] A combined analysis of all the available data is given in Table 22.1.

Family Data

Van Thiel et al.[6] reported a family of 43 individuals with 3 members affected by a variable expression of a syndrome consisting of immunoglobulin A deficiency, diabetes mellitus, malabsorption, and a common HLA haplotype, A2-B8-DW3.

Segregation of HLA haplotypes was studied in 10 families by Oen et al.[2] There was no evidence of linkage with the HLA complex.

References

1. Ambrus M, Hernadi E, Bajtai G: Prevalence of HLA-A1 and HLA-B8 antigens in selective IgA deficiency. Clin Immunol Immunopathol 7:311-314, 1977
2. Oen K, Petty RE, Schroeder ML: Immunoglobulin A deficiency: Genetic studies. Tissue Antigens 19:174-182, 1982
3. Hammarstrom L, Smith CIE: HLA-A, -B, -C and DR antigens in immunoglobulin A deficiency. Tissue Antigens 21:75-79, 1983
4. Jersild C, Staub-Nielsen L, Svejgaard A: HLA and IgA deficiency in blood donors. Tissue Antigens 21:80, 1983
5. Perez-Jimenez F, Lopez PB, Tallo EP, Guzman JR, Molina JS, Pereperez JAJ: Selective IgA deficiency and the HLA-B8 antigen. Arch Intern Med 141:509-510, 1981
6. Van Thiel DH, Smith WI Jr, Rabin BS, Fisher SE, Lester R: A syndrome of immunoglobulin A deficiency, diabetes mellitus, malabsorption, and a common HLA haplotype. Ann Intern Med 86:10-19, 1977

Immunodeficiency (Unspecified)

Population Association

Hors et al.[1] first published a report on 26 Caucasian children suffering from various types of immune deficiency. In this sample A1 was present in 17 patients (47%) as compared with 21% in a control population of unknown size (corrected $p < 0.02$). A second report from Germany by Evers et al.[2] on 13 patients with primary immunodeficiency disorders and 514 controls showed an increased frequency of A2 (92.3% in patients vs. 60.8% in controls) and decreased frequencies of A9 (7.6% vs. 25% in controls) and B8 (0.0% in patients vs. 21.0% in controls). None of these deviations was highly significant.

A third report by Buckley et al.[3] on 66 patients with various types of well-defined primary immunodeficiency revealed no significant difference between the patients and 210 controls.

Rimm and Bortin[4] also reported A and B loci antigen frequencies in 57 Caucasian patients with severe combined immunodeficiency disease. The frequency of B7 was 39% in the patients as compared with 18% in 855 controls (corrected $p = 0.0083$).

As these data indicate, the association with A1 reported by Hors et al.[1] and that with B7 by Rimm and Bortin[4] was not observed in other studies. Furthermore, in the combined data these associations would not be significant. Thus, in the existing data there is no evidence to suggest an association of A or B loci antigens with immunodeficiency diseases. It should be noted that these data represent a mixture of diseases and some discrepancies in the results may be due to the heterogeneity of the sample.

Family Data

Buckley et al.[3] reported data on 22 families with patients suffering from immunodeficiency diseases. Five families had 2 affected siblings who were also HLA-identical. In 4 families there were 2 or more haploidentical affected members, 3 had 2 haplotype-different affected members, and 10 of the families had normal siblings who were HLA-identical to the affected member. Thus, in these data there was no evidence in favor of linkage between HLA and a gene controlling the inheritance of primary immunodeficiency diseases.

See also refs. 5–15.

References

1. Hors J, Griscelli C, Schmid M, Dausset J: HL-A antigens and immune deficiency states. Br Med J 4:45, 1974
2. Evers KG, Kruger J, Hagele R, Haase W, Leven B: HLA frequencies in primary immunodeficiency diseases (PIDD). Eur J Pediatr 124:199-205, 1977
3. Buckley RH, MacQueen JM, Ward FE: HLA antigens in primary immunodeficiency diseases. Clin Immunol Immunopathol 7:305-310, 1977
4. Rimm AA, Bortin MM: HLA antigens and severe

combined immunodeficiency disease. Lancet i:1361-1362, 1977

5. Evers KG, Kruger J, Hagele R: Extraneous HLA antigens in severe combined immunodeficiency disease (SCID): Survey of the literature and report of one new case. Eur J Pediatr 125:39-43, 1977
6. Betuel H, Touraine JL, Souillet G, Jeune M: Absence of cell-membrane HLA antigens in an immunodeficient child. Tissue Antigens 11:68-70, 1978
7. Hansen JA, Good RA, Dupont B: HLA-D compatibility between parent and child. Transplantation 23:366-374, 1977
8. Noreen HJ, Van Der Hagen BA, Greenberg LJ, Kersey J, Emme L, Yunis EJ: Previously unexplained HLA antigens of combined immunodeficiency disease due to IA alloantigens. Transplant Proc 9:1717-1719, 1977
9. Stiehm ER, Lawlor GJ, Kaplan MS, Greenwald HL, Neerholt RC, Sengar DPS, Terasaki PI: Immunologic reconstitution in severe combined immunodeficiency without bone-marrow chromosomal chimerism. N Engl J Med 286:797-803, 1972
10. Terasaki PI, Miyajima T, Sengar DPS, Stiehm ER: Extraneous lymphocytic HL-A antigens in severe combined immunodeficiency disease. Transplantation 13:250-255, 1972
11. Touraine JL, Betuel H, Souillet G, Jeune M: Combined immunodeficiency disease associated with absence of cell-surface HLA-A and -B antigens. J Pediatr 93:47-51, 1978
12. O'Reilly RJ, Pahwa R, Dupont B, Good RA: Severe combined immunodeficiency: Transplantation approaches for patients lacking an HLA genotypically identical sibling. Transplant Proc 10:187-199, 1978
13. Touraine JL, Betuel H: Immunodeficiency diseases and expression of HLA antigens. Hum Immunol 2:147-153, 1981
14. Durandy A, Virelizier JL, Griscelli C: Enhancement by interferon of membrane HLA antigens in patients with combined immunodeficiency with defective HLA expression. Clin Exp Immunol 52:173-178, 1983
15. Pollack MS, Kirkpatrick D, Kapoor N, Dupont B, O'Reilly RJ: Identification by HLA typing of intrauterine-derived maternal T cells in four patients with severe combined immunodeficiency. N Engl J Med 307:662-666, 1982

CHAPTER 23

Immune Response

Immune Response to Influenza Virus

Population Association

Spencer et al.[1] investigated the association of HLA antigens with antibody response in a clinical trial with live, attenuated, serum-inhibitor resistant, recombinant intranasal influenza A vaccine ("Alice" strain). This vaccine had the antigenic characteristics of A/England/42/72. In the first clinical trial 99 individuals were administered intranasal "Alice" strain vaccine. Fifty volunteers were given a placebo solution in 2 doses 14 days apart. A group of 50 other volunteers received a single intramuscular injection of a standard bivalent inactivated influenza vaccine.

In the second clinical trial, 26 individuals received "Alice" strain vaccine. The specimens for nasal antibody titer studies were obtained on days 0, 13, and 30.

Convalescent phase titer in BW16 individuals ($n = 11$) was 14, the lowest, and that of BW5 ($n = 21$) was 26, the next lowest. There was a significant difference between these 2 groups ($t = 2.16$, $p < 0.05$). Also, there was a significant difference ($t = 4.11$, $p < 0.001$) between BW16 group and non-BW16 group (geometric mean titer = 36). There were 25 recipients with poor antibody response (acute or convalescent phase titer ≤ 8) and 8 (32%) were positive for BW16. Only 5% of the 62 recipients with good antibody response ($\geq$ 4-fold titer rise or acute titer ≥ 16 with 2-fold titer rise) were positive for BW16. This difference in frequency was significant ($p < 0.05$ by χ^2 test). The mean titers in nasal secretions of 5 BW16 subjects at 13 and 30 days were < 3 as compared with 8 and 9, respectively, in 22 subjects negative for BW16. The authors have suggested that the lower antibody response of BW16 individuals may be due to the increased cellular resistance to infection rather than to a suppressed immune response, since BW16 individuals vaccinated with killed influenza vaccine had normal antibody response.

In another report from Australia, Mackenzie et al.[2] studied antibody response to A/Hong Kong/68, A/England/72, and A/Port Chalmers/73 influenza viruses in serum samples from 111 BW16-positive and 107 BW16-negative individuals. There was no difference in the hemagglutinating inhibiting antibody titers or geometric mean antibody titers between the 2 groups. Furthermore, the authors[2] reported no difference in the capacity of influenza virus to attach to fractionated white blood cells from BW16 subjects compared with cells from subjects with other HLA antigens. In another set of data from a retrospective study of a clinical trial,[2] there was no evidence to suggest that BW16 subjects were resistant to live, attenuated influenza virus.

Cunningham-Rundles et al.[3] studied the response of lymphocytes *in vitro* to influenza antigens following immunization in 47 HLA-typed healthy individuals. Each person was given 1 dose of 0.5 ml of vaccine containing 200 CCA units each of influenza A/New Jersey/8/76 and influenza A/Victoria/3/75 intramuscularly. Analysis of lymphocyte response *in vitro* showed that BW35 individuals had maximum responses to 4 influenza antigen preparations at 3 weeks. These responses were 50% lower than those of individuals negative for BW35 ($p = 0.03$). (See also ref. 4.)

Cuthbertson et al.[5] studied association between HLA-A and B antigens and antibody to influenza A (Victoria strain) in 456 British Caucasian individuals undergoing routine tissue typing in the laboratory. No significant frequency difference between antibody-positive and -negative groups was found.

Family Data

Shaw and Biddison[6] reported a family of 10 individuals (2 parents and 8 siblings) in which influenza virus-immune cytotoxicity segregated with HLA haplotypes.

References

1. Spener MJ, Cherry JD, Terasaki PI: HL-A antigens and antibody response after influenza A vaccination. N Engl J Med 294:13-16, 1976
2. Mackenzie JS, Wethrall JD, Flower RLP, Fimmel PJ, Dawkins RL: HLA antigens and the response to influenza A virus. Vox Sang 37:201-208, 1979
3. Cunningham-Rundles S, Brown A, Gross D, Braun D, Hansen JA, Goor RA, et al: Association of HLA in immune response to influenza-A immunization. Transplant Proc 11:1849-1852, 1979
4. McMichael AJ, Ting A, Zweerink HJ, Askonas BA: HLA restriction of cell-mediated lysis of influenza virus-infected human cells. Nature 270:524-526, 1977
5. Cuthbertson B, Dick HM, Sommerville RG: Histocompatibility types and antiviral antibodies in a diverse group of individuals. Hum Immunol 4:259-264, 1982
6. Shaw S, Biddison WE: HLA-linked genetic control of the specificity of human cytotoxic T-cell responses to influenza virus. J Exp Med 149:565-575, 1979

Immune Response to Vaccinia Virus

Population Association

In a study of a group of healthy recruits from the Training Center of the Royal Dutch Navy who were vaccinated against smallpox (vaccinia-virus vaccine), De Vries et al.[1] reported an association with B40 and CW3 (Table 23.1). In 12 low and 37 high responders the frequencies of B40 were 67% and 19%, respectively. In the case of CW3 83% of the 12 low responders and 24% of the 37 high responders were positive. Thus, these 2 antigens were significantly increased in the low responder group. The frequencies of B40 and CW3 in a Dutch control population were reported to be 18% and 30%, respectively (see unpublished data in 1). The authors' analysis showed that the association with B40 was most probably secondary to that with CW3 through linkage disequilibrium between these 2 antigens.

Cuthbertson et al.[2] studied 456 British Caucasian individuals for A and B loci antigens. There was no significant difference between the antibody-positive and -negative groups (no frequency data are given).

References

1. De Vries RRP, Kreeftenberg HG, Loggen HG, Van Rood JJ: In vitro immune responsiveness to vaccinia virus and HLA. N Engl J Med 297:692-696, 1977
2. Cuthbertson B, Dick HM, Sommerville RG: Histocommpatibility types and antiviral antibodies in a diverse group of individuals. Hum Immunol 4:259-264, 1982

Immune Response to Cytomegalovirus

Population Association

Scott et al.[1] studied complement-fixing antibodies to cytomegalovirus in 35 B8-positive and 35 B8-negative individuals (56 patients with chronic liver disease and 14 healthy volunteers) from England. The 2 groups were exactly matched for age, disease, type and duration of treatment, and sex.

TABLE 23.1. Immune Response to Vaccinia Virus

	Patients		Controls				
Country/Population	n	%+	n	%+	RR	χ^2	Ref.
HLA-B40							
BENELUX	12	67	37	19	7.75	8.94	1
HLA-CW3							
BENELUX	12	83	37	24	12.57	11.53	1

No difference of antibody titers between the 2 groups was observed.

Cuthbertson et al.[2] studied A and B loci antigens in 456 British Caucasian individuals. When the sample was separated into antibody-positive and -negative subgroups, no significant differences in the antigen frequencies were found.

References

1. Scott B, Cooke EM, Hambling MH, Rajah SM, Swinburne ML, Losowsky MS: HL-A8 and the immune response to various antigens. J Immunogenet 3:185-189, 1976
2. Cuthbertson B, Dick HM, Sommerville RG: Histocompatibility types and antiviral antibodies in a diverse group of individuals. Hum Immunol 4:259-264, 1982

Immune Response to Measles

Population Association

Complement-fixing antibody to measles was measured in 35 B8-positive and 35 B8-negative English subjects (56 patients with chronic liver disease and 14 healthy volunteers) matched for age, sex, disease, and type and duration of treatment.[1] A comparison of antibody titers in the 2 groups did not show any significant difference.

Cuthbertson et al.[2] studied A and B loci antigens in 456 British Caucasian individuals who were also tested for antibody to measles. In this sample 165 individuals were found to be positive and 250 negative for the antibody. The frequency of B15 was 6.1% in the antibody-positive group and 15.2% in the antibody-negative group. The difference was significant with an uncorrected probability value of 0.007.

References

1. Scott B, Cooke EM, Hambling MH, Rajah SM, Swinburne ML, Losowsky MS: HL-A8 and the immune response to various antigens. J Immunogenet 3:185-189, 1976
2. Cuthbertson B, Dick HM, Sommerville RG: Histocompatibility types and antiviral antibodies in a diverse group of individuals. Hum Immunol 4:259-264, 1982

Immune Response to Rubella Virus

Population Association

High Responders vs. Low Responders

Spencer et al.[1,2] studied 232 rubella seronegative (antibody titer < 8) children from the United States who were immunized with RA27/3 vaccine. Of the vaccinees 94% were Caucasian, 4% Mexican-Americans, and 2% were Orientals and Blacks. There were 9 children with high (≥ 512) convalescent-phase hemagglutination-inhibiting antibody titers and 4 of these had A28. Only 8% of the total study population had this antigen. Thus, A28 was significantly increased in the group with high titers ($\chi^2 = 12.06$).

In a similar study on 75 individuals from England (67 of European origin, 5 Asian, 2 of Chinese origin, and 1 Black) Harcourt et al.[3] correlated antibody response with HLA antigens. All were seronegative adult women and were given RA27/3 vaccine subcutaneously. The antibody titers were determined 8 weeks after vaccination. There were 11 individuals with titers $> 1/64$, 15 with $< 1/64$, and 8 with titers equal to 1/64. When antigens of 11 volunteers with titers higher than the mean ($> 1/64$) and 15 volunteers with titers less than that ($< 1/64$) were compared with those of the total group tested, there was no association between the high and low titers and any of the antigens.

Scott et al.[4] measured hemagglutination-inhibiting antibodies to rubella in 37 B8-positive and 37 B8-negative English subjects (56 with chronic liver disease and 18 healthy volunteers). The subjects in both groups were matched for age, sex, disease, and type and duration of treatment. The antibody titers of the 2 groups did not differ significantly.

A study of 997 persons from Denmark by Hansen et al.[5] did not find any significant correlation between presence of a strong rubella specific antibody and A and B loci antigens.

Two reports were also available on Japanese populations. Kato et al.[6] studied 182 seronegative, unrelated, normal healthy Japanese schoolgirls immunized with a live, attenuated rubella vaccine (T0336 strain). The antibody levels were measured 6 weeks after vaccination. Forty-two (24%) were low responders (titer ≤ 32) and 28 (16%) were high responders (titer ≥ 256). There were 102 (59%) girls with intermediate titers ($64 \leq$ titer ≤ 128). The frequencies of A11 (21.4%) and B15 (32.1%) were higher in high responders as compared with 4.8% and 9.5%, respectively, in low responders. The difference between the 2 groups became insignificant after correction by multiplying with the number of antigens studied (n = 17).

Kato et al.[7] published a second study on 78 Japanese schoolgirls not included in the previous sample. In this sample B15 was found to be associated with high responders (n = 55). In addition, DR4 was found to be increased in this group (41.8% in high responders vs. 17.4% in 23 low responders, p = 0.03). In the low responder group the frequency of DR2 was 30.4% vs. 1.8% in high responders (p = 0.0006).

In another Japanese study by Ishii et al.,[8] 71 healthy, unrelated, and seronegative (titer < 8) females were immunized with GEF vaccine D-105. Antibody titers were measured 12 weeks after vaccination. Eleven of 44 (25%) with titers ≥ 32 (high responders) were positive for B15. On the other hand, only 1 of the 27 individuals (8.3%) with a titer ≤ 16 (low responders) was B15-positive. The difference was significant only before the probability values were corrected for multiple comparisons.

Thus, in the Japanese population the increased frequency of B15 in high responders was evident in 2 studies. The increased frequency of A28 was seen only in Spencer's[1] and not in the British studies.[3,4] In view of these data it is not certain that there is any HLA (A and B loci) association with immune response to rubella.

Antibody Response in Various HLA Types

Spencer et al.[1,2] calculated the geometric mean titers (GMT) of vaccinees positive for a specific HLA antigen. A significant difference ($p < 0.01$ by Student's t-test) was observed when combined B14 and BW22 titer (GMT = 152) was compared with the titer (GMT = 88) of all vaccinees negative for B14 and BW22. It should be noted that this difference will not be significant if adjustments in probability are made for multiple comparisons.

In the Japanese study by Kato et al.,[6] individuals with A11 and B15 had the highest and those with A24 and B5 had the lowest titers. The differences between the A11 and A24 groups and between the B15 and B5 groups were significant but only before the corrections for multiple comparisons were made. In the second report from Japan[8] the individuals with AW33 showed the highest and A9 showed the lowest titers. The difference, however, was not significant. B locus subjects with B15 showed the highest titer and those with B40 and BW51 showed the lowest. Again the difference was not significant.

Harcourt et al.[3] also reported no association between HLA-A and -B loci antigens and excretion of either high or low titers of RA27/3 vaccine among 26 volunteers. Also, there was no association between joint symptoms and HLA in the same study.

Family Data

Spencer et al.[1] compared the antibody titers in 37 sib-pairs with those in 71 randomly matched pairs of nonsiblings. Fifteen of the 37 sib-pairs had titers identical to each other. Only 18% of the 71 randomly matched pairs had identical titers. The difference between the 2 groups was significant ($p < 0.01$).

References

1. Spencer MJ, Cherry JD, Powell KR, Mickey MR, Terasaki PI, Marcy SM, et al: Antibody responses following rubella immunization analyzed by HLA and ABO types. J Immunogenet 4:365-373, 1977
2. Spencer MJ, Cherry JD, Terasaki PI, Powell KR, Sumaya CV, Marcy SM: Clinical and antibody response following immunization with RA27/3 rubella vaccine analyzed by HL-A type. Pediatr Res 10:393, 1976
3. Harcourt GC, Best JM, Banatvala JE, Kennedy LA: HLA antigens and responses to rubella vaccination. J Hyg 83:405-412, 1979
4. Scott B, Cooke EM, Hambling MH, Rajah SM, Swinburne ML, Losowsky MS: HL-A8 and the immune response to various antigens. J Immunogenet 3:185-189, 1976
5. Hansen HE, Larsen SO, Leerhoy J: Lack of correlation between the incidence of rubella antibody and the distribution of HLA antigens in a Danish population. Tissue Antigens 15:325-328, 1980
6. Kato S, Kimura M, Takakura I, Sakakibara T, Inouye H, Tsuji K: Possible associations between HLA antigens and the immune responsiveness to attenuated rubella vaccine. Tissue Antigens 11:475-478, 1978
7. Kato S, Muranaka S, Takakura I, Kimura M, Tsuji K. HLA-DR antigens and the rubella-specific immune response in man. Tissue Antigens 19:140-145, 1982
8. Ishii K, Nakazono N, Sawada H, Wakisaka A, Moriuchi J, Nakai Y, et al: Antibody response following rubella immunization analyzed by HLA types. Jpn J Med Sci Biol 33:103-106, 1980

Immune Response to Rotavirus

Population Association

The plasma samples of 456 British Caucasian individuals (211 healthy, 99 renal disease patients, and

136 patients with various other diseases) were tested for antibody to rotavirus by Cuthbertson et al.[1] For each HLA antigen (A and B loci) individuals were classified into 2 groups: positive (antibody at a titer of 1:8 or greater) or negative.

No significant correlation between HLA antigen and the presence or absence of the antibody was found.

Reference

1. Cuthbertson B, Dick HM, Sommerville RG: Histocompatibility types and antiviral antibodies in a diverse group of individuals. Hum Immunol 4:259-264, 1982

Immune Response to Varicella/Zoster Virus

Population Association

Cuthbertson et al.[1] tested the plasma samples of 456 British Caucasian individuals (221 healthy, 99 renal disease patients and 136 patients with other diseases) for antibody to varicella/zoster virus. All individuals were typed for A and B loci antigens.

No significant association between HLA antigens and the presence or absence of antiviral antibody was observed.

Rcference

1. Cuthbertson B, Dick HM, Sommerville RG: Histocompatibility types and antiviral antibodies in a diverse group of individuals. Hum Immunol 4:259-264, 1982

Immune Response to Tetanus Toxoid

Population Association

In a study by Sasazuki et al.[1] 92 Japanese premedical students were given a primary intramuscular immunization with tetanus toxoid. In this group there were 14 low responders and 78 high responders. The frequency of B5 was 71.4% (10/14) in low responders and 60.3% (47/78) in high responders ($\chi^2 = 4.52$). The frequency of DHO, a new D locus specificity, was 58.3% (7/12) in low responders compared with 11.3% (7/62) in high responders ($\chi^2 = 14.50$). The frequencies of these 2 antigens in low responders were also compared with those in 416 controls and the differences were similar to those obtained when low responders were compared with the high responder group. The association with B5 was not statistically significant. There is a strong linkage disequilibrium between B5 and DHO in the Japanese population (see ref. in 1) and thus the primary association was probably with DHO (Table 23.2).

These results, if confirmed, may provide an example of an immune response gene linked with the HLA-D locus.

See also ref. 2.

References

1. Sasazuki T, Kohno Y, Iwamoto I, Tanimura M, Naito S: Association between an HLA haplotype and low responsiveness to tetanus toxoid in man. Nature 272:359-361, 1978
2. Repo H, Leirsalo M, Laitenen O: A contribution to immunopathogenesis of B27-associated diseases. Scand J Rheumatol 42:12, 1982

Immune Response to Streptococcal Antigens

Population Association

In a study by Greenberg et al.[1] the lymphocytes from 217 randomly selected individuals having normal immune function were incubated *in vitro* with varying concentrations of streptococcal antigens (streptokinase-streptodornase, SK/SD). Fifty-two individuals responded over the entire antigen concentration range (responders), 118 responded only to the highest antigen concentrations (low responders), and 47 did not respond to any antigen concentration (nonre-

TABLE 23.2. Immune Response to Tetanus Toxoid

	Patients		Controls				
Country/Population	n	%+	n	%+	RR	χ^2	Ref.
HLA-DHO							
Japan	12	58	69	16	6.82	9.42	1

sponders). B5 was present in 30.8% of the responders, in 5.9% of the 118 low responders, and in 8.5% of the nonresponders. Thus, it was significantly increased in the responder group when compared with low responders ($\chi^2 = 19.03$), nonresponders ($\chi^2 = 7.59$), and low + nonresponders ($\chi^2 = 21.08$).

A similar study was done by Kawa et al.[2] on 90 healthy Japanese volunteers. There were 38 responders and 52 low responders + nonresponders. No association was found between B5 and response to SK/SD antigens. The authors reported a marginally significant increase ($\chi^2 = 7.52$) of BW22 in the responder group.

Itoh et al.[3] studied association between A and B loci antigens and antistreptolysin O titers in 150 Japanese individuals. No significant deviations were observed.

Family Data

Greenberg et al.[4] presented a linkage analysis of one 3-generation kindred and 8 nuclear families. The results showed that in the immune response at least 2 loci were involved in 1 of 2 ways: 1 locus closely linked to HLA and 1 locus that was unlinked or a 2-locus system of complementary alleles that were both tightly linked to HLA. In another report Greenberg et al.[5] presented some family data that seem to be compatible with the concept that the immune response is controlled by 2 HLA-linked complementary genes.

Sasazuki et al.[6] studied immune response to streptococcal cell wall antigen in 7 informative families typed for HLA-A, -B, -C, -D, and -DR loci antigens. The mode of inheritance for immune responsiveness to this antigen was studied by maximum likelihood scoring method and linkage with HLA complex was analyzed by the sequential test. The analysis showed that the high response to this antigen was controlled by a single recessive gene (i.e., the low response to the antigen was controlled by a single dominant gene). The maximum lod scores between HLA and low responsiveness to the antigen was 3.209 at a 0% recombination. Thus there was significant evidence in favor of linkage with the HLA complex (see also refs. 7, 8, 9).

References

1. Greenberg LJ, Gray ED, Yunis EJ: Association of HL-A5 and immune responsiveness in vitro to streptococcal antigens. J Exp Med 141:935-943, 1975
2. Kawa A, Matsuyama T, Fujii H, Nakamura S, Ogaki S, Ooe H, et al.: Relations between the HLA-antigens and immune responsiveness to SK/SD in healthy Japanese subjects. Tissue Antigens 12:236-237, 1978
3. Itoh C: Association of HLA with humoral immune responses. Tohoku J Exp Med 134:281-288, 1981
4. Greenberg LJ, Chopyk RL, Bradley PW, Lalouel JM: Immunogenetics of response to a purified antigen from group A streptococci. Immunogenetics 11:161-167, 1980
5. Greenberg LJ, Bradley PW, Chopyk RL, Lalouel JM: Genetic control of response to streptococcal antigens: Implication of two HLA-linked complementary loci. Transplant Proc 13:992-994, 1981
6. Sasazuki T, Kaneoka H, Nihimura Y, Kaneoka R, Hayama M, Ohkuni H: An HLA-linked immune suppression gene in man. J Exp Med 152:297s-313s, 1980
7. Nishimura Y, Sasazuki T: Suppressor T cells control the HLA-linked low responsiveness to streptococcal antigen in man. Nature 302:67-69, 1983
8. Sasazuki T, Nishimura Y, Muto M, Ohta N: HLA-linked genes controlling immune response and disease susceptibility. Immunol Rev 70:51-75, 1983
9. Nishimura Y: Genetic control of the immune response in man. Evidence for the HLA-linked immune suppression gene to streptococcal cell wall antigen. Fukuoka Igaku Zasshi 73:155-178, 1982

Immune Response to Tuberculin

Population Association

Buckley et al.[1] reported data on 63 melanoma patients (62 American Caucasians and 1 American Black) treated with bacilli Calmette-Guerin (BCG). Cutaneous responses to tuberculin were measured in 24 B7-positive and in 39 B7-negative patients before and 5–44 weeks after the BCG immunotherapy. The average area of induration detected in B7-positive patients was half the area of induration of B7-negative patients before and after BCG treatment. The difference was statistically significant. These results showed that B7 had a strong effect on delayed cutaneous tuberculin responsiveness.

It should be noted that the study group consisted of melanoma patients. The authors presented data in the report showing an association of melanoma (BCG-treated patients) with B7. The frequency of B7 in 63 patients was 19% compared with 11% in a control population of unknown size ($\chi^2 = 7.42$). Thus, the association of B7 with immune response to BCG in healthy individuals may not be present.

Reference

1. Buckley CE, White DH, Seigler HF: HLA-B7 associated tuberculin hyporesponsiveness in BCG treated melanoma patients. Monogr Allergy 11:97-105, 1977

Immune Response to *Schistosoma Japonicum*

Population Association

Sasazuki et al.[1] studied immune responsiveness to schistosomal worm antigen in 57 Japanese individuals infected with *Schistosoma japonicum* by measuring the antigen specific proliferative response of the peripheral T lymphocytes *in vitro*. For comparison 21 random healthy individuals without any prior infection were also studied. HLA-A, -B, -C, and -D loci antigens were typed in all of these individuals.

In the infected group there were 10 low responders and 47 high responders. When compared with the healthy group the frequencies of BW52 and DW12 were found to be increased in the low responder group (Table 23.3). Furthermore, the frequency of BW52 in the low responder group was also high (7/10 = 70%) as compared with that in the high responder group (7/47 = 14.9%, $p < 0.001$). Similarly, DW12 was also found in 70% of the low responders as compared with only 13.3% (6/45) of the high responders ($p < 0.0005$).

See also ref. 2.

References

1. Sasazuki T, Ohta N, Kaneoka R, Kojima S: Association between an HLA haplotype and low responsiveness to schistosomal worm antigens in man. J Exp Med 152:314s-318s, 1980
2. Sasazuki T, Nishimura Y, Muto M, Ohta N: HLA-linked genes controlling immune response and disease susceptibility. Immunol Rev 70:51-75, 1983

Immune Response to *Salmonella Adelaide*

Population Association

In a study by Whittingham et al.[1] from Australia 200 healthy adult volunteers were immunized with 1 μg of the bacterial antigen monomeric flagellin from *Salmonella adelaide*. All individuals were classified as responders and nonresponders on the basis of a rise in titer of antibody 2 weeks after immunization.

HLA-B12 was found to be more frequent in responders who made IgM antibody. This difference, however, would not be highly significant if probabilities are corrected for the large numbers of HLA-A, -B, and immunoglobulin allotypes that were compared in this study.

Reference

1. Whittingham S, Mathews JD, Schanfield MS, Mathews JV, Tait BD, Morris PJ, et al: Interactive effect of GM allotypes and HLA-B locus antigens on the human antibody response to a bacterial antigen. Clin Exp Immunol 40:8-15, 1980

Immune Response to *Candida* Allergen

Population Association

Nose et al.[1,2] tested 110 normal healthy Japanese adults (age 22-45). Injections of 0.02 ml of *Candida albicans* were given intracutaneously and after 48 h long and short diameters of induration with erythema were measured on each individual. All subjects were typed for A, B, D, and DR antigens.

The frequency of B7 was 2.27% in 44 low responders as compared with 28.13% in 32 high responders ($p < 0.0033$).[2]

Antigen DW1 was present in 34.38% of the 32 high responders as compared with 2.27% of the 44 in the low responder group ($p < 0.0005$). The fre-

TABLE 23.3. Immune Response to *Schistosoma Japonicum*

	Patients		Controls				
Country/Population	n	%+	n	%+	RR	χ^2	Ref.
HLA-BW52							
Japan	10	70	21	18	8.87	7.46	1
HLA-DW12							
Japan	10	70	21	21	7.46	6.55	1

quency of DR1 was identical to that of DW1 in both of these groups.[2] See also ref. 3.

References

1. Nose Y, Komori K, Inouye H, Nomura K, Yamamura M, Tsuji K: Relationship between HLA-D and *in vitro* and *in vivo* responsiveness to *Candida* allergen. Clin Exp Immunol 40:345-350, 1980
2. Tsuji K, Nose Y, Inouye H, Komori K, Yamamura M: HLA-D/DR linked immune response to *Candida* allergen : An *in vivo* and *in vitro* study in Japanese. Tokai J Exp Clin Med 6:113-120, 1981
3. Nose Y, Komori K, Inouye H, Nomura K, Yamamura M, Tsuji K: Role of macrophages in T lymphocyte response to *Candida* allergen in man with special reference to HLA-D and DR. Clin Exp Immunol 45:152-157, 1981

Immune Response to Milk

Population Association

Milk antibodies were studied in 38 B8-positive and 38 B8-negative English subjects (46 patients with chronic liver disease, 12 with celiac disease, and 18 healthy volunteers) by Scott et al.[1] The B8-positive and -negative groups were matched for age, disease, sex, and type and duration of treatment.

The antibody titers in these 2 groups did not differ significantly.

See also ref. 2.

References

1. Scott B, Cooke EM, Hambling MH, Rajah SM, Swinburne ML, Losowsky MS: HL-A8 and the immune response to various antigens. J Immunogenet 3:185-189, 1976
2. Scott BB, Swinburne ML, Rajah SM, Losowsky MS: HL-A8 and the immune response to gluten. Lancet ii:374-377, 1974

Immune Response to Gluten

Population Association

In a study of 101 British patients with various diseases (22 cirrhosis, 17 chronic active hepatitis, 23 celiac disease, 11 other liver diseases, etc.) and 23 normal individuals, Scott et al.[1-3] reported a significantly higher titer of gluten antibodies in B8-positive subjects. Fifteen of the 58 (26%) B8-positive individuals had gluten antibodies at a titer $> 1/128$ as compared with only 2 of the 66 (3%) B8-negative individuals. The difference between the 2 groups was highly significant ($p < 0.0005$).

If 23 celiac patients are excluded from the data (as B8 is associated with celiac disease), then gluten antibody titer exceeded 1/128 in 15% of the B8-positive subjects as compared with 0% in the B8 negative subjects. The difference was still highly significant ($p < 0.0005$) (see also comments by Hobart and Petrie[4]).

In another report, Simpson et al.[5] studied leucocyte migration inhibition as an indicator of cell-mediated immunity to gluten fraction III in 30 healthy controls. B8-positive controls showed significantly lower migration indices, indicating greater immune response, than B8-negative individuals ($p < 0.02$).

References

1. Scott BB, Swinburne ML, Rajah SM, Losowsky MS: HL-A8 and the immune response to gluten. Lancet ii:374-377, 1974
2. Scott B, Cooke EM, Hambling MH, Rajah SM, Swinburne ML, Losowsky MS: HL-A8 and the immune response to various antigens. J Immunogenet 3:185-189, 1976
3. Scott BB, Swinburne LM, Rajah SM, Losowsky MS: The HLA system and the immunological response to dietary antigens. Gut 15:823, 1974
4. Hobart MJ, Petrie A: HL-A8 and the immune response to gluten. Lancet ii:1573-1574, 1974
5. Simpson FG, Bullen AW, Robertson DAF, Losowsky MS: HLA-B8 and cell-mediated immunity to gluten. Gut 22:633-636, 1981

Immune Response to Egg

Population Association

Antibody to homogenized boiled egg white was measured in 42 English subjects (38 patients with chronic liver disease and 4 with celiac disease). The sample of 42 consisted of 21 B8-positive and 21 B8-negative individuals, matched for age, sex, disease, and type and duration of treatment.[1]

There was no difference in antibody titers between the 2 groups.

Reference

1. Scott B, Cooke EM, Hambling MH, Rajah SM, Swinburne ML, Losowsky MS: HL-A8 and the im-

mune response to various antigens. J Immunogenet 3:185-189, 1976

Immune Response to Rh(D) Antigen

Population Association

Brain and Hammond[1] compared HLA types of 2 groups of South African (all Caucasians of Western European origin) Rh-negative women: those who made Rh antibodies and those who did not. There were 96 Rh-negative women who made antibodies against factors included in the Rh system. In the control group there were 78 Rh-negative women whose husbands were all Rh-positive. They all had at least 2 pregnancies but Rh antibodies were not detected in any of the pregnancies. A1 was found to be increased and A2 and BW10 were decreased in the group with anti-Rh antibodies. None of these differences, however, was significant if the probabilities were adjusted for the number of antigens compared in the study.

Hors et al.[2] also studied 93 Rh-negative French individuals submitted to a planned schedule of anti-D immunization. Sixty-two were found to be immunologically responding and 31 were nonresponding. All were typed for 25 A and B loci antigens. There was no significant difference in the frequency of any of the antigens. Similar results were also reported by Reznikoff-Etievant et al.[3] in a sample of 83 French Rh(D)-negative mothers with anti-D antibodies. Twelve of these were also tested for DR antigens.

Darke[4] also found no significant difference in HLA-A and -B antigen frequencies between 36 Rh(D)-negative male volunteers who responded to the Rh(D) antigen during a deliberate immunization program, 22 who failed to respond, and 176 unrelated individuals in a control population. All individuals were English. He also studied 84 female donors undergoing plasmapheresis for the production of anti-Rh(D) immunoglobulin. These women had become immunized during pregnancy and all had been given injections of Rh(D)-positive red cells. In this group the albumin anti-Rh(D) titers were higher than 1:128. The frequency of A3 in this group was 39.3%, compared with 25.6% in 176 controls (χ^2 = 4.46).

In a second report Darke et al.[5] studied DR locus antigens in 39 female responders, 26 male responders, 26 male nonresponders, and 200 controls. No significant difference was found.

Murray et al.[6] also observed an increased incidence of A3 in immunized mothers. A combined analysis of all the data on A3 showed that this antigen was significantly increased in the immunized mothers known to have formed anti-Rh(D) antibodies.

See also refs. 7–9.

References

1. Brain P, Hammond MG: Association between histocompatibility type and the ability to make anti-Rh antibodies. Eur J Immunol 4:223-225, 1974
2. Hors J, Dausset J, Gerbal A, Salmon C, Ropartz C, Lanset S: HL-A phenotype and anti-Rh(D) immunization. Haematologia 8:217-221, 1974

TABLE 23.4. Immune Response to Rh(D) Antigen

Country/Population	Patients n	Patients %+	Controls n	Controls %+	RR	χ^2	Ref.
HLA-A3							
South Africa	96	40	454	30	1.56	3.73	1
England	288	36	246	26	1.60	6.11	6
England	84	39	176	26	1.82	4.58	4
	372	37	422	26	1.66	10.54	
	Heterogeneity χ^2 (1 df)					0.15	
France	62	26	152	24	1.12	0.12	2
France	83	33	100	26	1.40	1.08	3
	145	30	252	25	1.26	0.99	
	Heterogeneity χ^2 (1 df)					0.22	
	613	36	1128	27	1.53	14.28	
	Heterogeneity χ^2 (4 df)					1.34	

3. Reznikoff-Etievant MF, Muller JY, Julien F, Patereau C: An immune response gene linked to MHC in man. Tissue Antigens 22:312-314, 1983
4. Darke C: HLA types and the immune response to the Rh(D) antigen. Tissue Antigens 9:171-172, 1977
5. Darke C, Street J, Sargeant C, Dyer PA: HLA-DR antigens and properdin factor B allotypes in responders and nonresponders to the Rhesus-D antigen. Tissue Antigens 21:333-335, 1983
6. Murray S, Dewar PJ, Lee E, McNay RA, Collins AK: A study of HL-A types in Rh haemolytic disease of the newborn. Vox Sang 30:91-104, 1976
7. Turowski G, Morawska A, Turowska B: Alloimmunization to HL-A antigens and hemolytic disease of newborns on the background of incompatibility in the Rh system. Mater Med Pol 7:210-215, 1975
8. Moulinier J: Immunisation anti-HL-A et formes lethales de maladie hemolytique Rh. Pathologica 64:39-41, 1972
9. Moulinier J, Merle MC: Histo-compatibilite et maladie rhesus. Bordeaux Med 3:919-924, 1970

Immune Response to Synthetic Amino Acids

Population Association

Immune response to the synthetic amino acid terpolymer (L-glutamic acid^{55}-L-lysine^{33}-L-tyrosine^{15})n (GLT) was studied in 61 human volunteers (18–48 years) immunized by the intradermal injection of 0.1 ml of GLT at 2 sites on the forearm on days 0, 7, and 14.[1] Skin test reactivity to GLT was determined by measuring the maximum diameter of erythema and/or induration at the skin test site at 30 min, and at 24, and 48 h after immunization.

All volunteers were typed for A and B loci antigens and were grouped into 34 responders and 27 nonresponders.

Antigen frequencies were not significantly different in the 2 groups.

Family Data

Hsu et al.[2] studied lymphoproliferative response to poly(*L*-His, *L*-Glu)-poly(*DL*-Ala)-poly(*L*-Lys) and to poly(*L*-Tyr, *L*-Glu)-poly(*DL*-Ala)-poly(*L*-Lys) synthetic polypeptides. Subjects could be classified into high, intermediate, and nonresponders. In the families, high responses to these antigens were inherited as HLA-linked dominant traits. One family in which there was a recombination within the HLA complex provided evidence that this immune response gene was closer to the B and D region.

References

1. Scher I, Berning AK, Strong DM, Green I: The immune response to a synthetic amino acid terpolymer in man: relationship to HL-A type. J Immunol 115:36-40, 1975
2. Hsu SH, Chan MM, Bias WB: Genetic control of major histocompatibility complex-linked immune responses to synthetic polypeptides in man. Proc Natl Acad Sci USA 78:440-444, 1981

Immune Response to Penicillin

Population Association

Spengler and De Weck[1] typed 46 Swiss patients with allergy to penicillin for A and B loci antigens. When compared with a normal control population, no significant deviation in any of the antigen frequencies was observed.

Disease Heterogeneity

In the Swiss study[1] 36 of the 46 patients had positive skin tests to penicilloyl-polylysine and had therefore produced IgE antibodies against the penicilloyl determinant. The antigen frequencies in this subgroup were not significantly different from those in the control group.

Reference

1. Spengler H, De Weck AL: Evaluation of genetic control of the immune response to penicillin in man. Monogr Allergy 11:116-123, 1977

Immune Response to Collagen

Population Association

Solinger and Stobo[1] measured reactivity to denatured bovine collagen in 74 individuals typed for DR antigens. In 36 DR4-positive individuals percent inhibition of reactivity to collagen was 47 $\pm$ 4 as compared to only 8 $\pm$ 2 in 38 DR4-negative individuals. This difference was significant ($p < 0.001$). (For experimental details see the original paper.)

Reference

1. Solinger AM, Stobo JD: Immune response gene control of collagen reactivity in man: Collagen unresponsiveness in HLA-DR4 negative nonresponders is

due to the presence of T-dependent suppressive influences. J Immunol 129:1916-1920, 1982

Immune Response to Cold Agglutinin

Population Association

Itoh[1] measured cold agglutinin titers in 150 healthy Japanese individuals typed for HLA-A and -B antigens.

No significant association between cold agglutinin titer and any of the HLA antigens was found in this sample.

Reference

1. Itoh C: Association of HLA with humoral immune responses. Tohoku J Exp Med 134:281-288, 1981

Immune Response to Heterophil

Population Association

Itoh[1] did not find any association between heterophil antibody titers and A and B loci antigens in a sample of 150 healthy Japanese individuals.

Reference

1. Itoh C: Association of HLA with humoral immune responses. Tohoku J Exp Med 134:281-288, 1981

Immune Response to Platelet Group PL^{A1}

Population Association

In a study from France, Reznikoff-Etievant et al.[1,2] typed 26 Caucasian mothers who were negative for platelet group PL^{A1}. These mothers had anti-PL^{A1} antibodies and gave birth to children affected with neonatal thrombocytopenia.

In this sample significant increases of B8 and DR3 were observed (Table 23.5).

References

1. Reznikoff-Etievant MF, Dangu C, Lobet R: HLA-B8 antigen and anti-PL^{A1} allo-immunization. Tissue Antigens 18:66-68, 1981
2. Reznikoff-Etievant MF, Muller JY, Julien F, Patereau C: An immune response gene linked to MHC in man. Tissue Antigens 22:312-314, 1983

Measles Antibodies

Haverkorn and Norrby[1] examined the serum samples of 140 twin pairs from Sweden for the presence of antibodies against 3 different components of measles virus: hemagglutinating-inhibiting, hemolysis-inhibiting, and nucleocapsid complement-fixating antibodies. Each twin pair was of the same sex, living in the same household, and attending the same elementary school. Half of the twin pairs were monozygotic and half were dizygotic.

Population Association

To study the possible association between HLA antigen and antibody titers, a population sample was created by using only 1 member of the twin pairs. Comparison of mean antibody titer between groups with and without a particular HLA antigen did not reveal any significant difference.

Family Data

The authors measured the variability of antibody titers in dizygotic twin pairs with common HLA haplotypes. If there is a genetic linkage between HLA

TABLE 23.5. Immune Response to Platelet Group PL^{A1}

	Patients		Controls				
Country/Population	n	%+	n	%+	RR	χ^2	Ref.
HLA-B8							
France	26	62	100	17	7.64	18.98	2
HLA-DR3							
France	21	95	100	15	72.78	30.15	2

and a gene involved in the immune response associated with the observed titers, then one would expect relatively small variability of antibody titer in such comparisons. No indication of linkage was found in these data.

Reference

1. Haverkorn MJ, Norrby E: Measles antibodies and HLA. J Immunogenet 5:129-134, 1978

Antibodies to Native DNA

Population Association

Griffing et al.[1] reported a significant increase of DR3 antigen in 37 American Caucasian systemic lupus erythematosus patients with high titer antibodies to native DNA (Table 23.6).

In 15 patients without anti-DNA antibody the frequency of DR3 was 27%, not significantly different from that of the control group.

It should be noted, however, that this observed association may be an artifact, for DR3 is one of the antigens significantly associated with systemic lupus erythematosus.

Reference

1. Griffing WL, Moore SB, Luthra HS, McKenna CH, Fathman CG: Associations of antibodies native to DNA with HLA-DRw3. A possible major histocompatibility complex-linked human immune response gene. J Exp Med 152:319s-325s, 1980

Anti-Albumin Autoantibody

Population Association

Wager et al.[1] reported DR antigen frequency data in 126 Finnish patients with an abnormality of the albumin line (tailing albumin). This abnormality is due to the complexes formed by albumin and polyclonal IgG autoantibodies toward albumin.

The report noted an increase frequency of DR3 in the patients (50% vs. 25.3% in 83 controls, $p = 0.03$).

Reference

1. Wager O, Haltia K, Koskimies S, Tiilikainen A: HLA antigens and anti-albumin autoantibody response. Scand J Rheumatol 42:13, 1982

Inhibition of Mixed Lymphocyte Culture Reaction by Iron

Population Association

Bryan et al.[1] examined the lymphocyte response of 77 unrelated American Caucasian blood donors following pretreatment with 1.0 mM F-citrate. The mean percent response of individuals who were A2-positive was significantly higher ($0.005 < p < 0.01$) than the mean percent response of those who did not have this antigen.

To test the association between HLA antigens and lymphocyte sensitivity to iron the responder cells were classified into groups with "low sensitivity" and "high sensitivity." A responder cell was assigned to the low sensitivity group if the percent response of the cell was > 70% (the mean percent response for the total group) and to the high sensitivity group if it was < 70%.

A significant association was found between resistance to iron treatment in the mixed lymphocyte reaction and A2 antigen ($p = 0.00039$).

Reference

1. Bryan CF, Nishiya K, Pollack MS, Dupont BO, Sousa MD: Differential inhibition of the MLR by iron: Association with HLA phenotype. Immunogenetics 12:129-140, 1981

TABLE 23.6. Antibodies to Native DNA

	Patients		Controls				
Country/Population	n	%+	n	%+	RR	χ^2	Ref.
HLA-DR3							
U.S.A.	37	70	286	37	3.87	13.58	1

Concanavallin A-Induced Suppression

Population Association

Ambinder et al.[1] studied the number of Ig plaque-forming cells produced after a 6-day culture (without mitogen) in 18 DR3-positive and 24 DR3-negative normal volunteers. The former group showed a significantly greater number of plaque-forming cells (1039 ± 644 plaques per 106 mononuclear cells vs. 337 ± 341, $p < 0.001$).

In the presence of pokeweed mitogen there was no significant difference between the two groups.

Reference

1. Ambinder JM, Chiorazzi N, Gibofsky A, Fotino M, Kunkel HG: Special characteristics of cellular immune function in normal individuals of the HLA-DR3 type. Clin Immunol Immunopathol 23:269-274, 1982

IgD Level in Serum

Population Association

Fraser and Schur[1] typed A and B loci antigens and also measured serum IgD levels in 1549 Caucasian individuals (48 normals and the remainder with various rheumatic diseases). The antigen B8 was found to be significantly increased (Table 23.7) in 70 individuals with low serum IgD (< 0.002 mg/ml).

Family Data

See ref.1.

Reference

1. Fraser PA, Schur PH: Hypoimmunoglobulinemia D: Frequency, family studies, and association with HLA. Clin Immunol Immunopathol 19:67-74, 1981

IgM-Rheumatoid Factor in Serum

Population Association

The association of DR antigens and *in vitro* production of IgM-rheumatoid factor by lymphocytes from a group of 35 healthy young subjects was examined by Rodriguez et al.[1] No significant association was found.

Reference

1. Rodriguez MA, Bankhurst AD, Williams RC Jr, Troup GM, Stastny P: Studies on the relationship between HLA DR4 and *in vitro* IgM rheumatoid factor production. Clin Immunol Immunopathol 27:96-109, 1983

Defective F_c-Receptor Function

Population Association

F_c-receptor function (the rate of clearance from the circulation of antibody-coated ^{51}Cr-labeled autologous erythrocytes) of 8 B8-DR3-positive healthy individuals was studied by Lawley et al.[1] Four individuals had defective and the other 4 had normal F_c-receptor function. There appeared to be no difference between the two groups.

See also ref. 2.

References

1. Lawley TJ, Hall RP, Fauci AS, Katz SI, Hamburger MI, Frank MM: Defective Fc-receptor functions associated with the HLA-B8/DRw3 haplotype: Studies in patients with dermatitis herpetiformis and normal subjects. N Engl J Med 304:185-192, 1981
2. Bartolotti SR: Defective Fc-receptor functions with the HLA-B8/DRw3 haplotype. N Engl J Med 305:346, 1981

TABLE 23.7. IgD Level in Serum

	Patients		Controls				
Country/Population	n	%+	n	%+	RR	χ^2	Ref.
HLA-B8							
U.S.A.	70	40	48	20	2.58	5.07	1

Degradation Rate of Sheep Red Blood Cells Endocytized by Macrophages

Population Association

Legrand et al.[1] used sheep red blood cells to evaluate the speed of antigen degradation in human mononuclear phagocytes in culture. In 100 unrelated French blood donors HLA typing (A, B, C, and DR), phagocytosis, and catabolism of sheep red blood cells by peripheral blood phagocytes was studied (for experimental details see ref. 1).

The data were analyzed by grouping the subjects according to their phagocytosis or degradation indices and HLA (presence or absence of each antigen).

Seven of 14 "low degraders" (50%) had DR3 antigens as compared with 11 out of 86 other individuals (12.8%). This difference in the frequency of DR3 between the two groups was significant (P = 0.001). No other HLA antigens were significantly associated with the rate of degradation.

Also, there was no association between phagocytosis and the HLA antigens.

It is interesting to note that Gm phenotype 3, 23, 11 was also significantly increased in the subgroup of low degraders.

Reference

1. Legrand L, Perran-Rivat L, Huttin C, Dausset J: HLA-and Gm-linked genes affecting the degradation rate of antigens (sheep red blood cells) endocytized by macrophages. Hum Immunol 4:1-13, 1982

Lymphocyte Abnormality

Population Association

The lymphocyte abnormality, expressed as a decreased proliferative response to suboptimally stimulating concentrations of phytohemagglutinin (PHA) and concanavallin A (Con A), and its association with HLA antigens has been studied in healthy subjects by McCombs and Michalski.[1]

In three experiments (for details see the original paper) highly purified T cells proliferated less in response to a suboptimal concentration of PHA than did the original cell suspensions (unseparated cells). However, when subjects positive and negative for B8 were compared, in each experiment the T cells from B8-positive subjects showed impaired response compared with that of B8-negative subjects.

It should be noted that the response to optimally stimulating concentrations of PHA and Con A was not affected.

Reference

1. McCombs CC, Michalski JP: Lymphocyte abnormality associated with HLA-B8 in healthy young adults. J Exp Med 156:936-941, 1982

Interferon Production

Population Association Data

Andreotti and Cresswell[1] studied interferon production in mixed lymphocyte culture in 3 pairs of HLA-identical siblings, 3 pairs of unrelated individuals phenotypically identical for both DR and MB antigens and nonidentical for A and B antigens, and 5 pairs of unrelated individuals nonidentical for A, B, and DR antigens.

No detectable interferon was produced between HLA-identical siblings. However, interferon was produced in siblings and unrelated individual pairs who showed HLA-A, -B, or -DR locus incompatibility. The highest level of concentration of interferon was detected in the HLA-DR incompatible pairs. (For experimental details see the original paper).

Reference

1. Andreotti PE, Cresswell P: HLA control of interferon production in the human mixed lymphocyte culture. Hum Immunol 3:109-120, 1981

CHAPTER 24

Miscellaneous Diseases

Age

Population Association

Several studies have compared the A and B loci antigen frequencies in "old" and "young" population groups. However, the criteria for classifying these groups were not identical in all of the studies.

In the combined data from 8 independent studies the increase in the frequency of B40 was marginally significant (Table 24.1). However, this increase in the old group was primarily the result of to the data of Macurova et al.[1] and Yarnell et al.[2] There was also evidence of heterogeneity in the data.

In the report of Hodge and Walford[3] 103 Caucasians over 90 years of age were studied. The observed frequency of B40 was 14.6% as compared with 10.9% of the "expected frequency" of this antigen (no sample size for the control group is available). This difference in the frequency was not found to be significant. However, if the frequency of B40 in the control is greater than that in the aged population it will increase the χ^2 value in the table. This will contribute toward the significant increase of B40 in the combined sample.

In combining the data from these 6 studies, the "old group" was defined as age > 60 years.

The report by Pandey et al.[4] included data on 104 individuals in the 51–70-year age group and 46 individuals older than 70 years. We have treated both groups as old and have pooled the frequencies of B40 in Table 24.1.

The definition of "young group" was also variable in these studies. It ranged from 1 to 50 years. Thus, the increased frequency of B40 in the old group may be an artifact of classification criterion, sample size, HLA serology, and typing techniques. In the data of 4 of the studies shown in Table 24.1, there was no association with B40 and in 2 of the reports[5,6] B40 was found to be decreased in the old group.

Yasuda et al.[7] studied A and B loci antigens in 688 Japanese individuals. The total sample was divided into various age groups. There was no statistical evidence of difference in the antigen frequencies between these groups.

Heterozygosity

Gerkins et al.[8] first reported a significant increase in the heterozygosity (defined as the frequency of individuals with 2 detectable antigens at each locus) in the old group. Two subsequent reports by Macurova et al.[1] and Converse and Williams[9] also found a similar increase in heterozygosity. However, in the data of Bender et al.,[5] Hansen et al.,[6] Pandey et al.,[4] Proust et al.,[10] Hodge and Walford,[3] Blackwelder et al.,[11] and Yarnell et al.,[2] HLA heterozygosity was similar in the old and young groups.

Yasuda et al.[7] observed some evidence of difference in heterozygosity between old group (50-91 years) and young (0–9 years). (For analysis of the data, see the original paper, ref. 7).

Thus, available data did not provide very strong evidence in favor of HLA frequency differences between the age groups.

See also refs. 12–16.

References

1. Macurova H, Ivanyi P, Sajdlova H, Trojan J: HL-A antigens in aged persons. Tissue Antigens 6:269-271, 1975
2. Yarnell JWG, Leger ASST, Balfour IC, Russell RG: The distribution, age effects and disease associations of HLA antigens and other blood group

TABLE 24.1. Age

Country/Population	Patients n	Patients %+	Controls n	Controls %+	RR	χ^2	Ref.
HLA-B40							
U.S.A.	150	16	39	10	1.57	0.72	4
U.S.A.	95	4	228	8	0.53	1.49	11
U.S.A.	128	13	148	13	1.00	0.00	8
	373	12	415	10	0.96	0.03	
	Heterogeneity χ^2 (2 df)					2.19	
Czechoslovakia	83	29	350	10	3.67	19.35	1
England	356	20	403	9	2.51	18.06	2
France	155	11	312	9	1.26	0.54	10
West Germany	182	15	169	17	0.86	0.26	5
Denmark	162	12	708	18	0.63	3.20	6
	1311	16	2357	13	1.38	8.74	
	Heterogeneity χ^2 (7 df)					34.89	

markers in a random sample of an elderly population. J Chronic Dis 32:555-561, 1979
3. Hodge SE, Walford RL: HLA distribution in aged normals. In Terasaki PI (Ed): Histocompatibility Testing 1980. UCLA Tissue Typing Laboratory, Los Angeles, 1981, pp 722-726
4. Pandey JP, Fudenberg HH, Loadholt CB: HLA antigens in different age groups. Ric Clin Lab 7:220-223, 1977
5. Bender K, Mayerova A, Klotzbucher B, Burckhardt K, Hiller CH: No indication of postnatal selection at the HL-A loci. Tissue Antigens 7:118-121, 1976
6. Hansen HE, Sparck JV, Larsen SO: An examination of HLA frequencies in three age groups. Tissue Antigens 10:49-55, 1977
7. Yasuda N, Tsuji K, Itakura K: HLA heterozygosity in children and old people. Tokai J Exp Clin Med 5:165-169, 1980
8. Gerkins VR, Ting A, Menck HT, Casaggrande JT, Terasaki PI, Pike MC, et al: HL-A heterozygosity as a genetic marker of long-term survival. J Natl Cancer Inst 52:1909-1911,1974
9. Converse PJ, Williams DRR: Increased HLA-B heterozygosity with age. Tissue Antigens 12:275-278, 1978
10. Proust J, Moulias R, Fumeron F, Bekkhoucha F, Busson M, Schmid M, et al: HLA and longevity. Tissue Antigens 19:168-173, 1982
11. Blackwelder WC, Mittal KK, McNamara PM, Payne FJ: Lack of association between HLA and age in an aging population. Tissue Antigens 20:188-192, 1982
12. Walford RL: Multigene families, histocompatibility systems, transformation, meiosis, stem cells, and DNA repair. Mech Ageing Dev 9:19-26, 1979
13. Meredith PJ, Walford RL: Autoimmunity, histocompatibility, and aging. Mech Ageing Dev 9:61-77, 1979
14. Yunis EJ, Lane MA: Cellular immunity in aging. J Invest Dermatol 73:24-28, 1979
15. Walford RL: Antibody diversity, histocompatibility systems, disease states, and ageing. Lancet ii:1226-1229, 1970
16. Macurova H, Ivanyi P, Sajdlova H, Trojan J: HL-A antigens in old people. Cas Lek Cesk 114:835-837, 1975

Vasectomy

Population Association

Jennings et al.[1] found no HLA lymphocytotoxic antibodies in 19 vasectomized men followed for 21–42 months after surgery. Similar results were also reported by Law et al.[2] In the latter study, however, when 99 men before vasectomy and 184 after vasectomy were typed for A and B antigens, a strong association with A28 and head agglutinating antibody was found in the postvasectomy group.

References

1. Jennings PB, Wettlaufer JN, Paulsen CA: Absence of circulating HL-A lymphocytotoxic antibodies in men 21 to 44 months after vasectomy. Fertil Steril 28:446-447, 1977
2. Law HY, Bodmer WF, Mathews JD, Skegg DCG: The immune response to vasectomy and its relation to the HLA system. Tissue Antigens 14:115-139, 1979

Familial Mediterranean Fever

Population Association

Sixty-seven Israeli Jewish patients and 335 controls were typed for A and B antigens.[1] There was no significant difference between the 2 groups. Similar results for A and B loci antigens were also reported by Chaouat et al.[2,3] in a study of 31 patients from France (Israeli-Sephardic origin).

Family Data

In the French study,[2,3] 7 families with at least 2 affected siblings were also HLA-typed. In these families the inheritance of the disease was recessive but there was no evidence for linkage with HLA. Similar results have also been reported by Gazit et al.[1]

See also ref. 4.

References

1. Gazit E, Orgad S, Pras M: HLA antigens in familial Mediterranean fever. Tissue Antigens 9:273-275, 1977
2. Chaouat Y, Tormen JP, Godeau P, Camus JP, Kahn MF, Ryckewaert A, et al: Marqueurs HLA chez les sujets atteints de maladie periodique (fievre familiale mediterraneenne). Nouv Presse Med 6:2949-2953, 1977
3. Chaouat Y, Tormen JP, Hors J, Dausset J: HLA et maladie periodique. Rev Rhum Mal Osteoartic 44:703-708, 1977
4. Lehman TJA, Hanson V, Kornreich H, Peters RS, Schwabe AD: HLA-B27-negative sacroiliitis: A manifestation of familial Mediterranean fever in childhood. Pediatrics 61:423-426, 1978

Sudden Infant Death Syndrome

Population Association

Sixty-six parents of 33 sudden infant death syndrome (SIDS) cases were typed for A and B loci antigens by Tait et al.[1,2] When compared with normal controls the frequency of A10 was found to be increased (Table 24.2).

A10 was present in 9 of 26 parents of 13 infants classified as SIDS but with evidence of laryngitis. This value was significantly higher than 39 A10-positives in 375 controls ($p < 0.005$) and 6 A10-positives in 40 parents of infants with no evidence of laryngitis ($p < 0.05$).

The antigen A10 was also more frequent in mothers (9/33) than in controls ($p < 0.005$).

References

1. Tait BD, Williams AL, Mathews JD, Cowling DC: HLA and sudden infant death. Lancet 1:1178-1179, 1976
2. Tait BD, Williams AL, Mathews JD, Cowling DC: HLA and the sudden infant death syndrome. Monogr Allergy 11:55-59, 1977

Plasma Lipids

Family Data

Winata et al.[1] measured plasma lipids (free cholesterol, esterified cholesterol, total cholesterol, and triglycerides) in 71 pairs of dizygotic twins of the same sex. The pairs were separated into the groups sharing 0, 1, and 2 haplotypes.

The mean plasma lipids of the three groups was compared using a *t*-test. No significant difference between the groups was found and thus, in these data, there was no association between plasma lipid levels and the haplotype groups.

Reference

1. Winata SS, Biegel AA, Kang KW, Harmath F, Christian JC: A search for stratification-free association between plasma lipids and HLA using dizygotic twins. Acta Genet Med Germellol (Rome) 30:213-216, 1981

TABLE 24.2. Sudden Infant Death Syndrome

	Patients		Controls				
Country/Population	n	%+	n	%+	RR	χ^2	Ref.
HLA-A10							
Australia	66	23	375	10	2.72	9.08	1

Plasma Calcium Level

Population Association

Henrotte[1] measured plasma calcium concentrations in 84 healthy male French individuals. Average concentrations were calculated for all the individuals with a particular HLA antigen (e.g., B5, B7, B8, etc.). When the values were compared with the average values of all the individuals lacking that particular antigen (e.g., B5 vs. non-B5) there was no significant difference between the groups. Thus, calcium concentration in the plasma did not appear to be associated with the A and B loci antigens.

Reference

1. Henrotte JG: Relations entre magnesium, zinc erythrocytaires et groupes HLA. C R Acad Sci (Paris) 285:737-739, 1977

Cadmium Blood Level

Cadmium is a poisonous pollutant in industrial atmospheres. It accumulates in blood through smoking, food, and environmental pollutants.

Population Association

Gualde and Delage[1,2] HLA-typed 100 healthy French individuals who were occupationally not exposed to cadmium. Fifteen individuals had a high cadmium blood level (≥ 9 mg/ml) and 7 of these were positive for A3 (46.66%). Of the 85 subjects with low cadmium blood levels (< 9 mg/ml), 15 were positive for A3 (17.64%). This difference is significant ($\chi^2 = 5.80$) only if corrections for multiple comparisons are not taken into consideration.

Lymphocyte transformation tests with phytohemagglutinin and cadmium were performed on 5 different A3 and 10 non-A3 cells. The results indicated that A3 cells were more sensitive than others to inhibition by cadmium.

Family Data

In the aforementioned French study[1] there were also data on a 3-generation family of 9 individuals. All 4 smokers (40–60 cigarettes per day) in the second generation and 2 smokers in the third generation had high cadmium blood levels. The 2 grandparents and one sibling in the second generation, all nonsmokers, had low cadmium blood levels. The high cadmium blood level was not segregating with any specific haplotype. It seemed to be more dependent on the duration of nicotinism.

References

1. Gualde N, Delage C: HLA phenotypes and cadmium blood level. Tissue Antigens 14:303-308, 1979
2. Delage C, Gualde N, Malinvaud G, Guichard C: Mise en evidence d'un marqueur genetique predisposant au stockage du cadmium. Ann Pharm Fr 37:475-482, 1979

Red Blood Cell Zinc Level

Population Association

Levels of zinc in red blood cells were measured in 84 French Caucasian males.[1] The average concentration of Zn in B15-positive individuals (n = 7) was 14.59 mg/liter (standard deviation 1.12). This was significantly different from that in non-B15 individuals ($p < 0.01$). The concentration in a B5-positive group (n = 19) was 12.91 mg/liter (standard deviation 1.19) and this was also significant ($p < 0.05$). There was no difference between the 2 groups with respect to the Zn levels in plasma.

The authors have suggested the role of genetic factors in the regulation of Zn red blood cell concentration.

Reference

1. Henrotte JG: Relations entre magnesium, zinc erythrocytaires et groupes HLA. C R Acad Sci (Paris) 285:737-739, 1977

Red Blood Cell Magnesium Level

Population Association

Henrotte[1] (see also refs. 2, 3) measured red blood cell magnesium in 351 French male Caucasian blood donors of known HLA types. The average Mg concentration in 57 BW35-positive individuals was 50.58 mg/liter. This was significantly lower than the average level of all the other non-BW35 individuals (52.73 mg/liter) combined ($p < 0.001$). The results were significant even when corrected for the number of antigens compared in the study. The standard deviation of the BW35 group was 4.10 and this was also significantly different from that of the non-BW35 group (5.25) ($p < 0.05$).

In another analysis of the same data, the individuals were classified as BW4- or BW6- (or both) positive. The group positive for BW4 had a significantly higher Mg value than the group positive for BW6. The heterozygotes (BW4/BW6) showed intermediate values. The difference between the BW4 and BW6 groups appeared to be independent of the BW35 effect.

The author has suggested the role of genetic factors in the regulation of Mg concentrations in red blood cells (see also ref. 4).

References

1. Henrotte JG: The variability of human red blood cell magnesium level according to HLA groups. Tissue Antigens 15:419-430, 1980
2. Henrotte JG: Relations entre magnesium, zinc erythrocytaires et groupes HLA. C R Acad Sci (Paris) 285:737-739, 1977
3. Henrotte JG: Magnesium erythrocytaire et groupes HLA. C R Acad Sci Paris 289:445-447, 1979
4. Dausset J, Henrotte JG: HLA and BW35. Possible influence of Mg metabolism. Tissue Antigens 20:81-85, 1982

Hyperlipoproteinemia Type IIA

Population Association

In a study on 100 French patients by Raffoux et al.[1] a significant increase of B17 was reported (Table 24.3).

Family Data

In a family of 15 members covering 3 generations,[1] all 5 affected siblings had 1 haplotype in common that came from the affected father.

Reference

1. Raffoux C, Pointel JP, Drouin P, Streiff F, Derby G, Sauvanet JP: Type IIa hyperlipoproteinemia and the HLA system. Tissue Antigens 11:55-58, 1978

Hyperlipoproteinemia Type IIB

Population Association

One-hundred and thirty unrelated French patients were typed for HLA-A and -B loci antigens by Raffoux et al.[1] The comparison of frequencies with 340 controls did not reveal any significant differences between the 2 groups.

Reference

1. Raffoux C, Pointel JP, Sauvanet JP, Drouin P, Janot C, Streiff F, et al: Type IV and IIB hyperlipoproteinemia and the HLA system. Tissue Antigens 12:212-214, 1978

Hyperlipoproteinemia Type IV

Population Association

When a sample of 106 unrelated French patients was compared with 340 controls, no association with A and B antigens was observed by Raffoux et al.[1]

Reference

1. Raffoux C, Pointel JP, Sauvanet JP, Drouin P, Janot C, Streiff F, et al: Type IV and IIB hyperlipoproteinemia and the HLA system. Tissue Antigens 12:212-214, 1978

TABLE 24.3. Hyperlipoproteinemia Type IIA

	Patients		Controls				
Country/Population	n	%+	n	%+	RR	χ^2	Ref.
HLA-B17							
France	100	20	340	6	3.90	16.87	1
HLA-BW35							
France	100	25	340	14	2.06	6.88	1

Periodontitis

Population Association

Using the same data, Terasaki et al.[1] and Kaslick et al.[2] reported a significantly decreased frequency of A2 in the patient group (Table 24.4). This was confirmed in a followup study by Kaslick et al.[3] However, in a Danish study[4] this decreased frequency was not significant (Table 24.4). There was evidence of heterogeneity in the combined data from all 3 studies.

In comparison with periodontosis there was no difference in the frequencies of A28, A9, and B15 (Table 24.4).

See also ref. 5.

References

1. Terasaki PI, Kaslick RS, West TL, Chasens AI: Low HL-A2 frequency and periodontitis. Tissue Antigens 5:286-288, 1975
2. Kaslick RA, West TL, Chasens AI, Terasaki PI, Lazzara R, Weinberg S: Association between HL-A2 antigen and various periodontal diseases in young adults. J Dent Res 54:424, 1975
3. Kaslick RS, West TL, Chasens AI: Association between ABO blood groups, HL-A antigens and periodontal diseases in young adults: A follow-up study. J Periodontol 51:339-342, 1980
4. Reinholdt J, Bay I, Svejgaard A: Association between HLA-antigens and periodontal disease. J Dent Res 56:1261-1263, 1977
5. Grimoud AM, De Mouzon A, Lodter J-Ph, Duffaut D: The major histocompatibility complex in man. Possible opening in odonto-stomatology. Actual Odontostomatol (Paris) 35:683-692, 1981

Periodontosis

Population Association

Data are available for Caucasian populations from several studies.[1-4] The frequencies of A2, A28, A9, and B15 were reported to be deviating in the patient groups compared with the controls. The data and the combined analysis of these 4 antigens are given in Table 24.5. In the total sample B15 appeard to be significantly associated with this disease.

Cullinan et al.[2] also published data on 18 Black patients from England in whom BW35 was significantly increased (Table 24.5).

Family Data

The study by Cullinan et al.[2] included data on 8 families (7 Black and 1 Caucasian) with more than 1 affected member. There was some indication of joint segregation of the disease and HLA haplotypes. However, the authors did not present any formal analysis of this data.

See also ref. 5.

References

1. Reinholdt J, Bay I, Svejgaard A: Association between HLA-antigens and periodontal disease. J Dent Res 56:1261-1263, 1977
2. Cullinan MP, Sachs J, Wolf E, Seymour GJ: The distribution of HLA-A and -B antigens in patients and their families with periodontosis. J Periodont Res 15:177-184, 1980
3. Terasaki PI, Kaslick RS, West TL, Chasens AI:

TABLE 24.4. Periodontitis

Country/Population	Patients n	Patients %+	Controls n	Controls %+	RR	χ^2	Ref.
HLA-A2							
U.S.A.	28	21	41	61	0.18	10.13	1
U.S.A.	41	32	53	57	0.36	5.69	3
	69	28	94	59	0.28	14.80	
	Heterogeneity χ^2 (1 df)					1.03	
Denmark	29	59	1967	54	1.21	0.27	4
	98	37	2061	54	0.54	6.27	
	Heterogeneity χ^2 (2 df)					9.83	

TABLE 24.5. Periodontosis

Country/Population	Patients n	Patients %+	Controls n	Controls %+	RR	χ^2	Ref.
HLA-A2							
U.S.A.	19	32	41	61	0.32	4.25	3
U.S.A.	33	33	53	57	0.38	4.60	4
	52	33	94	59	0.35	8.78	
	Heterogeneity χ^2 (1 df)					0.07	
England	12	42	174	45	0.91	0.03	2
Denmark	39	44	1967	54	0.67	1.55	1
	103	38	2235	53	0.55	7.59	
	Heterogeneity χ^2 (3 df)					2.84	
HLA-A9							
U.S.A.	33	12	53	23	0.49	1.51	4
England	12	42	174	19	3.13	3.97	2
Denmark	39	39	1967	17	3.15	12.49	1
	84	29	2194	17	2.20	9.65	
	Heterogeneity χ^2 (2 df)					8.32	
HLA-B15							
U.S.A.	33	9	53	6	1.55	0.36	4
England	12	33	174	17	2.52	2.42	2
Denmark	39	39	1967	18	2.94	11.05	1
	84	26	2194	18	2.62	13.19	
	Heterogeneity χ^2 (2 df)					0.64	
HLA-BW35							
West Indies—Black	18	50	166	14	6.03	13.02	2

Low HL-A2 frequency and periodontitis. Tissue Antigens 5:286-288, 1975

4. Kaslick RS, West TL, Chasens AI: Association between ABO blood groups, HL-A antigens and periodontal diseases in young adults: A follow-up study. J Periodontol 51:339-342, 1980
5. Kaslick RA, West TL, Chasens AI, Terasaki PI, Lazzara R, Weinberg S: Association between HL-A2 antigen and various periodontal diseases in young adults. J Dent Res 54:424, 1975

Neonatal Hyperbilirubinemia

Population Association

See ref. 1.

Reference

1. Stampar-Plasaj B, Pfeifer S, Jeric J, Benic LJ, Vukadinovic S: Neonatal hyperbilirubinaemia and HLA sensibilisation. Blut 40:362, 1980

Healthy Fetus

Population Association

Johansen and Festenstein[1] published data on 960 pregnancies from England showing a significantly higher male-to-female birth ratio among primigravidas who developed HLA antibodies. The ratio of male to female was highest in women who had formed antibodies to A1 (4:1), A11 (4:1), B5 (6:1), B12 (7:3), and B13 (6:2). In another report from England on 901 pregnancies, Doughty[2] also found a significant increase in the male to female newborn ratio in primiparous women producing detectable HLA-A and -B cytotoxic antibodies.

Woodrow,[3] on the other hand, found no evidence in 279 first-term pregnancies from England that a first pregnancy in which the fetus was male was more likely to be associated with antibodies in the mother than one in which the fetus was female.

Doughty[2] also reported no significant effect of HLA-A and -B loci antigens and antibodies on the birth weight and placental weight of infants from 911 pregnancies.

References

1. Johansen K, Festenstein H: Maternal HL-A antibodies and fetal sex. Br Med J 4:202-203, 1974
2. Doughty RW: HLA-A and -B antigens and the human fetus. Tissue Antigens 13:314-316, 1979
3. Woodrow JC: Maternal HL-A antibodies and fetal sex. Br Med J 1:36, 1975

Triploid Conceptus

Population Association

Couillin et al.[1] typed fibroblasts grown from tissues of 16 triploid conceptuses for 28 A and B loci antigens. The authors reported that HLA typing was useful in identifying the origin of triploidy.

Family Data

In another report from the same group of authors[2] A and B loci markers were tested in 49 French couples who had one or more triploid abortions. The antigen frequencies were compared with those in 591 normal controls and 209 normal couples. No significant differences among these 3 groups were found. However, the authors observed a nonsignificant excess of antigens shared by both parents (as compared with the 209 normal couples).

References

1. Couillin P, Hors J, Boue J, Boue A: Identification of the origin of triploidy by HLA markers. Hum Genet 41:35-44, 1978
2. Couillin P, Boue A, Boue J, Ravise N, Feingold N, Hors J: HLA markers in parents of triploid conceptuses. Pathol Biol 25:647-650, 1977

Down's Syndrome

Down's syndrome is a disease associated with trisomy (an extra copy) of chromosome 21.

Population Association

Boxer and Yokoyama[1] first reported decreased frequencies of all 5 antigens measured in 36 patients compared with 126 normal controls. In a later report Segal et al.[2] found no deviations in any of the 25 A and B loci antigens in 76 Caucasian patients and 733 normal controls from Canada. These authors attributed the discrepancy to the small sample of patients and multispecific sera used by Boxer and Yokoyama.[3]

References

1. Boxer LA, Yokoyama M: Lymphocyte antigens in patients with Down's syndrome. Vox Sang 22:539-543, 1972
2. Segal DJ, Schlaut JW, Pabst HF, McCoy EE, Dossetor JB: HL-A frequencies in Down's syndrome. Hum Genetik 27:45-48, 1975

Turner's Syndrome

Population Association

Twenty-one American Caucasian patients with Turner's syndrome were typed for A and B loci antigens by Cassidy et al.[1] The antigen frequencies in the patients were compared with those of 200 controls (Caucasian cadaver donors) from the same geographic area. They observed no significant difference between the 2 groups.

Disease Heterogeneity

The patients were subdivided according to the type of karyotype anomaly: pure XO, X structural anomaly, and XO/euploid mosaic. There was no HLA difference between these 3 subgroups either when compared to each other or when compared with the control group.

Reference

1. Cassidy SB, Niblack GD, Lorber CA, Mann JM, Engel E: HLA frequencies, diabetes mellitus and autoimmunity in Turner's patients. Ann Genet 21:203-208, 1978

Cleft Lip and/or Cleft Palate

Population Association

Bonner et al.[1,2] typed 72 American Caucasian and 61 Mexican American patients with cleft lip and/or cleft palate for A and B loci antigens. The frequency of AW24 in 34 Caucasian males with cleft lip and cleft palate was 32% as compared with 14% in 756 controls ($p = 0.07$). In the Mexican American group of 35 males with cleft lip and/or cleft palate, the frequency of A28 was 37% as compared with 13% in 124 controls ($p = 0.07$). These differences, however, would not be significant if probabilities are corrected for 27 A and B loci antigen comparisons that were studied in these data. (See also ref.3.)

Disease Heterogeneity

Bonner's[1] report had data on 24 Caucasian and 26 Mexican American females with cleft lip and/or cleft palate. There was no HLA frequency deviation in these 2 groups.

In the same report,[1] all the Caucasian patients were classified according to sex and presence of cleft lip with cleft palate or isolated cleft palate. In 34 males and 13 females with cleft lip and cleft palate the frequency of A2 was 61.7% and 23%, respectively. The difference between the 2 sexes was significant ($\chi^2 = 4.24$). Similarly, in 11 males with isolated cleft palate the frequency of A2 was 91% and in 8 females in the same category the frequency was only 12.5%. This difference was also significant ($\chi^2 = 8.7$).

Family Data

Van Dyke et al.[4] studied 8 families with at least 2 siblings affected by cleft lip or cleft lip and palate. These families were typed for A, B, and C loci antigens. Three of the 8 affected siblings differed in both haplotypes and the segregation of HLA haplotypes was not significantly different from that expected on the basis of random Mendelian segregation. Thus, there was no evidence in support of close linkage between HLA and this disorder.

Rapaport et al.[3] analyzed the segregation of HLA-A, -B, and -C antigens in 104 families. There was no clearcut evidence of any significant association between HLA and craniofacial developmental anomalies.

See also refs. 5–7.

References

1. Bonner JJ, Terasaki PI, Thompson P, Holve LM, Wilson L, Ebbin AJ, et al: HLA phenotype frequencies in individuals with cleft lip and/or cleft palate. Tissue Antigens 12:228-232, 1978
2. Bonner JJ: Studies on the major histocompatibility complex and cleft lip and/or cleft palate. Prog Clin Biol Res 46:499-510, 1980
3. Rapaport FT, Converse JM, McCarthy JG, Bachvaroff RJ, Raisbeck AP, Bach FH: The current status of the major histocompatibility complex (HLA) in family studies of craniofacial developmental anomalies. Prog Clin Biol Res 46:491-498, 1980
4. Van Dyke DC, Goldman AS, Spielman RS, Zmijewski CM, Oka SW: Segregation of HLA in sibs with cleft lip or cleft lip and palate: Evidence against genetic linkage. Cleft Palate J 17:189-193, 1980
5. Rapaport FT, Bachvaroff R, Converse JM, Raisbeck AP, Ayvazian JH, Segall M, et al: Atypical patterns of inheritance of serologically detectable (SD) products of HL-A complex in human developmental anomalies. Transplant Proc 5:1817-1822, 1973
6. Rapaport FT, Bachvaroff R, Converse JM, Raisbeck AD, Ayvazian JH, Segall M, et al: Genetic studies of mixed leukocyte culture reactivity in human developmental anomalies. Transplant Proc 5:1823-1832, 1973
7. Slavkin HC: Major histocompatibility complex (H-2) linked genes affecting teratogen-induced congenital craniofacial malformations in mice. Prog Clin Biol Res 46:121-147, 1980

Recurrent Oral Aphthae

Population Association

In the data of Challacombe et al.[1] a significant increase of B12 in patients was observed. In other studies[2–4] on Caucasian populations this result was not confirmed. The data on B12 from all of these studies are given in Table 24.6. In the pooled sample the association with B12 appeared to be significant.

Lehner et al.[4] also reported an increased frequency of DR2 in 17 patients from England (Table 24.6).

Disease Heterogeneity

Dolby et al.[3] subdivided their 64 patients according to sex, family history, age at onset of ulceration, duration of ulceration, and maximum number of concurrent ulcers. No HLA association was found in any of the subgroups.

TABLE 24.6. Recurrent Oral Aphthae

Country/Population	Patients n	Patients %+	Controls n	Controls %+	RR	χ^2	Ref.
HLA-B12							
England	64	36	100	38	0.92	0.06	3
England	100	44	100	22	2.75	10.65	1
England	20	45	100	22	2.88	4.68	4
	184	41	300	27	1.81	8.42	
	Heterogeneity χ^2 (2 df)					6.98	
Denmark	38	32	1967	25	1.44	1.15	2
	222	40	2267	25	1.70	9.24	
	Heterogeneity χ^2 (3 df)					7.31	
HLA-DR2							
England	17	47	70	20	3.48	5.26	4

Family Data

Challacombe et al.[1] also published the HLA types of 3 small families. In 2 of these families the affected siblings shared 1 haplotype. In the third family the 2 affected individuals were father and son.

References

1. Challacombe SJ, Batchelor JR, Kennedy LA, Lehner T: HLA antigens in recurrent oral ulcerations. Arch Dermatol 113:1717-1719, 1977
2. Platz P, Ryder LP, Donatsky O: No deviations of HLA-A and -B antigens in patients with recurrent aphthous stomatitis. Tissue Antigens 8:279-280, 1976
3. Dolby AE, Walker DM, Slade M, Allan C: HL-A histocompatibility antigens in recurrent aphthous ulceration. J Dent Res 56:105-107, 1977
4. Lehner T, Welsh KI, Batchelor JR: The relationship of HLA-B and DR phenotypes to Behcet's syndrome, recurrent oral ulceration and the class of immune complexes. Immunology 47:581-587, 1982

Adductor Laryngeal Paralysis

Family Data

Mace et al.[1] reported a 3-generation family with hereditary bilateral adductor paralysis of the larynx. No other clinical abnormality was present. There were 4 males and 1 female with this disorder. The mode of inheritance appeared to be autosomal dominant.

Linkage analysis by the lod score method of this family gave a maximum lod score of 1.505 at 0% recombination. The maximum lod score with GLO was 1.440, again at 0% recombination (a maximum lod score of +3.00 is generally considered as evidence of linkage). Thus, this pedigree provides some evidence in favor of linkage between this disorder and HLA. (See also ref. 2.)

References

1. Mace M, Williamson E, Worgan D: Autosomal dominantly inherited adductor laryngeal paralysis—a new syndrome with a suggestion of linkage to HLA. Clin Genet 14:265-270, 1978
2. Brunner FX, Herrmann IF: Familial recurrent laryngeal nerve paralysis, a genetically fixed syndrome—additional remark on linkage deficiency gene and HLA. Laryngol Rhinol Otol (Stuttg) 61:186-188, 1982

Obesity

Population Association

Apfelbaum et al.[1] typed 86 unrelated obese subjects from France. The HLA-A and -B antigen frequencies, when compared with 591 controls, did not show any significant deviations.

Fumeron et al.[2] reported some evidence of association between B18 and the familial-obesity syndrome. In this study 24 French families with 2 or more obese siblings and obese parents were analyzed. The study sample consisted of 24 individuals (1 affected sibling from each family). The frequency of B18 in this group was 37% as compared with 12% in 591 French controls ($p < 0.005$).

Family Data

In the above French study,[1] the authors also typed 10 families with more than 1 obese subject in each family. Although no formal genetic analysis of this data was given, the inspection of the pedigrees provided no strong evidence of linkage with HLA.

References

1. Apfelbaum M, Fumeron F, Dunica S, Magnet M, Brigant L, Boulange A, et al: Genetic approach of family obesity: Study of HLA antigens in 10 families and 86 unrelated obese subjects. Biomedicine 33:98-100, 1980
2. Fumeron F, Apfelbaum M: Association between HLA-B18 and the familial-obesity syndrome. N Engl J Med 305:645, 1981

Hereditary Angioneurotic Edema (HANE)

Hereditary angioneurotic edema (HANE) is an autosomal dominantly inherited disease due to a deficiency of the inhibitor of the activated first component of complement. In this condition there are recurring episodes of edema of the skin, gastrointestinal tract, and larynx. The disease has incomplete penetrance.

Family Data

HLA data are available on 7 French,[1–3] 2 Finnish,[4] 2 Danish,[5] 3 American (2 Caucasian,[6] 1 Black[7]), and 2 Japanese[8] families. The results from these families were remarkably similar. The disease, within a family, did not segregate with the marker HLA haplotype. Thus there was no evidence of linkage between HANE and HLA. Lod score calculations, however, were given only for 3 American families studied by Jackson et al.[6] and Blumenthal et al.[7]

References

1. Reznikoff-Etievant MF, Richter N, Sylvestre R, Hors J, Interator L, Laurent J, et al.: Marqueurs genetiques HLA et erythrocytaires dans une famille atteinte d'oedeme angioneurotique hereditaire. Pathol Biol (Paris) 26:103-106, 1978
2. Goasguen J, Fauchet R, Guerin D, Genetet B, Brecy H, Ollier MP, et al: The gene(s) controlling the synthesis of C1 esterase inhibitor is not linked to the genes of the HLA system and is not on the 6th chromosome. Biomedicine 29:248-252, 1978
3. Seignalet C, Berthoux F, Seignalet J, Michel FB: Hereditary angio-oedema and C3 nephritic factor—HLA study. Clin Allergy 9:527-533, 1979
4. Ohela K, Tiilikainen A, Kaakinen A, Rasanen J: Hereditary angioneurotic edema (HANE): Lack of close linkage between HLA haplotypes and C1 esterase inhibitor deficiency. Tissue Antigens 9:90-95, 1977
5. Eggert J, Zachariae H, Svejgaard E, Svejgaard A, Kissmeyer-Nielsen F: Hereditary angioneurotic edema and HLA types in two Danish families. Arch Dermatol Res 273:347-348, 1982
6. Jackson CE, Sweet LC, Hayashi H, Paul TD: Evidence for nonlinkage of genes for HLA and hereditary angioedema. J Allergy Clin Immunol 61:331-333, 1978
7. Blumenthal MN, Dalmasso AP, Roitman B, Kelley J, Noreen H, Emmy L, et al: Lack of linkage between hereditary angioedema and the A and B loci of the HLA system. Vox Sang 35:132-136, 1978
8. Tanimoto K, Horiuchi Y, Juji T, Yamamoto K, Kodama J, Murata S, et al: HLA types in two families with hereditary angioneurotic edema. Clin Immunol Immunopathol 7:336-339, 1977

Secondary Amyloidosis of Nonrheumatoid Origin

Population Association

Pasternack and Tiilikainen[1] found no significant association in 11 Finnish patients with amyloidosis of nonrheumatoid origin. Only the A and B loci antigens were compared in this study, however.

Reference

1. Pasternack A, Tiilikainen A: HLA-B27 in rheumatoid arthritis and amyloidosis. Tissue Antigens 9:80-89, 1977

Cystic Fibrosis

Population Association

Frequency data on a total of 199 unselected Caucasian patients from Austria,[1,2] Sweden,[3] Hungary,[4] and France[5] showed no evidence of association of cystic fibrosis with A and B loci antigens.

Family Data

Lamm et al.[6] calculated lod scores in 14 families with cystic fibrosis. In these data there was no evidence of linkage between HLA and cystic fibrosis. However, there was weak evidence for linkage to the PGM3 locus.

Herrod et al.[7] studied 10 families with more than 1 affected member in each family. The segregation of HLA in these affected sib-pairs was no different from that expected based on the independent assortment of HLA and cystic fibrosis genes.

The lod score data from 7 families studied by Hennequet et al.[5] and from 60 families by Goodchild et al.[8] also showed no evidence of linkage between HLA and cystic fibrosis.

References

1. Polymenidis Z, Ludwig H, Gotz M: Cystic fibrosis and HL-A antigens. Lancet ii:1452, 1973
2. Gotz M, Ludwig H, Polymenidis Z: HL-A antigens in cystic fibrosis. Z Kinderheilk 117:183-186, 1974
3. Safwenberg J, Kollberg H, Lindblom JB: HLA frequencies in patients with cystic fibrosis. Tissue Antigens 10:287-290, 1977
4. Kaiser Gl, Laszlo A, Gyurkovits K: Cystic fibrosis: An HLA associated hereditary disease? Acta Paediatr Acad Sci Hung 18:27-29, 1977
5. Hennequet A, Jehanne M, Betuel H, Gilly R, Schmid M, Hors J: Cystic fibrosis and HLA. Tissue Antigens 12:159-162, 1978
6. Lamm LU, Thorsen I, Peterson GB, Jorgensen J, Hemmingsen K, Bech B, et al: Data on the HL-A linkage group. Ann Hum Genet 38:383-390, 1975
7. Herrod HG, Amos DB, Spock A: HLA determinants in families with more than one member with cystic fibrosis. J Pediatr 94:676, 1979
8. Goodchild MC, Edwards JH, Glenn KP, Grindey C, Harris R, Mackintosh P, et al: A search for linkage in cystic fibrosis. J Med Genet 13:417-419, 1976

Hypercholesterolemia

Population Association

Mathews and Tait[1] typed 27 men with high serum cholesterol (273 mg/dl or more) and 25 men with low serum cholesterol (202 mg/dl or less). In the high cholesterol group the frequency of B8 was lower than that in the controls (Table 24.7). Six of the 25 (24%) with low cholesterol levels were B8-positive.

Reference

1. Mathews JD, Tait BD: HLA-B8 and serum-cholesterol. Lancet ii:1215-1216, 1975

Alkaptonuria

Alkaptonuria is the first disease for which recessive inheritance was proposed, by A. E. Garrod in 1902.

Family Data

Gaucher et al.[1,2] published HLA haplotype data on 1 pedigree with 10 members affected by alkaptonuria. These data did not provide evidence for linkage between HLA and alkaptonuria. Similar results were also observed by Srsen et al.[3] in another family with 9 members affected by this condition.

References

1. Gaucher A, Pourel J, Raffoux C, Faure G, Netter P, Streiff F: HLA antigens and alkaptonuria. J Rheumatol 4(Suppl 3):97-100, 1977
2. Gaucher A, Netter P, Faure C, Raffoux C, Chanson B, Baumgartner J, et al: Antigene HLA-B27 et alcaptonurie. Rev Rhum Mal Osteoartic 44:273-277, 1977
3. Srsen S, Nyulassy S, Buc M, Srsnova K: Alkaptonuria and the HLA system. Cas Lek Cesk 117:1523-1525, 1978

TABLE 24.7. Hypercholesterolemia

	Patients		Controls				
Country/Population	n	%+	n	%+	RR	χ^2	Ref.
HLA-B8							
Australia	27	7	506	27	0.25	4.83	1

TABLE 24.8. Essential Homogeneous Immunoglobulinemia

	Patients		Controls				
Country/Population	n	%+	n	%+	RR	χ^2	Ref.
HLA-B7							
BENELUX	64	43	285	24	2.39	9.38	1
HLA-B15							
BENELUX	64	3	285	16	0.20	6.70	1

Osteomalacia

Population Association

Fifty-eight patients from Belgium were typed for A and B loci antigens by Weingast et al.[1] None of the antigen frequencies was significantly different from those in 136 controls.

Reference

1. Weingast J, Manicourt D, Govaerts A: Osteomalacia and HLA. Tissue Antigens 9:276, 1977

Essential Homogeneous Immunoglobulinemia

Population Association

The data reported by Van Camp et al.[1] on 64 patients from Belgium showed deviations in the frequencies of B7 and B15 (Table 24.8).

Disease Heterogeneity

In the Belgian study[1] 26 patients had low polyclonal immunoglobulin levels. In this subset the frequencies of B7 and B15 were 46% and 0%, respectively. Thus, the increase of B7 in this subgroup was similar to that of the total sample.

Reference

1. Van Camp BGK, Cole J, Peetermans ME: HLA antigens and homogeneous immunoglobulins. Clin Immun Immunopathol 7:315-318, 1977

Whipple's Disease

Population Association

In a small sample of 9 German patients,[1] the frequency of B27 was increased (Table 24.9). In another case report,[2] an American Caucasian male was positive for B27.

References

1. Feurle GE, Dorken B, Schopf E, Lenhard V: HLA B27 and defects in the T-cell system in Whipple's disease. Eur J Clin Invest 9:385-389, 1979
2. Canoso JJ, Saini M, Hermos JA: Whipple's disease and ankylosing spondylitis: Simultaneous occurrence in HLA-B27 positive male. J Rheumatol 5:79-84, 1978

Fletcher Factor Deficiency

Family Data

Raffoux et al.[1] published a large pedigree with several affected siblings. All individuals of this family were typed for the antigens of A, B, C, and DR loci.

TABLE 24.9. Whipple's Disease

	Patients		Controls				
Country/Population	n	%+	n	%+	RR	χ^2	Ref.
HLA-B27							
West Germany	9	44	964	10	7.21	10.31	1

The disease was not found to be segregating with any specific HLA haplotype.

Reference

1. Raffoux C, Alexandre P, Perrier P, Briquel ME, Streiff F: HLA typing in a new family with Fletcher factor deficiency. Hum Genet 60:71-73, 1982

Hemangioma

Population Association

Majsky et al.[1,2] reported an increased frequency of B40 in 48 Czechoslovakian patients (Table 24.10).

References

1. Majsky A, Abrahamova J, Bek V: Hemangioma and HLA-B40 antigen. Tissue Antigens 15:220-221, 1980
2. Abrahamova J, Majsky A, Bek V: HLA system a hemangiomy. Cas Lek Cesk 119:54-55, 1980

Cystinosis

Population Association

Steinherz et al.[1] reported an increased frequency of B7 and a decreased frequency of A9 in 41 American Caucasian patients (Table 24.11).

Disease Heterogeneity

The clinical course of the disease was not associated with B7.[2]

Family Data

The report by Steinherz et al.[1] also included data on 5 families with at least 1 affected child. The total lod score of these families was -2.042 at 1% recombination. Thus there was no evidence of close linkage of this disease with the HLA complex.

References

1. Steinherz R, Raiford D, Mittal KK, Schulman JD: Association of certain human leukocyte antigens with nephropathic cystinosis in the absence of linkage between these loci. Am J Hum Genet 33:227-233, 1981
2. Steinherz R, Schulman JD, Reed GF: HLA types and the clinical course of cystinosis. Isr J Med Sci 18:293, 1982

Cerebrotendinous Xanthomatosis

Family Data

Brautbar et al.[1] reported A, B, C, and DR typings of a large family from Israel. Four siblings were healthy and 3 were affected by the disease. However, there was no haplotype common to all 3 affected

TABLE 24.10. Hemangioma

	Patients		Controls				
Country/Population	n	%+	n	%+	RR	χ^2	Ref.
HLA-B40							
Czechoslovakia	48	23	301	8	3.48	10.16	1

TABLE 24.11. Cystinosis

	Patients		Controls				
Country/Population	n	%+	n	%+	RR	χ^2	Ref.
HLA-A9							
U.S.A.	41	2	1465	23	0.11	8.54	1
HLA-B7							
U.S.A.	41	44	1465	24	2.50	8.57	1

siblings. Thus in this family a close linkage of the disease with HLA appeared unlikely.

Reference

1. Brautbar C, Yehuda O, Eisenberg S, Cohen N, Amar A, Sharon R, et al: Study of a family with cerebrotendinous xanthomatosis. Tissue Antigens 21:233-237, 1983

Otosclerosis

Population Association

Forty-one Czechoslovakian patients and 100 healthy controls were typed for A and B loci antigens by Majsky et al.[1] The antigen frequencies did not differ significantly between the 2 groups.

Reference

1. Majsky A, Novotny Z, Fajstavr Y: HLA and otosclerosis. Tissue Antigens 20:306-307, 1982

Nasal Polyps

Population Association

No significant association with A and B loci antigens was found in a small sample of 29 British patients studied by Moloney and Oliver.[1]

Reference

1. Moloney JR, Oliver RTD: HLA antigens, nasal polyps and asthma. Clin Otolaryngol 5:183-189, 1980

Dental Caries

Population Association

In an interesting report, Lehner et al.[1] studied the relationship between HLA antigens and the release of helper factor activity by the purified streptococcal antigen SAI/II (*Streptococcal mutans*) from lymphocytes of caries prone subjects.

Stimulation of lymphocytes with 1–10 ng SAI/II released significant amounts of helper factor activity in 7/9 resistant subjects with DRW6, as compared with 1/10 with DR4 (p = 0.0097). The low-dose helper factor activity of lymphocytes was associated predominantly with the DRW6, 1, 2, 3 cross-reactive groups. The high-dose (1000 ng of SAI/II) helper activity was found to be associated with DR4 antigen.

Reference

1. Lehner T, Lamb JR, Welsh KL, Batchelor RJ: Association between HLA-DR antigens and helper cell activity in the control of dental caries. Nature 292:770-772, 1981

Muckle-Wells Syndrome

Family Data

A 3-generation family with 6 affected members was reported by Hedon et al.[1] HLA-A and -B antigens were typed in all of the 14 members available for the study. Three of the affected siblings shared 1 haplotype, also present in the affected mother. Two healthy siblings, however, had the marker haplotype present in the affected siblings. The fourth affected sibling did not share any haplotype with the other affected ones.

Thus in this family there is no evidence of a close linkage with HLA.

This syndrome segregates like an autosomal dominant disease.

Reference

1. Hedon V, Kaplan C, Vaudour G, Muller JY: The Muckle-Wells syndrome and the major histocompatibility complex. Tissue Antigens 21:318-319, 1983

Ectopic Ossification After Total Hip Replacement

Population Association

Mattingly and Mowat[1] studied A and B loci antigens in 16 English osteoarthritic patients (12 men and 4 women) with ectopic ossification after total hip replacement. When compared with the frequencies in 100 controls no significant deviations were found.

Reference

1. Mattingly PC, Mowat AG: HLA antigens in patients with ectopic ossification after total hip replacement. J Rheumatol 7:582, 1980

Ossification After Spinal Cord Injury

Population Association

Hunter et al.[1] typed 24 Canadian patients (21 with spinal cord injury and 3 with cerebral damage) and 740 healthy controls for A and B loci antigens. The antigen frequencies did not differ significantly between the 2 groups.

Another report by Larson et al.[2] in 43 American Caucasian patients showed an increase of B27 antigen. In the data of Hunter et al.[1] B27 was actually decreased in the patient group. Thus a combined analysis of these 2 sets of data would not show significant increase of this antigen in the patients.

References

1. Hunter T, Dubo HIC, Hildahl CR, Smith NJ, Schroeder ML: Histocompatibility antigens in patients with spinal cord injury or cerebral damage complicated by heterotopic ossification. Rheumatol Rehab 19:97-99, 1980
2. Larson JM, Michalski JP, Collacott EA, Eltorai D, McCombs CC, Madorsky JB: Increased prevalence of HLA-B27 in patients with ectopic ossification following traumatic spinal cord injury. Rheumatol Rehab 20:193-197, 1981

Relapsing Polychondritis

Population Association

Luthra et al.[1] reported A and B loci antigen frequencies in 25 American Caucasian patients and 876 controls. There was no significant difference between these 2 groups.

Reference

1. Luthra HS, McKenna CH, Terasaki PI: Lack of association of HLA-A and B locus antigens with relapsing polychondritis. Tissue Antigens 17:442-443, 1981

Clubfoot (Talipes)

Family Data

The HLA haplotypes of 3 families with at least 2 affected siblings in each have been published by Kane and Suciu-Foca.[1] An analysis of segregation of the haplotypes and the disease appeared to exclude close linkage in all 3 families.

Lod scores for linkage between a hypothetical clubfoot gene and HLA complex were also computed. The total lod scores were all negative up to a recombination frequency of 39%.

Reference

1. Kane R, Suciu-Foca N: HLA and clubfoot (idiopathic talipes equinovarus). Tissue Antigens 19:95-96, 1982

Sex of the Offspring

Family Data

Giphart and D'Amaro [1] analyzed the HLA phenotypes and the sex of the offspring of 3900 Dutch families. Families were grouped on the basis of HLA-A and -B phenotypes of the father and mother and then sex ratio was analyzed in each of these subgroups.

In the subgroup of families in which the father was positive for B18 there were 154 male and 98 female children. This male/female ratio was significantly different from the expected 1:1 ratio ($p = 0.013$ after correction for 31 comparisons). In a second independent study of the families in which the father was positive for B18 antigen 49 male and 26 female children were observed. This male/female ratio was also statistically significant ($p = 0.008$).

In both studies the male/female ratio in the subgroup of families with the mother positive for B18 was not significantly different from the expected 1:1 ratio. (For example, in the first study there were 138 male and 147 female offspring.)

The male/female ratios for other A, B, and C loci antigens were also not significantly different from 1:1.

On the basis of these data the authors have suggested a significant association of B18 with an increased number of male offspring.

It should be noted that in the report by Giphart and D'Amaro[1] there is an appendix by M. Busson from Paris, France. In this appendix male/female ratios were tabulated for 115 families classified as "with B18 fathers," "with B18 mothers," and "with fathers not B18." The percentages of male offspring in these 3 groups of families were 52, 54, and 55, respectively. There was no difference in the ratio where the father was B18 as compared with the families in which mother was B18.

Thus the author has remarked that in this small sample of French data it was not possible to confirm the result of Giphart and D'Amaro.[1]

Reference

1. Giphart MJ, D'Amaro J: The association of HLA-B18 with increased male offspring in paternal back-cross matings. Tissue Antigens 15:329-332, 1980

Women with Large-for-Dates Infants

Population Association

Persson et al.[1] typed A, B, and D loci antigens in 123 Swedish mothers with large-for-dates infants. This was a followup study done 7 years after delivery. The antigen frequencies of this group were compared with a reference group of 272 individuals. No significant difference was found.

Reference

1. Persson B, Moller E, Thunell S: Follow-up of women with large-for-dates infants. Early insulin and C-peptide response to intravenous glucose, blood lipids and HLA types. Acta Endocrinol 98:420-427, 1981

Mate Selection

Population Association

Giphart and D'Amaro[1] performed an interesting analysis of HLA frequency data to test the hypothesis that "there is no selection in the choice of partners based on traits which are coded for by genes which may be linked to those in the MHC region."

In the analysis, for each of the 30 A, B, and C loci antigens, couples were selected on the basis of the presence of that antigen in the maternal phenotype. The frequencies of all of the 30 antigens were determined in their spouses. The frequencies in this subset of the paternal population were compared with those in the total paternal population, the expected antigen frequency in the absence of any HLA associated selection. The same method was followed after the selection for the presence of each antigen in the paternal phenotype. In this analysis the frequencies of 4 antigens in the spouses were significantly different from their expected values: selected antigen CW4 in male and AW19 in the female spouse; selected antigens A2, AW19, and B7 in females and the corresponding antigens B40, CW4, and B40 in the male spouses. The probability values were corrected for the 1800 frequency comparisons performed in the analysis (for details see the data in the report).

On the basis of these results, the authors have suggested "preferential association" of some HLA antigens in males and females (e.g., female B7 and male B40). This may indicate a positive selection bias on traits determined by genes in the region of the HLA complex.

In another interesting report Rosenberg et al.[2] counted the frequency of co-occurrence of the same antigen in 1017 American couples. The sample was very heterogeneous and consisted of Orientals, American Blacks, Latin Americans, and Caucasians of European origin.

The observed frequency of co-occurrence of the same antigen of A and B loci in couples was found to be significantly higher than the expected number. However, the authors noted that the population under study was racially and ethnically heterogeneous, and the observed results of apparent self-preference for A and B loci antigens may be entirely explained by racial and ethnic self-preference of subpopulations characterized by distinctive HLA antigen frequencies.

In an interesting study of sensitivity to androstenone in 66 mating pairs (couples married or living together for a minimum of 3 years) Pollack et al.[3] analyzed the observed and expected frequencies of the combination of "male antigen" and "female antigen" (e.g., the combination of male A2 antigen with female A2, A3,. . . B5, B7, etc). No deviations from the expected frequencies were found for any of the possible antigen combinations. Furthermore, the frequency of antigen sharing in the couples was not different from that predicted from the frequency of each antigen in the separate male and female populations.

See also ref. 4.

References

1. Giphart MJ, D'Amaro J: HLA and reproduction? J Immunogenet 10:25-29, 1983
2. Rosenberg LT, Cooperman D, Payne R: HLA and mate selection. Immunogenetics 17:89-93, 1983
3. Pollack MS, Wysocki CJ, Beauchamp GK, Braun D Jr, Callaway C, Dupont B: Absence of HLA association or linkage for variations in sensitivity to the

odor of androstenone. Immunogenetics 15:579-589, 1982
4. Boyse EA, Beauchamp GK, Yamazaki K: The sensory perception of genotypic polymorphism of the major histocompatibility complex and other genes: Some physiological and phylogenetic implications. Hum Immunol 6:117-183, 1983

Malignant Hyperthermia

Family Data

Lutsky et al.[1] published the HLA haplotypes of a 3-generation family in which 2 individuals had died due to malignant hyperthermia and 2 were known as "reactors" (i.e., those who experienced a clinically recognized nonfatal malignant hyperthermia episode after receiving general anesthesia).

The affected individuals did not share any haplotype.

Reference

1. Lutsky I, Witkowski J, Henschel EO: HLA typing in a family prone to malignant hyperthermia. Anesthesiology 56:224-226, 1982

Hypokalemia

Family Data

Gullner et al.[1] described a family in which 3 of the 4 siblings were affected by hypokalemia (hypokalemic alkalosis, hyperreninemia, aldosterone, high urinary prostaglandin E_2 excretion, normal blood pressure, and resistance of blood pressure to angiotensis II). All 3 affected siblings had identical HLA haplotypes. The healthy sibling did not share any haplotype with the affected siblings.

Under the assumption of a recessive mode of inheritance the maximum lod score for this family was 1.322, suggesting probable linkage with the HLA complex.

Reference

1. Gullner H, Bartter FC, Gill JR Jr, Dickman PS, Wilson CB, Tiwari JL: A sibship with hypokalemic alkalosis and renal proximal tubulopathy. Arch Intern Med 143:1534-1540, 1983

Ferritin Secretion

Population Association

In a study reported by Pollack et al.[1] hemolytic plaque-forming assay was used to measure ferritin secretion *in vitro* by phytohemagglutinin-activated or nonactivated mononuclear cells in response to stimulation by ferric citrate. Cells from 55 unrelated healthy individuals typed for A, B, C, and DR antigens were studied.

There was a significant increase of A3 among "low responders." Also, in the analysis of the distribution of ferritin-secretion responses, A3-positive individuals were significantly more frequent in the lowest quarter segment of the plaque values. The level of significance was not very high and in fact would not be significant if the probabilities are corrected for the large number of A, B, C, and DR antigens compared in this study.

It should be noted that the antigen A3 is associated with hemochromatosis (excess iron). This disease is also linked with the HLA complex.

Reference

1. Pollack MS, Da Silva BM, Moshief RD, Groshen S, Bognacki J, Du Pont B, et al: Ferritin secretion by human mononuclear cells: Association with HLA phenotype. Clin Immunol Immunopathol 27:124-134, 1983

Rapeseed Oil Disease

Population Association

Vicario et al.[1,2] reported from Spain DR antigen data on 39 randomly chosen "chronic" patients with ra-

TABLE 24.12. Rapeseed Oil Disease

	Patients		Controls				
Country/Population	n	%+	n	%+	RR	χ^2	Ref.
HLA-DR4							
Spain	39	31	63	11	3.50	6.13	1

peseed oil disease (poisoning from adulterated rapeseed oil). (In the acute stage, immediately after ingestion of adulterated oil the disease resembled pneumonia and in the chronic stage, deaths and serious illness with neuromuscular and scleroderma-like symptoms resulted.)

In this sample an increased frequency of DR4 has been observed (Table 24.12).

Disease Heterogeneity

In the above study[1] when the patients were separated by sex, the frequency of DR3 was found to be increased in 28 females (32.1% vs. 18.1% in 11 males, and 17.4% in 63 controls; $p < 0.05$).

The frequency of DR4 was not increased in the 11 males (18.1% in males, 35.7% in 28 females, and 11.1% in 63 controls).

References

1. Vicario JL, Serrano-Rios M, San Andres F, Arnaiz-Villena: HLA-DR3, DR4 increase in chronic stage of Spanish oil disease. Lancet i:276, 1982
2. Arnaiz-Villena A, Vicario JL, Serrano-Rios M, Bellas C, Mampaso F: Glomerular basement-membrane antibodies and HLA-DR2 in Spanish rapeseed oil disease. N Engl J Med 307:1404-1405, 1982

Index

MIX
Papier aus verantwortungsvollen Quellen
Paper from responsible sources
FSC® C105338

If you have any concerns about our products,
you can contact us on
ProductSafety@springernature.com

In case Publisher is established outside the EU,
the EU authorized representative is:
Springer Nature Customer Service Center GmbH
Europaplatz 3, 69115 Heidelberg, Germany

Printed by Libri Plureos GmbH
in Hamburg, Germany